Neural Mechanisms of Anesthesia

Contemporary Clinical Neuroscience

Series Editors:
*Ralph Lydic and
Helen A. Baghdoyan*

NEURAL MECHANISMS OF ANESTHESIA

Edited by

JOSEPH F. ANTOGNINI, MD

University of California at Davis
School of Medicine, Davis, CA

EARL CARSTENS, PhD

University of California at Davis
School of Medicine, Davis, CA

DOUGLAS E. RAINES, MD

Harvard Medical School
and Massachusetts General Hospital, Boston, MA

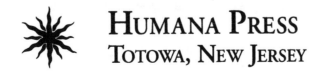

HUMANA PRESS
TOTOWA, NEW JERSEY

Cover design by Patricia F. Cleary.

Production Editor: Mark J. Breaugh.

For additional copies, pricing for bulk purchases, and/or information about other Humana titles, contact Humana at the above address or at any of the following numbers: Tel.: 973-256-1699;Fax: 973-256-8341; E-mail: humana@humanapr.com or visit our website: http://humanapress.com

This publication is printed on acid-free paper. ∞
ANSI Z39.48-1984 (American National Standards Institute) Permanence of Paper for Printed Library Materials.

Printed in the United States of America.   10 9 8 7 6 5 4 3 2 1

Library of Congress Cataloging-in-Publication Data

Neural mechanisms of anesthesia / [edited by] Joseph Antognini ; co-editors, Earl E.
Carstens, Douglas E. Raines.
    p. ; cm. -- (Contemporary clinical neuroscience)
  Includes bibliographical references and index.
  ISBN 0-89603-997-8 (alk. paper)
  1. Anesthesia. 2. Anesthetics--Physiological effect. 3. Anesthetics--Metabolism. 4.
Pharmacology. 5. Anesthesiology. I. Antognini, Joseph. II. Carstens, Earl E. III. Raines,
Douglas E. IV. Series.
  [DNLM: 1. Anesthetics--pharmacology. 2. Anesthesia--methods. 3. Nervous System
Physiology. QV 81 N494 2003]
RD82 .N476 2003
617.9'6--dc21
                                       2002068475

PREFACE

Although millions of people worldwide are anesthetized every year, we still have no true understanding of why the drugs we use do what they do. This remarkable lack of knowledge limits our ability to design drugs that would minimize or eliminate anesthetic side effects. Indeed, our anesthetic drugs are powerful poisons. The therapeutic index is defined as the lethal dose that kills 50% of the population divided by the effective dose for 50% of the population. For many drugs, the therapeutic index is several hundred or thousand fold; for anesthetics, the therapeutic index is only 3–4. This narrow margin of safety underscores the inherent danger of anesthetics. It is only because of the skill of well-trained anesthesiologists that anesthesia is relatively safe. Nonetheless, whereas serious complications such as death are rare, more bothersome complications (nausea, vomiting) are common, and are terribly distressing for patients. Only by thoroughly understanding how anesthetics exert their effects (good and bad) can we design drugs that will do one thing and one thing only—anesthetize patients, rendering them unconscious, amnestic, and insensible to noxious stimulation.

Neural Mechanisms of Anesthesia represents our current understanding of anesthetic mechanisms. Its emphasis is rather different from other books on the subject, which in the past focused primarily on molecular mechanisms. We have chosen to examine anesthetic mechanisms at multiple levels: the molecule, the cell, organ systems, and the whole body (Fig. 1). This broad overview is necessary, we believe, because it is difficult to grasp the impact and importance of an experimental finding in the absence of the context of the whole animal or human. For example, when a researcher reports that isoflurane enhances opening time of a particular channel, what does that mean to a clinician? How does that action result in the clinically relevant actions of anesthetics (such as unconsciousness)? Furthermore, how much effect on opening time is required to get the relevant result? If the researcher reports that isoflurane at one minimum alveolar concentration enhances channel opening time 10%, is that sufficient to achieve a clinical goal? One can see the fundamental flaw in not being able to link these specific experimental findings with clinical observations. If we knew through some independent means that 50% enhancement (exclusive of any other action, an important and probably incorrect caveat) was required to cause unconsciousness, then we could conclude that this effect on opening time is not relevant. Thus, we must synthesize all the experimental findings at multiple levels in order to determine the relevance of each. Claude Bernard, the eminent 19th century scientist, clearly recognized the folly of narrowly viewing experimental findings:

> ... If we break up a living organism by isolating its different parts, it is only for the sake of ease in analysis and by no means in order to conceive them separately. Indeed when we wish to ascribe to a physiological quality its value and true significance we must always refer it to this whole and draw our final conclusions only in relation to its effects in the whole—CLAUDE BERNARD, 1865

Each researcher clearly examines the problem of anesthetic mechanisms from a different perspective, not unlike the six blind men of Indostan, who "examined" the elephant, each having different ideas about the elephant's shape. In the end, though, the blind men had incomplete "visions" of the elephant:

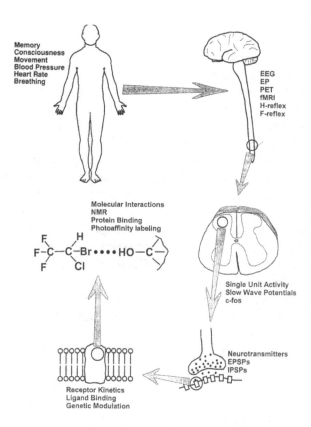

Fig. 1. Anesthesia results in clinically observable effects, such as amnesia, unconsciousness, and immobility. Anesthetic mechanisms must explain these endpoints, and are investigated by study of smaller and smaller components of the organism, such as the brain and spinal cord, the dorsal horn of the spinal cord, the synapse, the cell membrane with its associated receptors and proteins, individual receptors, and finally individual molecules, including molecular interactions between anesthetics and specific sites on proteins and other biological molecules. EEG = electroencephalogram; EP = evoked potentials; PET = positron emission tomography; fMRI = functional magnetic resonance imaging; EPSPs = excitatory postsynaptic potentials; IPSPs = inhibitory postsynaptic potentials; NMR = nuclear magnetic resonance. Other methods to investigate anesthetic mechanisms are available but have been omitted.

> And so these men of Indostan
> Disputed loud and long,
> Each in his own opinion
> Exceeding stiff and strong,
> Though each was partly in the right,
> And all were in the wrong!
> —JOHN G. SAXE, *The Blind Men and the Elephant*

So, too, is our understanding of anesthetic mechanisms incomplete. This book will hopefully bridge the gaps that exist between the various views and perspectives of the contributors.

We have separated *Neural Mechanisms of Anesthesia* into six sections. The first section discusses the history of research into mechanisms of anesthesia. The second section covers topics related to consciousness and memory. These chapters are important simply because before we can discuss how anesthetics work, we must decide what they affect. Ablation of nociceptive motor responses, a third critical anesthetic endpoint is included in Chapter 11. The third section includes chapters describing physiological (sleep) and pathophysiological (coma) states related to anesthesia. Section 4 (Neural Mechanisms) reviews the anatomic structures and physiological processes that are likely targets of anesthetics. A well-grounded knowledge of the cerebral cortex, thalamus, reticular formation, and spinal cord will aid the reader's understanding of chapters dealing with anesthetic action at these sites. The fifth section includes cellular and molecular mechanisms. We have included chapters on drugs that are not truly general anesthetics, but are used in clinical practice and can affect the action of general anesthetics (local anesthetics, opiates, neuromuscular blocking drugs). Lastly, we end with a chapter on the future of research into anesthetic mechanisms.

What is anesthesia? This simple question does not have a simple and straightforward answer. Ask any number of individuals and one is likely to get different answers. For the surgeon, general anesthesia consists of an immobile patient. For the patient, general anesthesia consists of amnesia, and not necessarily unconsciousness. That is, patients would likely choose the combination of amnesia and consciousness over the combination of recall and unconsciousness. The latter combination is possible, at least as regards implicit recall. For the anesthesiologist, general anesthesia entails immobility, amnesia, and unconsciousness. Other goals are desirable, but not necessary. Some argue that analgesia is needed, but we disagree. We defend this position first with a semantic argument. Analgesia, in its simplest form, is defined as relief of pain. Pain is the conscious awareness of a noxious stimulus (real or perceived) associated with certain emotional and behavioral patterns, such as withdrawal. Because anesthetized patients are usually unconscious, they do not perceive pain. Of course, they may develop physiological responses to the noxious stimulus (increased heart rate, blood pressure, catecholamine concentrations, etc.). But when awakened and asked if they "felt any pain" they would say: "None—I was completely knocked out." In some patients, amelioration of these physiological responses is desirable (such as those with coronary heart disease). However, in a healthy young patient, a heart rate of 130 bpm and blood pressure of 180/90 mmHg is not injurious. And, whether or not this response is harmful because of a failure to obtain pre-emptive analgesia is open to debate.

Figure 2 summarizes the sensitivities of various anesthetic goals or endpoints. It is important to point out that the sensitivities of memory and consciousness are similar, but that available evidence suggests that memory is more sensitive to anesthetics. These data, however, were developed in human volunteers who were not subjected to noxious stimuli. It is possible that noxious stimulation would shift both the memory and consciousness curves to the right. Because of ethical concerns, these studies have not been performed, and are not likely to be performed. The greater sensitivity of memory parallels the greater sensitivity of memory to other insults, such as trauma and ischemia. For example, minor head trauma can lead to just a few minutes of unconsciousness but hours of amnesia (both retrograde and antegrade). Both memory and unconsciousness are more sensitive than the movement response to noxious stimulation. This is in keeping with the importance of the withdrawal (flight) response. From an evolutionary perspec-

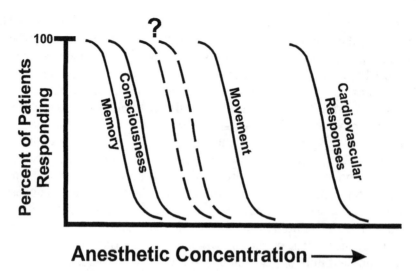

Fig. 2. Anesthetic endpoints have different sensitivities to anesthetics. Memory and consciousness are particularly sensitive, and ablated well below the concentrations needed to prevent movement. The effects on memory and consciousness have been examined primarily in human volunteers in the absence of noxious stimulation. It is quite possible that noxious stimulation shifts the memory and consciousness response curves to the right, although this is not known with certainty (thus, the question mark). Cardiovascular responses to noxious stimulation are very resistant, and require anesthetic concentrations well above those needed to ensure immobility.

tive, the withdrawal response to a noxious stimulus should be hardy and most resistant to physiological insults, as compared to consciousness and memory. Indeed, simple organisms have nociceptive withdrawal responses, but it is unclear whether they experience consciousness in a way similar to humans. These organisms probably do not have memory (as we know it), but they are capable of "learning," which means that classical conditioning can occur.

Neural Mechanisms of Anesthesia represents the most recent advances in research of anesthetic mechanisms. In part, progress in this research has advanced as a result of our increasing understanding of whole-body, cellular, and molecular processes. The mechanisms of anesthesia are still elusive, but we are closing in. Soon we will be able to design drugs that have specific desired actions, with no undesirable effects. We must continue to carefully judge the risks and benefits of the powerful and dangerous drugs that we use. When describing Morton's use of ether in Boston, Bigelow wrote: "Its action is not thoroughly understood, and its use should be restricted to responsible persons." This statement still rings true 150 years later.

The editors wish to thank the contributing authors who have been generous with their expertise, time, and effort. We are also grateful for the expert editorial assistance of Serena Reid at the University of California, Davis. Finally, we thank the staff at Humana Press, including Craig Adams, Paul Dolgert, and Mark Breaugh—we may write the words, but they put the words on paper for the world to read.

Joseph Antognini, MD
Earl Carstens, PhD
Douglas E. Raines, MD

CONTENTS

CONTRIBUTORS

ANTHONY ANGEL, PhD • *Department of Biomedical Science, University of Sheffield, Sheffield, UK*

JOSEPH F. ANTOGNINI, MD • *Department of Anesthesiology, University of California at Davis School of Medicine, Davis, CA*

THOMAS J. J. BLANCK, MD, PhD • *Department of Anesthesiology, New York University School of Medicine, New York, NY*

GARY J. BRENNER, MD, PhD • *Department of Anesthesia and Critical Care, Harvard Medical School, Massachusetts General Hospital, Boston, MA*

EARL CARSTENS, PhD • *Department of Neurobiology, Physiology and Behavior, University of California at Davis School of Medicine, Davis, CA*

DONALD CATON, MD • *Department of Anesthesiology and Obstetrics and Gynecology, University of Florida College of Medicine, Gainesville, FL*

J. G. COLLINS, PhD • *Department of Anesthesiology, Yale University School of Medicine, New Haven, CT*

STEPHEN DANIELS, PhD • *Welsh School of Pharmacy, Cardiff University, Cardiff, UK*

RODERIC G. ECKENHOFF, MD • *Department of Anesthesia, University of Pennsylvania School of Medicine, Philadelphia, PA*

LEONARD L. FIRESTONE, MD • *Departments of Anesthesiology/Critical Care Medicine and Pharmacology, University of Pittsburgh Medical Center, Pittsburgh, PA*

PAMELA FLOOD, MD • *Department of Anesthesia, Columbia University College of Physicians and Surgeons, New York, NY*

STUART A. FORMAN, MD, PhD • *Department of Anesthesia and Critical Care, Harvard Medical School, Massachusetts General Hospital, Boston, MA*

SCOTT GREENWALD, PhD • *Aspect Medical Systems, Newton, MA*

GERALD A. GRONERT, MD • *Department of Anesthesiology and Pain Medicine, University of California at Davis School of Medicine, Davis, CA*

FERENC E. GYULAI, MD • *Department of Anesthesiology, University of Pittsburgh Medical Center, Pittsburgh, PA*

HUGH C. HEMMINGS, JR., MD, PhD • *Department of Anesthesiology and Pharmacology, Weill Medical College of Cornell University, New York, NY*

GREGG E. HOMANICS, PhD • *Departments of Anesthesiology/Critical Care Medicine and Pharmacology, University of Pittsburgh Medical Center, Pittsburgh, PA*

JONAS S. JOHANSSON, MD, PhD • *Department of Anesthesia, University of Pennsylvania School of Medicine, Philadelphia, PA*

JOHN KEIFER, MD • *Department of Anesthesiology, Duke University Medical Center, Durham, NC*

JOAN J. KENDIG, PhD • *Department of Anesthesia, Stanford University School of Medicine, Stanford, CA*

HEATH LUKATCH, PhD • *Piper Jaffray Ventures, Redwood City, CA*

BRUCE MACIVER, MSc, PhD • *Department of Anesthesia, Stanford University School of Medicine, Stanford, CA*

JIANREN MAO, MD, PhD • *Department of Anesthesia and Critical Care, Harvard Medical School, Massachusetts General Hospital, Boston, MA*

KEITH W. MILLER, PhD • *Department of Anesthesia and Critical Care, Harvard Medical School, Massachusetts General Hospital, Boston, MA*

PHILIP G. MORGAN, MD • *Department of Anesthesiology, Case Western Reserve University Hospital, Cleveland, OH*

ROBERT A. PEARCE, MD, PhD • *Department of Anesthesiology, University of Wisconsin Medical School, Madison, WI*

MISHA PEROUANSKY, MD • *Department of Anesthesiology, University of Wisconsin School of Medicine, Madison, WI*

FRED PLUM, MD • *Departments of Neurology and Neuroscience, Weil Medical College of Cornell University, New York, NY*

DOUGLAS E. RAINES, MD • *Department of Anesthesia and Critical Care, Harvard Medical School, Massachusetts General Hospital, Boston, MA*

ESPERANZA RECIO-PINTO, PhD • *Hospital for Special Surgery, Department of Anesthesiology, Weill Medical College of Cornell University, New York, NY*

CARL ROSOW, MD, PhD • *Department of Anesthesia and Critical Care, Harvard Medical School, Massachusetts General Hospital, Boston, MA*

WARREN S. SANDBERG, MD, PhD • *Department of Anesthesia and Critical Care, Harvard Medical School, Massachusetts General Hospital, Boston, MA*

NICHOLAS D. SCHIFF, MD • *Departments of Neurology and Neuroscience, Weill Medical College of Cornell University, New York, NY*

MARGARET SEDENSKY, MD • *Department of Anesthesiology, Case Western Reserve University Hospital, Cleveland, OH*

TIMOTHY TAUTZ, MD • *Department of Anesthesiology and Pain Medicine, University of California at Davis School of Medicine, Davis, CA*

NORBERT TOPF, MD, PhD • *CV Starr Laboratory for Molecular Neuropharmacology, Department of Anesthesiology, New York Presbyterian Hospital, Weill Medical College of Cornell University, New York, NY*

ROBERT A. VESELIS, MD • *Department of Anesthesiology and Critical Care Medicine, Memorial Sloan-Kettering Cancer Center, New York, NY*

GING KUO WANG, PhD • *Department of Anesthesiology, Harvard Medical School, Brigham and Women's Hospital, Boston, MA*

G. BRYAN YOUNG, MD, FRCPC • *Department of Clinical Neurological Sciences, The University of Western Ontario, London, Ontario, Canada*

I   Introduction

1

The Development of Concepts of Mechanisms of Anesthesia

Donald Caton and Joseph F. Antognini

INTRODUCTION

Even before Morton's demonstration of surgical anesthesia in Boston, on October 16, 1846, physicians and scientists had begun to explore mechanisms by which drugs affect the central nervous system. In large part, this was an outgrowth of a revolution in therapeutics that had begun in wake of the Enlightenment. As philosophers and politicians threw out old patterns of religious, political, and economic thought, so physicians discarded a system of medical practice that had been in place for almost fifteen hundred years. Modern medicine began during this era and with it new disciplines such as physiology, pharmacology, and biochemistry *(1)*.

The discarded system of practice, called "Galenic Medicine", for the early Greek physician who established it, maintained that the body was composed of four elements (earth, air, fire, and water), which combined in various proportions to produce four humours (blood, black bile, yellow bile, and phlegm). Health was a state in which humours stayed in proper balance: disease a condition in which that balance had been upset by some internal or external disturbance. Physicians were to discern the character of the imbalance and institute appropriate restorative measures such as bleeding, purging, or cupping *(2,3)*.

In the centuries following Galen's death, physicians modified his original scheme in response to new discoveries in other areas of science. As engineers began to exploit hydraulics, for example, physicians attributed all disease to fluctuations of hydrostatic pressure. After the discovery of electricity, they exchanged hydraulics for energy imbalance to explain disease. Despite changing theory, however, therapy remained the same. Even at the beginning of the nineteenth century, physicians recommended many methods familiar to Galen, modified only in that they used them with less restraint. At the time of the American Revolution, for example, physician Benjamin Rush became known for his propensity to bleed patients to the point of death *(4)*.

The movement away from Galenic medicine began with French physicians. Early in the nineteenth century, they began to question and then discard Galenic concepts of disease and therapy. Coincidentally, they created a new system based on careful clinical observation, supplemented by post mortem dissection and statistical analysis *(5)*. From this, they developed the idea that disruptions in the structure of specific organs would induce functional changes recognizable to a clinician as distinctive patterns of signs and symptoms. In the context of this discussion, studies of neurological disorders proved to be particularly important. The association of localized lesions with specific

From: *Contemporary Clinical Neuroscience: Neural Mechanisms of Anesthesia*
Edited by: Joseph F. Antognini et al. © Humana Press Inc., Totowa, NJ

deficits led them to reject the concept that the central nervous system was a homogenous mass in favor of the concept that it consisted of many components, each with a different function. Physiologic data soon confirmed this.

Scottish physician Charles Bell showed, and French physiologist François Magendie demonstrated, that dorsal and ventral nerve roots of the spinal cord have different functions. Legallois recognized the importance of the cerebellum for the coordination of motor activity. Johannes Müller established the idea that different receptors respond to different stimuli–pain, light touch, or temperature, for example. Coincidentally, anatomists showed the nervous system to be a collection of highly differentiated cells, ganglia, and pathways. These concepts influenced physiologists and physicians who were just beginning their studies of drug action *(6)*.

Significant among early studies of drug action was work by French physiologist François Magendie (1783–1855). In 1810 he began experiments on the plant *upas tieuté*, a member of the styrchnos family *(7,8)*. Natives of Borneo and Java used a dried extract of the plant, which caused convulsions and cardio-pulmonary arrest, on the points of their arrows to kill small game much as Indians of South America used curare. Magendie showed:

- That the poison worked most quickly when placed directly on the spinal cord or brain rather than on a peripheral nerve.
- That the onset of action varied directly with the time it took for the drug to reach the brain. For example an intravenous injection killed more rapidly than intra-muscular injection.
- That the circulation had to be intact for poison to work. Dogs died quickly after an injection of the poison into a severed limb, but only when he left its arterial and venous connections intact.

Magendie's experiments influenced the next generation of physicians when they began to study mechanisms of anesthetic drugs.

EARLY STUDIES IN ANESTHESIA: ATTEMPTS TO ASCERTAIN ITS SITE OF ACTION

Important though they were, Magendie's experiments had little impact on the practical American physicians who first demonstrated the anesthetic effects of nitrous oxide and ether. Crawford Long, Horace Wells, and William Thomas Greene Morton simply wanted to relieve pain. They showed no particular interest in the mechanisms that brought this about. Their pragmatic approach was typical of early nineteenth century American physicians and scientists, who distrusted theory and had little interest in any innovation for which they could not find an immediate use. Accordingly, most early studies of mechanisms of anesthesia emerged not from the United States but from Europe among physicians and scientists who were better attuned to theory and scientific inquiry *(9,10)*.

At first, physicians appeared to be most concerned about establishing the site of action of anesthesia. They attacked this problem in much the same way that Magendie had dealt with strychnine. Here the influence of clinical and pathological studies of neurological disorders becomes apparent. As physicians used ether, for example, they recognized that anesthetized patients exhibit an orderly sequence of clinical signs, starting with a disturbance of consciousness, followed by a loss reflex activity, and finally a paralysis of respiratory and cardiac activity. From this they reasoned that some parts of the nervous system were more susceptible than others. In fact, within months of the announcement of Morton's demonstration in Boston, French physiologist Pierre Flourens described anesthesia as a progressive depression of the nervous system beginning with the cortex, followed by the cerebellum, and finally the brain stem and spinal cord *(11)*. Others confirmed his findings, among them Nicolai Pirogoff *(12–14)*.

Born in Moscow, Pirogoff (1810–1881) trained there before moving to Dorpat, Estonia to continue his studies. The University in Dorpat, staffed at that time by German speaking physicians, was to have a seminal influence on the development of experimental pharmacology and on early concepts of mechanisms of anesthesia. From Dorpat, Pirogoff moved to Saint Petersburg, where he became chief surgeon in the medical school. He was teaching there when he first learned about Morton's work with ether *(15)*. Within a year, Pirogoff published a book about anesthesia. In it he describes his use of ether, but he also describes more than forty-five experiments that he performed to elucidate its site and mechanism of action. For example, Pirogoff demonstrated that direct application of ether on a peripheral nerve caused partial anesthesia. He speculated, however, that this response might be due less to the pharmacological action of the drug than to a temperature change in the nerve caused by direct application of the liquid. Pirogoff then proceeded to demonstrate that ether had a more potent effect on the brain than on peripheral nerves, and that it worked better when distributed by the circulation rather than by direct application to the cortex. Pirogoff examined individual nerves looking for microscopic anatomical changes that might explain how ether blocked the conduction of impulses *(14)*. He suggested two possibilities. First, that ether might have some "chemical action on nervous tissue." Second, he thought that "ether vapor in the capillary system surrounding nervous tissue" might exert a "greater or lesser degree of compression on the component fibers of the brain and nerves, partly by the force of expansion or partly by passage into the cerebrospinal fluid." In fact, neither of Pirogoff's suggestions was particularly new. Pharmacology textbooks from the eighteenth century had speculated that morphine induced some physical change in nerve fibers, thereby inhibiting function *(16)*. Similarly, surgeons had long known that pressure on a nerve could render a limb anesthetic. In fact, one English surgeon, James Moore, tried to popularize this method for painless amputations *(17,18)*. In effect, Pirogoff simply substituted gaseous pressure for the mechanical force that Moore had used *(19)*.

Establishing the central nervous system as the primary target of anesthesia was no small achievement. Even after Magendie's work with strychnine, physicians continued to debate the primary site of action of morphine. Most believed that it affected the brain, but others believed that morphine had its most profound effect on peripheral nerves. For this reason, textbooks recommended that morphine be administered as close as possible to an injured part. In fact, it was for this purpose that Alexander Wood introduced hypodermic injections in 1855 *(20)*.

Perhaps the most extensive and sustained series of studies, during this early period, came from the laboratory of Claude Bernard. Bernard, who had been a student of Magendie, summarized his work in the book, *"Lectures on Anesthetics and on Asphyxia"(21)*. In the book, Bernard made several points. First, he defined anesthesia and distinguished it from narcotism, a state that he associated with morphine. Second, he sought to explain anesthesia in precise anatomical and physiological terms *(22)*. Third, he, too, sought to establish the primary site of action of anesthetic drugs. Towards this end, he performed a series of experiments on frogs not dissimilar from those used by Magendie in his studies of strychnine. Like Magendie and Pirogoff, Bernard concluded that anesthetics act on the brain rather than peripheral nerves. He also recognized, however, that anesthetic drugs suppress not just neurological activity of higher animals, but basic functions of many different kinds of cells, even those of plants. This led him, and others, to speculate that anesthetics may work by altering mechanisms common to the cells of many different tissues and species. Lastly, Bernard distinguished anesthesia from asphyxia, an important point about which more will be said in the Early Studies Section.

Among early contributors to studies of mechanisms of anesthesia, English physician John Snow also warrants mention. Snow also described clinical signs associated with different depths of anesthesia, but he went one step further. Whereas, experiments by Flourens, Bernard, and Pirogoff had largely been descriptive, Snow was among the first to establish a quantitative relationship between the concentration of inspired gas and the clinical response—a nineteenth century forerunner of the concept of minimum alveolar concentration (MAC). He did this by placing small animals in an enclosed chamber filled with air containing different concentrations of anesthetic. Snow made the gas mixtures himself by adding measured amounts of liquid chloroform to containers of known volume. After allowing time for the liquid anesthetic to vaporize, he placed animals in the container so that he could observe clinical signs associated with different concentrations of inspired gas. Snow used these data to argue for more precise control over concentrations of ether administered to patients, and even designed a temperature-controlled vaporizer to achieve this. His experiments demonstrate a remarkable understanding of the gas laws, which had only recently been described, but also an appreciation of the significance of these laws to theory and practice. Most important, by describing and measuring a dose-response relationship, he developed an approach that would become important for later studies *(23)*.

THE EMERGENCE OF MODERN PHARMACOLOGY

Coincident with the studies of the site of action of anesthesia, scientists also began to study mechanisms. An important stimulus for this work was the emergence of experimental pharmacology. In part this was an outgrowth of Magendie's work with strychnine, but there were other factors. By 1850, for example, chemists had identified nitrogen, carbon dioxide, oxygen, and nitrous oxide. Dalton and Henry had described the gas laws. By 1811, German pharmacist, Sertürner, had isolated two active principles of opium, morphine and codeine. By 1832, Samuel Guthrie and Justus von Liebig had synthesized chloral hydrate. Simultaneously, biologists began to shift their attention from descriptive to experimental work. For example, after the announcement of the cell theory by Schleiden and Schwann in 1838, pathologists and physiologists began to explore cellular mechanisms of disease. Simultaneously, Felix Hoppe-Seyler and others began to apply chemical analysis to the study of biological phenomena. In short, advances in many branches of science gave physicians tools and concepts that they could use to study drugs. Two men prominent in the emergence of experimental pharmacology were Rudolph Buchheim and Oswald Schmiedeberg. Both had sound training in experimental science. Directly, and indirectly, they shaped early studies of mechanisms of anesthesia. Curiously, both had strong ties to the medical school in Dorpat, the institution where Pirogoff once worked.

Historians often call Rudolph Buchheim (1820–1879) the founder of modern pharmacology. German by birth, Buchheim studied medicine first in Dresden and then in Leipzig, where he worked under E. H. Weber, a physiological chemist. Soon after completion of his studies, he became known as an editor of *Pharmazeutisches Zentralblatt*, and as the author of several chapters in Schmidt's *Jahrbüder der Medizin*. Not long thereafter, he won more praise for his translation into German of Pereira's *The Elements of Materia Medica*. Early in his career, Buchheim spent several productive years at the University of Dorpat, where he worked with Carl Schmidt and Friedrich Bidder. Later he moved to Giessen and finally, after the Franco-Prussian war of 1872, to Strassbourg, where he died *(24–27)*.

Buchheim made many contributions to pharmacology, among them the concept that drugs should be classified according to their mode of action. This signified a major departure from an earlier "Galenic" convention that simply classified drugs as stimulants or depressants. As late as 1793, for example, one major textbook included a long discussion about opium, whether it acted more as a stimulant or a depressant, that is to say as "hot" or as a "cold" form of therapy, using eighteenth century terminology *(16)*. To Buchheim, pharmacology meant identifying the effect of a drug on specific physiological processes—on liver metabolism or urine formation, for example. It meant understanding the relationship between a drug's structure and function, and it meant establishing how the body dealt with drugs, how they are metabolized and excreted. Buchheim borrowed experimental methods from many branches of science, but he also developed techniques widely used by subsequent generations of pharmacologists. Buchheim's research on chloral hydrate illustrates his approach.

Buchheim's interest in chloral hydrate grew from his studies of acid base balance. Noting the alkalinity of blood, he speculated that formic acid, a metabolite of chloral hydrate would "neutralize" blood, an effect that he believed might be clinically advantageous. Chloral hydrate did not have this effect, but Buchheim did observe that it made his subjects somnolent. He attributed their somnolence to the release of chloroform, another metabolite of the chloral hydrate. Unfortunately, when he failed to demonstrate this mechanism, Buchheim dropped the inquiry thereby missing the opportunity to introduce to clinical medicine the first synthesized hypnotic. Credit subsequently went to Oscar Lebereich of the University of Berlin, who did recognize the clinical implications of the observation *(28)*. Regardless, the story illustrates the shift in the approach to drug studies that was beginning to take shape.

Oswald Schmiedeberg (1838–1921), a student of Buchheim, further developed the systematic study of drug action. Born in Dorpat, Schmiedeberg studied there at the University under Buchheim. Schmiedeberg then moved to Leipzig, where he worked with Carl Ludwig, one of the most influential experimental physiologists of the nineteenth century. Schmiedeberg then returned to Dorpat, to take the chair once held by his mentor. Eventually, he too moved to the Kaiser Wilhelm Institute in Strassburg, where he ended his career *(29–30)*.

Schmiedeberg studied hypnotics and anesthetics at several different times during his career. As a student, he measured chloroform concentrations in blood, thereby making some of the first ever measurements of this kind. Shortly after the synthesis of paraldehyde and urethane, he performed pharmacological studies of these drugs. When Schmiedeberg was director of the pharmacology department in Strassburg, Joseph von Mering, another member of the faculty, introduced barbituric acid to clinical medicine. Like Buchheim, Schmiedeberg trained many students who made their own mark on pharmacology. One of them was H. H. Meyer, co-founder of the Meyer-Overton theory of narcosis *(31–33)*.

EARLY STUDIES OF MECHANISMS OF ANESTHESIA

As experimental pharmacology flourished, so did studies of mechanism of anesthesia. Theories also became increasingly sophisticated as clinicians and scientists brought to the problem principles and methods of physiology and biochemistry. Readers interested in a critical analysis of experimental data from this period should read the reviews by V. E. Henderson and G. H. W. Lucas *(34,35)*. In the remaining part of this chapter we will summarize some of the major ideas from this early era.

A popular and persistent theory attributed anesthesia to asphyxia. Initially, this concept arose among clinicians that observed the dark blood of anesthetized patients. They assumed a causal relationship. As mentioned earlier, Claude Bernard squelched this idea when he pointed out that patients remain anesthetized even when their blood was not dark. He concluded, therefore, that the asphyxia must be "merely an incident, a complication of anesthesia that arises because of the way in which the anesthetic was administered" *(21)*. Bernard's observation, though correct, did not dispel the idea. It simply reappeared in different forms. Some, noting a decrease in oxygen consumption and a rise in lactic acid and acetone, suggested that anesthesia might block a metabolic pathway. Others, who observed that the surface of the cortex turns pale during anesthesia, suggested that change in perfusion might limit the "asphyxia" to the brain. Over time each of these explanations lost favor.

Claude Bernard himself attributed anesthesia to a reversible "semi-coagulation" of cellular components. In support of this idea, he and others pointed to the fact that blood may turn "cloudy" and cells may become opaque and their nucleus indistinct, when they are exposed to solutions of chloroform, chloral hydrate, and morphine. This theory lost favor because the concentrations of drug needed to produce such changes far exceeded any dose used clinically. Perhaps it was coagulation and mechanical distortion of nerves that Pirogoff hoped to observe in his microscopic studies *(35)*.

Other investigators postulated that anesthetics cause cells to lose water, to the point that they shrink and become nonfunctional. Data supporting this idea came mostly from observations of microscopic alterations in protozoa exposed to anesthetics and from measurements of changes in their water content. Some investigators observed an inverse relationship between anesthetic potency and water solubility, although they were unable to suggest how this relationship might account for a loss of neurological activity.

The enduring theory of anesthesia to emerge from this period related potency to lipid solubility. An antecedent of the idea actually appeared as early as 1847, when Bibra and Harless suggested a relationship between a tissue's fat content, and its susceptibility to anesthesia. However, it was H. H. Meyer, Schmiedeberg's student, and C. E. Overton who developed the principle independently, and announced it simultaneously in 1899.

Like his mentor, Meyer served in Dorpat as professor of pharmacology. He then moved to the University of Marburg, and finally, to the University of Vienna where he became Chair of the Department of Experimental Pharmacology. Meyer developed his theory from work performed by three of his own students. They had been working with various narcotics for several years when he recognized:

1. That all fat soluble chemicals may act as narcotics in so far as they are absorbed;
2. That their effect is greatest in cells with the highest fat content;
3. That the activity of narcotics varies with their affinity to fat like compounds and to other constituents, such as water.

Overton arrived at the same conclusion through botanical studies, his original field of work. English by birth, and a distant relative of Charles Darwin, Overton grew up in Switzerland. He trained in botany at the University of Zürich. His interest in anesthesia developed from studies of osmosis. Working with different organic compounds, he observed that many were capable of inducing "narcosis" and that their potency was related to their lipid solubility, virtually the same conclusion as Meyer. Like Claude Bernard, Overton believed that narcosis was a fundamental biological phenomenon important to plants as well as animals *(32)*.

To a large extent, theories of anesthesia that emerged in the 20th century represent an outgrowth of this early work *(36)*. For example, whereas Bernard suggested that anesthetics "coagulated" nerves, a new generation of scientists suggested that they interfered with the movement of ions through "microtubules", or that that they altered surface tension at some critical site such as the extracellular/ cellular interface, e.g., the cell membrane. Later still, Nobel Laureate Linus Pauling postulated that certain anesthetics form microcrystals, or "clathrates," in the central nervous system *(37)*. Meanwhile, biochemists rephrased old questions as they discovered new mechanisms by which anesthetics might alter the metabolism of oxygen and other cellular processes. Similarly, anatomists revived Meyer-Overton's original hypothesis when they discovered that, for example, receptors interspersed in the bilipid layer of cell membranes *(38)*, might be a site of action of inhalation anesthetics. The development of the MAC concept stimulated other research, in as much as it permitted investigators to compare equipotent concentrations of anesthetics, and evaluate factors that altered anesthetic requirements *(39)*. Even this approach had pitfalls, however. Some investigators assumed a change in anesthetic requirement as evidence for a mechanism of anesthetic action. For example, some assumed that neuromuscular blocking agents had anesthetic properties because they depressed the muscular response to surgical stimuli.

CONCLUSION

Speculation about mechanisms of anesthesia flourished during the last half of the nineteenth century. To a large extent, development of these ideas reflected changes in science and medicine. Starting with descriptive work, scientists progressed rapidly to an analysis of underlying chemical and physical phenomena. Perhaps no one stated the motivation of these early scientists better than Claude Bernard:

"What should we think about the action of chloroform or ether on the central nervous cell? Any effect of whatever order on an anatomical unit can take place only through a physical or chemical modification of the unit. Nowadays, it is no longer acceptable to hypothesize about mysterious actions dubbed vital. Use of the word means that nothing precise is known about the phenomenon under discussion. At the present time, the physical or chemical phenomena underlying toxic effects have been precisely delineated in a few cases. As an example, carbon monoxide acts on the red cell by combining chemically with the hemoglobin. Chemical demonstration of the action is easy in this case, and one can reproduce the reaction with hemato-globin outside as well as inside the organism. We have not advanced as far as that in regard to the action of anesthetics, but arguing from a careful analysis of the facts, we may be able to form a fairly clear idea of the physio-chemical action which they have on nerve units" *(21)*.

In half a century, scientists did just that. Many current concepts of the mechanism of anesthetic action originated during this period. To a large extent, progress since that time has been shaped by the modification of these original ideas by more complex and sophisticated methods of study.

REFERENCES

1. Caton, D. (1985) The secularization of pain. *Anesthesiology* **62,** 493–501.
2. Smith, W. D. (1979) The Hippocratic Tradition. Cornell, Ithaca.
3. King, L. S. (1978) The Philosophy of Medicine: The Early Eighteenth Century. Harvard University Press, Cambridge.
4. Warner, J. H. (1986) The Therapeutic Perspective: Medical Practice, Knowledge and Identity in America Harvard University Press, Cambridge, MA, 1820–1885.
5. Ackerknecht, E. H. (1967) Medicine at the Paris Hospitals 1794–1846. Johns Hopkins Press, Baltimore.
6. Livingston, W. K. (1998) Pain and Suffering. (Fields H. L., ed.) IASF Press, Seattle.
7. Leake, C. D. (1975) An Historical Account of Pharmacology to the Twentieth Century. University of California, Charles C. Thomas, Springfield, pp. 140–169.
8. Holmstedt, B. G., Liljestrand, G. (1963) Readings in Pharmacology. MacMillan Company, New York.
9. Daniels, G. H. (1968) American Science in the Age of Jackson. Columbia University Press, New York.
10. Lesch, J. E. (1984) Science and Medicine in France: The Emergence of Experimental Physiology. Harvard University Press, Cambridge.
11. Flourens, M. J. P. (1847) Note touchant les effets de l'inhalation de l'éther sur la moelle allongée. *CR. Acad. Sci.* **24,** 253–258.
12. Anonymous. (1847) Physiological effects of ether. *Lancet* 411.
13. Brown, B. (1847) The pathological and physiological effects of ethereal inhalation. *Boston Med. Surg. J.* XXXVI, 369–378.
14. Pirogoff, N. (1992) Researches Practical and Physiological on Etherization. Translated by Fink, B. R. Wood Library Museum, Park Ridge, Illinois.
15. Secher, O. Biographical Note: Nikolai Ivanovitch Pirogoff. in Pirogoff, pp. 13–28.
16. Crumpe, S. (1793) An Inquiry into the Nature and Properties of Opium. G. G. and J. Robinson. 1793. Crumpe wrote: "With respect, however, to the immediate operation of the medicine on the nerves, after its arrival at their origin, we find a variety of opinions....In general, (most) suppose that its ultimate particle, entering the minute cavities of the nervous fibers, disturb, or totally impeded the free and equitable motion of the nervous fluid, or animal spirit.... By many it was attributed to the adhesive nature...by which the cavities of the nerves for a time were completely obstructed...that it drew the sides of the nerves together and therefore occluded passages, or "nervous fluids (necessary for nerve action) was condensed or coagulated." (pp. 90–93).
17. Moore, J. (1784) A Method of Preventing or Diminishing Pain in Several Operations of Surgery. T. Cadell, London.
18. Bergman, N.A. (1994) James Moore, an 18th Century advocate of mitigation of pain during surgery. *Anesthesiology* **80,** 657–662.
19. "Either it is the ether vapor in the capillary system surrounding nervous tissue that exerts a greater or lesser degree of compression on the component fibers of the brain and nerves, partly by the force of expansion or partly by passage into the cerebrospinal fluid....or else it is the chemical action of ether vapor on nervous tissue." Pirogoff pp. 56.
20. Wood, A. (1855) New method of treating neuralgia by the direct application of opiates to the painful points. *Edinburgh Med. Surg. J.* **82,** 265–267.
21. Lectures on Anesthetics and on Asphyxia by Claude Bernard. (1989) translated by B. Raymond Fink. Wood Library Museum of Anesthesiology, Park Ridge, Illinois.
22. "The nature of the physiological action of morphine is not yet fully known, but we may say that it selectively affects nerve centers and perhaps also the sensory units. All the same, it is far from totally suppressing consciousness as chloroform does, but in animals produces a kind of exaggerated excitability, or more exactly some sort of special sensitivity to sound. Bernard, C. pp. 133.
23. Snow, J. (1858) On Chloroform and Other Anaesthetics. John Churchill, London.
24. Kuschinsky, G. (1968) The influence of Dorpat on the emergence of pharmacology as a distinct discipline. *J. History Med.* **23,** 258–271.
25. Oelssner, W. (1969) Buchheim, R. Leben und Werk. *Ver. Deut. Gesell. für Exp. Med.* **22,** 364–370
26. Habermann, E. (1969) Üeinige Beziehungen zwischen Theorie und Experiment im Lebenswerk Rudolf Buchheims. *Ver. Deut. Gesell. für Exp. Med.* **22,** 371–377.
27. Rossbach, M. J. (1880) Rudolf Buchheim. *Berliner klinische Wochenschrift.* L, 477–479.
28. Leberich, O. (1874) Das Chloralhydrat, ein neues Hynoticum an Anaestheticum, und dessen Anwendung in der Medicin. *Berlin klin. Wochschr.* **11,** 50–52.
29. Meyer, H. H. (1903) Zu, O. Schmiedebergs siebzigstem Geburtstage. *Munch. Med. Woch.* **55,** 2192–2193.
30. Meyer, H. H. (1922) Schmiedebergs Werk. *Arch. Expt. Path. Pharmak.* **92,** I–XVII.
31. Lipnick, R. L. (1985) Hans Horst Meyer and the lipoid theory of Narcosis. *Trends in Pharmocologic Sci.* **10,** 265–269.

32. Lipnick, R. L. Charles Ernest Overton: narcosis studies and a contribution to general pharmacology in Overton, pp. 14–23.
33. Overton, C. E. (1991) Studies of narcosis, translated and edited by Lipnick, R. L., Wood Library-Museum, Park Ridge, Illinois.
34. Henderson, V. D. (1930) The present status of the theories of narcosis. *Physiol. Rev.* **101,** 171–267.
35. Henderson, V. E. and Lucas, G. H. W. (1932) Claude Bernard's theory of narcosis. *J. Pharmacol. Exp. Therap.* **44,** 253–267.
36. Cohen, P. J. (1975) History and theories of general anesthesia. In: Goodman L. S, Gilman A. The pharmacological basis of therapeutics. MacMillan, New York, pp. 53–59.
37. Pauling, L. (1961) A molecular theory of general anesthesia. *Science* **134,** 15–21.
38. Singer, S. J. and Nicolson, G. L. (1972) The fluid mosaic model of the structure of cell membranes. *Science* **175,** 720–731.
39. Eger, E. I., Saidman, L. J., Brandstater, B. (1965): Minimum alveolar anesthetic concentration: a standard of anesthetic potency. *Anesthesiology* **26,** 756–763.

II   Anesthesia, Consciousness, and Memory

2

Mechanisms of Consciousness with Emphasis on the Cerebral Cortical Component

G. Bryan Young

INTRODUCTION

Concepts of Consciousness

Consciousness has been defined as an awareness of oneself and one's environment *(1)*. This simple definition fails to account for the many discrete yet interrelated components of conscious awareness. We still do not have a complete understanding of how these components are integrated to produce conscious awareness, partly because consciousness is such a subjective, ephemeral subject. Nonetheless, considerable gains have been made in revealing details of the components and their interaction, e.g., alertness, attention, sensory processing and perception, memory mechanisms and executive functions. Neurophysiological techniques and functional neuro-imaging have helped understand the normal brain. Disease states and the differential effects of drugs (including anesthetics) have also provided insights into components of consciousness and how these elements contribute to integrated brain function.

The main components of consciousness are alertness and awareness. Each of these has subcomponents.

Alertness

Alertness refers to simple wakefulness behavior: the eyes are open in wakefulness; the patient can be roused from a sleep-like state to an eyes-open state; spontaneous wake and sleep cycles usually occur. The absence of this capacity–unarousable unconsciousness–is referred to as coma. Although a considerable amount of processing may occur in the comatose brain, alertness is essential for apperception, conscious appreciation and, usually, for later recall of this activity.

Many years ago, Morruzi and Magoun *(2)* demonstrated that the arousal component of consciousness, including (cerebral cortical) EEG activation, was dependent on the ascending reticular activating system (ARAS). The ARAS was first thought to be an undifferentiated collection or network of neurons with interconnections and projections from the rostral brainstem reticular formation through the thalamus to the cerebral cortex. This concept has been refined. There are not only some alternative pathways that produce EEG activation, but this "network" is composed of discrete systems with various neurotransmitters. Selective gating takes place in subcortical structures, allowing for the selection of information. Thus subcortical regions are important not only for primitive arousal and maintenance of the alert state, but also for components of awareness. This idea is discussed in detail in Chapter 8. Alertness and arousal are dependent on subcortical function (Fig. 1); indeed arousal can occur without a functioning cerebral cortex (*see* persistent vegetative state discussed below).

From: *Contemporary Clinical Neuroscience: Neural Mechanisms of Anesthesia*
Edited by: Joseph F. Antognini et al. © Humana Press Inc., Totowa, NJ

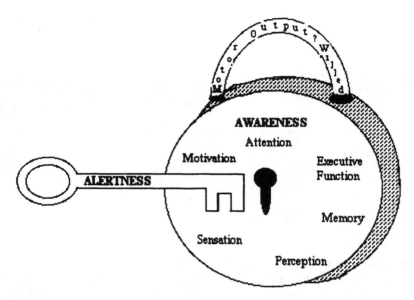

Fig. 1. This cartoon analogy illustrates the essential enabling effect of alertness (a function of the ascending reticular activating system) on awareness. Awareness (the body of the lock) has multiple associated components mainly represented in the cerebral cortex, but with subcortical interactions. The resultant motor output (the mobile shackle) results from processing in the cortical-subcortical system. Whether any action is truly willed or not is still debated.

Awareness

Unlike alertness and arousal, awareness is dependent on the cerebral cortex, but there are essential cortical-subcortical, especially cortical-thalamic, interactions for this more complex and higher form of consciousness. The persistent vegetative state represents alertness without awareness. In this condition the patient can be roused from sleep, shows spontaneous wake and sleep cycles but manifests no evidence of perception, comprehension, memory function or any meaningful reaction or purposeful behavioral response to internal or external stimuli. The persistent vegetative state is most commonly associated with diffuse cerebral cortical dysfunction (as from anoxic-ischemic or hypoglycemic damage). It may also be produced by white matter lesions that disconnect cortical regions from each other and the thalamus (as if diffuse axonal injury from trauma). It may also be produced by thalamic damage that preserves the arousal component, but prevents the transfer of other information to the cortex *(3)*.

There are a number of components of consciousness *(see* Fig. 1) that, in the intact, aware human, do not function in isolation. These are presented separately for purposes of discussion:

Sensation and Perception

Sensation relates to the awareness of a reception of signals from sensory receptors. Sensations have discrete or modular primary sensory receiving areas in the cerebral cortex and association areas for further processing. Primary sensory modalities include somatosensory, visual, auditory, vestibular, olfactory, gustatory, and visceral sensations *(see* Fig. 2). Sensations have temporal (timing relative to the present), spatial (reflecting part of the body plus or minus various regions of extrapersonal space) characteristics and are specific to certain modalities (e.g., visual sensation is separate from somatosensory and auditory senses, even when all refer to the same extrapersonal object). Each primary sensory area of the cerebral cortex has forward and backward connections with association areas; i.e., there is not a one-way mechanism of analysis. Furthermore, both serial and parallel processing of information occur within each sensory system.

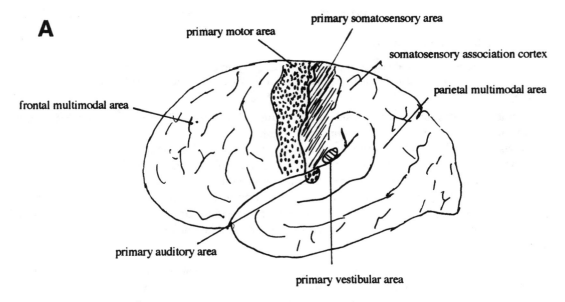

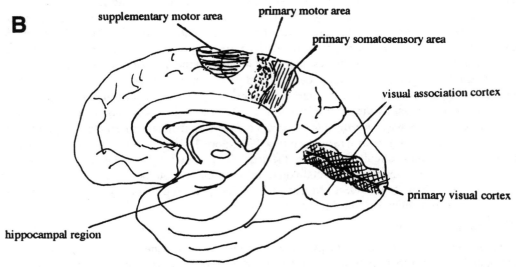

Fig. 2. Various cortical functions are represented in drawings of the convexity (**A**) and mesial (**B**) surfaces of the cerebral cerebral hemisphere.

Perception refers to the further processing of sensory information, providing a symbolic concept of what is happening in the external world. Usually, perception overrides sensation, so that we are aware of an external event or object rather than the fact that we are receiving a sensation. In object vision, the image is segmented into background and foreground and the impressions are fused into shapes and objects. The conscious appreciation of the object involves reception by the primary visual cortex, processing in the visual cortex, transfer to visual association areas and links with visual memory stores. In addition, the focusing of attention is necessary for awareness to occur. If the primary visual cortex is destroyed or isolated (even though it may be activated), conscious awareness does not occur. This is not to deny the occurrence of blindsight (a meaningful response to the visual stimulus, even though the patient denies the awareness of the stimulus). This illustrates the necessary interaction of a number of cortical areas for awareness.

Attention

Moscovitch *(4)* defined attention as

"a control process that enables the individual to select, form a number of alternatives, the task he will perform or the stimulus he will process, and the cognitive strategy he will adopt to carry out these operations."

Attention includes directivity and selectivity of mental processes. There is a close physiological relationship among attention, alertness and perception.

The anatomical location of cortical regions involved in attention include the anterior cingulate cortex and the inferior parietal lobule, with strong links to subcortical regions, including the thalamus, the reticular formation, and the superior colliculus. Motor inattention occurs with lesions of the dorsolateral frontal region. Akinetic mutism, a condition in which the patient appears awake and visually tracks moving objects, but does not otherwise respond to stimuli, may result from lesions of the mesial frontal cortex or the centromedian-parafascicular thalamic nuclei.

Memory

The neurophysiological basis of memory is unsettled, but enhancement of synaptic connections (either by facilitated neurotransmitter release by long term potentiation or by the physical increase in numbers and locations of synapses) underlies various forms of memory and learning *(5)*. *Working memory* refers to the short term retention of mental activities held in consciousness for immediate use; lesions of the dorsolateral prefrontal cortex have been found to alter visual working memory in monkeys *(6)*. *Anterograde memory*, the laying down of new explicit or declarative memories, and the appropriate retrieval of stored memories, appear to depend on the integrity of function of the mesial temporal structures, probably the hippocampus and/or the entorhinal and perirhinal cortex. Other structures form part of the circuit for anterograde memory: the parahippocampal gyri, the fornices, the medial dorsal or possibly the anterior thalamic nuclei, the cingulum or cingulate cortex and links of these structures. *Remote* or *retrograde memories* are stored outside the mesial temporal regions, as these are preserved in patients with newly acquired bitemporal lesions. *Implicit* and *procedural memories* do not require limbic circuits, at least for the acquisition of motor skills. Patients with bitemporal lesions can learn to play tennis or can retain other information without being able to verbally declare this knowledge without cues. Indeed, Moscovitch *(7)* has proposed that only explicit, not implicit, memories are accompanied by conscious awareness.

Motivation and Emotion

Motivation refers to a drive that helps to determine behavior. It depends on perception, attention, memory, and emotions that function in an interrelated fashion. Important structures in the generation of internal feelings and motivation are the amygdala, the hypothalamus, and associated limbic structures. The hippocampus consolidates information received from regions where sensory and perceptual processing has occurred. The amygdala, by its connections with various cortical and limbic structures, gives the information an affective tone. The posterior insula is also important in the interpretation of the significance of painful stimuli *(8)*.

Language and Other Extended Aspects of Consciousness

Language function, like mathematical ability, is a highly developed cognitive activity of great human importance. The temporal-parietal region of the dominant cerebral hemisphere converts processed information into symbols, allowing an "internal conversation" and conceptual formulation. However, individuals with destruction of this region can still interact with others and show awareness as demonstrated (e.g., by expression in art or other means of nonverbal communication). Thus, language function is not essential for consciousness, although it provides an important dimension to conscious activity.

Extended consciousness is a term that applies to meaningful cognitive function that gives the person a sense of self and a perspective of place and time *(9)*. It is built upon alertness and the various elements of awareness that have been discussed above. Such a process—integrating the previously discussed elements of awareness—involves coordinated function of various cerebral cortical regions in concert with subcortical structures, especially the thalamus. Some areas that are involved in attention, such as the anterior cingulate cortex, may play an essential or initiatory role.

Covert Processing in the Brain

It should be acknowledged that not all processing of information or resultant behavior is consciously directed. Indeed, there is a "phenomenal consciousness," in which the brain registers internal or external phenomena without this mode of processing, demanding attention, or entering into cognitive awareness and decision-making. There is, therefore, a covert or implicit awareness in the brain that is not apparent to the individual at the time. At least, the individual would not admit to it being in his/her awareness! Such phenomena may come into consciousness when they achieve a threshold of meaningful significance that demands our attention. For example, while driving a car, one is not consciously aware of all the stimuli in their fields of vision. However, the individual makes adjustments in speed and steering "without thinking". When, however, something appears that has special significance, e.g., a flashing red light, it receives conscious attention. A chain of events is initiated because of the symbolic importance of the flashing red light. Thus, much processing involving visual, memory areas, the amygdala, somatosensory, motor and other regions goes on without our conscious awareness, but full conscious awareness is called upon when our attention is demanded for important decisions.

Anatomical, Physiological, and Neurochemical Aspects

The cerebral cortex is anatomically and physiologically arranged in a modular fashion of radial columns at right angles to the surface, approx 3 mm in diameter (*see* Fig. 3). Within these vertical columns, pyramidal cells are the most prominent neurons, with basal dendrites extending horizontally, apical dendrites extending vertically, and axons projecting downwards. The latter have recurrent collaterals that excite other pyramidal cells in the same column, producing excitatory post synaptic potentials or EPSPs. The main intrinsic excitatory neurotransmitter is glutamate. Inhibition is an intracortical phenomenon produced by inhibitory interneurons that release gamma-amino-butyric acid (GABA). GABA acts on receptors linked to chloride channels, causing neurons to become hyperpolarized and producing inhibitory post-synaptic potentials (IPSPs). GABA receptors are on or near the neuronal cell body and the axon hillock where action potentials are generated. Since post-synaptic potentials decline spatially and because the net polarity of the neuronal membrane at the axon hillock (the site where action potentials are generated) relates to the net summation and subtraction of post-synaptic potentials, the inhibitory process is strategically placed and potent.

Cortical columns are interconnected by horizontal, laminar connections of neuronal processes. In addition, various cortical regions are interconnected by subcortical fibers of various lengths. The strength of cortical interconnections is greatest for nearby areas, and falls off with distance. Thus interconnection density is inversely related to distance. The axons interconnecting adjacent cortex are mostly of small diameter, allowing a conduction velocity on average of only 5.5 m/s. This results in a limiting of synchronous activity (resonance) of 50–100 ms or 10–20/s. However, some axons have larger diameters and greater conduction velocity. Many are dedicated for longer interconnections, e.g., to homologous regions in the opposite cerebral hemisphere via the corpus callosum. This allows for some rhythms of greater frequency.

The main afferents to the cerebral cortex come from the thalamus. There is an elaborate gating mechanism for this projection (*see* Chapter 8). The main output from the cortex is from pyramidal

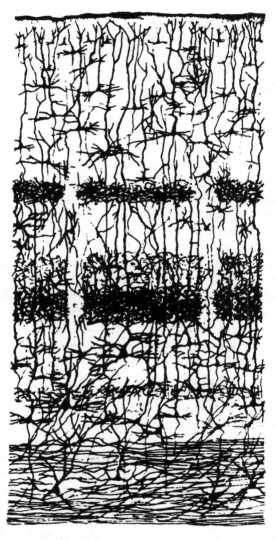

Fig. 3. This is a composite drawing of neurons with their dendrites and superimposed axonal plexuses, illustrating both the vertical columnar arrangement as well as the laminar interconnections of neurons. (Modified from F. O. Schmidt and F. G. Worden [eds.] (1979) *The Neurosciences 4th Study Program* MIT Press, Cambridge, with permission).

cells that project to the basal ganglia and to a lesser extent, the thalamus, brainstem and spinal cord structures.

Steriade and colleagues *(10)* have shown that most cortical rhythms, except for sleep spindles, are generated intrinsically in the cortex. The thalamus plays a modulating or facilitatory role in these rhythms. It has been proposed that a 40 Hz or gamma rhythm is important in allowing for consciousness and integrated brain function. This is produced by circuits during attention and sensory processing tasks that require attention and the "binding" of processed sensory information with memory, attention, and motor responses *(11)*. This rhythm is synchronous across various regions linking thalamocortical networks as well as the hippocampus and neocortex. It has been proposed that such coherent rhythms provide a timing reference that fosters simultaneous or parallel brain activity in a networked rather than purely hierarchical fashion. In this way, for example, all modalities of an

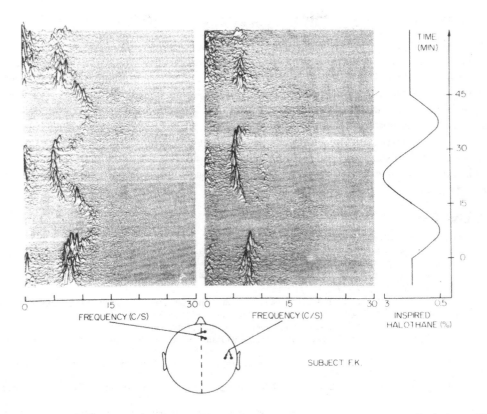

Fig. 4. The power spectrum of the human EEG with different inspired concentrations of halothane. Note the shift to lower frequencies, especially in the frontal region, when the halothane concentration is increased. (reproduced from Nunez, P. Electrical Fields of the Brain. The Neurophysics of EEG. Oxford:Oxford University Press, 1981, with permission.)

object held in memory can be appreciated. It has been found, however, that low voltage fast EEG activity patterns, similar to the gamma rhythm, occur in sleep and in the anesthetized state *(12)*. It may be, however, that there are different types of gamma rhythms (e.g., with varied degrees of synchrony, each with a different physiological significance) or that such unified activity is essential for awareness even though it may occur at other times.

CEREBRAL CORTICAL EFFECTS ON CONSCIOUSNESS PRODUCED BY ANESTHETICS

Most anesthetics decrease net neuronal activity; EPSPs are reduced or blocked in the anesthetic state. Small changes in synaptic gain can have marked effects over large neural systems prior to major blocking effects on individual neurons. Thus, the effects of anesthetics are noted in global or integrated brain function, before individual neurons are silenced.

Many anesthetics have a significant effect on the cerebral cortex, in addition to their profound subcortical effects *(13,14)*. Indeed, Kellaway et al. *(15)* showed that the effects of anesthetics on the isolated cerebral cortex were similar to those on the intact brain. Cortical rhythms of higher frequency affect a wider region of cortex in the normal brain; this high frequency "resonance" is inhibited by anesthetics, causing a coordinated shift to lower frequency spectra (Fig. 4) *(16)*. One high frequency resonance to be affected is the previously mentioned 40-Hz gamma rhythm. With increasing anesthetic dose, rhythmicity is lost altogether.

TOWARDS AN INTEGRATED MODEL OF CONSCIOUSNESS

Consciousness is likely the result of integrated function of multimodal states of the brain. While anyone who attempts to explain consciousness is doomed to be considered reductionalistic, certain aspects can be explained. These isolated components provide at least a glimpse into brain organization and allow for hypotheses about how consciousness arises out of the various processes. There are certain prerequisites to conscious awareness; these include alertness and the ability to attend to certain functions. It is essential that there are interconnections of the various processes or components of awareness. When inter-regional coactivations have not been shown by functional neuro-imaging, it might be that these tools are too crude to note the various subtle but essential interconnections. The mystery is that consciousness is more than the sum of its parts. Strategies are needed that go beyond existing approaches.

REFERENCES

1. James, W. (1890) The Principles of Psychology. Macmillan, London.
2. Moruzzi, G. and Magoun, H. W. (1949) Brain stem reticular formation and activation of the EEG. *Electroenceph. Clin. Neurophysiol.* **1,** 455–473.
3. Kinney, H. C., Korein, J., Panigraphy, A., Dikkes, P., and Goode, R. (1994). Neuropathological findings in the brain of Karen Ann Quinlan. *N. Eng. J. Med.* **330,** 1469–1475.
4. Moscovitch, M. (1979) Information processing and the cerebral hemispheres. (Gazzinga, M. S., ed.), Handbook of Clinical Behavioral Neurobiology, Vol 2: Neuropsychology, Plenum, New York, pp. 379–446.
5. Hebb, D. O. (1964) Organization of Behavior. John Wiley and Sons, New York.
6. Goldman-Rakic, P. S. (1990) Cellular and circuit basis of working memory in the prefrontal cortex of subhuman primates. *Prog. Brain Res.* **85,** 325–336.
7. Moscovitch, M. (1995) Models of consciousness and memory. (Gazzinga, M. S., ed.) The Cognitive Neurosciences. MIT Press: Cambridge, pp. 1341–1356.
8. Bertheier, M., Starkstein, S., and Leiguarda, R. (1988). Asymbolia for pain: a sensory-limbic disconnection syndrome. *Ann. Neurol.* **24,** 41–49.
9. Damasio, A. R. (2000) A neurobiology of consciousness. (Metzinger, T., ed.) Neural Correlates of Consciousness. MIT Press:Cambridge, pp. 111–120.
10. Steriade, M., Gloor, P., Llinas, R. R., Lopes da Silva, F. H., and Musalam, M. M. (1990). Report of IFCN Committee on Basic Mechanisms. Basic mechanisms or cerebral rhythmic activities. *Electoenceph. Clin. Neurophysiol.* **76,** 481–508.
11. Jeffreys, J. G. R., Traub, R. D., and Whittington, M. A. (1996) Neuronal networks for induced "40 Hz" rhythms. *TINS* **19,** 202–204.
12. Vanderwolf, C. H. (2000) Are neocortical gamma waves related to consciousness? *Brain Res.* **855,** 217–224.
13. Ries, C. R. and Puil, E. (1999) Mechanism of anesthesia revealed by shunting actions of isoflurane on thalamocortical neurons. *J. Neurophysiol.* **81,** 1795–1801.
14. Antognini, J. F., Carstens, E., Sudo, M., and Sudo, S. (2000) Isolflurane depresses electroencephalographic and medial thalamic responses to noxious stimulation via an indirect spinal action. *Anesth. Analg.* **91,** 1282–1288.
15. Kellaway, P., Gol, A., and Proler, M. (1966) Electrical activity of the isolated cerebral hemisphere and isolated thalamus. *Exp. Neurol.* **14,** 281–304.
16. Katznelson, R. D. (1980) Normal modes of the brain: neuroanatomical basis and a physiological theoretical model. (Nunez, P. L., ed.) Electric Fields of the Brain. Oxford, Oxford University Press, pp. 401–442.

3

Anesthesia Meets Memory

Tools for Critical Appraisal

Robert A. Veselis

GOALS

The singular, most overriding concern of this chapter is to provide the reader with a framework in which to interpret the exponentially increasing quantity of memory research, with emphasis on the interaction of memory with drugs. Pharmacologic manipulations of memory are used to either (1) understand how drugs affect memory or (2) understand how memory works. Beyond the classic concepts of memory, it is somewhat fruitless to provide a detailed description of the current state of understanding of memory processes, as undoubtedly they will be modified, if not outrightly changed, by the time this book is published. Currently, neurobiologic investigations in humans involve powerful, technologically and/or analytically complex methods to define memory processes. These techniques involve, but are certainly not limited to:

- Electrophysiology (electroencephalography [EEG], event-related potentials [ERPs]),
- Magnetoencephalographay (MEG),
- Detection of neuronal activation responses,
- Regional cerebral blood flow (rCBF) measured using positron electron tomography (PET), and
- Brain oxygen level dependent response (BOLD) as measured by functional magnetic resonance imaging (fMRI).

Basic concepts of functional neuroimaging (FNI) will not be systematically reviewed here, and is done so in other chapters. The emphasis will be on the application of these techniques to understand memory function.

INTRODUCTION

Memory is inextricably linked with arousal and attention. Anesthetics affect memory via changes in arousal and attention, as well as specific effects on memory. This chapter will outline methods and evidence used in separating these effects. We will term the anesthetic effects on attention and arousal systems as their *hypnotic* effects, while effects on memory per se will be termed their *amnesic* effects. Sedation can be considered a lighter level of hypnotic effect than loss of responsiveness, both of which can be considered as a spectrum of the hypnotic effect. There may be a discontinuity at the point of loss of consciousness rather than a smooth graded response *(1)*. Most of the literature reviewed in this chapter specifically involves human subjects. Occasional references will be made to the animal literature where appropriate, but the question always arises as to how a particular paradigm in animals (e.g., inhibitory avoidance behavior) relates to human memory processes.

From: *Contemporary Clinical Neuroscience: Neural Mechanisms of Anesthesia*
Edited by: Joseph F. Antognini et al. © Humana Press Inc., Totowa, NJ

The following definitions, based on original definitions of Posner, are useful *(2,3)*:

- *Arousal (alertness)*: level of alertness; ability to maintain an awake state; endogenous, sustained activation of the cerebral cortex.
- *Attention*: enhancement of task-relevant signals, and inhibition of irrelevant signals, within specific cortical areas processing input from sensory systems.
- *Memory*: retention and retrieval of previously processed information.

Changes in attention and arousal will affect memory performance. This is particularly true when drugs are administered. The methods used to separate the memory and hypnotic effects will be discussed in a separate section below.

Memory can be conceptualized in *cognitive* terms or in *anatomical* terms, which also include receptor mechanisms. There is a close interaction between these two conceptualizations, as will be seen in this chapter. Anesthesiologists may not be as familiar with non-anatomical models, as much of anesthetic research is closely tied to an anatomical constrict—for instance the neuromuscular junction, the respiratory or cardiovascular system, and the autonomic nervous system. Memory in its cognitive sense is NOT tied to a discrete anatomical substrate. A cognitive model of memory has discrete components and testable properties but there is no necessary requirement to elucidate a particular structure/neural network, etc. that embodies these aspects of memory. Current memory research thus has a two pronged emphasis—one investigating memory in a pure behavioral or cognitive sense, and the other elucidating discrete anatomical locations of various memory processes by using the neuro-localizing FNI techniques described previously.

This chapter will initially briefly present the classic model of memory, followed by discussion of various methodologic issues regarding memory research. A more thorough discussion of the cognitive and anatomical models of memory is then presented, followed by the electrophysiologic correlates of memory processes. The use of FNI to investigate memory processes will be highlighted throughout the chapter. The anesthesiologist will be of course most interested in the pharmacologic effects on memory processes, and these are emphasized throughout the chapter, with a discussion of learning during anesthesia near the end.

MEMORY—BASIC CONCEPTS AND ANATOMICAL CONSTRUCTS

Classic Concepts

There are many excellent reviews regarding classic constructs of memory *(4–7)*. These are briefly mentioned here to provide a framework for the rest of the chapter. The concept that memory has multiple, dissociable components rather than different manifestations of a single process under differing circumstances, has developed over time and is now fairly well accepted *(8–12)*. Many of these processes have electrophysiologic correlates, which have been studied intensively for quite some time *(13)*. Memory can be divided conceptually on the basis of time (short and long-term memory *[14]*), its contents (semantic—episodic, procedural *[12]*), and method of encoding and retrieval (explicit vs implicit *[10]*).

Short-Term or Working Memory

Short-term memory is now termed "working memory," and is on the order of a few seconds. It represents transient storage buffers for sensory information that is held and manipulated as part of other cognitive functions such as speech or attention, under the direction of a "central executive" control system. Working memory is composed of two subcomponents, a "visuospatial scratchpad" for temporary storage of visual images, and the "phonological loop" for articulatory rehearsal of verbal material *(15)*.

Long-Term Memory

Information remembered longer than a few seconds involves long-term memory. Transfer of information from working memory to long-term memory appears to be critically dependent on the integrity of medial temporal lobe (MTL) structures. Long-term memory can be further sub-divided.

EPISODIC AND SEMANTIC MEMORY

Episodic memory is that of specific events, people, places etc. This is the memory tested by later recall of, for instance, a list of words or pictures. Episodic memory is further divided into explicit and implicit memory. Explicit memory is memory as we normally think of it, that is, conscious recollection of how and where the events occurred. Implicit memory, on the other hand, does not require conscious recollection; it is manifested as a subtle, unconscious influence on behavior by stimuli that were previously presented, but not consciously remembered.

Semantic memory represents general knowledge, which is formed from multiple unrecallable events—knowledge such as geography and the working rules of a language, etc.

PROCEDURAL MEMORY

Procedural memory represents memory for tasks such as mirror writing, or learning to solve a complex problem such as the Tower of Hanoi, skating, bicycle riding, etc. This form of memory is dissociable from explicit episodic memory.

Methodologic Considerations in Memory Studies

The Classic Ebbinghausan Paradigm

Most memory studies are of a simple "Ebbinghausian" nature: discrete test items are presented for later recall. The circumstances of encoding are modified (e.g., give a drug), and the effect on memory performance is measured. Using this simple approach much useful information has been obtained, and represents a large body of literature on the anesthetic effects of drugs. These types of studies are the easiest to do, to quantitate, and to interpret. However, much information can also be obtained by measurements of other factors (order of recall, clustering of information by categories, memory for source of information, etc.).

Cognitive Memory Models: Double Dissociations

This is a most important concept in memory and behavioral research and thus will be discussed in quite some detail. A double dissociation is used to identify a unique form of memory or cognitive behavior. In itself, a dissociation is not firm evidence of a unique form of memory, and evidence from diverse investigations (behavioral, imaging, lesion studies, etc.) must converge to the conclusion that a separate form of memory exists. Until such a weight of evidence is accumulated, doubts regarding the separateness of different forms of memory exist (an example regarding explicit/implicit memory distinction is provided by *(16)* and *(17)*.

A double dissociation is a necessary, but not sufficient criterion to indicate a certain mechanism of memory exists *(18)*. Briefly—one postulates two memory systems A and B. It is unclear if A is distinct from B, or if A and B are manifestations of a single system under differing circumstances. A double dissociation of A from B essentially means that A and B can be manipulated, or affected, independently of each other. For instance, one can perform an experiment that demonstrates an enhancement of A without any change in B (preferably, an inhibition of B will be found). However, this is not entirely sufficient, and the second step is the demonstration of an inhibition of A with enhancement of B, thus the term "double". Double dissociations can be found in the following circumstances:

1. Anatomical: pathologic lesions (stroke, surgery, brain injury) that affect a certain type of memory. Much information can be obtained from a patient such as Phineas Gage, who survived a steel rod traversing his pre-frontal cortex *(19–21)*[*]. This patient demonstrated a very particular set of behaviors after this injury. The damaged area of the brain is postulated to control these behaviors. Other patients may perform poorly on a test of explicit memory while obtaining normal levels of priming for word stems or perceptually fragmented images *(18,22)*. These findings led to the hypothesis that implicit and explicit memory systems were separate. However, lesion studies alone cannot demonstrate with certainty the anatomical site for these behaviors. Lesions only affecting certain components of memory may be rare (e.g., an isolated short term memory deficit). Thus when a patient with a certain set of findings is located (such as *[23]*), this can be very significant for support of a certain memory model.

2. *Developmental*: effect of age. Children demonstrate adult behavior in certain memory systems as early as age 3, and elderly patients loose certain forms of memory out of proportion to others.

3. *Drug induced*: Many drugs, such as anticholinergics, alcohol and the benzodiazepines, can affect one form of memory and leave the other intact (for example *see [24–27]*).

4. *Manipulation of testing* procedures in normal subjects *(28)*. For example, reducing the exposure time of stimuli presented to normal subjects can reduce their memory performance to the level of amnesic patients. Alternatively, having normal subjects process the stimuli by searching for specific letters in the words, rather than by encoding the meaning of the words, will impair their ability to explicitly recall the words while maintaining the ability to complete word fragments with the correct word.

5. *Statistical independence* of an effect seen in B from A, even though the effects seen in memory tests can be mediated by both the A and B. Support is provided for two distinct memory systems if the performance on B is statistically unrelated to the performance on A.

Methodologic Considerations in Drug Studies

The most important consideration in memory—drug interaction studies is the confounding sedative effect invariably produced by the drugs administered. To isolate a sedative effect from an amnesic effect is difficult, but can be done using careful analysis. Similar dissociations to those described above can be used to define the separate nature of hypnosis (sedation) and amnesia in the case of drug effects, as follows:

1. *Anatomical (in animals)*: Lesion studies are limited, as there are no cases of people with decreased arousal, but normal memory. Lesion studies in animals are eminently possible, and much information is potentially available using these models. Some exciting possibilities regarding anesthetic drug actions have arisen in this situation. Examples include the apparent lack of amnesic effect with propofol and other benzodiazepines when the basolateral amygdala complex is absent, *(29–32)* or the cholinergic influence on the amnesic effects of propofol *(33)*. Caution is warranted in interpreting these data (p. 767 of *[34]*):

   "First, if a brain lesion fails to affect a learning task, it cannot be stated that this part of the brain is unimportant in normal animals. Second, if the lesion does influence performance of the task, it does not necessarily mean that it is the only neural structure involved. Third, the aim of the ablation methods is in a way never attainable, for it throws away the object (a region of the brain) one wishes to study."

   These points are exemplified when an attempt is made to relate neuropathologic findings to cognitive effects (*see* ref. *[35]* for a good example of this in patients with Korsafoff's syndrome). Care needs to be taken to distinguish between a system involved in memory processing, and one that affects a memory process. One needs to be cautious in extrapolating results in lesioned animals to functioning of human memory. For example, lesioned animals may respond entirely differently when only slight modification of testing procedures occurs. (for example, *see* refs. *[36,37]*) How does Pavlovian fear conditioning, or inhibitory avoidance relate to human memory? Even though humans and primates are very close evolutionarily, substantial difficulties are present in translating results from primate studies into humans *(38)*. Obviously, these types of problems are more critical in the case of rats and mice.

2. *Developmental*: not applicable.

3. *Drug induced*: A number of examples of drugs with hypnotic, but no or little amnesic effects are present, e.g. opioids, barbiturates, diphenhydramine. As changes in arousal affect memory, frequently the disso-

---

[*]*See* http://www.deakin.edu.au/hbs/GAGEPAGE/ for further interesting information relating to Phineas Gage, including historical information regarding lobotomy for treatment of psychiatric disease.

ciation is not pure. The memory effects of these drugs can be directly compared with amnesic drugs, and conclusions drawn regarding memory specific drug actions *(39,40)*. A specific antagonist can be used in partial doses to reverse hypnotic and memory effects differentially, though this is not always possible *(41,42)*. Similarly, repeated doses of drug may induce differential tolerance (hypnotic effects are more sensitive than memory effects), or different dose-response curves can be constructed *(43)*.

4. *Manipulation of testing procedures*: Various behavioral measures are more or less sensitive to the hypnotic vs. amnesic effects of drugs.

5. *Statistical Independence*: These methods are frequently used to dissociate sedative from amnesic effects, with varying degrees of success. Testing for correlations between sedation and memory scores can be performed, (for example *see* refs. *[44,45]*) or corrections for sedative effects can be performed using partial correlations.

There is always the question of the relevancy of volunteer memory studies to clinical situations. Stimuli are recalled based on their initial "depth of processing", or presence of concurrent orienting stimuli, such as pain, etc. *(46,47)*. Thus, the amnesic effect of drugs for a word list will be quite different than the amnesic effects for the injection of local anesthetic or bone drilling.

There are many influences on the encoding of verbal information that are already well known, and similar considerations probably apply to other classes of stimuli. Such factors include better memory when processes engaged during retrieval are the same as during encoding, deep or semantic processing during encoding, or retrieval based on context (associations regarding the retrieved stimulus) *(13)*. Such effects explain differences in memory for a list of real words versus a list of pseudowords. Three pseudo-words (no semantic processing) are as difficult to memorize as 5 real words (with automatic semantic processing) *(48)*. A similar phenomenon occurs when recalling unrelated words (5 words) vs a sentence containing a string of words that makes semantic sense (16 or more words) *(49)*. Short term memory involves "chunking" of related material, with each chunk acting as one item, even though that item may contain multiple words *(50)*. Such observations are still refining models of working memory *(49)*. Alternatively, if a person does not want to remember an unpleasant event, they can actively repress recall of such information, an ability which improves with repetition *(51)*. Such confounding factors must be considered in the interpretation of results from memory studies.

The most sensitive test for drug effects on memory are tasks that involve learning of new information beyond the capacity of short-term memory *(52)*. Thus, memorization of a single picture, or a few words may not be very informative, though it is likely that short-term or working memory processes are centrally involved in initial encoding of long term memory. Despite prior evidence that amnesic drugs have little effect on short term memory (as assessed by digit span *[52–54]*), other investigations reveal that the capacity of working memory is impaired by various sedative drugs *(55)*. As well, information in the working memory buffer or that which is recently encoded, is easily lost.

It is frequently difficult, particularly in older studies investigating memory-drug interactions, to obtain enough data to critically appraise confounding influences. Though drug effects on memory are clearly related to serum concentrations, few studies measure actual serum concentrations. Frequently, estimated serum concentrations are reported, but even in the best of situations, there is probably a 30% variance associated with these values. As well, especially with drugs such as propofol, it is important to obtain arterial concentrations, more representative of brain concentration *(56)*. Especially when only a single dose of drug is administered (some studies omit the dose administered!), a dose-effect response cannot be determined. Recently, more studies are measuring appropriate serum concentrations (i.e., arterial blood sampling, multiple doses), and are ensuring constant serum concentrations during the presentation of material to be learned using pharmacokinetically modeled infusion devices *(57–60)*. Though actual versus target concentrations maybe quite variable, these devices ensure relatively constant serum concentrations *(57)*.

In terms of psychometrics, differing methodologies are frequently used and reported with varying amounts of detail. Results may be difficult to interpret if non-standard tests are used without an appropriate control group, or development of norms. The psychopharmacologic literature seems less affected by this than the anesthesia literature *(61)*. Important details frequently not reported include the time of testing compared to drug administration, demographics of the study population, and the adequacy of memory testing to detect the type of memory being studied. Thus, caution is warranted regarding isolated findings in one or a few studies. Even though relating to ERP studies, an overview of publication standards for cognitive research using ERPs is very applicable to cognitive studies using drugs *(62)*. The interested reader is referred to sections A (formulation of the study), B (subjects), L (Statistical Analysis), and M (Discussion of Results) in that publication.

Anatomical Localization of Memory Processes

Multiplicity of Techniques and Converging Evidence

It is generally well accepted that specific memory processes are located in discrete, though possibly widely distributed, brain regions *(63)*. Thus, though there is no one "seat of memory," specific neuroanatomical constructs can be developed. Earlier understanding of memory processes was based primarily on careful study of patients with anatomically definable lesions. This understanding of memory was revolutionized using modern neuroimaging techniques, starting about 1990. The following discussion presents an example of the rapid progress in understanding the neuroanatomical underpinnings of cognitive behavior when both old and new investigative techniques are simultaneously used. This example presents an evolution of knowledge of a cognitively interesting region of the brain, the prefrontal cortex (PFC) in relation to memory processes.

Overwhelming evidence from human, animal, and lesion studies point to the medial temporal lobe (MTL) structures for the normal function of explicit episodic memory (remembering what one did or experienced past short term memory span for a few seconds to minutes *[7]*). This evidence strongly supports the ability to localize a given process to the MTL that is involved in explicit memory. (*See* ref. *[13]*). With the advent of FNI, numerous studies using explicit memory paradigms previously used in patients were undertaken. Surprisingly, the hippocampus, or even nearby MTL regions, were rarely identified as being active in these studies (a few notable exceptions are *[64,65]*). Alternatively, a great deal more studies found activations in the PFC with these episodic memory processes *(66,67)*(*see* Figs. 1 and 2) A number of explanations were advanced for this apparent inconsistency *(68)*. Based on these findings, a substantial and important role for the PFCs was advanced in memory encoding and retrieval *(69)*. This HERA model (hemispheric encoding and retrieval asymmetry) synthesized information from various FNI studies of memory and retrieval of visually presented words. The hypothesis stated that the left PFC was active during encoding, while the right PFC was active during retrieval of verbal information.

Yet, study of patients with lesions in the PFC revealed quite different results from the dramatic memory impairments seen in patients with MTL lesions. Based on the seemingly incongruous results of FNI studies, new memory paradigms were tested in patients with lesions in the PFC. The results of these further clarified the role of PFC in memory processing *(70)* (*see* Fig. 2) A new, testable, hypothesis was proposed where primarily the left PFC was involved in the selection of appropriate responses from competing possibilities, and that retrieval per se was likely a hippocampal/MTL function. This hypothesis was much more in keeping with the "executive" functions previously ascribed to PFC. These "executive" processes include inhibition of automatic responses, selection of appropriate response from competing alternatives, retrieval of contextual information about the stimulus ("remember" vs "know" memory), and imagining of complex mental processes in others *(71–74)*.

Episodic memory paradigms were developed to test these "executive" hypotheses for the PFC in memory processing. In sum, the results of these studies support the supervisory role of the PFC in episodic memory processes *(75–81)*. Recent availability of higher-resolution FNI techniques,

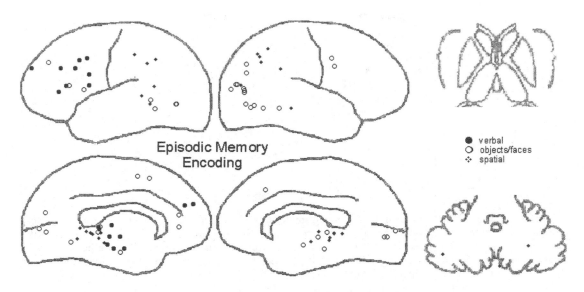

Fig 1. Locations of activations in PET imaging studies of rCBF during episodic memory encoding tasks. *(67)* Memory for personally experienced events (episodic memory) involves encoding, storage, and retrieval processes. Note the primarily left lateralization of verbal encoding processes. (Reproduced with permission, Fig. 9 from Cabeza,, R. and Nyberg, L (2000). Imaging cognition II: An empirical review of 275 PET and fMRI studies. *J. Cogn. Neurosci.* **12(1)**: p. 22.)

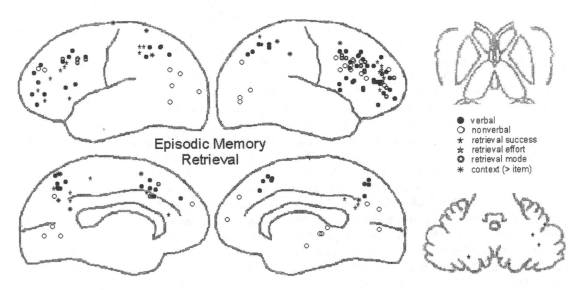

Fig 2. Locations of activations in PET imaging studies of rCBF during episodic memory retrieval tasks. *(67)* Note the greater right lateralization of verbal retrieval processes. This asymmetry (*see* Fig. 1) was the basis for the original HERA hypothesis. Further refinements of this hypothesis were necessary based on multiple experiments examining various aspects of retrieval processes (e.g., retrieval effort vs retrieval success, the nature of the retrieval task, type of material involved, etc.) (Reproduced with permission, Fig. 10 from Cabeza, R. and Nyberg, L. (2000). Imaging cognition II: An empirical review of 275 PET and fMRI studies. *J. Cogn. Neurosci.* **12(1)**: p. 25.)

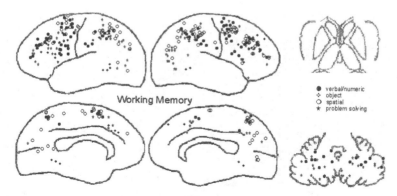

Fig. 3. Locations of activations in PET imaging studies of rCBF during working memory tasks. *(67)* Most working memory tasks activate prefrontal and parietal regions. Storage of material may occur primarily in the parietal regions, whereas rehearsal processes occur in the frontal regions. Communications between these regions may be mediated by oscillatory EEG activity in theta and gamma ranges. Problem solving represents the executive processes in the Braddeley model of working memory. (Reproduced with permission, Fig. 7. from Cabeza,, R. and Nyberg, L. (2000). Imaging cognition II: An empirical review of 275 PET and fMRI studies. *J. cogn. Neurosci.* **12(1)**: p. 17.

including analytic methods to ascertain the functional connectivity between brain regions, have in fact been able to identify hippocampal activity in memory processes *(82–85)*.

Careful ERP studies have also helped to define the role of PFC versus MTL in memory processes *(13)*. The left PFC is involved with encoding of new material, but the hippocampus retrieves semantic material during this encoding process, while the PFC plays a supervisory role (*see* Dm effect in the Section on Encoding). Encoding of new material in conjunction with the semantic attributes retrieved by the hippocampus (memorizing real words) results in deeper encoding, and thus more likely success at subsequent retrieval. Real words are more likely to be freely recalled with a "remember" judgment (knowing when the word was seen) than material encoded without this semantic benefit, such as pseudo-words. This more shallowly encoded material may only be recognized as a familiar item with a "know" judgment *(86–90)*.

Based on this large body of literature, a new synthesis of information incorporating the role of PFCs in episodic memory processes is made *(91)*. The original HERA model thus has been modified to a episodic memory retrieval mode (REMO) model, wherein retrieval is associated with an "on-line" neurocognitive state of previous experience, that is matched to incoming sensory stimuli *(80)*.

This "back and forth" scientific enquiry between different neuroimaging methodologies and older, more established investigative methods is rapidly refining what is known about memory processes. Advancement of knowledge is now so rapid that a detailed description of memory processes in this chapter is somewhat counter-productive, as by the publication date, understanding of these could be quite different. It is emphasized that the reader should concentrate on the principles presented here rather than specific details. The example regarding the PFC demonstrates the importance of obtaining evidence from multiple lines of inquiry to formulate an accurate assessment of the true nature of the memory process under investigation.

A Cognitive Model of Human Memory

Most constructs of memory that the reader will come across are described in cognitive terms. These describe memory processes without reference to specific anatomical substrates, other than localization to somewhere in the CNS. The seminal studies of Karl Lashley appeared to show that massive amounts of cortex could be removed from an experimental animal without abolishing a specific memory. Until recently, it was very difficult to locate the structures involved in particular aspects of memory. Thus, for many years it was felt that a specific memory "engram" was not localized to any particular part of the brain. Historically, the concept that memory processes were specific to certain neuroanatomical regions were based first on careful study of patients with defined neurologic lesions. This hypothesis was further strengthened by electrophysiologic investigations, though these were of poor spatial resolution (*see* Section on Elecrophysiologic Markers). More elegant animal studies provided further support for anatomical based memory processes *(92)*. The recent availability of FNI has provided strong corroboration of anatomical localization of specific memory processes in humans. Anatomical regions are discussed following this section describing memory processes in cognitive terms.

The Multiple Components of Memory

As discussed briefly above, the original division into short-term and long-term memory has now expanded to include numerous storage buffers ranging from the very temporary "working memory," to the long term stores of episodic (memory for events), and semantic (general knowledge) memory, which can preserve information for many years. A third category of memory is procedural memory, which includes classical conditioning, and memory for motor skills (e.g.; writing, swimming, riding a bicycle). Relevant aspects of these different forms of memory will be discussed in more detail in this section. As language processing is currently not a large area of research regarding anesthetic drug action, semantic memory is only briefly discussed.

Working Memory

The concept of working memory is becoming more important in understanding memory processes, and it is a topic of intense investigation (179 publications in 2000). Working memory (WM) as used in this chapter is defined in the cognitive sense:

> "a limited capacity system allowing the temporary storage and manipulation of information necessary for such complex tasks as comprehension, learning and reasoning."

WM maintains a limited amount of information in an active state for a brief period of time. Initial understanding of this cognitive process began with a "short term memory" of 7 plus or minus two items *(50)* held active for a period of 0–60 s. The neurophysiologic implementation of working memory is in reverberatory neuronal oscillations, first proposed by Hebb *(93)*.

The hallmark of WM is sustained neuronal activity over a "prolonged" time span (on the order of longer than a few seconds, for instance *see [48,94,95]*). Information in WM is held and manipulated in service of other behavioral goals, such as speech or attention, under the direction of a "central executive" control system *(96)*. Baddeley and Hitch were the first to propose this multi-component model of working memory, addressing inconsistencies of the original concept of a unitary short-term memory with observed results *(14,15,97)*.

The current model of WM is one of multiple interacting components. These are a "visuospatial scratchpad" for temporary storage of visual images, and a "phonological loop" for articulatory rehearsal of verbal material *(49)*. This model proposed over 25 yr ago, has been remarkably durable. Results from recent FNI studies still continue to validate the basic properties of this model *(98,99)*. Many of the properties of WM have been developed using dual task strategies, where a competing task interferes with the functioning of one of the components of WM. As an example, if articulatory rehearsal is repressed by having the subject constantly repeat "the," recall of items is markedly depressed, a behavioral effect now visualizable in the brain *(100)*.

The phonologic loop is the best understood component of WM. The purpose of phonological loop is to rehearse acoustic and verbal items in an articulatory rehearsal system. This rehearsal refreshes items in WM that begin to decay in a matter of seconds, and improves later recall of this material. The phonologic loop implements self-monitoring of both receptive and expressive speech to maintain coherency and comprehension, and have evolved to support language. The loop is particularly adapted for retention of sequential material, such as a digit span. The phonologic loop model explains the following observations: (1) phonologic similarity effect—items similar in sound are more difficult to recall accurately, (2) word-length effect—it's easier to recall a list of short words than long words, (3) transfer of information between codes—"non-verbal" material (e.g., pictures, sounds) are frequently named, and the verbal representation of this material is rehearsed for subsequent recall rather than the object itself. The visuospatial scratchpad is less well defined. Though similar rehearsal type processes can occur as with words, this ability seems less well developed. Frequently, these objects are named and handled in the phonologic loop.

The storage of material vs the manipulation of that material in working memory are dissociable *(101–103)*. Storage processes seem to occur in posterior, parietal regions, whereas manipulation of information occurs in anterior, prefrontal regions. There is a right/left asymmetry for spatial vs verbal material. Coherent EEG activity in the theta range "binds" information in separate brain regions involved with working memory into a cognitive whole *(104)*. This represents the neuroanatomical implementation of the cognitive concept of working memory, which was developed and tested independently of neuroanatomical understanding of this model. The neuroanatomical data add substantial support to the veracity of the cognitive model. In the cognitive model, it makes little difference where individual processes are located or how they communicate with each other.

As with any model, actual results may require the model to be modified. In the case of WM, such a result is the finding that it is much easier to remember 16 words contained in a meaningful sentence than it is to remember 16 unrelated words. This is not easily incorporated into the classic working memory model, and to explain these results an additional component of WM has been proposed. An episodic buffer of limited capacity is proposed to integrate information from a variety of sources. This refined model provides explanations for the impact of visual similarity between words on verbal recall, or the impact of meaning on the immediate recall of prose and sentences *(49)*.

WM is not only used to memorize lists of items. It is centrally important, being a cornerstone of higher cognitive processes such as reasoning, decision-making, problem solving, and language comprehension *(105,106)*. In fact, it is likely a key component of consciousness as well *(1,49)*. The additional episodic buffer in Baddeley's classic model of working memory provides a method of integrating information from various sources and expressing a conscious awareness of this multisensory perception *(49)*.

Long-term Memory

Transfer of most information from short-term working memory of limited capacity to long-term memory of essentially unlimited capacity appears to be critically dependent on the integrity of medial temporal lobe structures for episodic memories *(7,107)*. This process can be disrupted by various events including head injury, electric shock, extreme stress, and certain drugs (such as possibly propofol that inhibit protein synthesis) or REM sleep *(108–110)*. Careful studies in patients with specific neurologic lesions have demonstrated that encoding into long term memory is not necessarily dependent on short term memory processes. In fact, MTL structures are not needed for encoding of semantic memories *(111)*.

Episodic Memory: Explicit and Implicit

Episodic memory can be divided into explicit and implicit memory. Explicit memory is memory as we normally think of it, that is, conscious recollection of how and where the events occurred. In the terminology of consciousness, this type of memory has been termed autonoetic (being able to travel back in time and remember the exact context of a memory) *(90,106)*(*see* Figs. 1 and 2) Implicit memory, on the other hand, does not require conscious recollection; it is manifested as a subtle, unconscious influence on behavior by stimuli that were previously presented, but which are not consciously remembered. For instance, if a person is shown a series of letters that form a grammar (a set of rules defining which letters can occur following a given letter) that person will learn that knowledge, and tend to preferentially select correct letters according to those grammatical rules without any conscious knowledge of that grammar, even if the rules are quite complex *(112,113)*. Another form of implicit memory is the ability to be influenced by previous, subliminal, exposure to a stimulus (priming), and is discussed in more detail below.

A distinct type of memory has been termed noetic consciousness *(90,106)*. This memory occurs as a "familiarity", a feeling different than a distinct "remember" recollective response. "I remember dinner with you last night," for instance, is contrasted with the familiarity response of "I know you from somewhere ... what's your name?" *(90,114–116)*. Most likely, this type of memory is an explicit form of memory. The distinction between implicit, weak explicit, and semantic memory (e.g. knowledge about the world) can become a little blurry, especially when the time frame of stimulus presentation is that contained in most cognitive studies. For example, the memory demonstrated in the subjects above learning an artificial grammar over the short time frame of a study situation has been termed implicit *(112,113)*. But the grammatical rules of our native language are considered semantic memory. When does this implicit memory become a semantic memory? Another example of this blurriness is the difficulty in distinguishing weak explicit memory from implicit memory in studies of learning during anesthesia *(117–120)*. Various dichotomies have been proposed, and the interrelation of these still need to be sorted out. These include (1) remembering vs knowing, (2) explicit vs implicit memory, (3) conscious vs unconscious processes, (4) controlled vs automatic processes *(121)*.

Despite this indistinct division, numerous studies have demonstrated, in both patients and normals, that explicit memory can be impaired while implicit memory is unaffected *(16,122)*. Such effects have also been found with pharmacological agents, including diazepam, midazolam, and scopolamine *(24,25,42,123–130)*.

PRIMING: A FORM OF IMPLICIT MEMORY

This category of long-term memory is of particular interest to anesthesiologists, because it has been postulated as a possible mechanism for learning during anesthesia. This form of memory is demonstrated by certain testing procedures termed priming tests *(18)*. Priming is demonstrated when the probability of choosing the previously experienced stimulus is increased by the occurrence of some prior event that is not consciously recollected. Examples include faster relearning of information which had been encountered before, completion of word stems or word fragments with words from a previously presented list, perceptual priming (enhanced perception of visually degraded words or pictures, which were presented previously in their complete form), or preference for the subliminal stimulus (in terms of choice, familiarity or liking).

Perceptual priming is frequently studied; here the priming is based on physical aspects of the stimuli, such as visually degraded pictures, which are identified more quickly after having been previously viewed, or the increased reading speed of a previously presented story *(131,132)*. The factors underlying priming on perceptual tests are complex, including modality of encoding and semantic relationship *(133)*. *Conceptual priming* is based on semantic processing, e.g., category generation or word stem completion *(117–119)*. Faster relearning or recognition of information that has been encountered before is termed *repetition priming (134)*.

Methodologic issues regarding priming tests are discussed more thoroughly in the Section on Learning during Anesthesia.

PROCEDURAL MEMORY

Procedural memory is also dissociable from explicit or episodic memory *(12)*(*see* Fig. 4). Patients with severe anterograde amnesia may be trained to acquire a new motor skill (e.g., mirror writing, or learning to solve a complex problem such as the Tower of Hanoi, which requires manipulating objects using many steps in a particular sequence). These patients may have no conscious memory of ever having performed the test before, or indeed of having ever met the tester, yet their performance on the task shows significant gains over time *(12,124,135)*.

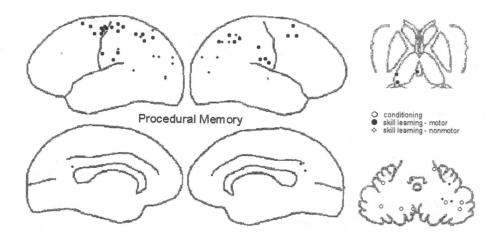

Fig. 4. Locations of activations in PET imaging studies of rCBF during procedural memory tasks. *(67)* These involve not only learning motor skills, but also the classic conditioning response. (Reproduced with permission, Fig. 11 from Cabeza, R. and Nyberg, L. (2000). Imagining cognition II: An empirical review of 275 PET and fMRI studies. *J. Cogn. Neurosci.* **12**(1): p. 30.)

IMPLICIT MEMORY—ANATOMICAL CORRELATES

No discrete anatomical structure or network embodies implicit or procedural memory mechanisms. It appears that a number of regions act in concert during this memory process. This section demonstrates the overlap between cognitive and neuroanatomical concepts, illustrating the somewhat artificial structure of this chapter. One of the best ways to distinguish implicit from explicit memory is by neuroanatomical separation. Behavioral distinctions may be difficult to demonstrate convincingly, but the combination of the two provides good evidence for the action of separate implicit memory mechanisms. Neuroanatomical separation between explicit and implicit memory is difficult to achieve with electrophysiology because of its limited spatial resolution (*see* the implicit memory section under Electrophysiologic correlates below). However, FNI techniques are ideally suited to this purpose, and there has been renewed interest in studies of implicit memory processes.

Priming effects are widespread in prefrontal, precuneus, angular gyrus, parietal, and occiptal regions, and is somewhat dependent on the modality of presentation/recall and the specific learning paradigm *(113,136–141)*. The temporal lobes seem important in face memory *(142)*, especially the amygdalar region when emotive responses are associated with the stimuli *(143,144)*. MTL activity seems related to retrieval of previously encoded information, and relates to awareness in subjects while learning the task *(85,139,141)*. These studies provide increasingly firm evidence for the separate existence of implicit memory from explicit memory processes.

An Anatomical Model of Memory

Traditionally, a small number of neuroanatomical regions were regarded as the "seat if memory," primarily the hippocampus and MTL structures. Studies of amnesic patients whose temporal lobes had been extensively removed to control their epileptic seizures, underlined the importance of these structures in the permanent acquisition of new information. However, once material has been encoded into long term memories, which are widely distributed through the cortex, they can still be retrieved despite the absence of MTL structures *(7,145–148)*. The nature of the old memory appears critical as to whether it is affected or not by hippocampal pathology *(149,150)*. The critical MTL regions can be thought of as "bottleneck" structures involved in memory. The hippocampus not only is active only during encoding of new memories, but also serves to "update" or "refresh" old memories *(149)*.

Because of notable clinical effects of MTL lesions, early memory research was focused on this neuroanatomical region first, and regions such as the PFC, for example, were identified as important in memory processes much later when more advanced techniques were used to study them. As current concepts of memory embody widespread networks, any anatomical division will be arbitrary. It must be remembered that in FNI studies, deactivations (inhibition of neuronal processing) are as important to look at as are activations (enhanced neuronal processing), and help understand cortical network dynamics *(151)*.

Systems and Processing Approaches to Neural Substrates of Memory

A fusion of two seemingly contradictory approaches to memory processes is occurring. These concepts are one of multiple distinct neural memory systems in the brain—the "systems" approach *(152)*—and the other of a single neural network, whose functionality is expressed in different ways— the "process" approach *(153,154)*. Functional neuroimaging studies have provided key insights leading to the fusion of these two concepts. The systems interpretation of data is supported by observations that different memory tasks activate different regions of the brain *(155,156)*, while the process approach is strengthened by the repeated observation that many regions of the brain work together in a distributed network to accomplish even simple tasks of mnemonic processing *(157)*. As an example, direct contrast between explicit and implicit memory reveals that many regions of activation are common to both tasks *(141)*.

Neuroanatomical Regions With Consistently Defined Roles in Memory Processes

MEDIAL TEMPORAL LOBE STRUCTURES (MTL): HIPPOCAMPUS; PARAHIPPOCAMPUS, ENTORHINAL AND PERIRHINAL CORTEX, AND AMYGDALA

These regions have been discussed extensively throughout this chapter already, and will be further discussed in other sections because of their key role in memory. Patients with lesions in MTL areas have severe memory loss for episodic or context sensitive events, such as, where one's house is (unless this is a very old memory *[148]*), the time of day, etc. Animal models of amnesia have confirmed these patient studies, and have added further insights into specific neuroanatomical features in the MTL *(158–162)*. Normal functioning of the MTL *(163,164)*, the diencephalon (thalamus, mammillary nuclei, and fornix) *(35,165)*, and the basal forebrain *(166,167)* is essential for the ability to remember *(see* Fig. 5 and 6). Both the hippocampus and amygdala are important in episodic memory formation, and one needs the destruction of both for severe and lasting amnesia *(111)*. The surrounding cortical masses, which include the entorhinal and perirhinal cortex, are critical to the transfer of episodic information to long-term memory, the location of which is still not understood, but probably is widespread throughout the cortex.

AMYGDALA

Animal lesion studies have demonstrated the importance of amygdala in emotive modulation of memories *(168,169)*. With the advent of FNI, the role of the amygdala in humans is becoming more clear *(144,170–175)*. The amygdala has been implied in priming processes, especially with visual face stimuli, supporting the separate role of amygdala and its connections in memory formation. Lesions in animals in the baso-lateral amygdala complex impair the memory effects of GABAergic agents such as the benzodiazepines and propofol, at least, in the memory paradigms used in these studies (e.g., inhibitory avoidance) *(29,30,32,176–179)*.

FRONTAL LOBES—PREFRONTAL CORTEX

As discussed previously, the role of the frontal lobes in memory is more complex than apparent on initial FNI studies using traditional memory paradigms. These more complex functions, correspond well to the traditional roles of frontal lobes in inhibition of automatic behavior, response selection, and other "executive" control functions *(180–184)*. Patients with frontal lobe lesions have difficulty

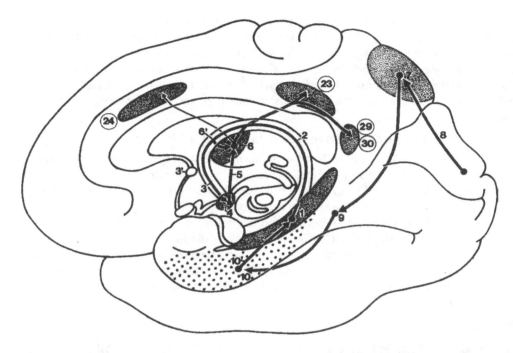

Fig. 5. Cortical connenctions of the polysynaptic intrahippocampal pathway. Note the wide dispersion of connections from the hippocampus to many brain regions involved with cognition and memory. This provides a neuroanatomical basis for the hippocampus being a bottleneck structure in memory processes. (1) hippocampus, (2) body, and (3) column of fornix (3 anterior commissure), (4) mamillary body, (5) mamilothalamic tract, (6) anterior thalamic nucleus, (7) parietal association areas, (8) superior visual system, (9) parahippocampal gyrus, (10) entorhinal area (10 perforant fibers). Brodmann's areas 24 (cingulate cortex), 23 (posterior cingulate cortex), and 29, 30 (retrosplenial cortex). (Reproduced with permission, Fig. 16 p. 34 Duvernoy, H. M. and Bourgouin, P. (1998). The Human Hippocampus: functional anatomy, vascularization, and serial sections with MRI. Berlin; New York, Springer.)

making estimates or inferences from everyday experiences *(182)*. They show normal ability to learn new information, but later may not be able to identify the source or context of that information *(183,184)*. They have difficulty with the temporal ordering of memory; thus, they are impaired when making judgments of recency both for word lists and for real-world events *(183,184)*. They show normal recognition memory, but surprisingly have great difficulty with free recall tests, perhaps owing to a lack of ability to organize the material coherently during initial learning. These patients are also impaired at retrieval of semantic information, for example, on word fluency tests. Prefrontal lesions cause severe problems when irrelevant information must be ignored, since they are particularly disrupted by irrelevant or extraneous details. These patients have problems shifting between different strategies; they will often persevere in using an inappropriate response, or interject elements from a previous task *(182,185)*.

CEREBELLUM

Recently, there has been an accumulation of evidence that the cerebellum makes a far more important contribution to cognition than was previously thought *(186,187)*(*see* Figs. 1–4). Far from being exclusively a motor organ, the cerebellum appears to be involved in some cognitive, linguistic, and emotional functions through links to the limbic system and the prefrontal cortex. Specifically, it appears to control verb generation, affecting linguistic fluency, and in the monkey, it is involved in

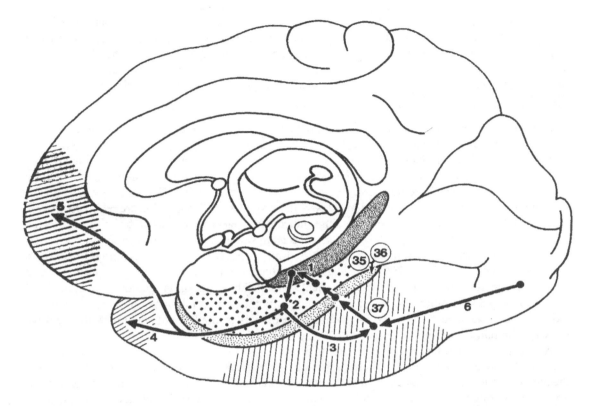

Fig. 6. Cortical connenctions of the direct intraippocamal pathway. (1) Hippocampus, (2) entorhinal cortex, (3) inferior temporal lobe association areas, (4) temporal pole, (5) prefrontal cortex, (6) inferior visual system. Brodmann's areas 37 (temporal lobe association areas), and 35, 36 (perirhinal cortex). (Reproduced with permission, Fig. 18 p. 35 Duvernoy, H. M. and Bourgoiun, P. (1998). The Human Hippocampus: functional anatomy, vascularization and serial sections with MRI. Berlin; New York, Springer.)

response inhibition in "go-no go" decisions *(186)*. A detailed anatomical description of the circuitry linking cerebellum to other brain structures in primates is presented by Schmahmann *(187)*. His model associates cognitive, linguistic, and some memory functions with the cerebellar hemispheres and dentate nucleus, while autonomic regulation and emotionally relevant memory are linked with other areas of the cerebellum.

The circuits linking prefrontal cortex to the contralateral cerebellum have been identified in humans using positron emission tomography (PET) imaging *(188)*. Lesions in frontal or parietal cortex are often associated with depressed metabolism in the contralateral cerebellar hemisphere, a phenomenon known as crossed cerebellar diaschisis. In normal subjects, naturally occurring asymmetries of glucose metabolism between left and right frontal lobes were correlated with similar but opposite asymmetries between the cerebellar hemispheres.

The Brain is Richly Connected to Itself

It has been estimated that every cortical area is connected to 10–20 other cortical areas *(189)*. Thus, it is no surprise that memory is dependent on many neural structures that interact with each other in interconnected networks as opposed to a linear, sequential fashion. *(4,103,164,190–193)*. Dissociable memory processes (e.g., spatial vs verbal memory), utilize overlapping, though distinct regions of the brain *(157,190,193,194)*. This concept of memory provides a neuroanatomical framework for the hypothesis that anesthetic drugs have specific effects on memory independent of their sedative/hypnotic effects, even though highly inter-correlated *(195,196)*. There are many possible neuroanatomical targets for the expression of amnesic effects of drugs other than the obvious target seemingly of the hippocampus and MTL structures. Recent FNI evidence indicates that amnesic drugs affect the thalamus, the pre-frontal cortices, and regions important in working memory.

Neuroanatomical Regions Affected by Drug Administration

A number of FNI studies have shown regional changes in glucose metabolism or cerebral blood flow in the presence of CNS active drugs *(197–206)*. The interesting finding across these studies is that discrete markers of changes in neuronal activity are located in neuroanatomically interesting regions. These regions coincide with those known to subserve cognitive functions affected by the particular drug studied. Note that most drugs studied will affect global CBF and metabolism. The markers of neuronal activity identified in many of these studies are changes that are relatively greater than the global changes induced. These findings indicate that selective regions of the brain are affected to a larger extent by these drugs, and could serve as a physiologic basis for the action of these drugs. FNI techniques localize cognitive processes based on changes in regional physiology coupled to neuronal activity *(66,67,207–209)*. The logical conclusion is that FNI techniques can be used to identify the neuroanatomical structures specifically affected by drug administration by imaging local changes in physiology related to drug administration. As most drugs inhibit neuronal activity, FNI is likely to be more successful if the interaction of a drug is studied in conjunction with cognitive activity stimulating neuronal activity *(205,206,210–214)*.

As a concrete example of this in relation to memory processes, some data relating to changes in rCBF with midazolam and propofol are presented. As both these drugs cause memory impairment, the hypothesis is that these drugs would inhibit neuronal activity. The neuroanatomical regions preferentially inhibited by these drugs would be identified by decreases in rCBF. First, it must be demonstrated that inhibition of neuronal activity is not representative of a generalized drug-induced impairment of neuronal responses. This is not the case for tactile stimulation, at least at low drug concentrations affecting memory, *(215)* and the expected increase in rCBF with increasing word stimulus rate is preserved during heavy propofol sedation *(see* Fig. 7*)*. It is interesting to note that cortical response to tactile stimulation is shut off when propofol concentration is approx 1.5 µg/mL, *(215)* whereas, a similar concentration appears not to affect auditory sensation (Fig. 7). This apparent contradictory observation may be explained by the fact that touch sensation is mediated via the ventral posterior thalamic nuclei, whereas sound is mediated via the medial geniculate body of the thalamus. These observations may point to the neuroanatomical basis for the clinical anecdotal observation that during induction and emergence from anesthesia hearing is the last thing to go, and the first thing to come back. This may also provide the basis for the influence of external auditory input on dream material in REM sleep.

Sedative drugs will decrease global CBF by approx 15% *(198)*. Decreases in rCBF greater than this global drug effect can be identified using voxel-based statistical techniques that test the entire brain image space with appropriate correction for multiple comparisons *(216,217)*. The results are shown in Fig. 8 for both midazolam and propofol. Both drugs cause localized decreases in rCBF. These changes are lateralized at low doses of drug, and become more widespread as the dose of drug increases. One can identify regions of the brain affected by the larger dose in comparison to the lower dose, and these are shown in Fig. 9 *(218)*. The regions of the brain preferentially inhibited by these drugs include the PFC and high parietal areas*, and correspond closely to areas previously identified as being involved in memory processes, particularly working memory *(102,219,220)*.

The relationship of these drug induced changes in rCBF and their relationship to changes in cognitive function need to be investigated and clarified more precisely using a process similar to that

---

*The studies done with midazolam were on an older scanner that did not allow imaging of the uppermost parietal regions.

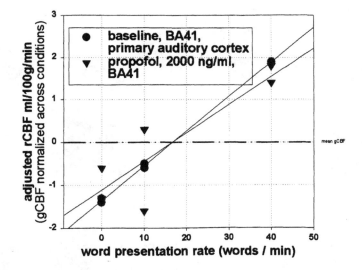

Fig. 7. Plot of relative regional cerebal blood flow in a discrete location (voxel) in primary auditory cortex during differing word stimulation rates. CBF values were normalized across conditions by SPM analysis to a mean value of 50 mL/100 g/min. A normal increase in rCBF as stimulation frequency increases (*circles*) is preserved during deep propofol sedation (*triangles*). The voxel chosen is located in the standard Talairach brain atlas at co-ordinates (x, y, z in mm) 50, –22, 12 in baseline condition and 54, –22, 14 during propofol ($Z = 3.61$, $p < 0.001$). The subject was unresponsive at this concentration of propofol. These data indicate that propofol sedation does not impair the ability of rCBF to respond to increases in neuronal activity as induced by autitory stimulation.

described above regarding the function of the pre-frontal cortices in memory processes. Traditional memory tests used in drug studies need to be modified based on current knowledge of memory processes, and preliminary FNI results from drug studies. For example, it would be crucial to closely examine the effects of these drugs on working memory, as assessed by tasks such as the n-back task or the continuous recognition task.

ELECTROPHYSIOLOGIC MARKERS OF MEMORY PROCESSES

Ever since anesthesiologists could monitor the EEG relatively easily in the operating theater, there has been hope that this technology will objectify the art of administering anesthesia *(221,222)*. This endeavor is fueled by the still present problem of awareness during anesthesia, which clearly demonstrates the still empirical nature of anesthetic administration *(223)*. As indicated in the previous section above, anesthetic effects on memory are closely intertwined with the hypnotic—sedative effects. The endpoint of the hypnotic effect (loss of responsiveness to verbal command) is much more distinct, and easily measurable in real-time than the onset of amnesia. Modeling the EEG effects of the hypnotic component of anesthesia has met with reasonable success *(224,225)*. This type of monitor is empirically based and designed, and it is difficult to determine if observations such as those of Alkire represent physiologic underpinnings of such a monitor, or rather represent strong inter-correlations of diverse anesthetic actions *(226)*. Currently, there are a number of emerging methods of modelling EEG effects in relation to depth of the hypnotic component of anesthesia *(227,228)*.

EEG monitors of the hypnotic effect of anesthesia are being used increasingly in studies of learning and memory during anesthesia to document the "depth of anesthesia" *(118,119)*. The next challenge is to utilize the EEG to measure the amnesic effects of anesthetic drugs. In order to achieve this goal, one must understand the relationship of the EEG and event related potentials (ERP) with memory processes in humans who have not received drug. The following section will address this.

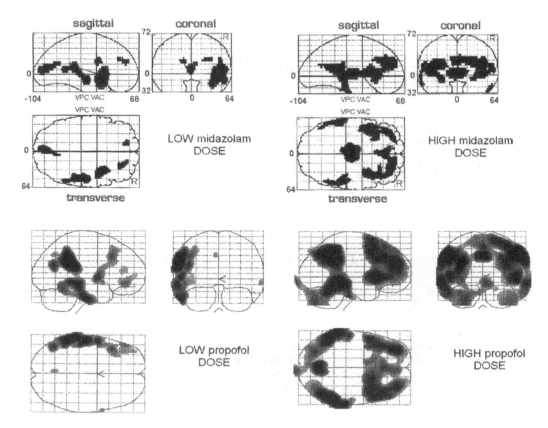

Fig. 8. Distribution of *relative* rCBF decreases at differing concentrations of midazolam or propofol (global blood flow changes normalized across conditions). The views of the brain are glass brains, meaning that one sees all activity in a given view whether it is on the front or back of the image. Thus, all three images must be considered simultaneously. Activity may appear outside the brain margins as all data are warped to a standard brain (the Talairach brain (425), or the Montreal Neurologic Institute (MNI) brain; for a discussion of these issues *see* http://www.mrc-cbu.cam.ac.uk/Imaging/mnispace.html and http://www.bic.mni.mcgill.ca/brainweb/ [426, 427]). As most cognitive brain activity occurs in the cortical layer (428), and sedative doses of drugs affect these processes, it is not surprising that drug induced decreases in rCBF may occur close to the surface of the brain. Small variations in individual anatomy may result in activity appearing outside the standard brain image. Note that at low concentrations, lateralized changes in rCBF occur, which become more widespread a serum concentration increases. The peak effects of these changes (i.e., the darkest regions in the propofol images) are very close to regions activated during working memory tasks (for example, *see* Fig. 3 of [102]). The midazolam images (top part of figure) were obtained on an older PET scanner using a previous version of SPM software (SPM95). The PET image has a limited axial field of view, and the top portion of the cerebrum is not imaged. The lower images are obtained with a more sensitive PET scanner and analyzed using a later version of SPM software (SPM99), thus accounting for some of the differences in images.

The Electrical Activity of the Brain and Event-Related Potentials

Brain activity entails multiple neurons acting in concert to produce measurable electrical currents from the summation of postsynaptic potentials of primarily pyramidal cells located in the neocortex.*
As these pyramidal cells are oriented in parallel, their individual activities sum to produce a record-

---

*There is good evidence that deep neural generators affect the surface recorded electrical activity. This can be demonstrated by differences in the surface voltage map versus the second spatial derivative of the scalp field (the Current Source Density; *[13,229]*).

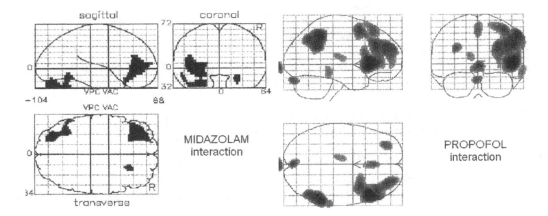

Fig. 9. An interaction analysis, where regions of significantly greater decreases in rCBF in one condition (*high dose*) vs another (*low dose*) can help identify regions of the brain that may be preferentially affected by the increase in drug concentration. This can help focus investigative attention on cognitive behaviors identified with these brain regions. For these drugs, one may be interested in response selection and encoding/retrieval processes (prefrontal regions), and storage of information in working memory (parietal regions).

able signal at the scalp, as opposed to other cells that are randomly oriented with respect to each other. Neural signaling occurs by movement of charges over space. Neurons are bathed in an electrically conductive media that can transmit current, and thus can support diffuse electrical fields (clouds) with measurable statistical properties *(1)*. These electromagnetic fields can be recorded from the surface of the head—EEG in the case of electrical charge, and MEG in the case of magnetic fields. In a physics analogy, neurons are the molecules or atoms comprising a gas (electromagnetic field). Though the atoms and molecules comprising a gas deterministically decide its properties, computational complexity and quantal uncertainty, preclude a bottom-up approach to definition of the properties of the system based solely on a thorough knowledge of molecular properties. The study of the statistical properties of the gas (EEG or MEG of the electromagnetic fields) may be the best, and possibly only way to quantify behavior of the system. Thus, an understanding of the EEG and ERP correlates of memory processes and their relationship to anesthetics may be the only way to understand anesthetic induced amnesia, no matter how much we know about anesthetic effects at receptors and synapses.

The simplest and longest studied electrical field property of the brain are evoked potentials, which represent the electrical activity of the brain in relation to an event such as hearing a sound, seeing a word, or feeling a stimulus. Each stimulus produces a fairly reproducible brain response with a unique electrical signature. Because of the continuous electrical activity of the brain, activity related to one stimulus is difficult, though not impossible, to discern *(230–235)*. To improve the signal to noise ratio, averaging of the time-locked response is undertaken, with the reproducible electrical activity becoming prominent over the unsynchronized background electrical activity, which tends to zero with repetitive averaging. Note that synchronized electrical activity (e.g., alpha oscillations) may be difficult to remove using this method, especially if oscillatory activity is in phase with stimulus presentation. The number of repetitive stimuli needed to obtain a reliable signal varies, but about 40 seems necessary for traditional averaging techniques in paradigms examining cognitive behavior.

Studies of cognition using ERP present a number of advantages. One is excellent time resolution, which can help dissect out sequential versus network memory mechanisms *(236)*. Though spatial resolution has been poor compared with other FNI techniques, it is constantly improving *(237,238)*. Another not insignificant advantage is the much lesser cost of ERP studies than other FNI techniques.

can then provide valuable clues to the design of FNI experiments. In fact, recent understanding of many memory processes are enhanced by the use of event-related fMRI (efMRI) using analogous paradigms to previous ERP studies *(239)*. For instance, the electrophysiologic response to subsequently remembered vs nonremembered material is different (the old/new effect), and seems to be located in the PFC *(240,241)*. Intracranial ERP recordings in humans indicate that the hippocampal and parahippocampal regions are also important in genesis of this effect *(242)*. Based on this robust ERP phenomenon, seminal efMRI studies were performed *(114,243)*, confirming and enhancing previous ERP data. Thus, an understanding of the ERP literature will aid interpretation of new FNI literature.

The Auditory ERP Waveform

The auditory event-related potential (ERP) is described by various positive and negative microvoltage deflections, or "peaks", occurring in a particular temporal relationship to an auditory event or stimulus *(244)*. Each ERP peak represents the synchronized electrical activity of a population(s) of neurons that is recordable at the scalp. The amplitude and shape of each peak is determined by the location and orientation of the activated neurons, as well as by the properties of the stimulus and the subject's task. Groups of neurons can be modeled as dipoles (a positive and negative charge separated by a distance), and the orientation of this dipole in relation to a surface electrode will determine the size of the ERP waveform, and the relation of CSD to voltage maps *(13)*. Positive and negative peaks occurring at progressively longer time intervals after stimulation are measured as latencies in milliseconds (ms) and may track successive stages of information processing through the nervous system *(241)*. Sequential processing is more evident in the early components of the ERP*, while later occurring components may embody significant information in terms of spatio-temporal patterns ("field" properties) *(244)*.

Methodologic Considerations

Drug Administration

Components of an ERP waveform are defined by three important properties: 1) their timing, 2) scalp distribution, and 3) pattern of sensitivity to experimental manipulations. For example, the most studied ERP in cognitive processing is the P300, which represents the response of the brain to a deviant stimulus *(245)*. In normal subjects, the P300 occurs approx 300 ms following the stimulus. It is maximal over the parietal cortex, and its amplitude is inversely related to the probability of the deviant stimulus, becoming larger as the probability of the stimulus decreases *(246)*. Traditional ERP components may be difficult to ascertain in the presence of drug administration, or other pathology. One cannot rely on latencies to identify components, as these can be significantly altered in the presence of drug. This is particularly true of the later occurring components (with normal latencies greater than about 200 ms). Thus, the investigator needs to concentrate on scalp distribution and response to experimental variables in determining the identity of a particular component *(13)*. As well, drug administration may increase the variability in latency of ERP components ("latency jitter"), which makes evaluation of ERP effects more difficult. This is particularly true in the case where the differences in waveforms (e.g., Dm [*see* Section on Encoding]) are highlighted by subtracting one ERP waveform from another (*see* ref. *(88)* for a discussion and example of this). This increased variability will make the use of grand average waveforms less desirable to interpret ERP changes. With drug administration, signal to noise ratios become less desirable, and frequently larger trial blocks are needed. Teasing out what the effect of a drug is on the brain as informed by ERP changes may be difficult, and behavioral data may be key to sorting this out. For example, ERPs may reveal quite different information in a drug state if the ERP is determined by stimulus locking (hearing a sound at $t = 0$) vs response locking (pushing a button in response to the sound at $t = 0$).

*For example, the following electrophysiologic–anatomical relationship exists for an auditory stimulus in the first 10 ms as recorded in a mid-latency auditory evoked response paradigm (MLAEP): wave I–distal CNVIII; wave II–proximal CNVIII; wave III–cochelar nucleus; wave IV superior olivary complex; wave V–inferior colliculus.

STIMULI FOR COGNITIVE STUDIES

Most EP studies with drugs involve the use of auditory stimuli, whereas, almost all cognitive EP studies in subjects not receiving drug involve visual stimuli. Visual stimuli have the advantage of being precisely localizable in time (discrete onset, and constant stimulus duration), but are unable to be presented to heavily sedated or anesthetized subjects. Auditory stimuli are discrete in time only if they consist of tones (such as mid-latency auditory evoked potentials, or the P3 oddball paradigm using tones). Word stimuli are more problematic as frequently stimuli last hundreds of msec, and it is difficult to determine the onset time of stimulus, though most commonly the beginning of the word is taken as stimulus onset *(247,248)*. There is some evidence that cognitive processing is similar regardless of visual or auditory presentation *(249)*. As fMRI will be an important modality for future investigations using drug administration, the problem of scanner noise is an important one *(250–253)*.

Auditory ERP Components

Early components (e.g., P1, N1), are influenced primarily by stimulus characteristics and automatic processing *(254,255)*, while later components (e.g., N2, P3) are influenced by arousal *(3)*, voluntary manipulations of attention *(256,257)*, and other cognitive processes such as stimulus evaluation and task demands *(258,259)*. The N1 and N2 components of the auditory ERP are representative of early and relatively automatic auditory processing, and are less likely to be rendered unrecognizable by increasing concentrations of propofol, as may occur with the P3. The N1 and N2 components are particularly sensitive to small deviations in the characteristics of a repetitive stimulus, even when the subject is not paying attention to it *(260,261)*. Subtracting the average ERP waveform for the frequent stimulus from the deviant one produces the "mismatch negativity" with a latency of about 100–200 ms. This may provide a useful way of exploring the ERP as an index of sedation, since conscious attention is not required for its production *(262)*.

Localization of ERP Components

Variations in location of the ERP peaks across the scalp reflect differences in the neural populations which generate a particular peak. Changes in ERP amplitude caused by task manipulation or drug administration may thus indicate fluctuations in the activity of the neural assemblies responsible for the observed scalp electrical activity. Inspection of topographical differences in the ERP waveform across the head may provide valuable information about changes in regional brain activity *(263,264)*. The most robust method for localization of ERP generators is direct cortical recordings *(242,265–269)*. Obviously, these techniques are only very selectively applicable, and other methods are needed to examine the total brain space in relation to ERP measures. These include mathematical modeling of surface EEG activity *(270)*, and magnetoencephalographic studies *(271)*. Modeling the surface EEG based on source generators in the brain falls into two broad categories: 1) methods that assume multiple discrete dipole generators (e.g., brain electrical source analysis [BESA] *[272–274]*), or 2) ones that assume distributed currents in the brain (e.g., low resolution tomographic analysis LORETA or VARETA *[238,275]*). Direct comparison of the two methods reveals similar results in certain applications *(276)*. Both methods are computationally complex, have no unique solutions (the so-called "inverse problem"), and thus require constraints on possible solutions to obtain interpretable results. For instance, discrete source localization works well when the dipoles are "seeded", frequently using coordinates from other FNI studies *(277–280)*. Similarly, LORETA requires assumptions regarding the degree of current density changes between adjacent regions of the brain, and solutions need to be confined to white or grey matter of the brain. This can be done using a normative MRI scan (for instance *see [228]*). ERP data can be similarly used to "seed" temporal components of images of brain glucose metabolism, which are averaged images obtained over many minutes *(281,282)*.

In response to auditory stimuli, the MLAEP components represent sequential activity occurring from the ear to the primary auditory cortex. The P1 (latency approx 50 ms) is generated in primary auditory cortex, while N1 and N2 (latency approx 100 and 200 ms respectively) are generated in the superior temporal plane *(244)*. The presence of wave V in the MLAEP can be used as a robust indicator that the central nervous system (CNS) detected an auditory stimulus during general anesthesia *(117)*. This type of evidence is important in clarifying confusing results from studies of learning during anesthesia. Later components of the auditory ERP are produced in more distributed brain regions, and may have more than one neural generator. These components index automatic orienting responses, or may represent high level cognitive, including memory, processes.

Relationship of ERP and Bispectral Index to Arousal vs Memory

In general, changes in arousal affect the early components of the ERP *(283,284)*. Various studies have examined auditory ERPs during anesthesia, and all indicate that auditory stimuli are registered during various anesthetic regimens, particularly components of the auditory ERP occurring within 100 ms of stimulus. A dose-dependent increase in latency and decrease in amplitude are found, with latencies being less variable than amplitude measures between individuals *(285,286)*. During anesthesia, particularly during cardiac surgery, the late positive components *(287,288)* or the mid-latency components *(117,289,290)* of the ERP seem to indicate the possibility of implicit memory formation or awareness. A study by Curran and colleagues *(39)* found decreased N1 amplitude with lorazepam and scopolamine sedation. We have found similar relationships with other sedative drugs *(40)*.

The late components of the ERP, such as the P3 or the Late Positive Complex (LPC), closely relate to whether a stimulus is remembered or not *(90,291–296)*. Other late components of the ERP, such as the N2b *(297)* MisMatch Negativity (MMN) *(298)*, and the N400 *(299)* also occur in this time range in response to incongruous stimuli, but have not been as well studied in relation to memory processes. Identification of these components and differentiation among them depend on details of the task paradigm, changes of the ERP with changes in parameters of the paradigm, and topographic analysis of the ERP waveform *(62,298,300)*. The earlier of these late components seem to relate to automatic detection of deviant stimuli (the "orienting" reflex). Subsequent ERP components index processes matching this deviant stimulus with an internally held template *(301)*, possibly maintained in working memory.

The Bispectral index (BIS) has been modeled against the point of hypnosis (loss of responsiveness) for a number of anesthetic agents using an extensive database of EEG data *(224)*. Before unresponsiveness is obtained, the BIS varies little as sedative levels vary considerably. A number of studies have shown that recall is severely impaired by a number of anesthetic drugs even at BIS values greater than 85 *(58,59,302,303)*. BIS values these high cannot reliably track changes in sedative level. However, after the loss of consciousness, the BIS is a good measure of hypnosis, and certain values have been shown to allow implicit memory formation during anesthesia *(119)*. The relationship of BIS to evoked potentials has not been studied to date.

Mid-Latency Auditory Evoked Potential (MLAEP)

The MLAEP represents early components of the ERP, and are the most frequently investigated during the administration of anesthesia, though they are too early to represent any memory processes. The typical MLAEP response consists of three major peaks: Na at 16–30 ms, Pa at 30–45 ms, and Nb at 40–60 ms. Smaller peaks may also be seen at shorter latencies after the stimulus (No at 8–10 ms, Po at 10–13 ms) and are usually identified with the brainstem auditory evoked potential. The MLAEP may possibly originate in or near auditory cortex, although the earliest peaks are probably generated by structures in the brainstem. Peak amplitudes are approx 1 microvolt or less, and are maximal over frontocentral scalp. An increase in stimulus intensity increases the amplitude and decreases the latency of the MLAEP, that is unchanged by maturation, variations in attention, light sleep, and sedative levels of anesthesia, when large changes in memory performance may occur *(304,305)*. MLAEPs may be particularly useful to dissociate the sedation component of anesthetics as opposed to the memory effect *(306)*. MLAEP components though not indexing memory processes, seem to relate closely to the possibility of memory formation during general anesthesia *(244)*. The auditory steady state response (ASSR) is a repetitive, overlapping stimulus paradigm that produces a summed or resonant response of the CNS, and seems to correlate with depth of anesthesia *(307–314)*. The ability of the MLAEP to detect auditory sensation (as opposed to perception, which involves cognitive and memory processes), which is abolished with sufficiently deep anesthesia, lends itself to a possibly reliable monitor of depth of anesthesia *(244)*.

Indexing of Memory Processes with Specific ERP Components

Different ERPs are obtained to material that has been seen before versus new material (the "repetition" effect), and is a positivity from 200–1500 ms occurring with repeated material. These differences can be more closely examined in relation to memory processes by looking at subsequent memory performance. Different ERPs to subsequently remembered material are obtained both at the time of encoding, and at the time of retrieval.

Long Term Memory

ENCODING—DIFFERENCE IN SUBSEQUENT MEMORY EFFECT

Material that is subsequently remembered is characterized by a different ERP at encoding than material that is not. This difference was initially demonstrated by Sanquist *(240)* and later refined by Paller *(295)* who subtracted the ERP waveforms from each other to isolate differences. A larger positive amplitude in the midline parietal region for subsequently remembered material was demonstrated. In these studies only a relatively few midline electrodes were utilized. Subsequent studies using dense arrays (at least 32 electrodes) revealed more precisely the topographical distribution of this effect *(13,47,87)*. Semantic (e.g., living vs nonliving judgment) is associated with a large negative current density over the left inferior frontal scalp between 400 and 1100 ms. Further refinements of this Dm response have been investigated using Remember (confident recall) vs Know (familiarity) judgments. The left inferior frontal negativity was demonstrated to be associated with Remember and not Know judgments. A Dm effect is sometimes also evident over the left temporal region starting at 400 ms, and may correspond to an N400 effect. This effect is evident when semantic incongruity occurs (e.g., He had blue for dinner vs He had pizza for dinner) *(299)*. This component is likely to be a semantic process component, as it occurs when environmental sounds can be named, but not when they cannot *(315)*. Remember judgments associated with successful free recall have larger Dm effects during the 1000–2000 ms range compared with successfully remembered, but not freely recalled items.

When a voltage map of the Dm effect is compared with a current source density map differences are evident. This indicates that deep subcortical structures are involved in the ERP waveforms of this effect. Direct, intracranial recordings reveal a Dm like effect starting about 300–500 ms in the hippocampal and medial temporal lobe structures, but not Wernicke's region *(242,316)*. This Dm effect appears to be closely associated with the N400 response, evoked with semantic processing *(299)*. These findings have been supported by recent FNI studies *(114,243,317)*.

RETRIEVAL—THE EPISODIC MEMORY EFFECT (EM) *(13)*

During recognition paradigms, viewing of "old," previously presented words, elicits a different ERP response that viewing of "new" words. Retrieval of information is associated with two processes (dual process theories)—an aspect associated with familiarity and one associated with context. The "the face is familiar, but I can't remember the name" effect demonstrates the dissociation of these two processes *(318)*. The familiarity process is associated with a negativity over the left prefrontal-central scalp at a latency of about 400 ms *(263,319)*. Familiarity processes have been equated with implicit memory (i.e., unconscious processes) *(320,321)*. However, this particular familiarity process involves the MTL, and thus indicates that it is explicit in nature *(322,323)*.

Following this early component, a characteristic, late positive component over parietal areas in the 400–800 ms interval, earlier in onset and associated with a shorter reaction time occurs to old material. This effect represents the retrieval of previously stored episodic memories (as opposed to new words that retrieve semantic memories), and this effect has been labeled as the "old/new" episodic memory effect or Em *(13)*. The Em effect appears to have a different scalp distribution depending on the nature of the material retrieved (spatial location vs verbal material) *(324,325)*. Verbal material has a left sided asymmetry. This parietal Em effect probably has some MTL components, as evidenced by intracranial recordings *(316,326,327)*.

Overlapping this process is a left parietal-occipital positivity, extending to 800 ms or so. This component has been extensively studied in terms of study-test repetition *(263)*, conscious recall *(328)*, and associative and contextual recognition *(296,329)*. These studies have shown that this component is associated with recollection, and retrieval success is associated with a larger amplitude of this component. Despite the correlation with correct contextual associations, source memory (e.g., words spoken in a male or female voice, or temporal information), do not seem to relate to this component *(86)*.

A right prefrontal component of the Em effect starts soon after the parietal component, and lasts for a much longer time. This activity may represent retrieval of source information, or may specifically index successful retrieval of information *(296)*. Contradictory results are reported, where this component is still present during unsuccessful retrieval *(86,330)*. Because of the long time frame for this component, it is unclear if this ERP component represents one or multiple cognitive processes *(13)*. The prolonged Em activity may reflect post-retrieval monitoring operations *(331)*.

THE P3 OR P300—RESPONSE TO NOVELTY

Various investigators label this ERP component as "P300" as it occurs approx 300 ms following a deviant stimulus, or the "P3" as it is the third large positive peak occurring in long latency ERPs (after 100 ms). This terminology is used interchangeably. The P3 is the longest studied ERP component *(245)*, and its great interest arises from the fact that this response occurs when a repetitive stimulus is deviant from previous stimuli (the "orienting reflex," a measure of phasic arousal). This type of response is crucial for animal species to survive, as they are constantly bombarded with relatively monotonous stimuli, but must react rapidly to deviant, potentially threatening or interesting ones. Though the P3 is very distantly related to this type of response, it does incorporate a memory process, as a template of how the world should be (the monotonous repetitive stimuli) must be compared with the incoming stimulus *(332)*. If the incoming stimulus is deviant, then a marked electrophysiologic response of large amplitude occurs, the P3 of 10–20 μV *(3)*. In fact, there is a temporally close relationship between the onset of working memory processes and the P3 *(191,325,333–335)*. However, the hallmark of working memory is sustained activity over a delay interval, and this is embodied in slow positive wave activity over the retention interval *(241,336)*.

Thus, even though the P3 is a response to a deviant stimulus, it is of great interest to investigators studying memory. Other electrophysiologic responses occur to deviant* stimuli, the earliest being the mismatch negativity (MMN) occurring 100–200 ms after the deviant stimulus *(261,298,337)*. The P3 response is defined by the following properties : maximal amplitude at parietal electrodes, increasing amplitude with decreasing deviant stimulus frequency, and latency values from 250–800 ms *(338)*. Because it is such a late occurring ERP component, it is particularly prone to "latency jitter"— the apparent change in amplitude when summed across conditions or subjects owing to variability in latency. Thus individual subject waveforms need to be considered.

The P3 has been on occasion divided into two components, the P3a and P3b, (which may be the same as what is originally labeled as the P3) *(339)*, though this distinction is difficult to define precisely, as the P3a is observable in only 20% of normal subjects *(3)*. The P3a is reflective of an early orienting process *(340)*, explaining its earlier latency than the P3b, and probably originates in the frontal lobe *(265,341,342)*. Thus, its maximal amplitude is more anterior at central or frontal electrodes. The P3a seems to be a response to unanticipated novel stimuli, and can be evident when novel tones are interspersed in a standard oddball paradigm that elicits a traditional P3 response to rare

---

*Deviance is noted in approx 200 ms "refractory" periods—only one MMN component occurs if the deviant stimuli are closer than approx 200 ms in time *(337)*.

deviant tones that the subject is attending to *(315,343,344)*. Because of these properties, this P3 component has been labeled the "novelty P3" *(342)*. The attentional component is important, as if the subject is not attending to the deviant stimuli (e.g., counting them), then novel sounds do not elicit a differential response *(315)*.

The generators of the P3 are difficult to identify, and are likely to be diffuse cortical structures *(264,345)*. Intracranial recordings and studies in some patients with hippocampal pathology have related the P3 response closely to the hippocampal region *(346)*, though the P3 is still observable in patients with temporal lobectomies, often times without apparent changes in morphology or response to stimulus modification *(266,267,347–351)*.

There is a close relationship between P3 amplitude and memory, with a larger amplitude present during improved memory performance *(241,291–294,333,352–355)*. Resource allocation and arousal modulates this response, and is shown in the process of habituation of the response over time. The P3 latency is shorter in subjects who perform better on neuropsychological tests that require rapid and higher levels of attentional resource allocation *(292,356–360)*.

IMPLICIT MEMORY

There is much less literature on the electrophysiology of implicit memory *(47,361–364)*. There are indications that ERPs to word stimuli that are recognized as "new," when in fact they have been presented before (and thus are unrecognized "olds") have a distinctive morphology *(321)*. The maximal effect is more posterior, in the parietal regions, than the robust old/new effect (correctly recognized stimuli), which has maximal effects in the frontal regions. But these effects are not necessarily reproducible, even by the same group of investigators *(47)*. It seems that subtle changes in the study paradigm can obscure or eliminate the effect.

Note that this form of implicit memory is one that is primed by previous exposure to a stimulus that is consciously perceived, though not subsequently recognized. Reaction times to this class of stimuli are faster than to truly new words. This is in distinction to priming paradigms where the stimulus is presented without conscious perception (i.e., less than approx 50 ms stimulus duration for visual stimuli) *(140)*.

The ERP effects associated with familiarity (the "know" vs "remember" response), which is often equated with explicit memory processes *(86–88,90,116,322,365)*, and those associated with truly implicit memory are closely intertwined. Both effects seem to occur in the 300–500 ms range. The primary distinguishing features are: (1) familiarity effects are sensitive to recognition accuracy (i.e., there is a difference between recognized old and unrecognized old words), and (2) differences in topographical distribution.

EEG Correlates of Memory Processes

There are many components in the EEG that relate to memory processes that are not necessarily event related. As alluded to above in the section on working memory, representation of the sensory experience of the world in working memory may be a key component to the awareness of consciousness. The neurophysiologic problem is how this information is rapidly or instantaneously transmitted from one part of the brain to another, part of the so-called binding problem *(366)*. Another way of stating this is how information from a range of separate independent sensory channels is bound together to allow the world to be perceived as comprising a coherent array of objects *(49)*. High frequency oscillations in the gamma range (30–80 Hz) are likely contenders for implementation of this property of the brain *(367–369)*, though EEG rhythms in other frequencies may also serve this purpose *(370–372)*. Loss of this binding, coherent activity is associated with transition from one cognitive state to the other ("releasing" the brain from a task) *(369)*, or may be associated with the loss of consciousness *(1)*.

Synchronous EEG activity is elicited during working memory tasks, and persists during the delay interval of the working memory task *(104,373,374)*. Oscillatory rhythms can also be associated with memory processing *(375–378)*. Of particular interest are theta rhythms, as these can be produced by the hippocampus *(379,380)*, can be related to memory processes *(379,381)*, and correlate with a large animal literature that demonstrate these rhythms are necessary for integration/encoding of new information, particularly in the spatial realm *(382,383)*. Theta oscillations associated with spatial memory processing also occur in humans *(384)*. There are some interesting animal data to show that anesthetic administration to animals after learning may enhance retention *(385,386)*, possibly based on physiology similar to effects occurring during sleep *(387,388)*. The same processes may also occur in humans *(389)*.

The amnesic effects of some anesthetic drugs may be neuroanatomically expressed in thalamic—frontal cortical networks and indexed by oscillatory EEG activity. During sedative drug administration, beta oscillations become a prominent part of the EEG when subjects are amnesic and almost unresponsive, but not demonstrating the classic EEG criteria for sleep *(390)*. This oscillatory activity occurs in association with decreases in rCBF in the thalamus and prefrontal cortex *(198)*, which may correspond with the thalamo-cortical networks known to be involved with the production of EEG oscillatory activity *(391)* (*see* Fig. 10) Propofol and benzodiazepines seem to have specific effects on thalamic physiology *(202,392)*, which has been postulated as a key target component in the loss of consciousness with anesthetic drugs *(393)*, Frontal cortical—thalamic networks have been postulated as important in memory processes on evidence from diencephalic amnesia such as occurs in Korsakoff's syndorme *(35)*. The neuroanatomical basis for these observations is illustrated in Figs. 10 and 11.

MEMORY AND LEARNING DURING ANESTHESIA

As Lister so eloquently states:

"To state that a particular drug impairs memory conveys about as much information as a physician stating that a patient is unwell."

Until recently, the primary goal of anesthesia was to produce unconsciousness. Today sedation is frequently used, where consciousness is preserved, but memory is ablated. It is well documented that patients can follow commands intra-operatively, but usually have no recollection of these events, even in the presence of pain *(394–396)*. On the other hand, electrophysiologic studies indicate that cognitive processing of auditory stimuli can occur under general anesthesia *(288,289,397)*. Are these "reflex" actions? The ability to follow complicated commands depends on the use of some form of memory as well as linguistic analysis. These processes are more complex than simple reflex phenomena. Similar responses occur when aroused from natural sleep, with the degree of memory reflecting the depth of sleep, or the length of time of awakening *(398)*. This effect was interpreted as an arousal phenomenon; subjects needed more time to wake up after deep (slow-wave) sleep. Thus, the degree and duration of cortical arousal will determine the degree to which information, or the episode itself, is later remembered.

Undoubtedly general anesthesia of sufficient degree completely ablates explicit memory *(119,399–401)*. No careful study to date has demonstrated the existence of fully explicit memory ("awareness") during adequate levels of general anesthesia. When awareness occurs, it is probably related to insufficient anesthetic being present *(223,402–405)*. Another intriguing phenomenon is that the incidence of dreaming associated with anesthesia is at least twice the incidence of awareness *(406–408)*. Dreaming is a poorly understood phenomenon in relationship to anesthesia, and there are few data regarding this *(117,409)*.

There is also little doubt that some type of memory formation can occur during general anesthesia, at least under some, yet to be defined, circumstances *(410–412)*. These circumstances may be defined by the depth of anesthesia, which until recently was difficult to quantify or control objectively *(119,196)*. The brain is capable of receiving auditory input during anesthesia (*see* Fig. 7 demonstrat-

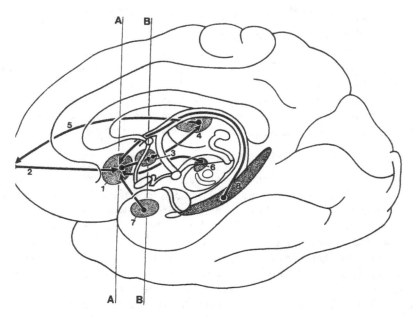

Fig. 10. Neuroanatomical basis for thalamocortical connections. These pathways are probably important in maintaining thalamically mediated EEG oscillatory activity. The ventral striatum (nucleus accumbens) (1) receives fibers from the prefrontal cortex (2) and controls the ventral pallidum (3), which projects to the dorsomedial thalamic nucleus (4), which completes the loop back to the prefrontal cortex (5). The nucleus accumbens receives inputs from the ventral tegmental area (6) (the dopaminergic mesolimbic system), the amygdala (7), and the hippocampus (8). Lines **A** and **B**, represent coronal sections corresponding to planes indicated in Fig. 11. (Reproduced with permission, Fig. 20, p. 37 Duvernoy, H. M. and Bourgouin, P. (1998). The Human Hippocampus: function anatomy, vascularization and serial sections with MRI. Berlin; New York, Springer.)

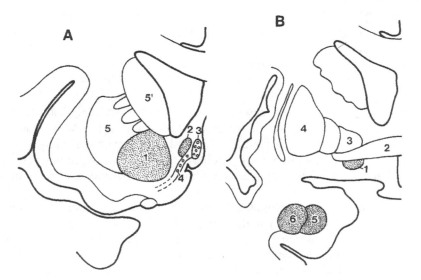

Fig. 11. (A) 1—nucleus accumbens, 2—lateralseptal nucleus, 3—medial septal nucleus, 4—nucleus of the vertical limb of the diagonal band, 5—caudate nucleus, 5—dorsal striatum; **(B)** 1—ventral palldium, 2—anterior commissure, 3—globus pallidus, 4—putamen, 5—basal nucleus amygdala, 5—lateral nucleus amygdala.

ing a neuronal response when the BIS level was 55–65), particularly in situations where "light" anesthesia is used. Information processing at a fairly high cognitive level has been demonstrated during general anesthesia *(289,397,413)*. Thus the encoding requirement for learning/memory during anesthesia is met. At least under some circumstances memories of these stimuli can be retrieved *(400,414–416)*. The implications of this type of memory are far from clear.

Thus, there is a whole milieu of peri-anesthetic phenomenon including explicit awareness, dreaming, implicit memory, hypnotically retrievable memories *(417)*, and weak explicit memory retrievable with strong repetitive cueing that need to be sorted out by careful study.

Methodology in "Learning During Anesthesia" Studies

In these studies, methodology is crucial in interpreting the results obtained. It would seem that a necessary requirement would be to determine the circumstances of memory formation during a state of sedation before it can be sorted out during general anesthesia, when the incidence is much lower. Memories formed during sedation are fragile, and could be termed weakly explicit. Others have labeled these as implicit, depending on the type of testing used to detect these memories. There is certainly controversy as to what "implicit" means, and how to differentiate these from "weak explicit" memories *(118,401)*. This distinction is of concern, as there is evidence that initially no memory on free recall or weak cueing may in fact be demonstrated if cueing for memories continues *(117,418)*. In this section, "implicit" refers to memory formation during drug administration, which is demonstrated in some fashion other than obvious explicit recall or recognition. Notable variables important to control in this type of study are:

- Depth of anesthesia,
- Anesthetic regimen,
- Type of memory test,
- Nature of stimuli (e.g., familiar stimuli seem to be recalled more than unfamiliar ones,
- The degree of repetition of stimuli *(419,420)*,
- Method of testing recall/recognition (timing of recall/recognition; modality of presentation/testing) *(117)*,
- Demonstration that the memory test used will reliably detect this type of memory formation in an appropriate control population, and
- Correction for chance results, (which can be done with the results from the control population above).

For example, people will complete word stems with a given set of words, based on frequency and usage in the English language (frequently at a "hit" rate of about 30%). Scoring of a priming effect requires correction for this chance factor. Thus "old" items must be supplemented with "new" distractor items *(421)*. Distractor items need to meet the same criteria as the "old" test items with regard to word frequency, imagery and meaningfulness value, et cetera.

Implicit memory may be sensitive to modality changes (auditory/visual) from stimulus presentation to recognition. Some research has shown that if the stimulus presentation is auditory but the word stems for completion are given visually, the number of stem completions may be severely decreased *(122)*, but this may not be a reliable finding *(136)*. Measures of priming may be influenced by perceptual characteristics of the individual stimuli more than traditional explicit memory testing *(55,422)*.

Investigators will often report a correlation between the explicit and implicit measures; a significant correlation is evidence of inability to differentiate the two types of memory. A more complex analysis of "stochastic independence" between the explicit and implicit measures computes the conditional probability of a given item being first correctly recalled on the explicit memory test, and later correctly completed on the implicit test *(423)*. Independence is demonstrated when this conditional probability is low. Other methods such as the process dissociation procedure have been used to dissociate explicit and implicit memories *(120,320)*. If the subjects become aware of the relationship between the implicit memory test and the prior presentation of words or pictures to be learned, they may well use their conscious explicit memory of these stimuli to guide their responses on the implicit memory test. This "test awareness" is another avenue wherein contamination of the results by explicit memory can occur *(127,424)*.

Thus, labeling memories formed during sedation or anesthesia, as explicit or implicit is difficult. An example is provided by the attempt to use the process dissociation procedure to perform this distinction for material learned during anesthesia. The difficulty in reliably interpreting these results may be partly owing to the fact that the effect being measured is small *(118,119)*. In terms of demonstrating that some memory may occur, this consideration may not be critical, but the opposite is true in terms of investigating the mechanisms of such memory formation, especially if neuroanatomical localization is considered.

As to the choice of which priming task should be used, consider that different tasks may be differentially vulnerable to disruption by sedative agents. For example, diazepam produced less priming on a category completion task, where the subject was asked to generate exemplars of a given category (e.g., animals) than on a word stem completion task *(123)*. This might occur because in generating exemplars of a particular category, there may be a greater number of possible answers that might be given, reducing the apparent effect of priming compared to the word stem completion, where the choice of possible correct answers is more constrained. Tasks based on perceptual priming may be more effective at detecting memory formation than conceptual priming. For example, Polster found robust priming effects with midazolam and propofol using a perceptual facilitation task (visually degraded words) that persisted after a 7 d retention interval *(131)*. Bennett has suggested the use of nonverbal response measures as being more robust to the effects of anesthesia and less likely than verbal stimuli to be influenced by explicit memory *(416)*.

In summary, detection of implicit or weak explicit memories is exquisitely sensitive to methodological considerations. These must be addressed fully before memory formation, particularly during administration of anesthetic agents, can be demonstrated. A more important consideration, considering the low incidence of memory formation during anesthesia, is the reliability of concluding in a particular study that no memory was formed.

CONCLUSION

Memory research is in an exciting, exponential growth stage. Drugs will become increasingly important as tools to further our investigations of memory, especially using powerful neuroimaging techniques. Concurrently, mechanisms of drug action in relation to memory processes will be clarified, also using these powerful neuroimaging tools. From these efforts, a more thorough understanding of how anesthesia affects memory should emerge. Monitors of memory processes will be as valuable as monitors of the hypnotic component of anesthesia, and are likely to be based on the EEG. Sophisticated analytic techniques will be required to develop these measures. There is good evidence that the hypnotic and amnesic effects of anesthetic drugs are separate, and that this dissociation can be demonstrated in the EEG. With the ability to monitor the amnesic and hypnotic effect of drugs objectively, the understanding of the mechanisms of anesthesia will increase dramatically. The key to unlocking how anesthesia works may very well rest on understanding the emergent field properties expressed by a multitude of neuronal activities and interactions present in the brain. These properties seem to be the substrate that explains consciousness awareness. As the fundamental property of anesthesia is the reversible collapse of this "field", the state of anesthesia will need to be understood in these terms.

REFERENCES

1. John, E. R. (2001) A field theory of consciousness. *Consciousness and Cognition* **10**, 184–213.
2. Oken, B. S. and Salinsky M. (1992) Alertness and attention: basic science and electrophysiologic correlates. *J. Clin. Neurophys.* **9**, 480–494.
3. Polich, J. and Kok A. (1995) Cognitive and biological determinants of P300: An integrative review. *Biol. Psychol.* **41**, 103–146.
4. Gabrieli, J. D. (1998) Cognitive neuroscience of human memory. *Ann. Rev. Psychol.* **49**, 87–115.

5. Tulving, E. (1992) Memory systems and the brain. *Clin. Neuropharm.* **15 Suppl. 1 Pt A,** 327A–328A.
6. Squire, L. R., Knowlton, B., and Musen G. (1993) The structure and organization of memory. *Ann. Rev. Psychol.* **44,** 453–495.
7. Squire, L. R. and Zola-Morgan, S. (1991) The medial temporal lobe memory system. *Science* **253,** 1380–1386.
8. Horner, M. D. (1990) Psychobiological evidence for the distinction between episodic and semantic memory. *Neuropsychol. Rev.* **1,** 281–321.
9. Nadel, L. (1994) Multiple Memory Systems: What and Why, an Update. In Schacter, D. L. and Tulving, E. L. (eds.), Memory Systems, MIT Press, Cambridge, MA. pp. 39–63.
10. Cohen, N. J. and Squire, L. R. (1980). Preserved learning and retention of pattern-analyzing skill in amnesia: dissociation of knowing how and knowing that. *Science* **210,** 207–210.
11. Schacter, D. L. (1985) Multiple forms of memory in humans and animals. In Weinberger, N. M., McGaugh, J. L., and Lynch, G. (eds.), Memory systems of the brain: Animal and human cognitive processes. Guilford Press, New York, pp. 351–379.
12. Tulving, E. (1987) Multiple memory systems and consciousness. *Hum. Neurobiol.* **6,** 67–80.
13. Friedman, D. and Johnson, R. (2000) Event-related potential (ERP) studies of memory encoding and retrieval: A selective review. *Microsc. Res. Tech.* **51,** 6–28.
14. Atkinson, R. C. and Shiffrin, R. M. (1971) The control of short-term memory. *Sci. Am.* **225,** 82–90.
15. Baddeley, A. D. (1992) Working memory. *Science* **255,** 556–559.
16. Roediger, H. L. I. (1990) Implicit memory: Retention without remembering. *Am. Psychol.* **45,** 1043–1056.
17. Torres, I. J. and Raz, N. (1994) Toward the neural basis of verbal priming: A cognitive-neuropsychological synthesis. *Neuropsychol. Rev.* **4,** 1–30.
18. Tulving, E. and Schacter, D. L. (1990) Priming and human memory systems. *Science* **247,** 301–306.
19. Harlow, J. M. (1868) Recovery from the passage of an iron bar through the head. *Publ. Mass. Med. Soc.* **2,** 327–347.
20. Damasio, H., Grabowski, T., Frank, R., Galaburda, A. M., and Damasio, A. R. (1994) The return of Phineas Gage: clues about the brain from the skull of a famous patient [published erratum appears in *Science* (1994) Aug 26;265(5176):1159]. *Science* **264,** 1102–1105.
21. Macmillan, M. (2000) An odd kind of fame : stories of Phineas Gage. MIT Press, Cambridge, MA.
22. Rugg, M. D. (1995) Memory and consciousness: a selective review of issues and data. *Neuropsychologia* **33,** 1131–1141.
23. Gabrieli, J. D. E., Fleischman, D. A., Keane, M. M., Reminger, S. L., and Morrell, F. (1995) Double dissociation between memory systems underlying explicit and implicit memory in the human brain. *Psychol. Sci.* **6,** 76–82.
24. Danion, J. M., Zimmermann, M. A., Willard-Schroeder, D., Grange, D., and Singer, L. (1989) Diazepam induces a dissociation between explicit and implicit memory. *Psychopharmacology* **99,** 238–243.
25. Danion, J. M., Zimmermann, M. A., Willard-Schroeder, D., et al. (1990) Effects of scopolamine, trimipramine and diazepam on explicit memory and repetition priming in healthy volunteers. *Psychopharmacology* **102,** 422–424.
26. Weingartner, H. (1985) Models of memory dysfunctions. *Ann. NY Acad. Sci.* **444,** 359–369.
27. Wolkowitz, O. M., Tinklenberg, J. R., and Weingartner, H. (1985) A psychopharmacological perspective of cognitive functions. II. Specific pharmacologic agents. *Neuropsychobiology* **14,** 133–156.
28. Graf, P., Mandler, G., and Haden, P. E. (1982) Simulating amnesic symptoms in normal subjects. *Science* **218,** 1243–1244.
29. Alkire, M. T., Vazdarjanova, A., Dickinson-Anson, H., White, N. S., and Cahill, L. (2001) Basolateral amygdala complex lesions block propofol-induced amnesia for inhibitory avoidance learning in rats. *Anesthesiology* **95,** 708–715.
30. Tomaz, C., Dickinson-Anson, H., McGaugh, J. L., Souza-Silva, M. A., Viana, M. B., and Graeff, F. G. (1993) Localization in the amygdala of the amnestic action of diazepam on emotional memory. *Behav. Brain Res.* **58,** 99–105.
31. Dickinson-Anson, H. and McGaugh, J. L. (1997) Bicuculline administered into the amygdala after training blocks benzodiazepine-induced amnesia. *Brain Res.* **752,** 197–202.
32. Dickinson-Anson, H., Mesches, M. H., Coleman, K., and McGaugh, J. L. (1993) Bicuculline administered into the amygdala blocks benzodiazepine- induced amnesia. *Behav. Neural. Biol.* **60,** 1–4.
33. Lehmann, O., Jeltsch, H., Lehnardt, O., Pain, L., Lazarus, C., and Cassel, J. C. (2000) Combined lesions of cholinergic and serotonergic neurons in the rat brain using 192 IgG-saporin and 5,7-dihydroxytryptamine: neurochemical and behavioural characterization. *Eur. J. Neurosci.* **12,** 67–79.
34. Gazzaniga, M. S. and Bizzi, E. (1995) The cognitive neurosciences. MIT Press, Cambridge, MA, pp. 767.
35. Paller, K. A., Acharya, A., Richardson, B. C., Plaisant, O., Shimamura, A. P., Reed, B. R., and Jagust, W. J. (1997) Functional neuroimaging of cortical dysfunction in alcoholic Korsakoff's syndrome. *J. Cogn. Neurosci.* **9,** 277–293.
36. Wilensky, A. E., Schafe, G. E., and LeDoux, J. E. (2000) The amygdala modulates memory consolidation of fear-motivated inhibitory avoidance learning but not classical fear conditioning. *J. Neurosci.* **20,** 7059–7066.
37. Wilensky, A. E., Schafe, G. E., and LeDoux, J. E. (1999) Functional inactivation of the amygdala before but not after auditory fear conditioning prevents memory formation. *J. Neurosci.* **19,** RC48.
38. Goldman-Rakic, P. (2000) Localization of function all over again. *Neuroimage* **11,** 451–457.
39. Curran, H. V., Pooviboonsuk, P., Dalton, J. A., and Lader, M. H. (1998) Differentiating the effects of centrally acting drugs on arousal and memory: an event-related potential study of scopolamine, lorazepam and diphenhydramine. *Psychopharmacology* (Berl) **135,** 27–36.
40. Veselis, R. A., Reinsel, R. A., and Feshchenko, V. A. (2001) Drug-induced amnesia is a separate phenomenon from sedation : electrophysiologic evidence. *Anesthesiology* **94,** 896–907.
41. Ghoneim, M. Block., M., R. I., Ping, S. T., el-Zahaby, H. M., and Hinrichs, J. V. (1993) The interactions of midazolam and flumazenil on human memory and cognition. *Anesthesiology* **79,** 1183–1192.
42. Bishop, K. I. and Curran, H. V. (1995) Psychopharmacological analysis of implicit and explicit memory: a study with lorazepam and the benzodiazepine antagonist flumazenil. *Psychopharmacology* **121,** 267–278.

43. Curran, H. V. (2000) Psychopharmacological Perspectives on Memory. In Tulving, E. and Craik, F. I. M. (eds.), The Oxford handbook of memory. Oxford University Press, Oxford; New York. pp. 539–554.
44. Reinsel, R., Veselis, R., Wronski, M., Marino, P., Heino, R., and Alagesan, R. (1993) Memory impairment during conscious sedation: A comparison of midazolam, propofol and thiopental. In Sebel, P. S., Bonke, B., and Winograd, E. (eds.), Memory and Awareness in Anesthesia. Prentice-Hall, Englewood, N.J. 127–140.
45. Curran, H. V., Shine, P., and Lader, M. (1986) Effects of repeated doses of fluvoxamine, mianserin, and placebo on memory and measures of sedation. *Psychopharmacology* **89**, 360–363.
46. Craik, F. I. M. and Lockhart, R. S. (1972) Levels of processing: a framework for memory research. *J. Verb. Learn. Verb. Beh.* **11**, 671–684.
47. Rugg, M. D., Allan, K., and Birch, C. S. (2000) Electrophysiological evidence for the modulation of retrieval orientation by depth of study processing. *J. Cogn. Neurosci.* **12**, 664–678.
48. Ruchkin, D. S., Berndt, R. S., Johnson, R., Grafman, J., Ritter, W., and Canoune, H. L. (1999) Lexical Contributions to Retention of Verbal Information in Working Memory : Event-Related Brain Potential Evidence. *J. Mem. Lang.* **41**, 345–364.
49. Baddeley, A. (2000) The episodic buffer: a new component of working memory? *Trends Cogn. Sci.* **4**, 417–423.
50. Miller, G. A. (1956) The magical number seven, plus or minus two: some limits on our capacity for processing information. *Pschol. Rev.* **63**, 81–97.
51. Anderson, M. C. and Green, C. (2001) Suppressing unwanted memories by executive control. *Nature* **410**, 366–369.
52. Ghoneim, M. M. and Mewaldt, S. P. (1990) Benzodiazepines and human memory: a review. *Anesthesiology* **72**, 926–938.
53. Curran, H. V. (1986) Tranquillising memories: a review of the effects of benzodiazepines on human memory. *Biol. Psychol.* **23**, 179–213.
54. Lister, R. G. (1985) The amnesic action of benzodiazepines in man. *Neurosci. Biobehav. Rev.* **9**, 87–94.
55. Reinsel, R. A., Veselis, R. A., Duff, M., and Feshchenko, V. (1996) Comparison of implicit and explicit memory during conscious sedation with four sedative-hypnotic agents. In Bonke, B., Bovill, J. G., and Moerman, N. (eds.), Memory and Awareness in Anaesthesia III. van Gorcum, Assen, Netherlands. pp. 41–56.
56. Coetzee, J. F., Glen, J. B., Wium, C. A., and Boshoff, L. (1995) Pharmacokinetic model selection for target controlled infusions of propofol. Assessment of three parameter sets. *Anesthesiology* **82**, 1328–1345.
57. Veselis, R. A., Glass, P., Dnistrian, A., and Reinsel, R. (1997) Performance of computer-assisted continuous infusion at low concentrations of intravenous sedatives. *Anesth. Analg.* **84**, 1049–1057.
58. Glass, P. S., Bloom, M., Kearse, L., Rosow, C., Sebel, P., and Manberg, P. (1997) Bispectral analysis measures sedation and memory effects of propofol, midazolam, isoflurane, and alfentanil in healthy volunteers. *Anesthesiology* **86**, 836–847.
59. Leslie, K., Sessler, D. I., Schroeder, M., and Walters, K. (1995) Propofol blood concentration and the Bispectral Index predict suppression of learning during propofol/epidural anesthesia in volunteers. *Anesth. Analg.* **81**, 1269–1274.
60. Chortkoff, B. S., Eger, II, E. I., Crankshaw, D. P., Gonsowski, C. T., Dutton, R. C., and Ionescu, P. (1995) Concentrations of desflurane and propofol that suppress response to command in humans. *Anesth. Analg.* **81**, 737–743.
61. Ghoneim, M. M., Ali, M. A., and Block, R. I. (1990) Appraisal of the quality of assessment of memory in anesthesia and psychopharmacology literature. *Anesthesiology* **73**, 815–820.
62. Picton, T. W., Bentin, S., Berg, P., et al. (2000) Guidelines for using human event-related potentials to study cognition: recording standards and publication criteria. *Psychophysiology* **37**, 127–152.
63. Posner, M. I. (1999) Localizing cognitive operations. *Brain Res. Bull.* **50**, 413.
64. Squire, L. R., Ojemann, J. G., Miezin, F. M., Petersen, S. E., Videen, T. O., and Raichle, M. E. (1992) Activation of the hippocampus in normal humans: A functional anatomical study of memory. *Proc. Natl. Acad. Sci. USA* **89**, 1837–1841.
65. Grasby, P. M., Frith, C. D., Friston, K., Frackowiak, R. S., and Dolan, R. J. (1993) Activation of the human hippocampal formation during auditory-verbal long-term memory function. *Neurosci. Lett.* **163**, 185–188.
66. Cabeza, R. and Nyberg, L. (1997) Imaging cognition : An empirical review of PET studies with normal subjects. *J. Cogn. Neurosci.* **9**, 1–26.
67. Cabeza, R. and Nyberg, L. (2000) Imaging cognition II: An empirical review of 275 PET and fMRI studies. *J. Cogn. Neurosci.* **12**, 1–47.
68. Fletcher, P. C., Frith, C. D., and Rugg, M. D. (1997) The functional neuroanatomy of episodic memory. *Trends Neurosci.* **20**, 213–218.
69. Tulving, E., Kapur, S., Craik, F. I., Moscovitch, M., and Houle, S. (1994) Hemispheric encoding/retrieval asymmetry in episodic memory: positron emission tomography findings. *Proc. Natl. Acad. Sci. USA* **91**, 2016–2020.
70. Thompson-Schill, S. L., Swick, D., Farah, M. J., D'Esposito, M., Kan, I. P., and Knight, R. T. (1998) Verb generation in patients with focal frontal lesions: A neuropsychological test of neuroimaging findings. *Proc. Natl. Acad. Sci. USA* **95**, 15,855–15,860.
71. Fine, C., Lumsden, J., and Blair, R. J. (2001) Dissociation between "theory of mind" and executive functions in a patient with early left amygdala damage. *Brain* **124**, 287–298.
72. Savage, C. R., Deckersbach, T., Heckers, S., et al. (2001) Prefrontal regions supporting spontaneous and directed application of verbal learning strategies: Evidence from PET. *Brain* **124**, 219–231.
73. Shallice, T. (2001) "Theory of mind" and the prefrontal cortex. *Brain* **124**, 247–248.
74. Stuss, D. T., Gallup, G. G., and Alexander, M. P. (2001) The frontal lobes are necessary for "theory of mind". *Brain* **124**, 279–286.
75. Thompson-Schill, S. L., D'Esposito, M., and Kan, I. P. (1999) Effects of repetition and competition on activity in left prefrontal cortex during word generation. *Neuron* **23**, 513–522.

76. Thompson-Schill, S. L., D'Esposito, M., Aguirre, G. K., and Farah, M. J. (1997) Role of left inferior prefrontal cortex in retrieval of semantic knowledge: a reevaluation. *Proc. Natl. Acad. Sci. USA* **94**, 14,792–14,797.

77. Dolan, R. J. and Fletcher, P. C. (1997) Dissociating prefrontal and hippocampal function in episodic memory encoding. *Nature* **388**, 582–585.

78. Klingberg, T. and Roland, P. E. (1998) Right prefrontal activation during encoding, but not during retrieval, in a nonverbal paired-associates task. *Cereb. Cortex* **8**, 73–79.

79. Rugg, M. D., Fletcher, P. C., Chua, P. M., and Dolan, R. J. (1999) The role of the prefrontal cortex in recognition memory and memory for source: an fMRI study. *Neuroimage* **10**, 520–529.

80. Lepage, M., Ghaffar, O., Nyberg, L., and Tulving, E. (2000) Prefrontal cortex and episodic memory retrieval mode. *Proc. Natl. Acad. Sci. USA* **97**, 506–511.

81. Opitz, B., Mecklinger, A., and Friederici, A. D. (2000) Functional asymmetry of human prefrontal cortex: encoding and retrieval of verbally and nonverbally coded information. *Learn. Mem.* **7**, 85–96.

82. Kapur, N., Friston, K. J., Young, A., Frith, C. D., and Frackowiak, R. S. (1995) Activation of human hippocampal formation during memory for faces: a PET study. *Cortex* **31**, 99–108.

83. Haxby, J. V., Ungerleider, L. G., Horwitz, B., Maisog, J. M., Rapoport, S. I., and Grady, C. L. (1996) Face encoding and recognition in the human brain. *Proc. Natl. Acad. Sci. USA* **93**, 922–927.

84. McIntosh, A. R., Nyberg, L., Bookstein, F. L., and Tulving, E. (1997) Differential functional connectivity of prefrontal and medial temporal cortices during episodic memory retrieval. *Hum. Brain Mapp.* **5**, 323–327.

85. Gabrieli, J. D. E., Brewer, J. B., Desmond, J. E., and Glover, G. H. (1997) Separate neural bases of two fundamental memory processes in the human medial temporal lobe. *Science* **276**, 264–266.

86. Trott, C. T., Friedman, D., Ritter, W., Fabiani, M., and Snodgrass, J. G. (1999) Episodic priming and memory for temporal source: event-related potentials reveal age-related differences in prefrontal functioning. *Psychol. Aging* **14**, 390–413.

87. Friedman, D. and Trott, C. (2000) An event-related potential study of encoding in young and older adults. *Neuropsychologia* **38**, 542–557.

88. Spencer, K. M., Vila Abad, E., and Donchin, E. (2000) On the search for the neurophysiological manifestation of recollective experience. *Psychophysiology* **37**, 494–506.

89. Nyberg, L., McIntosh, A. R., and Tulving, E. (1998) Functional brain imaging of episodic and semantic memory with positron emission tomography. *J. Mol. Med.* **76**, 48–53.

90. Duzel, E., Yonelinas, A. P., Mangun, G. R., Heinze, H. J., and Tulving, E. (1997) Event-related brain potential correlates of two states of conscious awareness in memory. *Proc. Natl. Acad. Sci. USA* **94**, 5973–5978.

91. Rugg, M. D. (1998) Memories are made of this. *Science* **281**, 1151–1152.

92. Ledoux, J. E. (1993) Emotional memory: In search of systems and synapses. *Ann. NY Acad. Sci.* **702**, 149–157.

93. Hebb, D. O. (1949) The organization of behavior; a neuropsychological theory. Wiley, New York.

94. Haxby, J. V., Petit, L., Ungerleider, L. G., and Courtney, S. M. (2000) Distinguishing the functional roles of multiple regions in distributed neural systems for visual working memory. *Neuroimage* **11**, 145–156.

95. Petit, L., Courtney, S. M., Ungerleider, L. G., and Haxby, J. V. (1998) Sustained activity in the medial wall during working memory delays. *J. Neurosci.* **18**, 9429–9437.

96. Baddeley, A. (1995) Working memory. In Gazzaniga, M. S. (ed.), The Cognitive Neurosciences. The MIT Press, Cambridge, MA. pp. 755–764.

97. Baddeley, A. (1996) The fractionation of working memory. *Proc. Natl. Acad. Sci. USA* **93**, 13,468–13,472.

98. Jonides, J., Smith, E. E., Koeppe, R. A., Awh, E., Minoshima, S., and Mintun, M. A. (1993) Spatial working memory in humans as revealed by PET. *Nature* **363**, 623–625.

99. Paulesu, E., Frith, C. D., and Frackowiak, R. S. (1993) The neural correlates of the verbal component of working memory. *Nature* **362**, 342–345.

100. Goldberg, T. E., Berman, K. F., Fleming, K., et al. (1998) Uncoupling cognitive workload and prefrontal cortical physiology: a PET rCBF study. *Neuroimage* **7**, 296–303.

101. Postle, B. R., Berger, J. S., and D'Esposito, M. (19990 Functional neuroanatomical double dissociation of mnemonic and executive control processes contributing to working memory performance. *Proc. Natl. Acad. Sci. USA* **96**, 12,959–12,964.

102. Smith, E. E., Jonides, J., Marshuetz, C., and Koeppe, R. A. (1998) Components of verbal working memory: evidence from neuroimaging. *Proc. Natl. Acad. Sci. USA* **95**, 876–882.

103. Smith, E. E. and Jonides, J. (1998) Neuroimaging analyses of human working memory. *Proc. Natl. Acad. Sci. USA* **95**, 12,061–12,068.

104. Sarnthein, J., Petsche, H., Rappelsberger, P., Shaw, G. L., and von Stein, A. (1998) Synchronization between prefrontal and posterior association cortex during human working memory. *Proc. Natl. Acad. Sci. USA* **95**, 7092–7096.

105. Koechlin, E., Basso, G., Pietrini, P., Panzer, S., and Grafman, J. (1999) The role of the anterior prefrontal cortex in human cognition. *Nature* **399**, 148–151.

106. Wheeler, M. A., Stuss, D. T., and Tulving, E. (1997) Toward a theory of episodic memory: the frontal lobes and autonoetic consciousness. *Psychol. Bull.* **121**, 331–354.

107. Gabrieli, J. D., Brewer, J. B., and Poldrack, R. A. (1998) Images of medial temporal lobe functions in human learning and memory. *Neurobiol. Learn. Mem.* **70**, 275–283.

108. Idzikowski, C. (1984) Sleep and memory. *Brit. J. Psychol.* **75**, 439–449.

109. Smith, E. E. and Jonides, J. (1995) Working memory in humans: Neuropsychological evidence. In Gazzaniga, M. S. (ed.), The Cognitive Neurosciences. The MIT Press, Cambridge, MA. pp. 1009–1020.

110. O'Gorman, D. A., O'Connell, A. W., Murphy, K. J., Moriarty, D. C., Shiotani, T., and Regan, C. M. (1998) Nefiracetam prevents propofol-induced anterograde and retrograde amnesia in the rodent without compromising quality of anesthesia. *Anesthesiology* **89**, 699–706.

111. Bechara, A., Tranel, D., Damasio, H., Adolphs, R., Rockland, C., and Damasio, A. R. (1995) Double dissociation of conditioning and declarative knowledge relative to the amygdala and hippocampus in humans. *Science* **269**, 1115–1118.

112. Fletcher, P., Buchel, C., Josephs, O., Friston, K., and Dolan, R. (1999) Learning-related neuronal responses in prefrontal cortex studied with functional neuroimaging. *Cereb. Cortex* **9**, 168–178.

113. Berns, G. S., Cohen, J. D., and Mintun, M. A. (1997) Brain regions responsive to novelty in the absence of awareness. *Science* **276**, 1272–1275.

114. Henson, R. N., Rugg, M. D., Shallice, T., Josephs, O., and Dolan, R. J. (1999) Recollection and familiarity in recognition memory: an event-related functional magnetic resonance imaging study. *J. Neurosci.* **19**, 3962–3972.

115. Henson, R. N., Rugg, M. D., Shallice, T., and Dolan, R. J. (2000) Confidence in Recognition Memory for Words: Dissociating Right Prefrontal Roles in Episodic Retrieval. *J. Cogn. Neurosci.* **12**, 913–923.

116. Otten, L. J., Henson, R. N., and Rugg, M. D. (2001) Depth of processing effects on neural correlates of memory encoding: Relationship between findings from across- and within-task comparisons. *Brain* **124**, 399–412.

117. Ghoneim, M. M., Block, R. I., Dhanaraj, V. J., Todd, M. M., Choi, W. W., and Brown, C. K. (2000) Auditory evoked responses and learning and awareness during general anesthesia. *Acta Anaesthesiol. Scand.* **44**, 133–143.

118. Lubke, G. H., Kerssens, C., Gershon, R. Y., and Sebel, P. S. (2000) Memory formation during general anesthesia for emergency cesarean sections. *Anesthesiology* **92**, 1029–1034.

119. Lubke, G. H., Kerssens, C., Phaf, H., and Sebel, P. S. (1999) Dependence of explicit and implicit memory on hypnotic state in trauma patients. *Anesthesiology* **90**, 670–680.

120. Toth, J. P., Reingold, E. M., and Jacoby, L. L. (1994) Toward a redefinition of implicit memory: process dissociations following elaborative processing and self-generation. *J. Exp. Psychol. Learn. Mem. Cogn.* **20**, 290–303.

121. Gardiner, J. M. and Richardson-Klavehn, A. (2000) Remebering and Knowing. In Tulving, E. and Craik, F. I. M. (eds.), The Oxford handbook of memory. Oxford University Press, Oxford; New York. pp. 229–244.

122. Schacter, D. L., Chiu, C.-Y. P., and Ochsner, K. N. (1993) Implicit memory: A selective review. *Ann. Rev. Neurosci.* **16**, 159–182.

123. Fang, J. C., Hinrichs, J. V., and Ghoneim, M. M. (1987) Diazepam and memory: evidence for spared memory function. *Pharmacol., Biochem. Behav.* **28**, 347–352.

124. Danion, J. M., Peretti, S., Grange, D., Bilik, M., Imbs, J. L., and Singer, L. (1992) Effects of chlorpromazine and lorazepam on explicit memory, repetition priming and cognitive skill learning in healthy volunteers. *Psychopharmacology* **108**, 345–351.

125. Sellal, F., Danion, J. M., Kauffmann-Muller, F., et al. (1992) Differential effects of diazepam and lorazepam on repetition priming in healthy volunteers. *Psychopharmacology* **108**, 371–379.

126. Curran, H. V., Barrow, S., Weingartner, H., Lader, M., and Bernik, M. (1995) Encoding, remembering and awareness in lorazepam-induced amnesia. *Psychopharmacology* **122**, 187–193.

127. Legrand, F., Vidailhet, P., Danion, J. M., et al. (1995) Time course of the effects of diazepam and lorazepam on perceptual priming and explicit memory. *Psychopharmacology* **118**, 475–479.

128. Cork, R. C., Heaton, J. F., Campbell, C. E., and Kihlstrom, J. F. (1996) Is there implicit memory after propofol sedation? *Brit. J. Anaesth.* **76**, 492–498.

129. Polster, M. R., McCarthy, R. A., O'Sullivan, G., Gray, P. A., and Park, G. R. (1993) Midazolam-induced amnesia: implications for the implicit/explicit memory distinction. *Brain Cogn.* **22**, 244–265.

130. Schifano, F. and Curran, H. V. (1994) Pharmacological models of memory dysfunction? A comparison of the effects of scopolamine and lorazepam on word valence ratings, priming and recall. *Psychopharmacology* **115**, 430–434.

131. Polster, M. R., Gray, P. A., O'Sullivan, G., McCarthy, R. A., and Park, G. R. (1993) Comparison of the sedative and amnesic effects of midazolam and propofol. *Brit. J. Anaesth.* **70**, 612–616.

132. Munte, S., Kobbe, I., Demertzis, A., et al. (1999) Increased reading speed for stories presented during general anesthesia. *Anesthesiology* **90**, 662–669.

133. Weldon, M. S. (1991) Mechanisms underlying priming on perceptual tests. *J. Exp. Psychol.: Learn. Mem. Cogn.* **17**, 526–541.

134. Henson, R., Shallice, T., and Dolan, R. (2000) Neuroimaging evidence for dissociable forms of repetition priming. *Science* **287**, 1269–1272.

135. Saint-Cyr, J. A., Taylor, A. E., and Lang, A. E. (1988) Procedural learning and neostriatal dysfunction in man. *Brain* **111**, 941–959.

136. Badgaiyan, R. D., Schacter, D. L., and Alpert, N. M. (1999) Auditory priming within and across modalities: evidence from positron emission tomography. *J. Cogn. Neurosci.* **11**, 337–348.

137. Schacter, D. L., Badgaiyan, R. D., and Alpert, N. M. (1999) Visual word stem completion priming within and across modalities: a PET study. *Neuroreport* **10**, 2061–2065.

138. Elliott, R. and Dolan, R. J. (1998) Neural response during preference and memory judgments for subliminally presented stimuli: a functional neuroimaging study. *J. Neurosci.* **18**, 4697–4704.

139. McIntosh, A. R., Rajah, M. N., and Lobaugh, N. J. (1999) Interactions of prefrontal cortex in relation to awareness in sensory learning. *Science* **284**, 1531–1533.

140. Dehaene, S., Naccache, L., Le Clec, H. G., et al. (1998) Imaging unconscious semantic priming. *Nature* **395**, 597–600.

141. Buckner, R. L., Petersen, S. E., Ojemann, J. G., Miezin, F. M., Squire, L. R., and Raichle, M. E. (1995) Functional anatomical studies of explicit and implicit memory retrieval tasks. *J. Neurosci.* **15**, 12–29.

142. Leveroni, C. L., Seidenberg, M., Mayer, A. R., Mead, L. A., Binder, J. R., and Rao, S. M. (2000) Neural systems underlying the recognition of familiar and newly learned faces. *J. Neurosci.* **20,** 878–886.
143. Dolan, R. J., Fink, G. R., Rolls, E., et al. (1997) How the brain learns to see objects and faces in an impoverished context. *Nature* **389,** 596–599.
144. Morris, J. S., Ohman, A., and Dolan, R. J. (1998) Conscious and unconscious emotional learning in the human amygdala. *Nature* **393,** 467–470.
145. Damasio, A. R. and Tranel, D. (1992) Knowledge systems. *Curr. Opin. Neurobiol.* **2,** 186–190.
146. Squire, L. R. and Alvarez, P. (1995) Retrograde amnesia and memory consolidation: a neurobiological perspective. *Curr. Opin. Neurobiol.* **5,** 169–177.
147. Zola Morgan, S. M. and Squire, L. R. (1990) The primate hippocampal formation : evidence for a time-limited role in memory storage. *Science* **250,** 288–290.
148. Teng, E. and Squire, L. R. (1999) Memory for places learned long ago is intact after hippocampal damage. *Nature* **400,** 675–677.
149. Nadel, L. and Moscovitch, M. (1997) Memory consolidation, retrograde amnesia and the hippocampal complex. *Curr. Opin. Neurobiol.* **7,** 217–227.
150. Viskontas, I. V., McAndrews, M. P., and Moscovitch, M. (2000) Remote episodic memory deficits in patients with unilateral temporal lobe epilepsy and excisions. *J. Neurosci.* **20,** 5853–5857.
151. Nyberg, L., McIntosh, A. R., Cabeza, R., et al. (1996) Network analysis of positron emission tomography regional cerebral blood flow data: ensemble inhibition during episodic memory retrieval. *J. Neurosci.* **16,** 3753–3759.
152. Gabrieli, J. D. E. (1995) A systematic view of human memory processes. *J. Int. Neuropsych. Soc.* **1,** 115–118.
153. Blaxton, T. A. (1995) A process-based view of memory. *J. Int. Neuropsych. Soc.* **1,** 112–114.
154. Roediger, H. L. I., Rajaram, S., and Srinivas, K. (1990) Specifying criteria for postulating memory systems. *Ann. NY Acad. Sci.* **608,** 572–595.
155. Perani, D., Bressi, S., Cappa, S. F., et al. (1993) Evidence of multiple memory systems in the human brain. A [18F]FDG PET metabolic study. *Brain* **116,** 903–919.
156. Nyberg, L., McIntosh, A. R., Houle, S., Nilsson, L.-G., and Tulving, E. (1996) Activation of medial temporal structures during episodic memory retrieval. *Nature* **380,** 715–717.
157. Ungerleider, L. G. (1995) Functional brain imaging studies of cortical mechanisms for memory. *Science* **270,** 769–775.
158. Buffalo, E. A., Ramus, S. J., Squire, L. R., and Zola, S. M. (2000) Perception and recognition memory in monkeys following lesions of area TE and perirhinal cortex. *Learn. Mem.* **7,** 375–382.
159. Clark, R. E., Zola, S. M., and Squire, L. R. (2000) Impaired recognition memory in rats after damage to the hippocampus. *J. Neurosci.* **20,** 8853–8860.
160. Teng, E., Stefanacci, L., Squire, L. R., and Zola, S. M. (2000) Contrasting effects on discrimination learning after hippocampal lesions and conjoint hippocampal-caudate lesions in monkeys. *J. Neurosci.* **20,** 3853–3863.
161. Zola, S. M., Squire, L. R., Teng, E., Stefanacci, L., Buffalo, E. A., and Clark, R. E. (2000) Impaired recognition memory in monkeys after damage limited to the hippocampal region. *J. Neurosci.* **20,** 451–463.
162. Zola-Morgan, S. and Squire, L. R. (1993) Neuroanatomy of memory. *Ann. Rev. Neurosci.* **16,** 547–563.
163. Eichenbaum, H. (1999) The hippocampus and mechanisms of declarative memory. *Behav. Brain Res.* **103,** 123–133.
164. Eichenbaum, H. (2000) A cortical-hippocampal system for declarative memory. *Nat. Rev. Neurosci.* **1,** 41–50.
165. Aggleton, J. P., McMackin, D., Carpenter, K., et al. (2000) Differential cognitive effects of colloid cysts in the third ventricle that spare or compromise the fornix. *Brain* **123,** 800–815.
166. Beiser, D. G., Hua, S. E., and Houk, J. C. (1997) Network models of the basal ganglia. *Curr. Opin. Neurobiol.* **7,** 185–190.
167. Lombardi, W. J., Gross, R. E., Trepanier, L. L., Lang, A. E., Lozano, A. M., and Saint-Cyr, J. A. (2000) Relationship of lesion location to cognitive outcome following microelectrode-guided pallidotomy for Parkinson's disease: support for the existence of cognitive circuits in the human pallidum. *Brain* **123,** 746–758.
168. LeDoux, J. E. (1996) The emotional brain : the mysterious underpinnings of emotional life. Simon & Schuster, New York, pp.138–178.
169. McGaugh, J. L. and Introini-Collison, I. B. (1987) Hormonal and neurotransmitter interactions in the modulation of memory storage: involvement of the amygdala. *Int. J. Neurol.* **21–22,** 58–72.
170. Buchel, C. and Dolan, R. J. (2000) Classical fear conditioning in functional neuroimaging. *Curr. Opin. Neurobiol.* **10,** 219–223.
171. Bechara, A., Damasio, H., and Damasio, A. R. (2000) Emotion, decision making and the orbitofrontal cortex. *Cereb. Cortex* **10,** 295–307.
172. Johnsrude, I. S., Owen, A. M., White, N. M., Zhao, W. V., and Bohbot, V. (2000) Impaired preference conditioning after anterior temporal lobe resection in humans. *J. Neurosci.* **20,** 2649–2656.
173. Cahill, L., Haier, R. J., White, N. S., et al. (2001) Sex-related difference in amygdala activity during emotionally influenced memory storage. *Neurobiol. Learn. Mem.* **75,** 1–9.
174. Morris, J. S., Friston, K. J., Buchel, C., et al. (1998) A neuromodulatory role for the human amygdala in processing emotional facial expressions. *Brain* **121,** 47–57.
175. Buchel, C., Dolan, R. J., Armony, J. L., and Friston, K. J. (1999) Amygdala-hippocampal involvement in human aversive trace conditioning revealed through event-related functional magnetic resonance imaging. *J. Neurosci.* **19,** 10,869–10,876.
176. Dickinson-Anson, H. and McGaugh, J. L. (1994) Infusion of the GABAergic antagonist bicuculline into the medial septal area does not block the impairing effects of systemically administered midazolam on inhibitory avoidance retention. *Behav. Neural. Biol.* **62,** 253–258.

177. Dickinson-Anson, H. and McGaugh, J. L. (1993) Midazolam administered into the amygdala impairs retention of an inhibitory avoidance task. *Behav. Neural. Biol.* **60,** 84–87.
178. Tomaz, C., Dickinson-Anson, H., and McGaugh, J. L. (1992) Basolateral amygdala lesions block diazepam-induced anterograde amnesia in an inhibitory avoidance task. *Proc. Natl. Acad. Sci. USA* **89,** 3615–3619.
179. Tomaz, C., Dickinson-Anson, H., and McGaugh, J. L. (1991) Amygdala lesions block the amnestic effects of diazepam. *Brain Res.* **568,** 85–91.
180. Malloy, P. F. and Richardson, E. D. (1994) Assessment of frontal lobe functions. *J. Neuropsych. Clin. Neurosci.* **6,** 399–410.
181. Shimamura, A. P. (1995) Memory and the prefrontal cortex. *Ann. NY Acad. Sci.* **769,** 151–159.
182. Rowe, A. D., Bullock, P. R., Polkey, C. E., and Morris, R. G. (2001) 'Theory of mind' impairments and their relationship to executive functioning following frontal lobe excisions. *Brain* **124,** 600–616.
183. Schnider, A. (2000) Spontaneous confabulations, disorientation, and the processing of "now". *Neuropsychologia* **38,** 175–185.
184. Schnider, A., Treyer, V., and Buck, A. (2000) Selection of currently relevant memories by the human posterior medial orbitofrontal cortex. *J. Neurosci.* **20,** 5880–5884.
185. Oscar-Berman, M. (1991) Clinical and experimental approaches to varieties of memory. *Int. J. Neurosci.* **58,** 135–150.
186. Leiner, H. C., Leiner, A. L., and Dow, R. S. (1995) The underestimated cerebellum. *Hum. Brain Mapp.* **2,** 244–254.
187. Schmahmann, J. D. (1996) From movement to thought: Anatomic substrates of the cerebellar contribution to cognitive processing. *Hum. Brain Mapp.* **4,** 174–198.
188. Junck, L., Gilman, S., Rothley, J. R., Betley, A. T., Koeppe, R. A., and Hichwa, R. D. (1988) A relationship between metabolism in frontal lobes and cerebellum in normal subjects studied with PET. *J. Cereb. Blood F. Met.* **8,** 774–782.
189. Felleman, D. J. and Van Essen, D. C. (1991) Distributed hierarchical processing in the primate cerebral cortex. *Cereb. Cortex* **1,** 1–47.
190. Nyberg, L., Persson, J., Habib, R., et al. (2000) Large scale neurocognitive networks underlying episodic memory. *J. Cogn. Neurosci.* **12,** 163–173.
191. McEvoy, L. K., Smith, M. E., and Gevins, A. (1998) Dynamic cortical networks of verbal and spatial working memory: effects of memory load and task practice. *Cereb. Cortex* **8,** 563–574.
192. Harrington, D. L., Haaland, K. Y., and Knight, R. T. (19980 Cortical networks underlying mechanisms of time perception. *J. Neurosci.* **18,** 1085–1095.
193. Fuster, J. M. (1997) Network Memory. *Trends Neurosci.* **20,** 451–459.
194. Tulving, E. and Markowitsch, H. J. (1997) Memory beyond the hippocampus. *Curr. Opin. Neurobiol.* **7,** 209–216.
195. Ghoneim, M. M. and Hinrichs, J. V. (1997) Drugs, memory and sedation: specificity of effects. *Anesthesiology* **87,** 734–736.
196. Veselis, R. A. (1999) Memory function during anesthesia (editorial). *Anesthesiology* **90,** 648–650.
197. Alkire, M. T., Pomfrett, C. J., Haier, R. J., et al. (1999) Functional brain imaging during anesthesia in humans: Effects of halothane on global and regional cerebral glucose metabolism. *Anesthesiology* **90,** 701–709.
198. Veselis, R. A., Reinsel, R. A., Beattie, B. J., et al. (1997) Midazolam changes cerebral blood flow in discrete brain regions: an H2(15)O positron emission tomography study. *Anesthesiology* **87,** 1106–1117.
199. Alkire, M. T., Haier, R. J., Shah, N. K., and Anderson, C. T. (1997) Positron emission tomography study of regional cerebral metabolism in humans during isoflurane anesthesia. *Anesthesiology* **86,** 549–557.
200. Gyulai, F. E., Firestone, L. L., Mintun, M. A., and Winter, P. M. (1996) In vivo imaging of human limbic responses to nitrous oxide inhalation. *Anesth. Analg.* **83,** 291–298.
201. Firestone, L. L., Gyulai, F., Mintun, M., Adler, L. J., Urso, K., and Winter, P. M. (1996) Human brain activity response to fentanyl imaged by positron emission tomography. *Anesth. Analg.* **82,** 1247–1251.
202. Volkow, N. D., Wang, G. J., Hitzemann, R., et al. (1995) Depression of thalamic metabolism by lorazepam is associated with sleepiness. *Neuropsychopharmacology* **12,** 123–132.
203. Hartvig, P., Valtysson, J., Lindner, K. J., et al. (1995) Central nervous system effects of subdissociative doses of (S)-ketamine are related to plasma and brain concentrations measured with positron emission tomography in healthy volunteers. *Clin. Pharmacol. Ther.* **58,** 165–173.
204. Grasby, P. M., Frith, C. D., Paulesu, E., Friston, K. J., Frackowiak, R. S., and Dolan, R. J. (1995) The effect of the muscarinic antagonist scopolamine on regional cerebral blood flow during the performance of a memory task. *Exp. Brain Res.* **104,** 337–348.
205. Grasby, P. M., Friston, K. J., Bench, C., et al. (19920 Effect of the 5-HT1A partial agonist buspirone on regional cerebral blood flow in man. *Psychopharmacology* **108,** 380–386.
206. Grasby, P. M., Friston, K. J., Bench, C. J., et al. (1993) The effect of the dopamine agonist, apomorphine, on regional cerebral blood flow in normal volunteers. *Psychol. Med.* **23,** 605–612.
207. Malonek, D. and Grinvald, A. (1997) Vascular regulation at sub millimeter range. Sources of intrinsic signals for high resolution optical imaging. *Adv. Exp. Med. Biol.* **413,** 215–220.
208. Malonek, D., Dirnagl, U., Lindauer, U., Yamada, K., Kanno, I., and Grinvald, A. (1997) Vascular imprints of neuronal activity: relationships between the dynamics of cortical blood flow, oxygenation, and volume changes following sensory stimulation. *Proc. Natl. Acad. Sci. USA* **94,** 14,826–14,831.
209. Shtoyerman, E., Arieli, A., Slovin, H., Vanzetta, I., and Grinvald, A. (2000) Long-term optical imaging and spectroscopy reveal mechanisms underlying the intrinsic signal and stability of cortical maps in V1 of behaving monkeys. *J. Neurosci.* **20,** 8111–8121.
210. Coull, J. T., Frith, C. D., Dolan, R. J., Frackowiak, R. S., and Grasby, P. M. (1997) The neural correlates of the noradrenergic modulation of human attention, arousal and learning. *Euro. J. Neurosci.* **9,** 589–598.

211. Friston, K. J., Grasby, P. M., Bench, C. J., et al. (1992) Measuring the neuromodulatory effects of drugs in man with positron emission tomography. *Neurosci. Lett.* **141,** 106–110.
212. Dolan, R. J., Fletcher, P., Frith, C. D., Friston, K. J., Frackowiak, R. S., and Grasby, P. M. (1995) Dopaminergic modulation of impaired cognitive activation in the anterior cingulate cortex in schizophrenia. *Nature* **378,** 180–182.
213. Friston, K. J., Grasby, P. M., Frith, C. D., et al. (1991) The neurotransmitter basis of cognition: psychopharmacological activation studies using positron emission tomography. *Ciba F. Symp.* **163,** 76–87; discussion pp. 87–92.
214. Bahro, M., Molchan, S. E., Sunderland, T., Herscovitch, P., and Schreurs, B. G. (1999) The Effects of Scopolamine on Changes in Regional Cerebral Blood Flow during Classical Conditioning of the Human Eyeblink Response. *Neuropsychobiology* **39,** 187–195.
215. Bonhomme, V., Fiset, P., Meuret, P., et al. (2001) Propofol Anesthesia and Cerebral Blood Flow Changes Elicited by Vibrotactile Stimulation: A Positron Emission Tomography Study. *J. Neurophysiol.* **85,** 1299–1308.
216. Friston, K. J., Frith, C. D., Liddle, P. F., and Frackowiak, R. S. (1991) Comparing functional (PET) images: the assessment of significant change. *J. Cereb. Blood F. Met.* **11,** 690–699.
217. Friston, K. J. (1994) Statistical parametric mapping. In Thatcher, R. W., Hallett, M., Zeffiro, T., John, E. R., and Huerta, M. (eds.), Functional Neuroimaging : Technical Foundations. Academic Press, San Diego. pp. 79–93.
218. Reinsel, R. A., Veselis, R. A., Dnistrian, A., Feshchenko, V. A., Beattie, B. J., and Duff, M. R. (2000) Midazolam decreases cerebral blood flow in the left prefrontal cortex in a dose-dependent fashion. *Int. J. Neuropsychopharm.* **3,** 117–128.
219. Jonides, J., Schumacher, E. H., Smith, E. E., et al. (1998) The role of parietal cortex in verbal working memory. *J. Neurosci.* **18,** 5026–5034.
220. Martinkauppi, S., Rama, P., Aronen, H. J., Korvenoja, A., and Carlson, S. (2000) Working memory of auditory localization. *Cereb. Cortex* **10,** 889–898.
221. Bickford, R. G. (1950) Automatic electroencephalographic control of general anesthesia. *Electroencephalogr. Clin. Neurophysiol.* **2,** 93–96.
222. Verzeano, M. (1951) Servo-motor integration of the electrical activity of the brain and its applications to the automatic control of narcosis. *Electroencephalogr. Clin. Neurophysiol.* **3,** 25–30.
223. Sandin, R. H., Enlund, G., Samuelsson, P., and Lennmarken, C. (2000) Awareness during anaesthesia: a prospective case study. *Lancet* **355,** 707–711.
224. Rampil, I. J. (1998) A primer for EEG signal processing in anesthesia. *Anesthesiology* **89,** 980–1002.
225. Sebel, P. S., Lang, E., Rampil, I. J., et al. (1997) A multicenter study of bispectral electroencephalogram analysis for monitoring anesthetic effect. *Anesth. Analg.* **84,** 891–899.
226. Alkire, M. T. (1998) Quantitative EEG correlations with brain glucose metabolic rate during anesthesia in volunteers. *Anesthesiology* **89,** 323–333.
227. Viertio-Oja, H., Sarkela, M., Talja, P., Tolvanen-Laakso, H., and Yli-Hankala, A. (2000) Entropy of the EEG Signal Is a Robust Index for Depth of Hypnosis. *Anesthesiology* **93,** A-1369.
228. John, E. R., Prichep, L. S., Valdes-Sosa, P., et al. (2001). Invariant Reversible QEEG effects of anesthetics. *Conscious. Cogn.* **10,** 184–213.
229. Picton, T. W., Lins, O. G., and Scherg, M. (1995) The recording and analysis of event-related potentials. In Boller, F. and Grafman, J. (eds.), Handbook of Neuropsychology, vol. 10. Elsevier Science B.V., Amsterdam. 3-73.
230. Effern, A., Lehnertz, K., Fernandez, G., Grunwald, T., David, P., and Elger, C. E. (2000) Single trial analysis of event related potentials: non-linear de- noising with wavelets. *Clin. Neurophysiol.* **111,** 2255–2263.
231. Demiralp, T., Ademoglu, A., Schurmann, M., Basar-Eroglu, C., and Basar, E. (1999) Detection of P300 waves in single trials by the wavelet transform (WT). *Brain Lang.* **66,** 108–128.
232. Effern, A., Lehnertz, K., Grunwald, T., Fernandez, G., David, P., and Elger, C. E. (2000) Time adaptive denoising of single trial event-related potentials in the wavelet domain. *Psychophysiology* **37,** 859–865.
233. Schurmann, M., Basar-Eroglu, C., Kolev, V., and Basar, E. (1995) A new metric for analyzing single-trial event-related potentials (ERPs): application to human visual P300 delta response. *Neurosci. Lett.* **197,** 167–170.
234. Arieli, A., Sterkin, A., Grinvald, A., and Aertsen, A. (1996) Dynamics of ongoing activity: explanation of the large variability in evoked cortical responses. *Science* **273,** 1868–1881.
235. Basar, E., Demiralp, T., Schurmann, M., Basar-Eroglu, C., and Ademoglu, A. (1999) Oscillatory brain dynamics, wavelet analysis, and cognition. *Brain Lang.* **66,** 146–183.
236. Rugg, M. D. (1998) Convergent approaches to electrophysiological and hemodynamic investigations of memory. *Hum. Brain Mapp.* **6,** 394–398.
237. Gevins, A., Smith, M. E., McEvoy, L. K., Leong, H., and Le, J. (1999) Electroencephalographic imaging of higher brain function. *Philos. Trans. R. Soc. Lond. B. Biol. Sci.* **354,** 1125–1133.
238. Pascual-Marqui, R. M. (1999) Review of methods for solving the EEG inverse problem. *Int. J. Bioelect.* **1,** 75–86.
239. Kirchhoff, B. A., Wagner, A. D., Maril, A., and Stern, C. E. (2000) Prefrontal-temporal circuitry for episodic encoding and subsequent memory. *J. Neurosci.* **20,** 6173–6180.
240. Sanquist, T. F., Rohrbaugh, J., Syndulko, K., and Lindsley, D. B. (1980) An event-related potential analysis of coding processes in human memory. *Prog. Brain Res.* **54,** 655–660.
241. Johnson, R., Jr. (1995) Event-related potential insights into the neurobiology of memory systems. In Boller, F. and Grafman, J. (eds.) Handbook of Neuropsychology, vol. 10. Elsevier Science B.V., Amsterdam. pp. 135–163.
242. Fernandez, G., Effern, A., Grunwald, T., et al. (1999) Real-time tracking of memory formation in the human rhinal cortex and hippocampus. *Science* **285,** 1582–1585.

243. Wagner, A. D., Schacter, D. L., Rotte, M., et al. (1998) Building memories: remembering and forgetting of verbal experiences as predicted by brain activity. *Science* **281**, 1188–1191.
244. Pockett, S. (1999) Anesthesia and the Electrophysiology of Auditory Consciousness. *Conscious. Cogn.* **8**, 45–61.
245. Sutton, S., Braren, M., Zubin, J., and John, E. R. (1965) Evoked-potential correlates of stimulus uncertainty. *Science* **150**, 1187–1188.
246. Polich, J. (1990) P300, probability, and interstimulus interval. *Psychophysiology* **27**, 396–403.
247. Attias, J. and Pratt, H. (1992) Auditory event related potentials during lexical categorization in the oddball paradigm. *Brain Lang.* **43**, 230–239.
248. Cobianchi, A. and Giaquinto, S. (1997) Event-related potentials to Italian spoken words. *Electroencephalogr. Clin. Neurophysiol.* **104**, 213–221.
249. Chee, M. W., O'Craven, K. M., Bergida, R., Rosen, B. R., and Savoy, R. L. (1999) Auditory and visual word processing studied with fMRI. *Hum. Brain Mapp.* **7**, 15–28.
250. Robson, M. D., Dorosz, J. L., and Gore, J. C. (1998) Measurements of the temporal fMRI response of the human auditory cortex to trains of tones [published erratum appears in Neuroimage 1998 Aug;8(2):228]. *Neuroimage* **7**, 185–98.
251. Edmister, W. B., Talavage, T. M., Ledden, P. J., and Weisskoff, R. M. (1999) Improved auditory cortex imaging using clustered volume acquisitions. *Hum. Brain Mapp.* **7**, 89–97.
252. Talavage, T. M., Edmister, W. B., Ledden, P. J., and Weisskoff, R. M. (1999) Quantitative assessment of auditory cortex responses induced by imager acoustic noise. *Hum. Brain Mapp.* **7**, 79–88.
253. Bandettini, P. A., Jesmanowicz, A., Van Kylen, J., Birn, R. M., and Hyde, J. S. (1998) Functional MRI of brain activation induced by scanner acoustic noise. *Magn. Reson. Med.* **39**, 410–416.
254. Picton, T. W. and Hillyard, S. A. (1974) Human auditory evoked potentials. II. Effects of attention. *Electroencephalogr. Clin. Neurophysiol.* **36**, 191–199.
255. Näätänen, R. (1992) Attention and brain function. L. Erlbaum, Hillsdale, NJ, pp. 103–133.
256. Donchin, E. and Alfred P. Sloan Foundation. (1984) Cognitive psychophysiology : Event-related potentials and the study of cognition, The Carmel conferences ; v. 1. L. Erlbaum, Hillsdale, N.J.
257. Johnson, R., Jr., Miltner, W., and Braun, C. (1991) Auditory and somatosensory event-related potentials: I. Effects of attention. *J. Psychophysiol.* **5**, 11–25.
258. Johnson, R. J. (1986) A triarchic model of P300 amplitude. *Psychophysiology* **23**, 367–384.
259. Verleger, R. (1997) On the utility of P3 latency as an index of mental chronometry. *Psychophysiology* **34**, 131–156.
260. Altenmueller, E. O. (1993) Psychophysiology and EEG. In Niedermeyer, E. and Lopes da Silva, F. (eds.), Electroencephalography, 3rd ed. Williams & Wilkins, Baltimore. pp. 597–613.
261. Ritter, W., Ford, J. M., Gailllard, A. W., et al. (1984) Cognition and event-related potentials. I. The relation of negative potentials and cognitive processes. In Karrer, R., Cohen, J. and Tueting, P. (eds.), Brain and Information. The New York Academy of Sciences, New York. pp. 24–38.
262. Alho, K. (1992) Selective attention in auditory processing as reflected by event-related brain potentials. *Psychophysiology* **29**, 274–263.
263. Johnson, R., Jr., Kreiter, K., Russo, B., and Zhu, J. (1998) A spatio-temporal analysis of recognition-related event-related brain potentials. *Int. J. Psychophysiol.* **29**, 83–104.
264. Johnson, R. 1993. On the neural generators of the P300 component of the event-related potential. *Psychophysiology* **30**, 90–97.
265. Baudena, P., Halgren, E., Heit, G., and Clarke, J. M. (1995) Intracerebral potentials to rare target and distractor auditory and visual stimuli. III. Frontal cortex. *Electroencephalogr. Clin. Neurophysiol.* **94**, 251–264.
266. Halgren, E., Baudena, P., Clarke, J. M., et al. (1995) Intracerebral potentials to rare target and distractor auditory and visual stimuli. II. Medial, lateral and posterior temporal lobe. *Electroencephalogr. Clin. Neurophysiol.* **94**, 229–250.
267. Halgren, E., Baudena, P., Clarke, J. M., et al. (1995) Intracerebral potentials to rare target and distractor auditory and visual stimuli. I. Superior temporal plane and parietal lobe. *Electroencephalogr. Clin. Neurophysiol.* **94**, 191–220.
268. Kropotov, J. D., Naatnen, R., Sevostianov, A. V., Alho, K., Reinikainen, K., and Kropotova, O. V. (1995) Mismatch negativity to auditory stimulus change recorded directly from the human temporal cortex. *Psychophysiology* **32**, 418–422.
269. Guillem, F., Rougier, A., and Claverie, B. (1999) Short- and long-delay intracranial ERP repetition effects dissociate memory systems in the human brain. *J. Cogn. Neurosci.* **11**, 437–458.
270. Tarkka, I. M., Stokic, D. S., Basile, L. F., and Papanicolaou, A. C. (1995) Electric source localization of the auditory P300 agrees with magnetic source localization. *Electroencephalogr. Clin. Neurophysiol.* **96**, 538–545.
271. Huotilainen, M., Winkler, I., Alho, K., et al. (1998) Combined mapping of human auditory EEG and MEG responses. *Electroencephalogr. Clin. Neurophysiol.* **108**, 370–379.
272. Berg, P. and Scherg, M. (1994) A fast method for forward computation of multiple-shell spherical head models. *Electroencephalogr. Clin. Neurophysiol.* **90**, 58–64.
273. Scherg, M. and Ebersole, J. S. (1993) Models of brain sources. *Brain Topogr.* **5**, 419–423.
274. Scherg, M. and Berg, P. (1996) New concepts of brain source imaging and localization. *Electroencephalogr. Clin. Neurophysiol. Suppl.* **46**, 127–137.
275. Pascual-Marqui, R. D., Michel, C. M., and Lehmann, D. (1994) Low resolution electromagnetic tomography: a new method for localizing electrical activity in the brain. *Int. J. Psychophysiol.* **18**, 49–65.
276. Picton, T. W., Alain, C., Woods, D. L., John, M. S., Scherg, M., Valdes-Sosa, P., Bosch-Bayard, J., and Trujillo, N. J. (1999) Intracerebral sources of human auditory-evoked potentials. *Audiolo. Neuro-otology* **4**, 64–79.

277. Opitz, B., Mecklinger, A., Von Cramon, D. Y., and Kruggel, F. (1999) Combining electrophysiological and hemodynamic measures of the auditory oddball. *Psychophysiology* **36,** 142–147.
278. Opitz, B., Mecklinger, A., Friederici, A. D., and von Cramon, D. Y. (1999) The functional neuroanatomy of novelty processing: integrating ERP and fMRI results. *Cereb. Cortex* **9,** 379–391.
279. Menon, V., Ford, J. M., Lim, K. O., Glover, G. H., and Pfefferbaum, A. (1997) Combined event-related fMRI and EEG evidence for temporal-parietal cortex activation during target detection. *Neuroreport.* **8,** 3029–3037.
280. Abdullaev, Y. G. and Posner, M. I. (1998) Event-related brain potential imaging of semantic encoding during processing single words. *Neuroimage* **7,** 1–13.
281. Absher, J. R., Hart, L. A., Flowers, D. L., Dagenbach, D., and Wood, F. B. (2000) Event-related potentials correlate with task-dependent glucose metabolism. *Neuroimage* **11,** 517–531.
282. Nenov, V. I., Halgren, E., Smith, M. E., et al. (1991) Localized brain metabolic response correlated with potentials evoked by words. *Behav. Brain Res.* **44,** 101–104.
283. Sallinen, M. and Lyytinen, H. (1997) Mismatch negativity during objective and subjective sleepiness. *Psychophysiology* **34,** 694–702.
284. Winter, O., Kok, A., Kenemans, J. L., and Elton, M. (1995) Auditory event-related potentials to deviant stimuli during drowsiness and stage 2 sleep. *Electroencephalogr. Clin. Neurophysiol.* **96,** 398–412.
285. Schwender, D., Daunderer, M., Mulzer, S., Klasing, S., Finsterer, U., and Peter, K. (1997) Midlatency auditory evoked potentials predict movements during anesthesia with isoflurane or propofol. *Anesth. Analg.* **85,** 164–173.
286. Schwender, D., Weninger, E., Daunderer, M., Klasing, S., Poppel, E., and Peter, K. (1995) Anesthesia with increasing doses of sufentanil and midlatency auditory evoked potentials in humans. *Anesth. Analg.* **80,** 499–505.
287. Van Hooff, J. C., De Beer, N. A., Brunia, C. H., et al. (1995) Information processing during cardiac surgery: an event related potential study. *Electroencephalogr. Clin. Neurophysiol.* **96,** 433–452.
288. Plourde, G., Joffe, D., Villemure, C., and Trahan, M. (1993) The P3a wave of the auditory event-related potential reveals registration of pitch change during sufentanil anesthesia for cardiac surgery. *Anesthesiology* **78,** 498–509.
289. Schwender, D., Kaiser, A., Klasing, S., Peter, K., and Poppel, E. (1994) Midlatency auditory evoked potentials and explicit and implicit memory in patients undergoing cardiac surgery. *Anesthesiology* **80,** 493–501.
290. Schwender, D., Madler, C., Klasing, S., Poppel, E., and Peter, K. (1995) Mid-latency auditory evoked potentials and wakefulness during caesarean section. *Euro. J. Anaesth.* **12,** 171–179.
291. Fabiani, M., Karis, D., and Donchin, E. (1986) P300 and recall in an incidental memory paradigm. *Psychophysiology* **23,** 298–308.
292. Johnson, R. J., Pfefferbaum, A., and Kopell, B. S. (1985) P300 and long-term memory: latency predicts recognition performance. *Psychophysiology* **22,** 497–507.
293. Karis, D., M. Fabiani, and E. Donchin. 1984. "P300" and memory: individual differences in the Von Restorff effect. *Cogn. Psychol.* **16,** 177–216.
294. Patterson, J. V., Pratt, H., and Starr, A. (1991) Event-related potential correlates of the serial position effect in short-term memory. *Electroencephalogr. Clin. Neurophysiol.* **78,** 424–437.
295. Paller, K. A., Kutas, M., and Mayes, A. R. (1987) Neural correlates of encoding in an incidental learning paradigm. *Electroencephalogr. Clin. Neurophysiol.* **67,** 360–371.
296. Wilding, E. L. and Rugg, M. D. (1996) An event-related potential study of recognition memory with and without retrieval of source. *Brain* **119,** 889–905.
297. Ritter, W. and Ruchkin, D. S. (1992) A review of event-related potential components discovered in the context of studying P3. *Ann. NY Acad. Sci.* **658,** 1–32.
298. Escera, C., Alho, K., Winkler, I., and Naatanen, R. (1998) Neural mechanisms of involuntary attention to acoustic novelty and change. *J. Cogn. Neurosci.* **10,** 590–604.
299. Kutas, M. and Federmeier, K. D. (2000) Electrophysiology reveals semantic memory use in language comprehension. *Trends Cogn. Sci.* **4,** 463–470.
300. Ritter, W., Paavilainen, P., Lavikainen, J., et al. (1992) Event-related potentials to repetition and change of auditory stimuli. *Electroencephalogr. Clin. Neurophysiol.* **83,** 306–321.
301. Metcalfe, J. (1993) Novelty monitoring, metacognition, and control in a composite holographic associative recall model: implications for Korsakoff amnesia. *Psychol. Rev.* **100,** 3–22.
302. Liu, J., Singh, H., and White, P. F. (1997) Electroencephalographic bispectral index correlates with intraoperative recall and depth of propofol-induced sedation. *Anesth. Analg.* **84,** 185–189.
303. Iselin-Chaves, I. A., Flaishon, R., Sebel, P. S., et al. (1998) The effect of the interaction of propofol and alfentanil on recall, loss of consciousness, and the Bispectral Index. *Anesth. Analg.* **87,** 949–955.
304. Schwender, D., Rimkus, T., Haessler, R., Klasing, S., Poppel, E., and Peter, K. (1993) Effects of increasing doses of alfentanil, fentanyl and morphine on mid- latency auditory evoked potentials. *Brit. J. Anaesth.* **71,** 622–628.
305. McPherson, D. and Starr, A. (1992) Auditory evoked potentials in the clinic. In Halliday, A. M. (ed.), Evoked Potentials in Clinical Testing, 2nd ed. Churchill Livingstone, New York. pp. 359–381.
306. Dutton, R. C., Smith, W. D., Rampil, I. J., Chortkoff, B. S., and Eger, II, E. I. (1999) Forty-hertz midlatency auditory evoked potential activity predicts wakeful response during desflurane and propofol anesthesia in volunteers. *Anesthesiology* **91,** 1209–1220.
307. Stapells, D. R. and Picton, T. W. (1981) Technical aspects of brainstem evoked potential audiometry using tones. *Ear Hear.* **2,** 20–29.
308. Stapells, D. R., Linden, D., Suffield, J. B., Hamel, G., and Picton, T. W. (1984) Human auditory steady state potentials. *Ear Hear.* **5,** 105–113.

309. Picton, T. W., Skinner, C. R., Champagne, S. C., Kellett, A. J., and Maiste, A. C. (1987) Potentials evoked by the sinusoidal modulation of the amplitude or frequency of a tone. *J. Acoust. S. Am.* **82,** 165–178.
310. Picton, T. W., Vajsar, J., Rodriguez, R., and Campbell, K. B. (1987) Reliability estimates for steady-state evoked potentials. *Electroencephalogr. Clin. Neurophysiol.* **68,** 119–131.
311. Plourde, G. and Picton, T. W. (1990) Human auditory steady-state response during general anesthesia. *Anesth. Analg.* **71,** 460–468.
312. Plourde, G., Stapells, D. R., and Picton, T. W. (1991) The human auditory steady-state evoked potentials. *Acta Otolaryngol. Suppl. (Stockh)* **491,** 153–159.
313. Gutschalk, A., Mase, R., Roth, R., et al. (1999) Deconvolution of 40 Hz steady-state fields reveals two overlapping source activities of the human auditory cortex. *Clin. Neurophysiol.* **110,** 856–868.
314. Woldorff, M. G. (1993) Distortion of ERP averages due to overlap from temporally adjacent ERPs: Analysis and correction. *Psychophysiology* **30,** 98–119.
315. Mecklinger, A., Opitz, B., and Friederici, A. D. (1997) Semantic aspects of novelty detection in humans. *Neurosci. Lett.* **235,** 65–68.
316. Elger, C. E., Grunwald, T., Lehnertz, K., et al. 1997) Human temporal lobe potentials in verbal learning and memory processes. *Neuropsychologia* **35,** 657–667.
317. Brewer, J. B., Zhao, Z., Desmond, J. E., Glover, G. H., and Gabrieli, J. D. (1998) Making memories: brain activity that predicts how well visual experience will be remembered. *Science* **281,** 1185–1187.
318. Jacoby, L. L. and Dallas, M. (1981) On the relationship between autobiographical memory and perceptual learning. *J. Exp. Psychol. Gen.* **110,** 306–340.
319. Curran, T. (2000) Brain potentials of recollection and familiarity. *Mem. Cogn.* **28,** 923–938.
320. Jacoby, L. L. (1991) A process dissociation framework : Separating automatic from intentional uses of memory. *J. Mem. Lang.* **33,** 1–18.
321. Rugg, M. D., Mark, R. E., Walla, P., Schloerscheidt, A. M., Birch, C. S., and Allan, K. (1998) Dissociation of the neural correlates of implicit and explicit memory. *Nature* **392,** 595–598.
322. Knowlton, B. J. and Squire, L. R. (19950 Remembering and knowing: two different expressions of declarative memory. *J. Exp. Psychol. Learn. Mem. Cogn.* **21,** 699–710.
323. Smith, M. E. and Halgren, E. (1989) Dissociation of recognition memory components following temporal lobe lesions. *J. Exp. Psychol. Learn. Mem. Cogn.* **15,** 50–60.
324. Mecklinger, A. (1998) On the modularity of recognition memory for object form and spatial location: a topographic ERP analysis. *Neuropsychologia* **36,** 441–460.
325. Mecklinger, A. and Meinshausen, R. M. (1998) Recognition memory for object form and object location: an event-related potential study. *Mem. Cogn.* **26,** 1068–1088.
326. Smith, M. E., Stapleton, J. M., and Halgren, E. (1986) Human medial temporal lobe potentials evoked in memory and language tasks. *Electroencephalogr. Clin. Neurophysiol.* **63,** 145–159.
327. Guillem, F., N'Kaoua, B., Rougier, A., and Claverie, B. (1995) Effects of temporal versus temporal plus extra-temporal lobe epilepsies on hippocampal ERPs: physiopathological implications for recognition memory studies in humans. *Brain Res. Cogn. Brain Res.* **2,** 147–153.
328. Smith, M. E. and Guster, K. (1993) Decomposition of recognition memory event-related potentials yields target, repetition, and retrieval effects. *Electroencephalog. Clin. Neurophysiol.* **86,** 335–343.
329. Rugg, M. D., Schloerscheidt, A. M., Doyle, M. C., Cox, C. J., and Patching, G. R. (1996) Event-related potentials and the recollection of associative information. *Brain Res. Cogn. Brain Res.* **4,** 297–304.
330. Ranganath, C. and Paller, K. A. (1999) Frontal brain activity during episodic and semantic retrieval: insights from event-related potentials. *J. Cogn. Neurosci.* **11,** 598–609.
331. Wilding, E. L. (1999) Separating retrieval strategies from retrieval success: an event-related potential study of source memory. *Neuropsychologia* **37,** 441–454.
332. Donchin, E. and Coles, M. G. (1988) Is the P300 component a manifestation of context updating? *Behav. Brain Sci.* **11,** 357–374.
333. Grune, K., Metz, A. M., Hagendorf, H., and Fischer, S. (1996) Information processing in working memory and event-related brain potentials. *Int. J. Psychophysiol.* **23,** 111–120.
334. Gevins, A., Smith, M. E., Le, J., et al. (1996) High resolution evoked potential imaging of the cortical dynamics of human working memory. *Electroencephalogr. Clin. Neurophysiol.* **98,** 327–348.
335. Barcelo, F. and Rubia, F. J. (1998) Non-frontal P3b-like activity evoked by the Wisconsin Card Sorting Test. *Neuroreport.* **9,** 747–751.
336. Ruchkin, D. S., Johnson, R., Canoune, H., and Ritter, W. (1990) Short-term memory storage and retention: an event-related brain potential study. *Electroencephalogr. Clin. Neurophysiol.* **76,** 419–439.
337. Winkler, I., Czigler, I., Jaramillo, M., Paavilainen, P., and Naatanen, R. (1998) Temporal constraints of auditory event synthesis: evidence from ERPs. *Neuroreport.* **9,** 495–499.
338. Polich, J. and Bondurant, T. (1997) P300 sequence effects, probability, and interstimulus interval. *Physiol. Behav.* **61,** 843–849.
339. Rugg, M. D. (1995) Cognitive event-related potentials: intracranial and lesion studies. In Boller, F. and Grafman, J. (eds.), Handbook of Neuropsychology, vol. 10. Elsevier Science B.V., Amsterdam. pp. 165–185.
340. Naatanen, R. (1990) The role of attention in auditory information processing as revealed by event-related potentials and other brain measures of cognitive function. *Behav. Brain Sci.* **13,** 201–288.
341. Knight, R. T. (1984) Decreased response to novel stimuli after prefrontal lesions in man. *Electroencephalogr. Clin. Neurophysiol.* **59,** 9–20.

342. Spencer, K. M., Dien, J., and Donchin, E. (1999) A componential analysis of the ERP elicited by novel events using a dense electrode array. *Psychophysiology* **36**, 409–414.
343. Friedman, D. and Simpson, G. V. (1994) ERP amplitude and scalp distribution to target and novel events: effects of temporal order in young, middle-aged and older adults. *Brain Res. Cogn. Brain Res.* **2**, 49–63.
344. Mecklinger, A. and Ullsperger, P. (1995) The P300 to novel and target events: a spatiotemporal dipole model analysis. *Neuroreport.* **7**, 241–245.
345. Kiehl, K. A., Laurens, K. R., Duty, T. L., Forster, B. B., and Liddle, P. F. (2001) Neural sources involved in auditory target detection and novelty processing: an event-related fMRI study. *Psychophysiology* **38**, 133–142.
346. Knight, R. (1996) Contribution of human hippocampal region to novelty detection. *Nature* **383**, 256–259.
347. Johnson, R. (1988) Scalp-recorded P300 activity in patients following unilateral temporal lobectomy. *Brain* **111**, 1517–1529.
348. Johnson, R. (1989) Auditory and visual P300s in temporal lobectomy patients: evidence for modality-dependent generators. *Psychophysiology* **26**, 633–650.
349. Halgren, E., Squires, N. K., Wilson, C. L., Rohrbaugh, J. W., Babb, T. L., and Crandall, P. H. (1980) Endogenous potentials generated in the human hippocampal formation and amygdala by infrequent events. *Science* **210**, 803–805.
350. Stapleton, J. M. and Halgren, E. (1987) Endogenous potentials evoked in simple cognitive tasks: depth components and task correlates. *Electroencephalogr. Clin. Neurophysiol.* **67**, 44–52.
351. Stapleton, J. M., Halgren, E., and Moreno, K. A. (1987) Endogenous potentials after anterior temporal lobectomy. *Neuropsychologia* **25**, 549–557.
352. Otten, L. J. and Donchin, E. (2000) Relationship between P300 amplitude and subsequent recall for distinctive events: dependence on type of distinctiveness attribute. *Psychophysiology* **37**, 644–661.
353. Beydagi, H., Ozesmi, C., Yilmaz, A., Suer, C., and Ergenoglu, T. (2000) The relation between event related potential and working memory in healthy subjects. *Int. J. Neurosci.* **105**, 77–85.
354. Allen, J. J., Iacono, W. G., and Danielson, K. D. (1992) The identification of concealed memories using the event-related potential and implicit behavioral measures: A methodology for prediction in the face of individual differences. *Psychophysiology* **29**, 504–522.
355. Friedman, D. (1990) ERPs during continuous recognition memory for words. *Biol. Psychol.* **30**, 61–87.
356. Gevins, A. and Smith, M. E. (2000) Neurophysiological measures of working memory and individual differences in cognitive ability and cognitive style. *Cereb. Cortex* **10**, 829–839.
357. Magliero, A., Bashore, T. R., Coles, M. G., and Donchin, E. (1984) On the dependence of P300 latency on stimulus evaluation processes. *Psychophysiology* **21**, 171–186.
358. Sirevaag, E. J., Kramer, A. F., Coles, M. G., and Donchin, E. (1989) Resource reciprocity: an event-related brain potentials analysis. *Acta Psychol. (Amst)* **70**, 77–97.
359. Wickens, C., Kramer, A., Vanasse, L., and Donchin, E. (1983) Performance of concurrent tasks: a psychophysiological analysis of the reciprocity of information-processing resources. *Science* **221**, 1080–1082.
360. McCarthy, G. and Donchin, E. (1981) A metric for thought: A comparison of P300 latency and reaction time. *Science* **211**, 77–80.
361. Rugg, M. D., Fletcher, P. C., Allan, K., Frith, C. D., Frackowiak, R. S. J., and Dolan, R. J. (1998) Neural correlates of memory retrieval during recognition memory and cued recall. *NeuroImage* **8**, 262–273.
362. Allan, K., Wilding, E. L., and Rugg, M. D. (1998) Electrophysiological evidence for dissociable processes contributing to recollection. *Acta Psychol. (Amst)* **98**, 231–252.
363. Paller, K. A. and Gross, M. (1998) Brain potentials associated with perceptual priming vs explicit remembering during the repetition of visual word-form. *Neuropsychologia* **36**, 559–571.
364. Paller, K. A., Kutas, M., and McIsaac, H. K. (1998) An electrophysiological measure of priming of visual word-form. *Conscious. Cogn.* **7**, 54–66.
365. Paller, K. A., Bozic, V. S., Ranganath, C., Grabowecky, M., and Yamada, S. (1999) Brain waves following remembered faces index conscious recollection. *Brain Res. Cogn. Brain Res.* **7**, 519–531.
366. Gross, J., Kujala, J., Hamalainen, M., Timmermann, L., Schnitzler, A., and Salmelin, R. (2001) Dynamic imaging of coherent sources: Studying neural interactions in the human brain. *Proc. Natl. Acad. Sci. USA* **98**, 694–699.
367. Tallon-Baudry, C. and Bertrand, O. (1999) Oscillatory gamma activity n humans and its role in object representation. *Trends Cogn. Sci.* **3**, 151–162.
368. Miltner, W. H., Braun, C., Arnold, M., Witte, H., and Taub, E. (1999) Coherence of gamma-band EEG activity as a basis for associative learning. *Nature* **397**, 434–436.
369. Rodriguez, E., George, N., Lachaux, J. P., Martinerie, J., Renault, B., and Varela, F. J. (1999) Perception's shadow: long-distance synchronization of human brain activity. *Nature* **397**, 430–433.
370. Basar, E., Basar-Eroglu, C., Karakas, S., and Schurmann, M. (1999) Are cognitive processes manifested in event-related gamma, alpha, theta and delta oscillations in the EEG? *Neurosci. Lett.* **259**, 165–168.
371. von Stein, A. and Sarnthein, J. (2000) Different frequencies for different scales of cortical integration: from local gamma to long range alpha/theta synchronization. *Int. J. Psychophysiol.* **38**, 301–313.
372. von Stein, A., Rappelsberger, P., Sarnthein, J., and Petsche, H. (1999) Synchronization between temporal and parietal cortex during multimodal object processing in man. *Cereb. Cortex* **9**, 137–150.
373. Tallon-Baudry, C., Bertrand, O., Delpuech, C., and Permier, J. (1997) Oscillatory gamma-band (30–70 Hz) activity induced by a visual search task in humans. *J. Neurosci.* **17**, 722–734.
374. Tallon-Baudry, C., Bertrand, O., Peronnet, F., and Pernier, J. (1998) Induced gamma-band activity during the delay of a visual short-term memory task in humans. *J. Neurosci.* **18**, 4244–4254.

375. Klimesch, W., Doppelmayr, M., Russegger, H., and Pachinger, T. (1996) Theta band power in the human scalp EEG and the encoding of new information. *Neuroreport.* **7,** 1235–1240.

376. Klimesch, W., Doppelmayr, M., Pachinger, T., and Russegger, H. (1997) Event-related desynchronization in the alpha band and the processing of semantic information. *Brain Res. Cogn. Brain Res.* **6,** 83–94.

377. Klimesch, W. (1997) EEG-alpha rhythms and memory processes. *Int. J. Psychophysiol.* **26,** 319–340.

378. Klimesch, W., Doppelmayr, M., Schimke, H., and Ripper, B. (1997) Theta synchronization and alpha desynchronization in a memory task. *Psychophysiology* **34,** 169–176.

379. Tesche, C. D. and Karhu, J. (2000) Theta oscillations index human hippocampal activation during a working memory task. *Proc. Natl. Acad. Sci. USA* **97,** 919–924.

380. Tesche, C. D., Karhu, J., and Tissari, S. O. (1996) Non-invasive detection of neuronal population activity in human hippocampus. *Brain Res. Cogn. Brain Res.* **4,** 39–47.

381. Burgess, A. P. and Gruzelier, J. H. (1997) Short duration synchronization of human theta rhythm during recognition memory. *Neuroreport* **8,** 1039–1042.

382. Poucet, B., Save, E., and Lenck-Santini, P. P. (2000) Sensory and memory properties of hippocampal place cells. *Rev. Neurosci.* **11,** 95–111.

383. O'Keefe, J. (1993) Hippocampus, theta, and spatial memory. *Curr. Opin. Neurobiol.* **3,** 917–924.

384. Kahana, M. J., Sekuler, R., Caplan, J. B., Kirschen, M., and Madsen, J. R. (1999) Human theta oscillations exhibit task dependence during virtual maze navigation. *Nature* **399,** 781–784.

385. Komatsu, H., Nogaya, J., Anabuki, D., et al. (1993) Memory facilitation by posttraining exposure to halothane, enflurane, and isoflurane in ddN mice. *Anesth. Analg.* **76,** 609–612.

386. Komatsu, T. (1998) Repetitive post-training exposure to enflurane modifies spatial memory in mice. *Anesthesiology* **89,** 1184–1190.

387. Buzsaki, G. (1998) Memory consolidation during sleep: a neurophysiological perspective. *J. Sleep Res.* **7,** 17–23.

388. Sandyk, R. (1998) A neuromagnetic view of hippocampal memory functions. *Int. J. Neurosci.* **93,** 251–256.

389. Karni, A., Tanne, D., Rubenstein, B. S., Askenasy, J. J., and Sagi, D. (1994) Dependence on REM sleep of overnight improvement of a perceptual skill. *Science* **265,** 679–682.

390. Feshchenko, V. A., Veselis, R. A., and Reinsel, R. A. (1997) Comparison of the EEG effects of midazolam, thiopental, and propofol: The role of underlying oscillatory systems. *Neuropsychobiology* **35,** 211–220.

391. Steriade, M., McCormick, D. A., and Sejnowski, T. J. (1993) Thalamocortical oscillations in the sleeping and aroused brain. *Science* **262,** 679–685.

392. Fiset, P., Paus, T., Daloze, T., et al. (1999) Brain mechanisms of propofol-induced loss of consciousness in humans: a positron emission tomographic study. *J. Neurosci.* **19,** 5506–5513.

393. Alkire, M. T., Haier, R. J., and Fallon, J. H. (2000) Toward a unified theory of narcosis: Brain imaging evidence for a thalamocortical switch as the neurophysiologic basis of anesthetic-induced unconsciousness. *Conscious. Cogn.* **9,** 370–386.

394. Nordstrom, O. and Sandin, R (1996) Recall during intermittent propofol anaesthesia. *Brit. J. Anaesth.* **76,** 699–701.

395. Russell, I. F. (1993) Midazolam-alfentanil: an anaesthetic? An investigation using the isolated forearm technique. *Brit. J. Anaesth.* **70,** 42–46.

396. Russell, I. F. and Wang, M. (2001) Absence of memory for intraoperative information during surgery with total intravenous anaesthesia. *Brit. J. Anaesth.* **86,** 196–202.

397. Schwender, D., Klasing, S., Madler, C., Poppel, E., and Peter, K. (1993) Depth of anesthesia. Midlatency auditory evoked potentials and cognitive function during general anesthesia. *Int. Anesth. Clin.* **31,** 89–106.

398. Bonnett, M. H. (1983) Memory for events during arousal from sleep. *Psychophysiology* **20,** 81–87.

399. Ghoneim, M. M. and Block, R. I. (1992) Learning and consciousness during general anesthesia [published erratum appears in Anesthesiology 1992 Jul;77(1):222]. *Anesthesiology* **76,** 279–305.

400. Ghoneim, M. M. and Block, R. I. (1993) Depth of anesthesia. Learning during anesthesia. *Int. Anesth. Clin.* **31,** 53–65.

401. Andrade, J. (1995) Learning during anaesthesia: a review. *Brit. J. Psychol.* **86(Pt 4),** 479–506.

402. Glass, P. S. (1993) Prevention of awareness during total intravenous anesthesia. *Anesthesiology* **78,** 399–400.

403. Kelly, J. S. and Roy, R. C. (1992) Intraoperative awareness with propofol-oxygen total intravenous anesthesia for microlaryngeal surgery. *Anesthesiology* **77,** 207–209.

404. Moerman, N., Bonke, B., and Oosting, J. (1993) Awareness and recall during general anesthesia. Facts and feelings. *Anesthesiology* **79,** 454–464.

405. Payne, J. P. (1994) Awareness and its medicolegal implications. *Brit. J. Anaesth.* **73,** 38–45.

406. Wilson, S. L., Vaughan, R. W., and Stephen, C. R. (1975) Awareness, dreams, and hallucinations associated with general anesthesia. *Anesth. Analg.* **54,** 609–617.

407. Liu, W. H., Thorp, T. A., Graham, S. G., and Aitkenhead, A. R. (1991) Incidence of awareness with recall during general anaesthesia. *Anaesthesia* **46,** 435–437.

408. Lyons, G., and Macdonald, R. (1991) Awareness during caesarean section. *Anaesthesia* **46,** 62–64.

409. Rosenberg, J., Wildschiodtz, G., Pedersen, M. H., von Jessen, F., and Kehlet, H. (1994) Late postoperative nocturnal episodic hypoxaemia and associated sleep pattern. *Brit. J. Anaesth.* **72,** 145–150.

410. Jelicic, M. and Bonke, B. (1996) Learning during anaesthesia : a survey of expert opinion. In Bonke, B., Bovill, J. G. and Moerman, N. (eds.), Memory and Awareness in Anaesthesia III. Van Gorcum, Assen, The Netherlands. pp. 97–101.

411. Caseley-Rondi, G. (1996) Perceptual processing during general anaesthesia reconsidered within a neuropsychological framework. In Bonke, B., Bovill, J. G., and Moerman, N. (eds.), Memory and Awareness in Anaesthesia III. Van Gorcum, Assen, The Netherlands. pp. 103–107.

412. Merikle, P. M. and Daneman, M. (1996) Memory for events during anaesthesia : a meta-analysis. In Bonke, B., Bovill, J. G. and Moerman, N. (eds.), Memory and Awareness in Anaesthesia III. Van Gorcum, Assen, The Netherlands. pp. 108–121.

413. Plourde, G. (1993) Depth of anesthesia. Clinical use of the 40-Hz auditory steady state response. *Int. Anesth. Clin.* **31,** 107–120.

414. Merikle, P. M. and Rondi, G. (1993) Memory for events during anesthesia has not been demonstrated : a psychologist's viewpoint. In Sebel, P. S., Bonke, B., and Winograd, E. (eds.), Memory and Awareness in Anesthesia. Prentice-Hall, Englewood, N.J. pp. 476–497.

415. Chortkoff, B. S. and Eger, E. I. (1993) Memory for events during anesthesia has not been demonstrated: an anesthesiologist's viewpoint. In Sebel, P. S., Bonke, B. and Winograd, E. (eds.), Memory and Awareness in Anesthesia. Prentice-Hall, Englewood, N.J. pp. 467–475.

416. Bennett, H. L. (1993) Memory for events during anesthesia does occur: A psychologist's viewpoint. In Sebel, P. S., Bonke, B., and Winograd, E. (eds.), Memory and Awareness in Anesthesia. Prentice-Hall, Englewood, N.J. pp. 459–466.

417. Chortkoff, B. S., Gonsowski, C. T., Bennett, H. L., et al. (1995) Subanesthetic concentrations of desflurane and propofol suppress recall of emotionally charged information. *Anesth. Analg.* **81,** 728–736.

418. Russell, I. F. and Wang, M. (1997) Absence of memory for intraoperative information during surgery under adequate general anaesthesia. *Brit. J. Anaesth.* **78,** 3–9.

419. Challis, B. H. and Sidhu, R. (1993) Dissociative effect of massed repetition on implicit and explicit measures of memory. *J. Exp. Psychol. Learn. Mem. Cogn.* **19,** 115–127.

420. Musen, G. (1991) Effects of verbal labeling and exposure duration on implicit memory for visual patterns. *J. Exp. Psychol. Learn. Mem. Cogn.* **17,** 954–962.

421. Tulving, E. and Hayman, C. A. G. (1995) On the measurement of priming: What is the correct baseline? *Euro. J. Cogn. Psychol.* **7,** 13–18.

422. Hintzman, D. L. and Hartry, A. L. (1990) Item effects in recognition and fragment completion: contingency relations vary for different subsets of words. *J. Exp. Psychol. Learn. Mem. Cogn.* **16,** 955–969.

423. Tulving, E. and Hayman, C. A. G. (1993) Stochastic independence in the recognition/identification paradigm. *Euro. J. Cogn. Psychol.* **5,** 353–373.

424. Watkins, M. J. and Gibson, J. M. (1988) On the relation between perceptual priming and recognition memory. *J. Exp. Psychol. Learn. Mem. Cogn.* **14,** 477–483.

425. Talairach, J. and Tournoux, P. (1988) Co-Planar Stereotaxic Atlas of the Human Brain. Georg Thieme Verlag, Stuttgart.

426. Collins, D. L., Neelin, P., Peters, T. M., and Evans, A. C. (1994) Automatic 3D intersubject registration of MR volumetric data in standardized Talairach space. *J. Comput. Assist. Tomogr.* **18,** 192–205.

427. Collins, D. L., Zijdenbos, A. P., Kollokian, V., et al. (1998) Design and construction of a realistic digital brain phantom. *IEEE Trans. Med. Imaging* **17,** 463–468.

428. Markowitsch, H. J. and Tulving, E. (1994) Cognitive processes and cerebral cortical fundi: findings from positron-emission tomography studies. *Proc. Natl. Acad. Sci. USA* **91,** 10,507–10,511.

III Sleep, Coma, and Anesthesia—Similarities and Differences

4

Sleep and Anesthesia

John Keifer

INTRODUCTION

Natural sleep and general anesthesia are similar. They are not identical. Both states are characterized by a reversible alteration of normal waking consciousness. This alteration affects the ability to perceive and process external stimuli. Both conditions also modify life sustaining functions including the control of breathing, cardiovascular performance, temperature regulation, and muscle tone. The relationship between wakefulness and the altered state (i.e., general anesthesia or sleep) has been used to characterize a "depth" of anesthesia and a "stage" of sleep. The intensity of arousal stimuli required to revert to normal consciousness is thus used as a reproducible gauge of anesthetic effect. The degree of dissimilarity between waking and sleeping electroencephalogram (EEG) is used to assign sleep stage. Interestingly, attempts to judge anesthetic effect by electroencephalography depend on similar EEG changes as those observed in natural sleep.

Sleep and Anesthesia are not homogeneous physiologic states. Both conditions are characterized by changes in several physiologic processes. During sleep, the variability takes on a repeating cyclic pattern. During general anesthesia, once a stable level of anesthetic exposure is achieved, physiologic functions do not display the cycling variation of natural sleep. The physiologic variability of general anesthesia is generally confined to the induction of and emergence from a stable anesthetic state.

Careful delineation of the neuroanatomical and chemical substrates responsible for the physiologic changes of sleep and general anesthesia has revealed a great deal of overlap in the responsible neurons and neurochemicals. Given the broad area of sites of action for anesthetic agents, and the failure to identify a single sleep-promoting center, it is unlikely that general anesthesia can be easily explained as pharmacological induction of natural sleep. However, many of the similarities between general anesthesia and natural sleep, at clinical, neural, and molecular levels make it likely that general anesthesia causes changes in neural systems that are also responsible for natural alteration of waking consciousness. That is, general anesthesia does not simply result from a generalized, uniform alteration of neural activity, but results from a selective alteration of neural function. This selectivity depends on the activation or inhibition of neural systems, which are also responsible for the changes seen during natural sleep.

However, the overlap between sleep and anesthesia is not total. At higher levels of anesthetic exposure, the changes of neural and electrophysiologic function cease to resemble natural sleep. At these levels, the decrement in neural function is both profound and global, producing patterns of neural function and electrophysiology that are only observed in a damaged brain. Additionally, there does not appear to be a neurophysiologic correlate of rapid eye movement (REM) sleep during general anesthesia, even though there may be a relationship. Selective activation of brainstem systems, which

From: *Contemporary Clinical Neuroscience: Neural Mechanisms of Anesthesia*
Edited by: Joseph F. Antognini et al. © Humana Press Inc., Totowa, NJ

can create a REM sleep state in experimental animals, is also effective in counteracting the spindle sleep pattern of general anesthesia in experimental animals. Conversely, the specific application of narcotic to brain stem neurons responsible for REM sleep generation result in a decrement in REM sleep that is naloxone reversible and mu receptor specific. The increased cortical activity and abnormal eye position that accompany the "excitement phase" of anesthetic induction and emergence, may eventually prove to be based in neural systems responsible for the activated cortical function and eye movements of REM sleep.

Basic Sleep Mechanisms

The discovery of EEG changes characterizing different stages of sleep has been attributed to Loomis et al in 1937. Aerinsky and Kleitman subsequently described REM sleep in 1953. The technique of sleep scoring based on the EEG, electromyography (EMG) and electrooculography (EOG) was published in 1968 by Reckstaffen and Kales *(1)*. Therefore, the heterogeneous nature of sleep was first recognized in the EEG. The addition of muscle tone and eye movement helped to distinguish the EEG of wakefulness from the EEG of REM sleep.

Cortical EEG, Muscle Tone, and Eye Movements Enable Staging of Sleep

During transition between wakefulness and the various phases of sleep, reliable changes occur in 3 areas: cortical EEG, muscle tone, and eye movement. Rechstafen and Kales developed rules for grouping these changes, enabling a staging of sleep (Table 1).

To summarize the changes in the EEG as one passes from waking to Stage 4 non- REM (NREM) sleep, there is a progressive increase in the number of "slow wave" oscillations comprising the raw EEG. Upon entering REM sleep, the raw EEG loses slow wave oscillation and takes on the appearance of the awake EEG. Additionally, there are stereotype waveforms occur during Stage 2 NREM sleep that serve to uniquely identify this stage. As will be introduced subsequently, the neural machinery responsible for these waveforms is also active during deeper stages of NREM sleep.

Pichlmayer demonstrates a similar progression of EEG pattern during increasing exposure to general anesthesia, alpha and beta frequency progressing to delta and theta frequency. In distinction to the progressive pattern of sleep, the general anesthetic state continues toward a pattern of flat EEG interspersed with bursts of activity, i.e., burst suppression.

Applying the staging rules of Kales and Rechstaffen to sequential 30 s epochs during the course of an evening sleep results in a typical sleep hypnogram (Fig. 1). This demonstrates the recurring cyclical nature of NREM sleep, the repeated recurrence of REM, (which is more plentiful in the early morning hours) and a tendency for deep sleep stages early in the evening, followed by lighter stages in the early morning hours.

The first REM episode period usually occurs about 70 min after the onset of sleep. After this first episode, the sleep cycle repeats itself with the appearance of NREM sleep and then about 90 min after the appearance of the first REM period, another REM episode. Over the course of the night, delta wave activity tends to diminish and NREM sleep has waves of higher frequencies and lower amplitude.

SLEEP MECHANISMS

The neurologic functions of REM and NREM sleep are not established. However, impaired neurocognition following chronic sleep deprivation underscores the important role of these altered states of consciousness in maintaining normal neurologic function. The percentage of time spent in slow wave sleep is reported to be low in newborns, with an increase over the first years of life, reaching a maximum at 10 yr and declining thereafter. Feinberg et al. hypothesize that one function of sleep is to recover from some of the metabolic consequences of information processing during waking. In this model, the process of neural maturation is considered in terms of a proliferative phase

Table 1
Rechstafen and Kales Sleep Stages

Stage	EEG		Muscle tone	Eye movement
Waking	Low amplitude High frequency		High	
Stage 1 Non-REM	Alpha frequency*		High	Rolling eye movement
Stage 2 Non-REM	Mixed frequency	K complex Sleep Spindles	High	None
Stage 3 Non-REM	20–50% Theta frequency*		High	None
Stage 4 Non-REM	≥50% Theta frequency*		High	None
REM	Low amplitude High frequency		Low	Rapid eye movement

*Delta = 0–35 Hz, Theta = 3.5–7.5 Hz, Alpha = 7.5–12.5 Hz, Beta = 12.5–30 Hz.

characterized by the establishing of extensive synaptic connections in the brain. Subsequently in the maturation, an organizational phase is characterized by a reduction in synaptic connections and consequent reduction in cerebral metabolic requirements. A maturational study of brain development reported a coincident increase of cerebral metabolic rate, synaptic density, and delta sleep duration and amplitude during early childhood followed by, a parallel decline in these variables during adulthood. The reduction in these three variables may reflect a reduction of cortical synapses necessary for an organizational phase of brain development (3). The function of REM sleep is also not established. However, as with NREM sleep, the large proportion of REM sleep observed in mammals in utero and in early development is followed by a gradual decline after age 10. These findings suggest a role of REM sleep in the maturational development of the brain (4).

Historically, exploration of sleep mechanisms has received its greatest impetus through use of EEG and the measurement of muscle tone and eye movement. Variations in these parameters showed that sleep is not a stable homogeneous state but is dynamic and composed of cyclic variations in these parameters enabling the initial grading of sleep.

The Genesis of the EEG

Synchronized vs Desynchronized

Before considering the EEG patterns observed in sleep, a required preface should include the phenomena necessary to create an EEG. Rampil has written a very cogent presentation on the neural mechanisms underlying the recording of scalp electrical potentials known as the EEG (5). The macroscopic electrical potentials recorded at the scalp are a summation of the microscopic potentials generated by individual cellular elements. These cells include neurons, glial cells, and muscle cells from the scalp (hence the artefact that can be generated from scalp EMG). The neuronal contribution to the EEG comes from postsynaptic potentials (PSPs), not from action potentials. The pyramidal neurons of the cerebral cortex are arranged so that their apical dendrites extend through the cortex

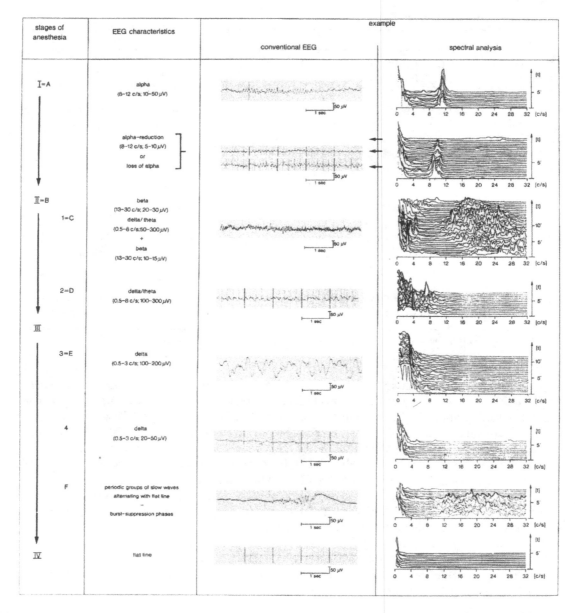

Fig. 1. Conventional EEG and accompanying EEG spectral analysis demonstrates the progressive "slowing" of EEG frequency with increasing anesthetic depth. Exposure to a greater concentration of anesthetic results in the EEG burst suppression, followed by "flatline" EEG.

and are oriented approximately at right angles to the pial surface. Therefore, dendrites from adjacent neurons are parallel to one another. This configuration allows for an additive combination of electrical potential enabling a detection of aggregate (PSPs) at the surface of the brain.

Synchrony is used to describe electrical activity among a group of neurons who have a similar change in membrane potential at similar locations of the cell and at a similar time, so that the individual potentials are additive and result in a large amplitude to the potential. In addition, because the orchestration of these individual neurons come from internal pacers, not from random changes in membrane potentials, the rate of these high amplitude waves tends to regular and slow. Therefore, synchronous EEG activity is recognized by high amplitude, slow frequency oscillations in the EEG, and reflect aggregate synchronous activity of neighboring cortical pyramidal cells, usually under the direction of another neural pacer. Conversely, a desynchronous combination of pyramidal cell PSPs is identified by a lower net amplitude and higher frequency of the scalp EEG oscillations. Anesthesia and other mechanisms that depress consciousness are associated with increasing cortical synchrony. Higher cortical function is usually associated with desynchronization as more neurons act independently in the creation of conscious human behavior *(5)*.

Additional themes have resulted from observations of the EEG during sleep.

1. The appearance of the cortical EEG during wakefulness and during REM are similar, both are desynchronous: This EEG is characterized by low amplitude, "high frequency, mixed frequency" oscillations. The low electrical amplitude and apparent randomness of this pattern is thought to be owing to a lack of additive synchrony among the variety of active cortical areas generating the potentials and has therefore come to be known as a desynchronized EEG.
2. The appearance of the cortical EEG during NREM sleep is characterized by a variety of waveforms: K complex, the spindle, and the delta wave: These EEG features are of sufficient amplitude and sufficient regularity as to suggest that they result from the synchronous activity of large portions of the cortex. The EEG features of NREM sleep have been collectively termed synchronized EEG.
3. Desynchronized EEG = perceiving brain, therefore synchronized EEG = non-perceiving brain: The association of desynchronized EEG with a brain that is able to consciously perceive (either during wakefulness or during dreaming in the REM state) led to the widely held notion that a desynchronized EEG was a necessary condition for perception. The association of synchronized EEG with a brain that is not consciously perceiving led to the converse notion that a synchronized EEG is a characteristic of a brain was not able to consciously perceive. The quality of recollected mental activity differs between NREM and REM sleep. Through use of dream reports, it is clear that more cogent mentation is obtained on awakening from REM than from NREM sleep. However, Nielsen summarized observations from 34 studies that addressed the rates of recall after subjects were aroused from various stages of NREM and REM sleep. The average rate of recall from stage 3 and 4 NREM sleep was 52.5 +/– 18.6%. The average rate of recall from REM sleep was 82.2 +/– 8.1% *(6)*. In summary, the presence of synchronous EEG activity does not eliminate the possibility of perception or mentation, although the ability to recall mental activity is increased with a desynchronous EEG.
4. The transition of an EEG from synchronized to desynchronized pattern is termed activation of the cortex. This electrical activation is confirmed in studies of cerebral metabolic rate: In a review of cerebral blood flow and metabolism during sleep *(7)*, Madsen and Vorstrup conclude,

"in contrast to the conflicting results regarding the global level of cerebral blood flow associated with REM sleep, measurements of cerebral metabolic rate seem to establish that the global level of cerebral metabolism during REM sleep is quite similar to the level associated with wakefulness"

NREM Sleep is most Similar to "Low Dose" General Anesthesia

EEG Correlates and Neural Substructure

Many of the electrophysiologic features of general anesthesia resemble those of NREM sleep (Fig. 2). These include spindles, K complexes, delta waves, and three characteristic features of NREM sleep. Interestingly, the cellular machinery responsible for these NREM rhythms are also induced by barbiturate anesthetics and inhaled agents.

NREM Sleep

The progression through the various stages of NREM sleep (i.e., Stages 1–4) is marked by three readily recognized EEG events:

1. Sleep spindles: short runs (0.5–3 s) of 12–14 Hz *(1)* waves or 7–14 Hz *(8)*.
2. K complexes: the occurrence of single, episodic, large amplitude waves. These K-complexes stand out from the background EEG in a fashion similar to the way a premature ventricular contraction stands out from a sinus EKG.

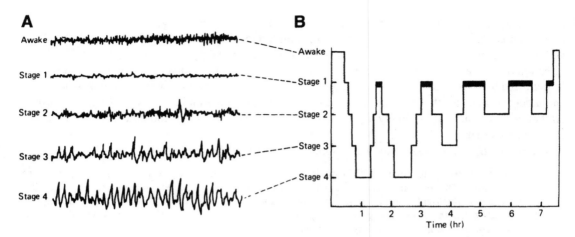

Fig. 2. A typical sleep hypnogram showing the cyclical nature of sleep stages during the course of an evening.

3. Slow waves: increased number of (i.e., oscillations that have a frequency of less than 8 Hz. These are named Delta waves for oscillations of 0.25–3.5 Hz and Theta waves for oscillations of 3.5–7.5 Hz).

Sleep Spindles

Initially demonstrated in 1945 by Morison and Bassett, spindles are a hallmark of early sleep stages in mammals. A waxing and waning envelope resulting in their name characterized the intermittent sequences of 8–12 Hz. Spindles could be recorded from the interlaminar thalamus in bilaterally decorticate animal, demonstrating that the spindle originates in the thalamus. Spindle activity became continuous in the thalamus when the decorticate animal additionally underwent a brain stem transection at the intercollicular level. This demonstrated that the brain stem while not the source of the spindle oscillation did possess the ability to modulate its occurrence *(9)*. Steriade et al. determined that spindle generation results from GABAergic reticular thalamic neurons generating prolonged inhibitory postsynaptic potentials (IPSP's) in thalamocortical neurons. Indeed, spindles are abolished in thalamocortical systems after disconnection from inputs arising in the reticular nucleus, and long lasting, cyclic IPSP's are transformed into short IPSPs without rhythmicity.

Why are spindles important? Steriade advances the view "Spindles precipitate brain disconnection from the outside world because synaptic transmission of incoming signals through the thalamus, en route to the cerebral cortex, is reduced during the cyclic inhibitory IPSPs that build up this rhythmic activity in thalamocortical neurons *(9)*. Steriade also pointed to the association between sleep spindles and absence seizures. Sleep spindles are associated with the spike and wave complexes observed with absence (petit mal) epileptic seizures. He referred to absence seizures as a perversion of spindle oscillations. He cited evidence that inhibition of thalamic reticular cell (the cells essential for sleep spindle generation) by direct thalamic injection of GABAB agonist into animals with genetic absence epilepsy increased the frequency of spike and wave discharges and that direct injection of GABAB antagonist decreased these seizures in a dose dependent manner *(10)*.

K Complex

The K complex (KC) was initially described by Loomis et al. *(11)* as an ample surface-positive transient followed by a slower, surface negative component characteristic of stage 2 slow wave sleep. This slow component may be followed by a spindle sequence. The cellular substrates of the KC are still unknown. The KC (also known as a vertex wave or biparietal hump) is a reliable sign for advanced drowsiness surviving in all stages of quiet sleep. During deep sleep, the presence of high amplitude delta waves (*see* next section) makes the identification of KCs difficult. However, careful signal analysis of sleep EEG from human and cat have demonstrated that the KC actually occurs with regular frequency in the deeper levels of NREM sleep and that the frequency of occurrence is 0–1 Hz. The appearance of the KC during natural sleep in humans resembles that of the cat during natural sleep. Moreover, both human and cat KC resemble the KC of cats while under ketamine and xylazine anesthesia *(12)*.

Slow Waves

The predominant EEG feature of progressive degrees of anesthesia is an increase in slow waves. This increase in slow waves has been studied in an attempt to correlate "anesthetic depth" with cortical EEG (e.g., decreasing spectral edge frequency). The bispectral index (BIS) monitor through its algorithm of identifying interfrequency correlation of component frequencies in the EEG succeeds in identifying the occurrence of slow waves in its algorithm *(5)*. It is of interest that the anesthesia literature makes no mention of sleep spindles or KC during induction or emergence from general anesthesia, nor during EEG monitoring of pharmacologically induced sedation. However, sleep researchers who have attempted to understand the neural machinery and neurotransmitters responsible for these naturally occurring events have done so using a variety of animal models studied under anesthesia *(8,12–19)*. This discrepancy may reflect variations in monitoring technique (use of bi-polar vs monopolar configurations or use of different frequency cut offs).

Burst Suppression

The One Anesthetic Pattern Without a Natural Sleep Corollary

Burst suppression is an EEG pattern consisting of intermittent sequences of high-voltage slow waves and sharp waves, alternating with periods of depressed background activity or complete electrographic flatness. Derbyshire reported this pattern in 1936 and demonstrated that this pattern may appear under different anesthetics. The name burst suppression was introduced by Swank in 1949 in deeply narcotized animals. Subsequently, burst suppression was reported in the isolated cerebral cortex, during coma, after trauma associated with cerebral anoxia, and in cortex infiltrated with tumoral tissue. Steriade et al. performed an experimental study using anesthetized cats to investigate the cellular correlates of EEG burst suppression. *(20)* Intracellular recordings of cortical, thalamocortical and reticular thalamic neurons as well as multi-site extracellular recordings were obtained. Burst suppression was elicited by the administration of a variety of anesthetic agents, including ketamine and xylazine, urethane, nitrous oxide and sodium pentobarbital. 60–70% of thalamic cells ceased firing before overt EEG burst-suppression and were completely silent during flat periods of EEG activity. The remaining 30–40% of thalamic cells discharged rhythmic (1–4 Hz) spike bursts during periods of EEG silence. However, with the deepening of burst-suppression, when silent EEG periods became longer than 30 s, thalamic cells also ceased firing. The study concluded that full-blown burst-suppression is achieved through virtually complete disconnection in brain circuits implicated in the genesis of the EEG.

ANATOMY RELEVANT TO SLEEP AND ANESTHESIA

Brain Stem

One of the similarities between sleep research and anesthesia research is that the brain stem is of essential importance for the manifestations of natural sleep and general anesthesia. Historically, the ablation work of Jouvet demonstrated that the brainstem was essential for generating the rhythms associated with activation of the cerebral cortex during wakefulness and dreaming. Further work showed that the portion of the brain stem responsible for this cerebral activation was the cholinergic (acetylcholine producing) reticular formation.

Brainstem Reticular Formation

Neurons that are outside the major nuclear groups of the brain stem comprise the reticular formation. It represents the rostral extension of the interneuronal network of the spinal cord but is considerably more extensive. The axons of the reticular formation are widely distributed throughout the neuraxis providing extensive control over many neurons.

In the 1940's, Moruzzi and Magoun demonstrated that stimulation of the reticular formation of deeply anesthetized animals produced changes in the overall electrical activity of the brain, transforming the EEG pattern from a state resembling sleep to the a wake state. Activation of the brain for behavioral arousal and for different levels of awareness is only one physiologic role for reticular neurons. The reticular formation controls the four features that are typically associated with anesthetic action: behavioral arousal, regulation of muscle tone, coordination of autonomic function (breathing and cardiac function), and modulation of pain sensation. Activity of neurons in LC and the dorsal raphe nuclei vary according to the arousal state. These cells are very active during waking periods, but fire at a slow rate during rest or slow wave sleep. These nuclei have projections to large areas of the CNS and thereby presumably modulate CNS activity *(21)*.

Locus Coeruleus and Raphe Nuclei (21–24)

The locus coeruleus, (LC) located in the rostral pontine central grey region, is one of the principle norepinepherine nuclei in the brainstem. LC neurons project axons rostrally and caudally.

Stages of the sleep/waking cycle are likely influenced by the LC, e.g., LC neuronal activity is highest during waking periods.

The raphe nucleus is located in the medial aspect of the caudal ventral- to-dorsal midbrain *(21,25)*. 5-HT is the primary neurotransmitter.

Neuronal activity in LC and dorsal raphe are similar during changes in vigilance (i.e., waking vs sleep). Activity is highest during waking and lower with rest or sleep.

IMPLICATIONS FROM THE FACT THAT GENERAL ANESTHESIA AND SLEEP SHARE SIMILAR SYSTEMS IN THE BRAIN STEM, THALAMUS AND CORTEX

Although the anesthetic state and natural sleep are not identical, the coincidence of their neuro-physiologic substrates become manifest in a variety of areas.

MORPHINE INHIBITION OF REM SLEEP

Acute and chronic exposure to narcotics decrease the amount of REM sleep in postoperative patients, healthy volunteers, and in human narcotic addicts. The cholinergic medial pontine reticular formation (mPRF) is an essential component for the generation of an "active" desynchronized EEG of REM sleep. The mPRF shows an increased release of acetylcholine during natural REM and responding to the exogenous administration of a cholinergic agonist, carbachol, by developing signs of a REM like state (including desynchronized EEG, hypotonia, and rapid eye movement). Because narcotic depresses acetylcholine release in various portions of the cat brain, a study of the effect of microinjection of morphine into the mPRF was undertaken. The purpose of the study was to test the hypothesis that the mPRF was responsible for the REM sleep altering effect of narcotic. Results of the study performed in cats showed a decrease of time spent in REM sleep following reticular formation microinjection of morphine. This effect was reversible with pretreatment with naloxone and was shown to be due to specific interaction at the mu receptor. These findings show that a cholinergic neural network, the pontine reticular formation, which is key to the generation of REM sleep, could be altered in a receptor specific fashion by a narcotic agent, and that this interaction may explain one of the neurologic side effects of this medication *(26)*.

CHOLINERGIC INHIBITION OF SLEEP SPINDLES

The pontine reticular formation is a potent stimulus to the development of REM sleep like state, in part by activation of cortical neurons, (i.e., converting a synchronized cortical EEG to a desynchronized EEG). The early stages of general anesthesia result in a synchronized cortical EEG. In fact, much of the work delineating the basic mechanisms of synchronized EEG development was performed in animals that were exposed to barbiturate, halogenated anesthetic agents, or ketamine and alpha-2 agonists. The interaction of sleep controlling brainstem networks and anesthetics was performed in cats anesthetized with halothane. At 1 MAC exposure, the EEG displayed spindles that were identical to EEG spindles recorded during natural sleep. During this anesthetic exposure, the cholinergic agonist, carbachol, was microinjected into the mPRF. Carbachol resulted in a decrease in sleep spindles showing that the anesthetically induced synchronized cortical EEG activity could be opposed through a neural network, which is responsible for a similar effect during natural sleep *(27)*.

BIS CHANGES IN SLEEP AS WELL AS IN ANESTHESIA

The bispectral index is a method of EEG signal analysis that identifies a degree of coherence among the sine wave frequencies of a Fourier transformed raw EEG. Because the synchronization of cortical EEG activity that occurs with natural sleep resembles that of lighter planes of general anesthesia, one might predict that the BIS index would reflect this degree of synchronization. Sleigh et al. *(28)* have reported the results of BIS monitoring in five healthy volunteers during natural sleep. They noted a change in the BIS index to a mean low of 59 during periods of slow wave sleep. During periods of probable REM, the BIS index reflected desynchronized cortical activity, with an increase to a mean of 83. Hypotonia was indicated by a decrease of frontalis muscle activity to 66. The authors concluded, that the similarity in BIS measurements indicate that the transition from consciousness to the naturally sleeping state is similar to the transition to the unconscious state caused by anesthesia.

THE USE OF ALPHA-2 AGONISTS AS SEDATIVES THAT MIMIC NATURAL SLEEP

The recent development of receptor specific sedatives appears after a longer use of these compounds as a component of veterinary medicine (xylazine). It is possible to demonstrate a deep sedative state by specifically depressing the sympathetic activity in a brainstem nucleus, the locus coeruleus. This brainstem nucleus is responsible for an arousing response, and lack of activity allows for the synchronization of natural sleep. It is also of interest that, this locus coeruleus effect is not associated with the respiratory depression seen with other sedative agents (hence its safety in veterinary medicine.)

CONCLUSION

Sleep and anesthesia are similar owing to an overlap in the neural and chemical substrates that mediate them. This overlap is probably best appreciated in the brain stem and thalamocortical systems, that are responsible for the electrical and physiologic manifestations of both alterations of state. Although incomplete, an increasing understanding of the neural mechanisms that mediate sleep will improve our understanding of the actions and side effects of anesthetic and sedative agents.

REFERENCES

1. Rechtschaffen, A. and Kales, A. (1968) A Manual of Standardized Terminology, Techniques and Scoring Systems for Sleep Stages of Human Subjects, Los Angeles, UCLA, Brain Information Service/Brain Research Institute.
2. IFSEC: (1974) A Glossary of Terms Most Commonly Used by Clinical Electroencephalographers. *Electroenceph. Clin. Neurophysiol.* **37,** 538–548.
3. Feinberg, I., Thode, H. C., Jr., Chugani, H. T., and March, J. D. (1990) Gamma distribution model describes maturational curves for delta wave amplitude, cortical metabolic rate and synaptic density. *J. Theo. Biol.* **142,** 149–161.

4. McCarley, R. (1995) Neurophysiology of Sleep: Basic Mechanisms Underlying Control of Wakefulness and Sleep, Sleep Disorders Medicine: Basic Science, Technical Considerations, and Clinical Aspects. Edited by Chokroverty S. Boston, London Oxford, Singapore Sydney, Toronto Wellington, Butterworth-Heinemann, pp. 17–36.

5. Rampil, I. (1998) A Primer for EEG Signal Processing in Anesthesia. *Anesthesiology* **89,** 980–1002.

6. Nielson, T. (1999) Mentation During Sleep, Handbook of Behavioral State Control, Cellular and Molecular Mechanisms. Edited by Lydic, R. and Baghdoyan, H. Boca Raton, London, New York, Washington, D.C., CRC Press, pp. 101–128.

7. Madsen, P. L. and Vorstrup, S. (1991) Cerebral blood flow and metabolism during sleep. *Cereb. Brain Met. Rev.* **3,** 281–296.

8. Bazhenov, M., Timofeev, I., Steriade, M., and Sejnowski, T. (2000) Spiking-bursting activity in the thalamic reticular nucleus initiates sequences of spindle oscillations in thalamic networks. *J. Neurophysiol.* **84,** 1076–1087.

9. Steriade, M. (1995) Thalamic origin of sleep spindles: Morison and Bassett (1945). *J. Neurophysiol.* **73,** 921–922.

10. Steriade, M., McCormick, D. A., and Sejnowski, T. J. (1993) Thalamocortical oscillations in the sleeping and aroused brain. *Science* **262,** 679–685

11. Loomis, A., Harvey N., and Hobart III, G. (1938) Distribution of Disturbance Patterns in the Human Electroencephalogram, with Special Reference to Sleep. *J. Neurophysiol.* **1,** 413–430.

12. Amzica, F. and Steriade, M. (1997) The K-complex: its slow (<1–Hz) rhythmicity and relation to delta waves. *Neurology* **49,** 952–959.

13. Amzica, F. and Steriade, M. (1998) Electrophysiological correlates of sleep delta waves. *Electroencephalog. Clin. Neurophysiol.* **107,** 69–83.

14. Feinberg, I., Floyd, T. C., and March, J. D. (1987) Effects of sleep loss on delta (0.3-3 Hz) EEG and eye movement density: new observations and hypotheses. *Electroencephalog. Clin. Neurophysiol.* **67,** 217–221.

15. Feinberg, I. and Campbell, I. G. (1993) Ketamine administration during waking increases delta EEG intensity in rat sleep. *Neuropsychopharmacol.* **9,** 41–48.

16. Feinberg, I. and Campbell, I. G. (1995) Stimulation of NREM delta EEG by ketamine administration during waking: demonstration of dose dependence. *Neuropsychopharmacol.* **12,** 89–90.

17. Feinberg, I. and Campbell, I. G. (1997) Coadministered pentobarbital anesthesia postpones but does not block the motor and sleep EEG responses to MK–801. Life *Sciences* **60,** L 217–222.

18. Feinberg, I. and Campbell, I. G. (1998) Haloperidol potentiates the EEG slowing of MK–801 despite blocking its motor effects: implications for the PCP model of schizophrenia. *Neuroreport* **9,** 2189–2193.

19. Feinberg, I. (1999) Delta homeostasis, stress, and sleep deprivation in the rat: a comment on Rechtschaffen et al. *Sleep* **22,** 1021–1030.

20. Steriade, M., Amzica, F., and Contreras, D. (1994) Cortical and thalamic cellular correlates of electroencephalographic burst suppression. *Electroencephalogr. Clin. Neurophysiol.* **90,** 1–16.

21. Williams, J. (1999) Synaptic and Intrinsic Properties Regulating Noradrenergic and Serotonergic Neurons During Sleep Wake Cycles, Handbook of Behavioral State Control, Cellular and Molecular Mechanisms. Edited by Lydic, R. and Baghdoyan, H. Boca Raton, London, New York, Washington, D.C., CRC Press, pp. 257–276.

22. Role, L. and Kelly, J. (1991) The Brain Stem: Cranial Nerve Nuclei and the Monoaminergic Systems, Principles of Neural Science, Third Edition. Edited by Kandel, E., Schwartz, J., and Jessell, T. New York, Amsterdam, London, Tokyo, Elsevier, pp. 683–699.

23. Moore, R. and Bloom, F. (1979) Central Catecholamine Neuron Systems: Anatomy and Physiology of the norepinepherine and epinepherine systems. *Ann. Rev. Neurosci.* **2,** 113–168.

24. Heimer, L. (1995) Brain Stem, Monoaminergic Pathways, and Reticular Formation, The Human Brain and Spinal Cord. New York, Berlin, Heidelberg, London, Paris, Tokyo, Hong Kong, Barcelona Budapest, Springer-Verlag, p. 506.

25. Nauta, W. and Feirtag, M. (1986) Midbrain, Fundamental Neuroanatomy. New York, W.H. Freeman and Company. pp. 340.

26. Keifer, J., Baghdoyan, H., and Lydic, R. (1992) Sleep Disruption and Increased Apneas after Pontine Microinjection of Morphine. *Anesthesiology* **77,** 973–982.

27. Keifer, J., Baghdoyan, H., and Lydic, R. (1996) Pontine Cholinergic Mechanisms Modulate the Cortical Electroencephalographic Spindles of Halothane Anesthesia. *Anesthesiology* **84,** 4.

28. Sleigh, J. W., Andrzejowski, J., Steyn-Ross, A., and Steyn-Ross, M. (1999) The bispectral index: a measure of depth of sleep? *Anesth. Analg.* **88,** 659–661.

5

Possible Relationships of Anesthetic Coma and Pathological Disorders of Consciousness

Nicholas D. Schiff and Fred Plum

INTRODUCTION

This chapter reviews pathological causes of coma and related global disorders of consciousness. We discuss these neurological disorders in the context of how contributions of subcortical arousal and gating systems relate to normal conscious states. We then briefly explore the possible overlap of mechanisms of different forms of anesthesia as compared to the reviewed pathological states.

Definition of Consciousness

We offer a definition of the psychological dimension of consciousness that closely follows that of James (1):

At its least, normal human consciousness consists of a serially time-ordered, organized, restricted and reflective awareness of self and the environment. Moreover, the experience is one of graded complexity and quantity.

Arousal, attention, intention, memory, awareness, and mood-emotion are primary neuropsychologic components of consciousness. Although it is self-evident that these components are interdependent, neuroimaging studies have increasingly confirmed classical neurological observations that particular brain systems develop to process or generate specific functions (2,3). Young, in Chapter 2, discusses these specific cortical contributions to neuropsychological components in greater detail.

Global disorders of human consciousness result from impairment of several neuropsychologic components and result in diffuse, severe, or total loss of meaningful behavior. We briefly review the anatomical substrates of these disorders placing special emphasis on the role of particular subcortical structures that contribute to consciousness. We also develop a distinction between arousal systems and "gating" systems. Arousal is identified with the different functional states that characterize forebrain activation on the basis of brainstem modulation of corticothalamic systems (4). We formulate gating as a set of selective processes that may facilitate transient long-range interactions of large-scale brain networks.

Global disorders of consciousness include stupor and coma, the vegetative state, akinetic mutism, absence and partial complex seizures, delirium, dementia, and a more recently defined state of hyperkinetic mutism (for broader review see ref. 5). However, we focus this chapter on coma, persistent vegetative state, akinetic mutism, and absence seizures (see Table 1) because all of these states bear close relationships to forms of pharmacologic anesthesia. We emphasize focal injuries that produce

From: *Contemporary Clinical Neuroscience: Neural Mechanisms of Anesthesia*
Edited by: Joseph F. Antognini et al. © Humana Press Inc., Totowa, NJ

Table 1
Global Disorders of Consciousness

	Coma*	PVS	ASZ	AKM
Arousal	–	+	+	+
Attention	–	–	–	+
Intention	–	–	–	–
Memory	–	–	–	–
Awareness	–	–	–	–/?

In addition to coma, generalized tonic-clonic seizures, post-ictal unconsciousness, concussion, and asystolic syncope may be included in the first column (*). PVS, persistent vegetative state, ASZ, absence seizure, AKM, akinetic mutism. –, absent; +, present, –/+; incompletely expressed, –/? Apparently absent.

global disorders for two reasons. One of these is that nonselective large cortical injuries or metabolic etiologies of coma usually shed little light on selective mechanisms of anesthesia. The other, as section IV will discuss, is an identifiable overlap between focal etiologies of global disorders and regional effects of several different anesthetic types.

PATHOLOGICAL STATES OF UNCONSCIOUSNESS

Coma

Coma reflects a totally unconscious and unarousable brain state that results from acute pharmacologic anesthesia, physical injuries, and a variety of serious medical disorders. All interfere with the brain's arousal mechanisms (*see* Plum and Posner *[6]* for a comprehensive review of causes). The most prominent behavioral state of coma may clinically resemble deep, sleep-like unconsciousness. Functionally, coma is characterized by unarousable unresponsiveness to internal or external stimuli. In pathologic coma, eyes are closed and even the most vigorous exogenous stimulation cannot evoke awakening. Comatose subjects express neither understandable words nor sounds, nor do they correctly localize specific noxious stimuli applied to any part of the body. While several components of the arousal system are identified (*see* section on Arousal and Gating Systems), only relatively large rostral dorsal-medial pontine, mesencephalic and paramedian thalamic lesions, or global damage to the cerebral hemispheres can produce sustained coma *(7)*. In the comatose state, no evidence exists of awareness of self or environment nor do cyclical state changes appear (*see* Fig. 1, column 1).

Most pathological coma derives from a relatively few causes. Following in order of incidence are: (1) Brain trauma; (2) Cerebral vascular damage, including: a. large cerebral and brain stem ischemic strokes; b. acute ruptured cerebral aneurisms; and c. large, critical cerebral or subtentorial hemorrhages (3). Severe anoxemia or asphyxia owing to cardiac asystole, drowning, immediate absence of atmospheric oxygen, carbon monoxide exposure, or abrupt, severe pulmonary dysfunction; (4) Acute intracranial inflammatory of infectious disease; (5) Intentional or accidentally inhaled or ingested sedative or street drugs, and (6) Several systemic or cerebral metabolic disorders.

Table 1 indicates a concomitant loss of all neuropsychologic components incurred with a coma. Stupor, is an imprecise term applied to patients with marked impairment of arousal who nevertheless, can be sufficiently stimulated from their sleep-like condition to express purposeful, but often inconsistent, responses to their environment. Forms of brief unconsciousness such as syncope, concussion, and brief generalized tonic-clonic seizures or post-ictal unconsciouness may also be included in the first column of Table 1.

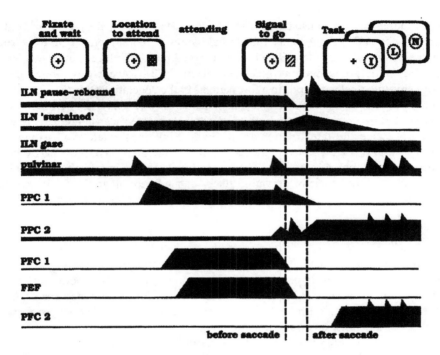

Fig. 1. Timing chart for cortical and subcortical activations during a visual attention task *(97)*. The figure schematizes extracellular unit activity in a hypothetical experiment in which a subject is asked to covertly attend to a target just lateral to a fixation cue and saccade to the target after a cue signal. The shaded regions represent absolute firing rates of neurons in several cortical and thalamic regions; PFC, pre-frontal cortex *(98)*; FEF, frontal eye field *(99)*; PPC; posterior parietal cortex *(118,119)*; pulvinar; and ILN, intralaminar nuclei (cells modeled from central lateral and paracentralis nucleus, Schlag and Schlag-Rey *[111,112]*). The gating role for the ILN is hypothesized to support and modulate such sustained activity across specific long-range corticocortical connections *(see* text).

Persistent Vegetative State

Among the most important contributions to our understanding of mechanisms generating arousal and sustained wakefulness in the past half century, have been the discovery of the physiology of arousal by Moruzzi and Magoun (1949 and others, see below) *(8)*, and Jennett and Plum's (1972) *(9)* clinical identification of the automatic and isolated sleep-wake function of the persistent vegetative state. The vegetative state presents the fundamental clinical dissociation of arousal from all other components of consciousness (Table 1). Patients in the vegetative state express irregular cyclic arousal which separate them from chronic coma. Nevertheless, they express no awareness of self or the environment. The structural anatomical damage that can precipitate a persistent vegetative state (PVS) varies widely *(10)*. Autopsy examinations in a large series of patients in a post-traumatic PVS *(10,11)* demonstrate varying degrees of destruction-degeneration that bilaterally affect the cerebral cortex, the cerebral white matter and, sometimes the mesencephalic tegmental structures, either independently or all together. The mesencephalic lesions mostly reflect damage secondary to early compression of the brainstem following swelling due to brain injury (tentorial herniation). Post-mortem studies of nontraumatically-induced PVS have been fewer but also disclose multifocal bilateral cerebral lesions with or without severe destruction of basal ganglia or thalamus *(12)*. In addition to cases of widespread damage owing to anoxic or traumatic brain injury, vegetative states may also result from focal injuries confined to the paramedian rostral brainstem and thalamus *(13–17)*.

The clinical judgment of unconsciousness in PVS has been supported by the results of positron emission tomography (PET) scan studies that reveal overall cerebral metabolism to be reduced by 50% or more below the normal rate *(18–21)*. The observed metabolic levels are equivalent to those found in persons undergoing deep surgical anesthesia) *(22)*. Recently, we have documented behavioral and physiological variations in a few patients in the vegetative state *(23–25)*. One of these patients randomly expressed occasional single, understandable words *(25)*. Her PET studies identified isolated islands of left frontotemporal cerebral structures that operated at an abnormally low metabolic rate but at nearly twice the rates of remaining brain. Similar isolated expressions have been encountered in several other vegetative patients. Typically, the patients express easily identifiable, stereotypical, emotional-limbic responses. These emotional expressions likely reflect distinct and isolated limbic mechanisms; their preservation likely depends on integrative brainstem structures that lie outside of the thalamocortical systems that typically undergo overwhelming injury in PVS patients.

Akinetic Mutism

The term akinetic mutism encompasses an uncommon unique behavior consisting of the appearance of constant wakeful hypervigilance, the making of only rare body movements, and, usually, a preservation of visual tracking in the form of smooth, slow pursuit movements. Classically, akinetic mutism as listed in Table 1 reflects the recovery of a crude wakeful attentiveness without the apparent recovery of any other neuropsychologic function.

Cairns, an English neurosurgeon, coined the term in 1941, to describe a young woman who, although appearing wakeful, became mute, rigidly motionless, not spastic and apparently unconscious, when a craniopharyngiomatous cyst expanded to compress the anterior walls of her third ventricle, plus the posterior medial-ventral surface of the frontal lobe *(26)*. When the cyst was drained, she recovered full awareness of the immediate present but possessed no memory of the previous event. Eye movements were not described in this girl, but almost all recent classic cases have been said to display rare, slow but seemingly attentive conjugate eye movements. Oculocephalic reflex stimulation may slowly evoke limited fractions of lateral gaze in akinetic mute patients.

Additional observers have somewhat widened the abnormal functional anatomy that relates to the syndrome, based on similar behavior. These include selective or associated injuries to the medial-basal prefrontal area including Cairn's zone, the medial forebrain bundle, the anterior cingulum; the general medial-prefrontal region supplied by the anterior cerebral arteries, and, the pallidum and caudate nuclei. The hyperattentive form of classic akinetic mutism typically occurs in patients with bilateral lesions affecting the anterior cingulate and mesial frontal cortices. Frequently, the state reflects medial frontal damage caused by rupture of an anterior communicating artery aneurysm *(27)*. The associated injury may sometimes be accompanied by injury to the hypothalamus and anterior pallidum. A similar picture, but not including absence of eye movements, can rarely be a feature of untreated, severely rigid Parkinson's disease. Recently, a few investigators reported finding strong clinical resemblances to the above syndrome in the terminal state of prion disease *(28)*.

A slightly different clinical expression of the disorder is seen with subcortical or upper brainstem damage. Patients with this form of akinetic mutism appear apathetic and hypersomnolent *(29)* but may speak with understandable words. Castainge et al. *(30)* emphasized that patients suffering structural injuries affecting the medial-dorsal thalamus extending into the mesencephalic tegmentum suffered severe memory loss and apathetic behavior. Segarra *(31)* described 7 more examples of combined damage to the medial caudal thalamus extending into the medial dorsal mesencephalon that appeared to him to cause the same signs and symptoms as having "akinetic mutism". Because of this unfortunate confusion in both behavior and structure, we have termed the behavior of Segarra's patients's as having "slow syndrome". Most of them, after they regain awareness, are able to move and speak, and despite their apathy and amnesia, they are not semi-rigid as are akinetic mute patients. They also slowly communicate, although usually at the edge of severe dementia and their motor system reflects classic corticospinal tract abnormalities. They also lack the appearance of vigilance.A persistent dementia characterizes the recovery phase of this disorder *(32)*. Subcortical lesions that may produce this state include bilateral lesions of the paramedian anterior or posterior thalamus and basal forebrain *(26,30)* the mesencephalic reticular formation including periaqueductal gray matter *(31)*, and caudate nuclei (or left caudate in isolation, *see* refs. *33–36*).

The common denominator of all akinetic mute states appears to be related to the disabling of several parallel, segregated cortico-straitopallidal-thalamocortical loops that involve the frontal lobes either directly or indirectly *(34)*. The most devastating injury is a bilateral loss of basal-mesial frontal cortical tissue, after which little further recovery develops. Bilateral lesions of the globus pallidus interna are unusual in that this structure contains each of the identified cortico-striato-pallidal-thalamocortical (CSPTC) circuits involving the frontal lobe, striatum, globus pallidus, substantia nigra, and thalamus *(34)*. Thus, a bilateral pallidal injury can disable all of the parallel networks. At least partial cognitive function can recover following some bilateral injuries to the paramedian thalamus and mesencephalon (*see* refs. *31,15,35,* and *36*), discussion in *(38)*. The akinetic mutism resulting from injury to these structures is likely to reflect their unique role along with the nucleus reticularis of the thalamus in gating both these parallel CSPTC loops *(39,40)* and specific long-range cortico-cortical interactions (*see* below). Isolated injury to the periaqueductal grey region has also been described in experimental models of akinetic mutism *(41,42)*. This structure may modulate regions of the paramedian mesodiencephalon. Selective injury to the medial forebrain bundle removes a strong dopaminergic modulation of medial frontal lobe structures functionally down-regulating these regions *(43)*. This loss of modulation is reversible, and can sometimes be corrected by giving patients dopaminergic agonists *(44)*.

Absence Seizures

Absence seizures reflect a unique global alteration of consciousness. These events exhibit attentional and intentional failure, loss of working memory and intra-ictal perceptual dissociation. In their classic form, absence seizures represent momentary vegetative states (c.f. Table 1). Although debate surrounds the underlying mechanism of absence seizures, thalamocortical generation is indicated by both clinical and experimental studies of absence seizures *(45–47)*. The key role of cortico-thalamic projections in organizing large scale coherent EEG patterns has been well demonstrated in recent studies *(48)*. Most current animal models include the nucleus reticularis of the thalamus (NRT) in conjunction with thalamocortical relay cells, and the cortex as the essential substrate for the cortical initiation of the seizure *(46,49)*. In addition, the passage from the thalamus to the cortex must rely on specific and nonspecific relay nuclei that project to the cortex (the NRT does not project to the cortex, [*see* ref. *50*]. Among these thalamic nuclei, the intralaminar nuclei play an important role in the genesis of these seizures. Experimental studies in guinea pig, cat, monkey, and man all demonstrate that generalized 3/s spike-waves and an associated behavioral absence may be elicited by electrical stimulation of the intralaminar nuclei and related nonspecific thalamic nuclei, primarily, the median dorsalis and ventral anterior nuclei, *(51–57)*. These studies show a robust reproducibility of the 3/s spike and wave phenomenon across species and behavioral state. In addition, an important role for brainstem reticular contributions to this seizure has also been argued *(58,59)*.

Taken together, an overlap exists between the anatomical structures involved in absence seizures and those that when injured, induce coma, vegetative states, and akinetic mutism. Absence seizures represent one of few conditions that may produce brief unconsciousness without any evidence of lasting structural injury. Unlike concussions, syncope, or pharmacologic anesthesia, arousal is preserved during the absence seizure demonstrating the selective loss of integrative functions with these events (*see* Section on Early Centrencephalic Theories).

AROUSAL AND GATING SYSTEMS

In all cases of selective injuries producing global disorders, unconsciousness appears to arise from either large bilateral damage to frontal or posterior association cortices or selective subcortical injuries. As noted in the Section on Absence Seizures, the expressed pattern of subcortical injuries suggests that the paramedian mesodiencephalic structures of the "classical" arousal system (the intralaminar nuclei of the thalamus and the mesencephalic reticular formation) may play a primary role in this loss of integration observed in the different pathological states described in Pathological States of Unconsciousness above. The following Section (Arousal Systems) discusses the current concepts of arousal mechanisms and their possible distinction from structures that may be more appropriately considered "gating" systems.

Arousal Systems

The concept of brainstem arousal systems was introduced by the pioneering work of Moruzzi, Magoun, Morrison, and Dempsey (*see* refs. *60–62* and *68*). Initially the role of the mesencephalic reticular formation (MRF) and the thalamic intralaminar nuclei (ILN) were emphasized as mediating arousal and setting the stage for sensory processing in higher integrative brain functions *(8,52) see* recent review *(63)*. Electrical stimulation of these mesodiencephalic structures demonstrated their role in both electroencephalographic desynchronization and behavioral arousal.

The classic interpretations of the arousal system have been incorporated into a present conception that identifies arousal as interdependent on the output of cholinergic, serotoninergic, adrenergic and histaminergic nuclei located predominantly in the brainstem, basal forebrain, and posterior hypothalamus *(64–66)*. Arousal is now viewed in terms of global modulations of the thalamocortical system that define specific functional states *(64)*. Several studies have sought to determine how necessary or sufficient other neuronal groups are for arousal without providing compelling evidence that any single group is indispensable *(65–67)*. Even within global modulatory states increasing evidence identifies the fine structure contributed by selective activation of interdependent arousal systems *(65,68,69)*. For example, varying effects of noradrenergic, dopaminergic, and cholinergic neuromodulators have been identified in visuospatial attention paradigms *(69)*. The nucleus basalis of the basal forebrain has also been partitioned into regions that can become selectively active in different behaviors *(71)*. The increasingly high degrees of interconnection identified in anatomical studies of these neuronal populations provide a substrate for complex interactions among these brainstem nuclei *(72)*.

Cholinergic pathways that originate in the laterodorsal tegmental and pedunculopontine nuclei project rostrally to various targets and play a prominent role in most discussions of arousal mechanisms *(see* ref. *66)* Their selective output is probably insufficient to generate normal arousal (which must require additional glutamatergic and other brainstem populations, *(73)*, although much evidence indicates that they play a role in sharpening attention and modulating conscious activity *(74,69)*. Well documented clinical reports indicate that selective damage to these pontine cholinergic nuclei, can prevent or greatly reduce REM and normal sleep patterns, thereby resulting in chronic hyposomnia, but not necessarily even a transient coma *(75,76)* for further discussion and related findings in olivopontocerebellar atrophy patients). Cognitive ability reportedly remains intact in such persons so long as they do not incur more rostral brainstem damage *(77)* Cholinergic nuclei located more rostrally in the basal forebrain influence cortical cognitive and memory functions as well as EEG desynchronization. Nevertheless, they seem to make no firmly established contribution to arousal per se. The selective contributions of dopaminergic (ventral tegmental area) and histaminergic (tubomammilary nucleus) agents have also been studied *(65)* and may strongly influence the expression of sleep and wake states.

Centrencephalic Integration and Early Models of Forebrain "Gating" Systems

Half a century ago, Penfield and Jasper, refs. *(79,80)* proposed a clinically engendered hypothesis involving brainstem arousal mechanisms and termed the process 'centrencephalic integration', *(see* refs. *59* and *63* for historical reviews). Penfield drew his speculation from observing the temporary loss of consciousness accompanying absence seizures and linked this unique paroxysmal event to interfering with a "highest level" brain mechanism that underlay conscious awareness. Importantly, he suggested that the observed loss of consciousness was the result of a specific failure of a generalized integrating mechanism. Penfield never precisely detailed the model in physiological terms or anatomical specificity, but he strongly emphasized the role of the thalamic intralaminar nuclei and the adjacent mesencephalic reticular formation in wakeful behavior. The theory was extensively, but nonscientifically, criticized by conflating the hypothetical system with a locus (a "centrencephalon") that would achieve such an integration underlying consciousness *(80–82)*. A close reading of Penfield's writings, however, clearly indicate his concept that these mesodiencephalic structures organized a process that enabled a

"synchronous central and cortical activity, activity in the brainstem and in those areas of the cortex of either hemisphere whose function is suited to the changing requirements of the moment"*(84)*.

Further extensions of centrencephalic models have been developed. Working with both alert and anaesthetized cats *(83)*, pioneered a series of experiments that examined the integrative physiology of the MRF, the NRT and the medial thalamic-mesial frontal cortical systems (these included the ILN and related nonspecific thalamic nuclei). These investigators proposed that gating of attention was achieved by medial thalamo-frontal cortical and MRF control of NRT inhibition of specific thalamic relay nuclei (*see* Fig. 1B). The model proposed that intentionally directed action emanated from the frontal cortical-thalamocortical projections together with reflex orienting responses able to interrupt via the MRF pathway to NRT, that otherwise remained under cortical direction. Schiebel *(84)* enlarged on this model with a more anatomically detailed treatment of the MRF and Crick *(85)* further proposed that the NRT focused the conscious "searchlight" of attention. Crick's proposal emphasized a role for the low threshold spike burst that results from NRT mediated hyperpolarization. This conductance inactivates, however, during the depolarized states associated with wakefulness and attentive behaviors, a factor that rules out this "searchlight" mechanism *(86)*. Recent anatomical studies have detailed specific sectors within the NRT that could partition thalamocortical activation along the lines envisioned by Crick and others *(87)*. A physiological study in rats recently demonstrated such a selective NRT role in attentional processing using a covert-attention paradigm (Posner task) *(88)*.

Physiological Studies of the Role of "Gating" Systems in Forebrain Integration

The concept of forebrain gating has been enlarged by several physiological investigations that provide evidence of interaction of functional states with selective integrative mechanisms. Recent human PET studies demonstrate that the MRF and ILN coactivate during attentional processing providing further support for the 'gating' concept of selective attention *(90)*. In Kinomura et al.'s studies, PET scans showed increased regional blood flow in the mesencephalic reticular formation, in ILN and, in prefrontal, frontal, parietal, and primary sensory cortices when quiet wakefulness was compared to simple reaction time tasks in a visual or somatosensory attentional paradigm. Along the same lines, Portas et al. *(93)* identified a specific role for the thalamus in mediating interactions of attention and arousal during careful, state-controlled studies using fMRI paradigms.

Recent studies have detailed the physiological connections between the ILN and MRF and further elucidated their essential role in both arousal *(91,92)* and attentive states *(93)*. Both the centromedian-parafascularis complex, Cm-Pf, (posterior intralaminar group) and the central lateral nucleus (CL, anterior intralaminar group), may desynchronize the EEG during arousal *(94,91)* and may play a role similar to the activation observed in Kinomura et al.'s studies. Tonic rapid firing in CL correlates with desynchronization of the EEG and responds to inputs from the MRF *(91)*. These studies demonstrate specific changes in the spectral content of background brain activity within different behavioral states, including natural awake attentive states that have been found to exhibit increased high frequency activity *(93)*.

Additional anatomical and physiological evidence suggests that the ILN may also contribute to the formation of specific "event-holding" functions that support attention and working memory *(95–97* and *see* below). Such event-holding functions may represent focal, sustained activations or amplifications of cortical activity *(98)* and also, may be associated with neuronal transient responses *(99,100)*, oscillatory activity *(94,101,102)*, or possibly other physiological signatures *(99,103,104)*, identified the possible role of these patterns of sustained cortical firing, supported by the ILN, in working memory. Several experimental results from Mair and colleagues, *(105,107)* have provided evidence that marked deficits in delayed match to sample performance are attributable to lesions specifically, of the intralaminar nuclei (paracentral, central lateral, and central medial, but not the median dorsalis nucleus). The investigators interpret the observed memory deficits primarily as a disabling of mnemonic functions of CSPTC loops by ILN injury.

Experimental studies also support a selective integrative role for the ILN. Integrative problems in visuospatial awareness associate with both anterior and posterior thalamic lesions involving the ILN. Circumscribed thalamic lesions thought to be restricted to the Cm-Pf complex result in specific impairments in trying to use extraretinal eye position signals to produce accurate memory-guided saccades (an example consists of following a truncal rotation or caloric stimulus, [*see* ref. *108*]). Studies of CL also demonstrate a role in visual awareness. In cats, contraversive head turning and conjugate and contraversive saccadic eye movements are elicited by stimulation of CL *(109)*. Similarly, unilateral lesions of CL in cats lead to contralateral visual neglect *(110)*.

Schlag-Rey and Schlag *(111,112)*, first described a role for the ILN in primate visuo-spatial awareness. They characterized visuomotor functions in the rostral intralaminar nuclei (primarily CL) of alert monkeys using single-unit recordings in animals performing behavioral tasks. One population of neurons ceased firing during a saccade and then rebounded with a burst of action potentials at the start of the next intersaccadic interval ("pause-rebound", *see* Fig. 2). Most of these neurons demonstrated this behavior for any saccade, with the direction or amplitude of the saccade having no effect on the dynamics of the response. Other neighboring visuomotor units in the ILN (eye position and saccadic burst cells) were highly sensitive to the parameters (amplitude, latency, direction) of the saccade ("gaze" and "sustained", *see* Fig. 2). Schlag and Schlag-Rey *(112)* interpreted their findings as antithetical to the concept of "mass action" in the ILN but rather hinting at "control signals" or a "clocking device synchronized on saccades used to pace operations at the next stage of (cortical processing)".

Based on Schlag and Schlag-Rey's pioneering studies, Purpura and Schiff *(97)* proposed that the CL firing responses, which are sensitive to levels of arousal, also have a multifunctional purpose in both setting up large areas of cortical activation and in facilitating more local activations related to visual awareness. ILN neurons are presumed to share intrinsic membrane properties that are common to all thalamic neurons *(113)*. This means that these neurons should be capable of two modes of firing behavior, i.e., when hyperpolarized they should fire a short high frequency burst superimposed on slower lower amplitude Ca^{2+} spikes; or, if depolarized, they should fire spikes at a regular rate determined by the level of depolarization. The temporal structure of firing patterns of CL neurons may be controlled both by levels of arousal and visuomotor behavior. Such local activations may be excited by the saccade related bursts identified by Schlag and Schlag-Rey *(111)* thereby facilitating processing, in separated cortical regions that receive input during the intersaccadic interval. One requirement of this proposal is that fast bursting neurons must be able to burst in the active depolarized states associated with wakefulness *(65)*. New evidence from in vivo intracellular recordings during natural sleep-wake cycles shows that such a mechanism may be available *(11)*.

Figure 2 illustrates a hypothesis by Purpura and Schiff *(97)* for how ILN populations may play a role in selectively gating forebrain activity in addition to facilitating tonic changes in arousal states.

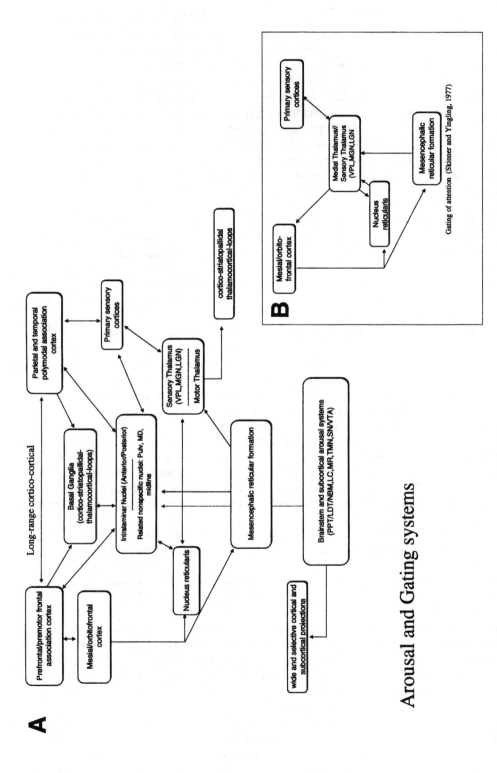

Arousal and Gating systems

Fig. 2. (A) A schematic overview of brainstem arousal and mesodiencephalic gating systems. (B) Early model of gating of attention by Skinner and Yingling ca. 1977 (83).

In this hypothetical experiment, recordings from several cortical and thalamic (ILN and pulvinar) sites are illustrated. The responses are modeled from recordings in the alert primate as reviewed above and below. Unlike neurons of the specific thalamic relay nuclei, neurons of the ILN make their synapse in layer I onto the apical dendrites of pyramidal cells in layers II–III, and layers V and VI *(114)*. Following this input pattern, ILN stimulation activates both the supragranular and infragranular layers of the cortical microcircuit *(115)*. During the tonic firing mode of ILN cells, activation of NMDA channels in the supragranular layers may support sustained activity in local populations of cortical pyramidal cells *(96,97,116)*. In primates that have learned selective attention paradigms, neuronal activity with these characteristics can be recorded from the prefrontal cortex (PFC) *(98)*, the frontal eye fields (FEF) *(117)*, and posterior parietal cortex (PPC) *(118,119)*. In such paradigms, a period of sustained activation in cortical neurons is observed between presentation of a peripheral target and a subsequent saccade to the target's location *(see* Fig. 2). Such shifts of attention relate closely to saccadic eye-movements and may reflect similar transient activation patterns in the forebrain. ILN subdivisions selectively project to PFC (Pf, CL and paralaminar MD), FEF (CL and paralaminar MD), and PPC (Cm-Pf, CL). Through these specific projections, they may facilitate, and possibly trigger such sustained activations or "event-holding functions" utilized in visuospatial attention. These sustained neuronal responses may act as "activity envelopes" that gate many different carriers generated by relatively independent local network processes *(120)*. The transient activation of such activity envelopes may be the basis for episodic cortical processing linking attention and working memory to oculomotor behavior and the intersaccadic interval *(97)*.

The model in Fig. 2 focuses on projections of the ILN to networks related to attention and oculomotor activity. Each cortical region in the example is identified with functions that are selectively vulnerable to anesthetics *(see* Young Chapter 2). In the PFC, neuronal activations would reflect working memory processing, whereas in the PPC these cortical activations would determine the dynamics of the attentional gate with the ILN facilitating the well-documented interdependence of these psychophysical variables *(121,122)*. In FEF, these activations would prepare saccadic eye-movements to attended targets. Though not illustrated, important projections to the basal ganglia and modulation of the cortico-striato-pallidal-thalamocortical components of the frontal cortices involved would significantly contribute to the performance of the hypothetical task. Thus, through the activation of widely separated local patches of cortex and subcortical structures, particular subdivisions of the ILN may facilitate specific long-range cortico-cortical interactions *(93,123,124)*. Thus, forebrain gating per se, would reflect the ongoing formation of episodic activity within these circuits organized around behaviorally significant events.

Other subdivisions of the ILN and related gating system components may engage in different behavioral states. Of note, some evidence exists for similarly selective single-unit behavior in the MRF *(125)*. Knowledge of the specific functional contributions of the thalamic reticular nucleus in alert humans or primates is very limited outside of interesting attentional and memory failures associated with somewhat selective injury to the NRT, following poisoning with domoic acid *(126,127)*, or anoxic injury *(128)*.

Taken together, the main role of the ILN, MRF, and NRT, following on the earlier models of Penfield and Jasper, Skinner and Yingling, and others as reviewed above, is to facilitate the gating of cortico-cortical information processing and not arousal, per se *(see* Fig. 1A and 1B). Several lines of evidence support a selective role for subcortical gating systems in the mechanism of global disorders, interdependent upon contributions from the arousal systems. The clinical expression of global disorders produced by subcortical injuries may thus depend on whether such selective gating processes are completely or only partially disabled. The specific gating processes may be identified with activity envelopes organized around important endogenous transient events. Examples include eye-movements or shifts of attention, that are used to facilitate long-range communication in the forebrain. The episodic dynamics of these activity envelopes, operating within the background arousal state, may be primarily facilitated by the gating systems and themselves may organize many different ongoing neuronal assembly processes.

POSSIBLE RELATIONSHIPS OF ANESTHETIC MECHANISMS AND PATHOLOGIC STATES OF UNCONSCIOUSNESS

Both subcortical arousal and gating systems play key roles in global disorders of consciousness. Whether or not these structures play such a role in selective mechanisms underlying anesthesia is unknown. A few recent studies have examined the regionally selective effects of pharmacologic anesthesia. While preliminary, these data do show some overlap between the areas of significant reduction in cerebral metabolic activity or blood flow that are associated with anesthesia and those selective areas that produce global disorders of consciousness following structural injury.

Veselis and colleagues *(129)* examined alterations in regional cerebral blood flow (rCBF) in normal subjects undergoing midzolam infusions of different concentrations. In their studies, that evaluated blood flow using 15-O positron emission tomography (PET) techniques (*see* Chapter 3), several cortical association areas and the thalamus demonstrated significant reductions of rCBF compared to the generalized decrease observed throughout the brain in each subject. The findings are consistent with similar observations of marked reduction of thalamic metabolism with other benzodiazepine agents *(130)*. These investigators interpret their findings in the context of coinactivation of both cortical and subcortical regions important for attention, working memory (*see* Chapters 2 and 3) and arousal.

Alkire and colleagues *(131)* have postulated a unified mechanism for anesthetics that involves a hyperpolarization block of thalamocortical transmission, they emphasize the role of both the thalamus and the MRF in activating specific populations of cortical neurons. In a recent FDG-PET study examining regional cerebral metabolic rates (rCMR), the investigators compared two inhalational anesthetics (halothane and isoflurane) for overlapping regions affected by both agents. A strong overlap was identified in rCMR reductions in the thalamus and MRF. These findings were noted to be consistent with rCMR studies and 15-O rCBF studies of benzodiazepine agents discussed in Veselis and colleagues' results. Their opinion closely follows that of Angel *(132)* who, in a comprehensive review of neuronal responses to anesthetic agents, identified suppression of thalamic activity (particularly the NRT and ILN), and a relatively stronger effect on cortical pyramidal cells in both layer III and layer V. These selective effects within the cortical microcircuit, particularly upon layer V cells, may be important and relate to several present theories of cellular underpinnings of the conscious state *(122,134,135,* and Chapter 8).

Other investigators have examined variations in depth of anesthesia and preservation of selected systems. Logothetis and colleagues recently demonstrated the partial preservation of perceptual sensorimotor integration in monkeys undergoing ketamine anesthesia *(136)*. They systematically varied anesthetic levels and tracked the optokinetic nystagmus (OKN) response; the results demonstrate that this elemental aspect of sensorimotor integration can remain despite low doses of ketamine anesthesia. The response; however, is changed to reflect an asymmetric activation pattern consistent with functional loss of top-down influences. This elegant model demonstrates that integrated circuits may remain functional even with substantial reductions of other modulatory forebrain activity. The OKN response is often preserved in akinetic mutism, and along with occasional isolated behavioral fragments seen in some PVS patients, may simply reflect very limited preservation of forebrain circuits.

These functional studies hint at an intersection of common action of anesthetics in MRF and thalamus. It is possible that, in general, anesthetics act first to disable selective integrative cerebral functions, followed by more global impairment of the cortico-thalamic system, as neuronal firing is suppressed. The patterns of behavior in the clinical syndromes reviewed above and the considerations of selective cellular effects of anesthetics on the basic corticothalamic microcircuit and brainstem (*see* Chapters 6–10) support such a view. A strict structure-function correlation, however, is difficult to identify between the loss of consciousness seen with anesthetic agents that produce widespread hemodynamic and metabolic changes, and regional physiological suppression of cerebral function. As Cariani *(137)* has argued, it is not clear whether anesthesia primarily overwhelms and suppresses neuronal firing rates, or whether it alters specific patterns of neuronal activity such as that engendered by alteration of gating mechanisms, as suggested in the section on Gating Systems. The further elucidation of the relative importance of the alteration of global cerebral activation vs specific patterns of forebrain activity associated with anesthetic agents, will strengthen our understanding of relationships between pathological and pharmacological forms of impaired consciousness.

REFERENCES

1. James, W. (1890) Principles of Psychology. Reprinted Dover Books, 1950.
2. Fracowiak, R. S. J., Friston, K., Frith, C., Dolan, R., and Mazziota, J. C. (1998) Human brain mapping. London: Academic Press.
3. Johnson, M (1997) Developmental Cognitive Neuroscience. Blackwell Press.
4. Steriade, M. and Llinas, R. R. (1988) The functional states of the thalamus and the associated neuronal interplay. *Physiol. Rev.* **68(3)**, 649–742.
5. Schiff and Plum, (2000) The Role of Arousal and "Gating" Systems in the Neurology of Impaired Consciousness. *J. Clin. Neurophysiol.* **17(5)**, 438–452.
6. Plum, F. and Posner, J. (1982) The Diagnosis of Stupor and Coma. Third Edition F. A. Davis, Philadelphia, PA.
7. Plum, F. (1991) Coma and related global disturbances of the human conscious state. In Jones, E. and Peters, P. (eds.), Cerebral Cortex, Vol. 9, Plenum Press.
8. Moruzzi, G. and Magoun, H. W. (1949) Brainstem reticular formation and activation of the EEG. *Electroencephalog. Clin. Neurophysiol.* **1**, 455–473.
9. Jennett, B. and Plum, F. (1972) Persistent vegetative state after brain damage. A syndrome in search of a name. *Lancet* **1**, 734–737.
10. Multisociety Task Force on PVS. (1994) Medical aspects of the persistent vegetative state. Part 1. *N. Engl. J. Med.* **330**, 1499–1508.
11. Danze, F., Brule, J. F., and Haddad, K. (1989) Chronic vegetative state after severe head injury; clinical study; electrophysiological investigations and CT scan in 15 cases. Neurosurg. Rev. **12 Suppl. 1**, 477–499
12. Dougherty, J. H., Jr, Rawlinson, D. G., Levy, D. E., and Plum, F. (1981) Hypoxic-ischemic brain injury and the vegetative state: clinical and neuropathologic correlation. *Neurology* **31(8)** 991–997.
13. Facon, M., Steriade, M., and Wertheim, N. (1958) Hypersomie prolonge engendere par des lesions bilatereles du systeme activateur medial. Le syndrome thrombotique de la bifurcation du tronc basilaire. *Rev. Neurol.* **98**, 117–133.
14. Plum, F. and Posner J. (1966) The diagnosis of stupor and coma. Philadelphia: Davis, F.A.
15. Castaigne, P. et al. (1981) Paramedian thalamic and midbrain infarcts: clinical and neuropathological study. *Ann. Neurol.* **10**, 127–148.
16. Kinney, HC et al. (1994) Neuropathological findings in the brain of Karen Ann Quinlan. *N. Engl. J. Med.* **330**, 1469–1475.
17. Relkin, N. R., Petito, C., and Plum, F. (1990) Coma and vegetative state secondary to severe anoxic-ischemic damage involving the thalamus. *Ann. Neurol.* **28**, 221–222.
18. Levy, D. E., Sidtis, J. J., and Rottenberg, D. A., (1987) Differences in cerebral blood flow and glucose utilization in vegetative versus locked-in patients. *Ann. Neurol.* **22**, 673–682.
19. DeVolder, A. G. et al. (1990) Brain glucose metabolism in postanoxic stroke. *Arch. Neurol.* **47**, 197–204.
20. Tomassino, C., Grana, C., Lucignani, G., Torri, G., and Ferrucio, F. (1995) Regional metabolism of comatose and vegetative state patients. *J. Neurosurg. Anesthesiol.* **7(2)**, 109–116.
21. Rudolf, J., Ghaemi, M., Ghaemi, M., Haupt, W. F., Szelies, B., and Heiss, W. D. (1999) Cerebral glucose metabolism in acute and persistent vegetative state. *J. Neurosurg. Anesthesiol.* **11(1)**, 17–24.
22. Blacklock, J. B. (1987) Effect of barbituate coma on glucose utilization in normal brain versus gliomas. Positron emission tomography studies. *J. Neurosurg.* **67**, 71–75.
23. Plum, F., Schiff, N., Ribary, U., and Llinas, R. (1998) Coordinated expression in chronically unconscious persons. *Trans. R. Soc. Lond.* **353**, 1929–1933.
24. Ribary, U., Schiff, N., Kronberg, E., Plum, F., and Llinas, R. (1998) Fractured brain function in unconscious humans: Functional brain imaging using MEG. *Neuroimage* **7(4)**, S106.
25. Schiff, N., D., Ribary, U., Plum, F., and Llinas, R. (1999a) Words without mind. *J. Cogn. Neurosci.* **11(6)**, 650–656.
26. Cairns, H., Olfield, R. C., Pennybacker, J. B., and Whitteridge, D. (1941) Akinetic mutism with an epidermoid cyst of the third ventricle. *Brain* **64**, 273–290.
27. Nemeth, G., Hegedus, K., and Molnar, L. (1988) Akinetic mutism associated with bicingular lesions: clinicopathological and functional anatomical correlates. *Eur. Arch. Psychiatry Neurol. Sci.* **237(4)**, 218–222.
28. Otto, A., Zerr, I., Lantsch, M., Weidehaas, K., Riedemann, C., and Poser, S. (1998) Akinetic mutism as a classification criterion for the diagnosis of Creutzfeldt-Jakob disease. *J. Neurol. Neurosurg. Psychiatry* **64(4)**, 524–528.
29. Fisher, C. M. (1983) Honored guest presentation: abulia minor vs. agitated behavior. *Clin. Neurosurg.* **31**, 9–31.
30. Castaigne, P. et al. (1966) Demence thalamique d'origine vasculaire par 'ramollissement bilateral limite au territorie du pedicle retro-mamillaire. *Rev. Neurol.* **114**, 89–107.
31. Segarra, J. M. (1970) Cerebral vascular disease and behavior. The syndrome of the mesencephalic artery (basilar artery bifurcation). *Arch. Neurol.* **22**, 408–418.
32. Katz, D. I., Alexander, M. P., and Mandell, A. M. (1987) Dementia following strokes in the mesencephalon and diencephalon. *Arch. Neurol.* **44**, 1127–1133

33. Bhatia, K. P. and Marsden, C. D. (1994) The behavioural and motor consequences of focal lesions of the basal ganglia in man. *Brain* **117(4)**, 859–876.
34. Mega, M. S. and Cohenour, R. C. (1997) Akinetic mutism: disconnection of frontal-subcortical circuits. *Neuropsychiatry Neuropsychol. Behav. Neurol.* **10(4)**, 254–259.
35. Stuss, D. T., Guberman, A., Nelson, R., and Larochelle, S. (1988) The neuropsychology of paramedial thalamic infarction. *Brain Cogn.* **8(3)**, 348–378.
36. van Domburg, P. H., ten Donkelaar, H. J., and Notermans, S. L. (1996) Akinetic mutism with bithalamic infarction. Neurophysiological correlates *J. Neurol. Sci.* **139**, 58–65.
38. Schiff, N. D. and Plum, F. (1999) Target article: The neurology of impaired consciousness: global disorders and implied models. Association for Scientific Study of Consciousness Electronic Seminar Series http://athena. english.vt.edu/cgi-bin/netforum/nic/a/1.
39. Groenewegen, H. and Berendse, H. (1994a) The specificity of the "nonspecific" midline and intralaminar thalamic nuclei. *Trends Neurosci.* **17**, 52–66.
40. Groenewegen, H. and Berendse, H. (1994b) Anatomical relationships between prefrontal cortex and basal ganglia in rat. In: Thierry, A.M. et al. (eds.), Motor and cognitive functions of the prefrontal cortex. Springer Verlag Berlin.
41. Panksepp J. (1998) Affective Neuroscience. Oxford UK: Oxford University Press.
42. Watt, D. (1998) Emotions and Consciousness: Implications of affective neuroscience for extended reticular thalamic activating system theories of consciousness. ASSC Eseminar Target article. http://server.phil.vt.edu/assc/watt/default.html.
43. Ross, E. D. and Stewart, R. M. (1981) Akinetic mutism from hypothalamic damage: successful treatment with dopamine agonists. *Neurology*, **31**, 1435–1439.
44. Fleet, W. S., Valenstein, E., and Watson, R. T. (1987) Dopamine agonist therapy for neglect in humans. *Neurology* **37(11)** 1765–1770.
45. Snead, O. C. (1995) Basic mechanisms of generalized absence seizures. *Ann. Neurol.* **37**, 146–157.
46. Steriade, M. and Contreras, D. (1995) Relations between cortical and thalamic cellular events during transition from sleep patterns to paroxysmal activity. *J. Neurosci.* **15(2)**, 623–642.
47. McCormick, D. A. and Bal, T. (1997) Sleep and arousal: thalamocortical mechanisms. *Ann. Rev Neurosci.* **20**, 185–215.
48. Contreras, D., Destexhe, A., Sejnowski, T. J., and Steriade, M. (1997) Spatiotemporal patterns of spindle oscillations in cortex and thalamus. *J. Neurosci.* Feb 1; **17(3)**, 1179–1196.
49. Huguenard, J. (1999) Neuronal circuitry of thalamocortical epilepsy and mechanisms of antiabsence drug action. In: Delgado-Escueta, A. V. et al. (eds.), Jasper's Basic Mechanisms of the Epilepsies, Third Edition. Advances in Neurology Vol 79.
50. Scheibel, M. E. and Schiebel, A. B. (1966) The organization of the nucleus reticularis: a golgi studu. *Brain Res.* **1**, 43–62.
51. Jasper, H. H. and Droogelever-Fortuyn, J. (1948) Experimental studies on the functional anatomy of petit mal epilepsy. *Rs. Pub. Assist. Nerv. Ment. Disord.* **26**, 272–298.
52. Hunter, J. and Jasper, H. H. (1949) Effects of thalamic stimulation in unanesthetized animals. *Electroencephalogr. Clin. Neurophysiol.* **1**, 305–324
53. Ingvar, D. H. (1955) Reproduction of 3 per second spike and wave EEG pattern by subcortical electrical stimulation in cats. *Acta Physiol. Scan.* **33**, 137–150.
54. Pollen, D. A., Perot, P., and Reid, K. H. (1963) Experimental bilateral wave and spike from thalamic stimulation in relation to level of arousal. *Electroencephalogr. Clin. Neurophysiol.* **15**, 1017–1028.
55. Steriade, M. (1974) Interneuronal epileptic discharges related to spike-and-wave conical seizure in behaving monkeys. *Electroencephalogr Clin. Neurophysiol.* **37**, 247–263.
56. David, J., Marathe, S. B., Patil, S. D., and Grewal, R. S. (1982) Behavioral and electrical correlates of absence seizures induced by thalamic stimulation in juvenile rhesus monkeys with frontal aluminum hydroxide implants: a pharmacologic evaluation. *J. Pharmacol. Meth.* **7**, 219–229.
57. Velasco, F., Velasco, M., Marquez, I., and Velasco, G. (1993) Role of centromedian thalamic nucleus in the genesis, propagation, and arrest of epileptic activity. An electrophysiological study in man. *Acta Neurochir. (Suppl).* **58**, 201–204.
58. Gloor, P., and Fariello, R. G. (1988) Generalized epilepsy: some of its cellular mechanisms differ from those of focal epilepsy. *Trends Neurosci.* **11(2)**, 63–68.
59. Jasper, H. H. (1991) Current evaluation of concepts of centrencephalic and corticoreticular seizures. *Electroencephalogr. Clin. Neurophysiol.* **78**, 2–12.
60. Morison, R. S. and Dempsey, E. W. (1942) A study of thalamo-cortical relationships. *Am. J. Physiology* **135**, 281–292.
61. Jasper, H. (1949) Diffuse projection systems. *Electronencephalogr. Clin. Neurophysiol.* **1**, 405–420.
62. Jasper, H. H. and Droogelever-Fortuyn, J. (1947) Experimental studies on the functional anatomy of petit mal epilepsy. *Res. Pub. Assist. Nerv. Ment. Disord.* **26**, 272–298.
63. Jasper, H. (1998) Consciousness and sensory processing. In: Consciouness at the frontiers of neurology. Advances in Neurology Vol. 77 Lippincott Raven Publishers, Philadelphia, PA, pp. 33–48.
64. McCormick (1992)
65. Marracco, R. T., Witte, E., and Davidson, M. C. (1994) Arousal systems. *Curr. Opin. Neurobiol.* **4**, 166–170.
66. Steriade, M. (1997) Thalamic substrates of disturbances in states of vigilance and consciousness in humans, In: Steriade, M., Jones, E. and McCormick, D. (eds.), Thalamus. Elsevier Publishers.
67. Dringenberg, H. C. and Vanderwolf, C. H. (1997) Neocortical activation: modulation by multiple pathways acting on central cholinergic and serotonergic systems. *Exp. Brain* **116(1)**, 160–174.

68. Silberstein, R. (1995) Neuromodulation of neocortical dynamics. In: Nunez, P. (ed.), Neocortical Dynamics and Human EEG Rhythms. Oxford University Press.

69. Marracco, R. T. and Davidson, M. C. (1998) Neurochemistry of attention. In: Parasuraman, R. (ed.), The attentive brain. Cambridge, MA: MIT Press, pp. 35–50.

70. Coull, J. T., Frith, C. D., Dolan, R. J., Frackowiak, R. S., and Grasby, P. M. (1997) The neural correlates of the noradrenergic modulation of human attention, arousal and learning. *Eur. J. Neurosci.* **9(3)**, 589–598.

71. Sarter, M. and Bruno, J. P. (2000) Cortical cholinergic imputs mediating arousal, attentional processing and dreaming: differential afferent regulation of the basal forebrain by telencephalic and brainstem afferents. *Neuroscience* **95,** 933–952.

72. Smiley, J. F., Subramanian, M., and Mesulam, M. M. (1999) Monaminergic-cholinergic interactions in the primate basal forebrain. *Neuroscience* **93(3)**, 817–829.

73. Steriade, M. (1999) Invited commentary. Disorders of Consciousness. Association for Scientific Study of consciousness Electronic Seminar Series. http://athena.englishh.vt.edu/cgi-bin/netforum/nic/a/14-1.2.2.

74. Posner, M. I. and Rothbart, M. K. (1998) Attention, self regulation and consciousness. *Trans. R. Soc. Lond.* **353**, 1915–1929.

75. Autret, A., Laffont, F., de Toffol, B., and Cathala, H. P. (1988) A syndrome of REM and non-REM sleep reduction and lateral gaze paresis after medial tegmental pontine stroke. Computed tomographic scans and anatomical correlations in four patients. *Arch. Neurol.* **45(11)**, 1236–1242.

76. Plum, F. (1991) Coma and related global disturbances of the human conscious state. In: Jones, E., Peters, P. (eds.), Cerebral cortex. Vol. 9. New York: Plenum Press.

77. Lavie, P., Pratt, H., Scharf, B., Peled, R., and Brown, J. (1984) Localized pontine lesion: nearly total absence of REM sleep. *Neurology* **34(1),** 118–120.

78. Penfield, W. (1952) Epileptic automatism and the centrencephalic integrating system. *Res. Ass. Nerv. Ment. Disc. Proc.* **30,** 513–528.

79. Penfield, W. G. and Jasper, H. H. (1954) Epilepsy and the functional anatomy of the human brain. Boston: Little Brown.

80. Walshe, F. M. R. (1957) The brainstem conceived as the "highest level" of function in the nervous system; with particular reference to the "automatic apparatus" of Carpenter (1850) and to the "centrencephalic integrating system" of Penfield. *Brain* **80,** 510–539.

81. Penfield, W. (1958) Centrencephalic integrating system. *Brain* **81,** 231–234.

82. Thompson, R. (1993) Centrencephalic theory, generalized learning system and subcortical dementia. In: Crinella, F. and Yu, J., (eds.), Brain Mechanisms. New York Academy of Sciences: **702** pp. 197–224.

83. Skinner, J. E. and Yingling, C. D. (1977) Central gating mechanisms that regulate event-related potentials and behavior. In: Desmedt, J. E. (ed.), Progress in clinical neurophysiology. Vol 1. Attention, voluntary contraction, and event-related cerebral potentials. Basel:Karger, pp. 70–96.

84. Schiebel, A. B. (1980) Anatomical and physiological substrates of arousal: view from the bridge. In: Hobson, J. A. and Brazier, M. A. B. (eds.), The Reticular Formation Revisted, (New York, Raven Press).

85. Crick, F. (1984) Function of the thalamic reticular complex: the searchlight hypothesis. *Proc. Natl. Acad. Sci. USA* **81,** 4586–4590.

86. Steriade, M, Timofeev, I., and Grenier, F. (1999) Intracellular activity of various neocortical cell-clasess during the natural sleep-wake cycle. Society for Neuroscience 29th Annual Meeting Abstract 664.14

87. Guillery, R. W., Feig, S. L., and Lozsadi, D. A. (1981) Paying attention to the thalamic reticular nucleus. *Trends Neurosci.* **21,** 28–32.

88. Weese, G. D., Phillips, J. M., and Brown, V. J. (1999) Attentional orienting is impaired by unilateral lesions of the thalamic reticular nucleus in the rat. *J. Neurosci.* **19(22),** 10,135–10,139.

89. Kinomura, S., Larssen, J., Gulyas, B., and Roland, P. E. (1996) Activation by attention of the human reticular formation and thalamic intralaminar nuclei. *Science* **271,** 512–515.

90. Portas, C. M., Rees, G., Howseman, A. M., Josephs, O., Turner, R., and Frith, C. D. (1998) A specific role for the thalamus in mediating the interaction of attention and arousal in humans. *J. Neurosci.* **18(21),** 8979–8989.

91. Glenn, L. L. and Steriade, M. (1982) Discharge rate and excitability of cortically projecting intralaminar neurons during waking and sleep states. *J. Neurosci.* **2(10),** 1387–1404.

92. Pare, D., Smith, Y., Parent, A., and Steriade, M. (1988) Projections of brainstem core cholinergic and non-cholinergic neurons of cat to intralaminar and reticular thalamic nuclei. *Neuroscience* **25(1),** 69–86.

93. Steriade, M., Amzica, F., and Contreras, D. (1996) Slynchronization of fast 30–40 Hz spontaneous cortical rhythms during brain activation. *J. Neurosci.* **16,** 392–417.

94. Steriade, M. and Buzsaki, G. (1990) Parallel activation of thalamic and cortical neurons by brainstem and basal forebrain cholinergic systems. In: Steriade, M., Bliesold, D., (eds.), Brain cholinergic system. New York: Oxford University Press.

95. Vogt, B. A. (1990) The role of layer 1 in cortical function. In: Jones, E. G., Peters, A., (eds.), Cerebral Cortex. Vol. 9. New York: Plenum Press, pp. 49–80.

96. Mair, R. (1994) On the role of thalamic pathology in diencephalic amnesia. *Rev. Neurosci.* **5,** 105–140.

97. Purpura, K. P. and Schiff, N. D. (1997) The thalamic intralaminar nuclei: role in visual awareness. *Neuroscientist* **3,** 8–14.

98. Fuster, J. M. (1973) Unit activity in prefrontal cortex during delayed-response performance: neuronal correlates of transient memory. *J. Neurophysiol.* **36,** 61–78.

99. Schall, J. D. (1991) Neuronal activity related to visually guided saccades in the frontal eye fields of rhesus monkeys: comparison with supplementary eye fields. *J. Neurophysiol.* **66,** 559–579.

100. Friston, K. (1995) Neuronal transients. *Proc. R. Soc. Lond. B.* **261,** 401–405.

101. Llinas, R. and Ribary, U. (1993)Coherent 40-Hz oscillation characterizes dream state in humans. *Proc. Natl. Acad. Sci. USA* **90(5),** 2078–2081.

102. Singer, W. and Gray, C. (1995) Visual feature integration and the temporal correlation hypothesis. *Ann. Rev. Physiol.* **55,** 349–374.
103. Vaadia, E. et al. (1995) Dynamics of neuronal interactions in monkey cortex in relation to behavioural events. *Nature* **373,** 515–518.
104. Schiff, N. D., Purpura, K. P., and Victor, J. D. (1999c) Gating of local network signals appear as stimulus-dependent activity envelopes in striate cortex. *J. Neurophysiol.* **82,** 2182–2196.
105. Mair, R. G., Burk, J. A., and Porter, M. C. (1998) Lesions of the frontal cortex, hippocampus, and intralaminar thalamic nuclei have distinct effects on remembering in rats. *Behav. Neurosci.* **112,** 772–791.
106. Burk, J. A. and Mair, R. G. (1998) Thalamic amnesia reconsidered: excitotoxic lesions of the intralaminar nuclei, but not the mediodorsal nucleus, disrupt place delayed matching-to-sample performance in rats (Rattus norvegicus). *Behav. Neurosci.* **112,** 54–67.
107. Zhang, Y., Burk, J. A., Glode, B. M., and Mair, R. G. (1998) Effects of thalamic and olfactory cortical lesions on contiuous olafactory delayed non-matching-to-sample and olfactory discriminationin rats (Rattus norvegicus). *Behav. Neurosci.* **112,** 39–53.
108. Gaymard, B., Rivaud, and S., Pierrot-Deseilligny (1994) Impairment of extraretinal eye position signals after central thalamic lesions in humans. *Exp. Brain Res.* **102,** 1–9.
109. Schlag, J. and Schlag-Rey, M. (1971) Induction of oculomotor responses from thalamic internal medullary lamina in the cat. *Exp. Neurol.* **33,** 498–508.
110. Orem, J., Schlag-Rey, M., and Schlag, J. (1973) Unilateral visual neglect and thalamic intralaminar lesions in the cat. *Exp. Neurol.* **40,** 784–797.
111. Schlag-Rey, M. and Schlag, J. (1984) Visuomotor functions of central thalamus in monkey. II unit activity related to visual events, targeting and fixation. *J. Neurophysiol.* **40,** 1175–1195.
112. Schlag-Rey, M. and Schlag, J. (1984b) Visuomotor functions of central thalamus in monkey. II. Unit activity related to visual events, targeting and fixation. *J. Neurophysiol.* **40,** 1175–1195.
113. Jahnsen, H. and Llinas, R. (1984) Electrophysiological properties of guinea-pig thalamic neurones: an in vitro study. *J. Physiol.* **349,** 205–226.
114. Macchi, G. and Bentivoglio, M. (1985) The thalamic intralaminar nuclei and the cerebral cortex. In: Jones, E. G. and Peters, A, (eds.), Cerebral Cortex. Vol. 5. New York, Plenum Press, pp. 355–389.
115. Sukov, W. and Barth, D. S. (1998) Three-dimensional analysis of spontaneous and thalamically evoked gamma oscillations in the auditory cortex. *J. Neurophysiol.* **79(6),** 2875–2884.
116. Larkum, M. E., Zhu, J. J., and Sakmann, B. (1999) A new cellular mechanism for coupling inputs arriving at different cortical layers. *Nature,* **398,** 338–341.
117. Schall, J. D. (1991) Neuronal activity related to visually guided saccades in the frontal eye fields of rhesus monkeys: comparison with supplementary eye fields. *J. Neurophysiol.* **66,** 559–579.
118. Andersen, R. (1989) Visual and eye movement functions of the posterior parietal cortex. *Ann. Rev. Neurosci.* **12,** 377–403.
119. Colby, C. L. (1991) The neuroanatomy and neurophysiology of attention. *J. Child Neurol.* **6,** S90–S118.
120. Schiff, N. D., Ribary, U. Plum, F., et al. (1999c) Words without mind. *J. Cogn. Neurosci.* **11,** 650–656.
121. Reeves, A. and Sperling, G. (1986) Attention gating in short-term visual memory. *Psychol. Rev.* **93(2),** 180–206.
122. Sperling, G. and Weichselgartner, E. (1995) Episodic theory of the dynamics of spatial attention. *Psychol. Rev.* **102(3),** 503–532.
123. Barth, D. S. and MacDonald, K. D. (1996) Thalamic modulation of high-frequency oscillating potentials in auditory cortex. *Nature* **383,** 78–81.
124. Amzica, F., Neckelmann, D., and Steriade, M. (1997) Instrumental conditioning of fast (20–50 Hz) oscillation in corticothalamic networks. *Proc. Natl. Acad. Sci. USA* **94,** 1985–1989.
125. Waitzman, D. M., Silakov, V. L., and Cohen, B. (1996) Central mesencephalic reticular formation (cMRF) neurons discharging before and during eye movements. *J. Neurophysiol.* **75(4),** 1546–1572.
126. Newman, J. (1997) Putting the puzzle together Part II. *J. Conscious. Stud.* **4(2),** 100–122.
127. Teitelbaum, J. S. et al. (1990) Neurologic sequelae of domoic acid intoxication due to the ingestion of contaminated mussels. *N. Engl. J. Med.* **322(25),** 1781–1787.
128. Ross, D. T. and Graham, D. I. (1993) Selective loss and selective sparing of neurons in the thalamic reticular nucleus following human cardiac arrest. *J. Cereb. Blood Flow Metab.* **13(4),** 558–567.
129. Veselis, R. A., Reinsel, R. A., Beattie, B. J., et al. (1997) Midazolam changes cerebral blood flow in discrete brain regions: an H2(15)O positron emission tomography study. *Anesthesiology* **87(5),** 1106–1117.
130. Volkow, N. D., Wang, G. J., Hitzemann, R., Fowler, J. S., Pappas, N., Lowrimore, P., Burr, G., Pascani, K., Overall, J., Wolf, A. P. (1995) Depression of thalamic metabolism by lorazepam is associated with sleepiness. *Neuropsychopharmacology* **12(2),** 123–132.
131. Alkire, M. T., Haier, R., and Fallon, J. H. (2000) Toward a unified theory of narcosis. *Conscious. Cogn.* **9,** 370–386.
132. Crick, F. and Koch, C. (1990) Foward a neurobiological theory of consciousness. *Sem. Neurosci.* **2,** 263–275.
133. Llinas, R., Ribary, U., Contreras, D., and Pedroarena, C. (1998) The neuronal basis for consciousness. *Philos. Trans. R. Soc. Lond. B. Biol. Sci.* **353(1377),** 1841–1849.
134. Steriade, M. (2000) Corticothalamic netwarks, oscillations, and plactiaty. *Adv. Neurol.* **77,** 105–134.
135. Plettenberg, H. K. W., Leopold, D. A., Smirnakis, S. M., and Logothetis, N. K. (2000) Perception—related optokinetic responses in the semi–conscious monkey. Society for Nuroscience abstract 2000 #250.11.
136. Angel, A. (1993) Central neuronal pathways and the process of anaesthesia. *Br. J. Anaesth.* **71(1),** 148–163.
137. Cariani, P. (2000) Anesthesia, neural information processing, and conscious awareness. *Conscious. Cogn.* **9,** 387–395.

IV Neural Mechanisms

6

Cerebral Cortex—Anesthetic Action
on the Electroencephalogram

Cellular and Synaptic Mechanisms and Clinical Monitoring

Heath Lukatch and Scott Greenwald

INTRODUCTION

No one will argue with the statement that general anesthetics exert their action by affecting normal brain function. This then begs the question: what exactly is "normal brain function" and how is it affected by general anesthetics? At a reductionist level one may attempt to understand anesthetic effects on the brain by examining anesthetic actions on individual neurons (e.g., spike train frequency), synapses (e.g., amplitude and time course of synaptic currents), and/or ion channels (e.g., activation and inactivation kinetics). While this mode of study will no doubt yield a plethora of useful information (as is documented in *Neural Mechanisms of Anesthesia*), it is likely to tell only part of the story of how general anesthetics evoke their myriad of consciousness altering effects. A more complete understanding of anesthetic effects on the brain will necessitate hypotheses that explain how anesthetics disrupt synchronous and coordinate neuronal network activities that are thought to give rise to emergent brain properties such as consciousness, learning and memory, and the perception of pain.

While our ability to link emergent brain properties with neural network activity and cellular, synaptic and molecular mechanisms is still in its infancy, the arsenal of tools and technologies for elucidating these linkages continues to grow. At the network level, these tools include electroencephalogram (EEG) and magnetoencephalogram (MEG) activity monitoring, as well as functional magnetic resonance imaging (MRI) and position emission tomography (PET) scanning *(1)*. At the cellular and molecular level, these techniques include patch-clamping, single and multi-unit recording, field recording and micro-EEG recording. This chapter will focus on linking anesthetic induced changes in patterned neural network activity (as represented by the EEG) with anesthetic effects on single cell properties (*see* overview). In addition, this chapter will review EEG monitoring techniques for detecting and characterizing behavioral depth of anesthesia in humans as discussed in the section on Methods of Quantifying EEG.

OVERVIEW OF ANESTHETIC EFFECTS ON EEG ACTIVITY
AND SINGLE CELL PROPERTIES

Modern medicine uses multiple agents to invoke clinical anesthesia (e.g., analgesics, sedative-hypnotics and general anesthetics). These agents are known to have unique and stereotypical effects on EEG activity *(2,3)*. For example, opiods at hypnotic levels evoke large amplitude low frequency delta oscillations *(4)*. Alternatively, many volatile and intravenous general anesthetics, as well as

From: *Contemporary Clinical Neuroscience: Neural Mechanisms of Anesthesia*
Edited by: Joseph F. Antognini et al. © Humana Press Inc., Totowa, NJ

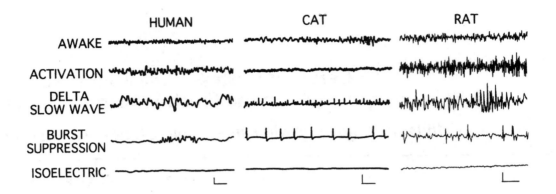

Fig. 1. Anesthetics produce characteristic changes in EEG activity. Thiopental evokes EEG activation, delta activity, burst suppression, and isoelectric activity in multiple species. Calibration bars are 50 μV, 1 s for human; 200 μV, 2 s for cat; 200 μV, 500 ms for rat. (Data adapted from [refs. *9,13,142*]).

benzodiazepines, have been shown to produce biphasic alterations in patterned EEG activity *(5–13)*. These concentration-dependent biphasic EEG changes are characterized by an initial activation period (i.e., increased high frequency activity) followed by EEG slowing, burst suppression and then isoelectric activity* (Fig. 1). Using well-defined clinical end points, this progression of EEG states has been correlated with anesthetic depth *(12–15)*. Specifically for halothane, isoflurane, propofol and barbiturates: Administration of subanesthetic drug concentrations causes EEG activation, characterized by increased power in frequency bands >4 Hz. At anesthetic concentrations that produce sedation and light anesthesia, slow wave delta frequency (1–4 Hz) EEG power is elevated, while power in higher frequency bands (theta 4–8 Hz, alpha 8–13 Hz, beta 13–30 Hz and gamma >30 Hz) is depressed. Anesthetic concentrations capable of producing surgical anesthesia are associated with burst suppression EEG activity, and the highest anesthetic concentrations cause EEG signals to become isoelectric (or "flat-line"). A reverse progression of these EEG states is observed following removal of anesthetic agents.

At the cellular level anesthetics have been shown to produce multiple effects, including: enhanced inhibition *(16–19)*, depressed excitation *(20)*, neuronal hyperpolarization *(21,22)*, and modulation of calcium *(23,24)* and potassium *(25,26)* conductances. Unfortunately little is known about how these anesthetic-induced cellular actions result in altered EEG states such as those described previously. An understanding of the mechanisms responsible for anesthetic-induced alterations in patterned EEG activity will provide insight into basic mechanisms of neuronal synchronization, and it may also help to identify common sites of action important for anesthetic-induced amnesia, unconsciousness and analgesia *(3,27,28)*.

EEG Mechanism Basics

To begin to understand how anesthetic-induced changes in EEG activity may result from anesthetic effects on single neurons and synchronized neuronal activity, it is first necessary to understand the basics of EEG generation. The following four points, while highly simplified, represent key concepts in EEG generation. (1) EEG signals recorded at the skull surface represent the summated activity of hundreds of thousands to millions of neocortical neurons. (2) While EEG rhythms recorded at the

---

*These anesthetic-induced EEG states reflect the effects of individual anesthetic agents on patterned neuronal activity. In many clinical situations, multiple agents are used in combination resulting in more complex and difficult to interpret EEG signals. For simplicity, the remainder of this chapter focusing on anesthetic mechanisms will primarily examine effects of *individual* anesthetic agents on EEG activity and single cell properties.

skull surface are generated by neocortical neurons, these rhythms may originate either in the neocortex itself, or they may be "imposed on" the neocortex by subcortical structures which "pace" the activity of neocortical neurons. (3) Multiple neurotransmitter systems can be involved in generating different types of EEG activity. (4) EEG activity within individual frequency bands (i.e., delta, theta, alpha, beta or gamma) likely represents more than one phenomenon *(29)*.

EPITIDE Theory of Anesthetic Action on Patterned Brain Activity

Ultimately, the specific mechanisms underlying each type of EEG signal will depend on which cell types, anatomical connections and neurotransmitter systems are involved. That being recognized, I (Heath Lukatch) believe that enough evidence exists to piece together a high level hypothesis regarding how anesthetic effects at the cellular level give rise to large scale changes in patterned neuronal network (EEG) activity observed during progressively deeper anesthetic states. I propose that the progressive changes in EEG states associated with increasing levels of anesthesia (i.e., EEG slowing, burst suppression and isoelectric activity*) result from a progressive recruitment of cellular effects beginning with increased phasic inhibition, followed by increased tonic inhibition that is followed by depressed excitatory transmission. I call this hypothesis the EPITIDE (Enhanced Phasic Inhibition, Tonic Inhibition and Depressed Excitation) theory of anesthetic action on patterned brain activity (an outline of this hypothesis was first put forth in Lukatch and MacIver 1996) *(30)*. The remainder of this chapter will expand on, and provide support for the EPITIDE theory.

EGG Slowing

Anesthetic concentrations that produce EEG slowing, (characterized by rising delta [1–4 Hz] power and decreasing power in higher frequency bands), have been shown to increase phasic inhibition. Specifically, these anesthetic concentrations prolong GABA$_A$-mediated inhibitory postsynaptic currents (IPSCs) *(16,19,31,32)*, but they do not directly activate GABAergic currents in the absence of GABA, nor do they change GABA$_A$-mediated IPSC amplitudes. Previous authors have suggested that prolongation of inhibitory currents (which represents enhanced phasic inhibition) may contribute to EEG slowing *(33–35)*. The EPITIDE model of anesthetic action on patterned brain activity expands on these suggestions via the following proposal: Anesthetic-induced prolongation of inhibitory currents may slow EEG activity by limiting neuronal discharge frequencies of EEG-generating neurons (Fig. 2). It is hypothesized that at the network level, this cellular effect could produce a state in which low frequency EEG oscillations (e.g., delta activity) are supported by the network, while higher frequency oscillations are filtered out (much like the activity of a low pass filter in an electronics circuit).

To further understand how prolongation of inhibitory currents may slow EEG activity it is necessary to delve into the neural population dynamics that underlie synchronous oscillatory EEG activity. It has been shown that a majority of neurons discharge preferentially during EEG oscillation peak negativities and are silent during peak positivities (Fig. 2a) *(36)*. Thus, one full EEG oscillation (approximated by 360° of a sine wave), likely represents the synchronous discharge, quiescence and secondary discharge of a neuronal population. Stated another way, the length of time between neuronal population discharges determines the periodicity of an EEG oscillation. What then determines neuronal inter-discharge time intervals? One likely candidate is the time course of GABA$_A$-mediated inhibition (or potentially, a potassium-mediated inhibitory current). As neurons behave in a non-linear fashion (in regard to discharge properties), it is hypothesized that when inhibitory influences on EEG generating neurons are above a certain critical threshold, these neurons will have a low probability of firing. However, as inhibitory currents fall below this threshold, EEG-generating

---

*Early EEG activation associated with low anesthetic concentrations is not addressed in the EPITIDE hypothesis because this EEG state is not associated with clinical levels of anesthesia evoked by halothane, isoflurane, propofol or barbiturates.

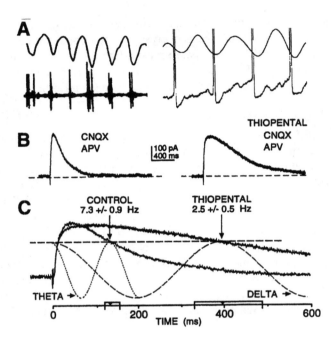

Fig. 2. Mechanisms of EEG slowing: Enhanced Phasic Inhibition **(A)** Neurons typically discharge at the peak negativities of EEG oscillations, with one full EEG oscillation (360°) associated with neural firing, quiescence and secondary discharge. *Left* EEG oscillations (*top*) and extracellular single unit activity (*bottom*: adapted from [ref. *143*]). *Right* EEG oscillations (*top*), and intracellularly recorded neural discharges (*bottom*: adapted from [ref. *144*]) **(B)** Anesthetics prolong evoked inhibitory postsynaptic currents (IPSCs) that have been isolated using glutamate receptor antagonists CNQX and APV (adapted from [ref. *30*]). **(C)** Comparison of IPSC time courses and micro-EEG periodicities. When theta and delta waveforms were plotted against control and thiopental-prolonged IPSCs, it becomes clear that one full oscillation of each waveform intercepts its appropriate IPSC at similar amplitudes (*dashed line*). This amplitude may represent a critical degree of inhibition, above which EEG generating cells may be unable to discharge. Plotted on the time bar below is the mean and standard deviation for each micro-EEG waveform (adapted from [ref. *30*]).

neurons become much more likely to fire action potentials in response to excitatory inputs. This leads to the prediction that the degree of anesthetic-induced EEG slowing should relate to the degree anesthetic-induced prolongation of inhibitory currents (Fig. 2B,C). In support of this hypothesis, it has been demonstrated in brain slices that concentrations of anesthetics that produce a threefold slowing in micro-EEG activity (from theta to delta frequencies) also cause a threefold prolongation in $GABA_A$-mediated currents *(19,30)*. While conceptually intriguing, more experiments will be required to confirm these results.

It should be noted that the focus of this section has been on the effects of general anesthetics on intrinsic neocortical circuitry, however, cortico-thalamo-cortical circuits are known to be involved in generating delta activity during slow wave sleep *(29,37)*. Specifically, transitions from "awake" to "asleep" EEG states have been associated with the hyperpolarization of thalamic neuronal sub-populations thought to participate in "pacing" delta EEG activity *(29)*. Thus, it is possible that in addition to their effects on local neocortical circuitry, anesthetics may contribute to the induction and maintenance of delta EEG oscillations by transiently hyperpolarizing key thalamic (and potentially neocortical) neurons.

Burst Suppression

Previous studies have shown that EEG burst suppression activity occurs during surgical anesthesia *(2,8,9,12,14,38)*. This anesthetic-induced burst suppression activity has been shown to be associated with enhanced tonic inhibition, as demonstrated by increased neocortical neuron hyperpo-

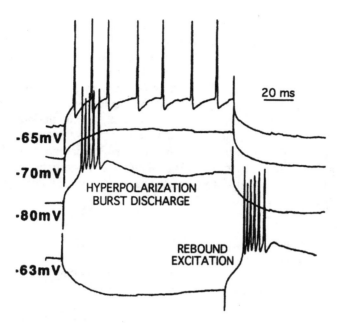

Fig. 3. Mechanisms of EEG burst suppression: Enhanced Tonic Inhibition. Cellular responses to depolarizing and hyperpolarizing current pulses at different membrane potentials. Tonic firing (at –65 mV) was transformed into burst firing as the neuron is hyperpolarized. Burst firing was also triggered at the break of a hyperpolarizing pulse (*bottom trace* –63 mV), likely as a result of removal of membrane potential inactivation from sodium and calcium channels. (adapted from [ref. *126*])

larizations (~10 mV), and reduced neural input resistances observed during anesthetic-induced burst suppression activity in vivo *(39)*. In vitro studies have further elucidated the mechanisms by which anesthetics enhance tonic inhibition. Specifically, anesthetic concentrations that produce burst suppression activity have been shown to hyperpolarize neurons *(21,22)* by increasing chloride *(17,40)* and potassium conductances *(41,42)*.

In the EPITIDE theory of anesthetic action on patterned brain activity, it is hypothesized that hyperpolarization of EEG generating neurons via direct activation of chloride and/or potassium currents *(43)* (which represents enhanced tonic inhibition) produces burst suppression EEG activity by creating conditions in the neural network where EEG generating neurons become *quiescent yet hyperexcitable*. Specifically, the EPITIDE model predicts that hyperpolarization of EEG generating neurons should cause EEG burst suppression activity by way of a combination of the following three mechanisms (Fig. 3): (1) Removal of membrane potential-dependent inactivation from low threshold, voltage-activated calcium and sodium channels *(44)* should make neurons more responsive to excitatory inputs. (2) Decreased tonic discharge frequencies of EEG generating neurons should lead to EEG quiescent periods in which excitatory synaptic transmission between cortical neurons is diminished. During these quiescent periods, fewer neurons should be refractory to firing in response to excitatory inputs. (3) Neuronal discharge patterns should shift from single spikes to burst discharges *(45–47)*, which in turn should provide more concentrated and less frequent excitatory drive for triggering EEG burst events. To summarize, the combination of these three effects (which result from neuronal hyperpolarization brought on by enhanced tonic inhibition) likely evokes burst suppression EEG activity by creating a state in which EEG generating neurons become both quiescent, (leading to periods of suppressed EEG activity), and hyperexcitable, (leading to large amplitude bursts in response to excitatory inputs).

Although it still remains to be proven where the excitatory drive comes from (neocortex versus subcortical structures) that triggers anesthetic-induced EEG bursts during clinical anesthesia, both in vivo *(48)* and in vitro *(30)* studies have clearly demonstrated that neocortex alone is capable of producing and sustaining anesthetic-induced burst suppression activity. Specifically, thiopental-induced burst suppression activity in vivo has been shown to persist in neocortex which has been isolated from ascending inputs by undercutting the white matter, while leaving the blood supply intact *(48,49)*. In addition, the demonstration of thiopental-induced micro-EEG burst suppression activity in a neocortical brain slice preparation in which all ascending glutamatergic afferents were severed strongly suggests that micro-EEG bursts can be triggered by spontaneously active local excitatory neurons within neocortex *(30)*. Work by Steriade has also suggested that anesthetic-induced hyperpolaization of neocortical cells can functionally uncouple the neocortex from thalamic inputs *(39)*. Thus, the evidence strongly suggests that neocortical cells are involved in burst genesis. However, it remains an open question whether there are specific sub-populations of neocortical neurons that are responsible for generating EEG burst events during anesthesia, or if any excitatory neocortical neuron is capable of eliciting this activity.

Isoelectric Activity

At progressively higher anesthetic concentrations in vivo, burst frequencies decrease while interburst EEG suppression durations increase, until such point in time that an isoelectric EEG signal dominates *(2,9,13)*. The EPITIDE model predicts that decreased bursting activity during the transition to isoelectric activity results from an anesthetic-induced depression of excitatory transmission. This mechanism of action is supported by studies showing that clinically relevant anesthetic concentrations depress excitatory transmission (Fig. 4A) in various brain regions *(20,30,50–52)*. In addition, glutamate receptor antagonists have been shown to force transitions from burst suppression to isoelectric micro-EEG activity in a neocortical brain slice model system (Fig. 4B) *(30)*. This mechanism of action is further supported by the finding that isoflurane concentrations that produce isoelectric micro-EEG activity also significantly depress glutamate-mediated excitatory postsynaptic current (EPSC) amplitudes and frequencies (unpublished observations). In summary, the current evidence strongly suggests that depression of excitatory transmission plays a significant role in facilitating the transition from EEG burst suppression activity to EEG isoelectric activity. Further studies will be required to solidify this perspective.

Reconciliation of the EPITIDE Model With Other Theories of Anesthetic Action

The EPITIDE theory of anesthetic action on patterned brain activity is consistent with previous authors' proposals that anesthesia may result from increased inhibitory transmission *(16,18,31,53)* decreased action potential generation via membrane hyperpolarization *(21,41,42)* and/or decreased excitatory transmission *(54–56)*. The EPITIDE theory, by providing a mechanistic description of how anesthetics alter patterned brain activity, also compliments the Multi-site Agent Specific (MAS) theory of anesthetic action *(28,57–59)*, which predicts that concentration-dependent recruitment of separate synaptic and membrane actions leads to deepening levels of anesthesia.

METHODS OF QUANTIFYING EEG

As an introduction to the analysis of EEG, consider the analogous process of analyzing piano music. Notes generated by striking keys on the piano keyboard increase in pitch from left to right (i.e., from lower to higher frequencies.) Imagine that piano notes are pure tones (i.e., sinusoidal waveforms) like those generated by tuning forks. The harder a key is struck, the louder the note and the larger the magnitude and power of that component in the music. If a computer analyzing music kept track of the loudness of each note over some epoch (e.g., 30 s), then it could produce a plot showing the loudness (i.e., power) for each note (i.e., frequency) within the range of the entire keyboard (i.e., spectrum). Such a representation of power vs frequency is a "power spectrum." The loudest notes contributed the greatest power to the music and would have the largest peaks in the power spectrum. A musician, without listening to the music, could look at the power spectrum and discern whether the music was predominantly bass, treble or a mix. "Synthesis" is the process of

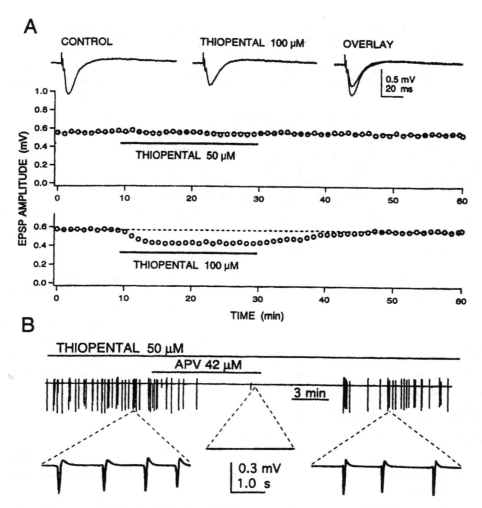

Fig. 4. Mechanisms of EEG isoelectric activity: Depressed Excitation. (**A**) Data traces (*top*) show that 100 μ*M* thiopental depresses evoked field excitatory postsynaptic potentials (EPSPs). Plots (*bottom*) display time course of thiopental effects on EPSPs. Note that 50 μ*M* thiopental (which produces burst suppression micro-EEG activity) does not depress EPSPs, while 100 μ*M* thiopental (which evokes isoelectric EEG activity) does depress EPSPs. (**B**) Anesthetic-induced steady state burst suppression activity can be forced to isoelectric activity with the glutamate receptor antagonist APV.

generating a signal from components, like music from notes. Fourier Analysis is one mathematical tool used for the reverse process of extracting the components from a given signal.

Power spectral analysis, based upon Fourier Analysis, is a traditional method used to analyze segments of EEG signals. Frequency ranges that predominate during specific behavioral states have been identified. For example, beta patterns (13–30 Hz) predominate during mental concentration, while alpha patterns (8–13 Hz) predominate in relaxed states (with eyes closed), or in sleep stage 1. Theta activity (4–8 Hz) occurs in sleep stage 2 and during learning, and delta patterns (<4 Hz) in the deepest stages (3 and 4) of sleep.

Traditional power based methods used to quantify the EEG state include:

1. Calculate absolute power of the delta, theta, alpha and beta bands as well as total power across all these bands.
2. Normalize band powers by total power to generate relative delta, theta, alpha and beta power.

3. Determine uppermost significant EEG frequency (i.e., the upper edge of the spectrum). For example, the frequency below which 95% of the EEG power is contained is called the "95% Spectral Edge Frequency" (i.e., SEF95).
4. Determine central frequency of the EEG (i.e., the frequency that divides the spectrum in half, separating half the power above and below the "median frequency" (MF). MF is equivalent to the 50% spectral edge frequency.

A useful, but limited, approximation of changes in the EEG under anesthesia is that the EEG changes from a predominantly small amplitude, high frequency signal in the awake patient to a large amplitude, low frequency signal in the deeply unconscious patient. The asynchronous activity among the pyramidal cells in the cortical layer of the awake, thinking subject causes spatial cancellation resulting in a low amplitude, high frequency signal (*see* Section on Mechanisms of EEG Generation for more details). Conversely, synchronous activity of cells in the deeply unconscious subject summates creating a large amplitude, low frequency signal. Consequently, as sedated patients become hypnotically deeper, their EEG "slows" resulting in decreased beta power, increased delta power, and the resultant decrease in spectral edge and median frequency.

Exceptions to this simple approximation occur at the lightest and deepest hypnotic levels. At the light hypnotic range, initial low doses of many anesthetic agents (e.g., inhalational agents, benzodiazipines, and barbiturates) elicit EEG activation, subsequently followed by slowing as agent concentration increases. This results in a biphasic dose response of many power-based metrics rendering them useless at the light anesthetic range *(60)*. For example, the same SEF95 value will occur at two different clinical states (e.g., awake and unconscious.) In addition, power-based variables are typically unstable during periods of burst-suppression EEG activity because of the intermittent changes in distribution of power. Consequently, power based methods historically have been unsuccessful in quantifying the full range of anesthesia.

EEG Activity Clinical Correlates

Consciousness and Memory vs Analgesia

The first reported observation by Gibbs et al. *(61)*, in 1937 of anesthetic-induced changes in spontaneous EEG activity raised a fundamental question: What clinically relevant information was reflected by the change in EEG? That is, does the EEG state reflect the patient's analgesic state, hypnotic state, or something else? Results from both human and animal studies demonstrate that changes in EEG with anesthesia primarily reflect hypnotic, not analgesic, information. For example, administration of low dose opioids to patients increases analgesia but not hypnosis. Such doses profoundly affect the probability of movement or hemodynamic response to skin incision (i.e., a classic analgesic endpoint), but do not affect the EEG *(62)*. Conversely, small doses of hypnotic agents (e.g., propofol) profoundly affect the EEG, but marginally affect the probability of response to skin incision. Moreover, in the absence of painful stimulation, changes in EEG are predictive of reawakening from anesthesia, but blood pressure and heart rate are not predictive *(63)*.

Corroborating evidence from two animal studies support these conclusions. Antognini *(64)* surgically prepared 6 goats in which the circulation to the head could be isolated from the rest of body. He determined minimum alveolar concentration (MAC) when administering isoflurane to the whole animal ($1.2 \pm 1.3\%$) and to the head alone ($2.9 \pm 0.7\%$). The exaggerated anesthetic requirement when anesthetizing the brain alone demonstrates that subcortical structures are important in the response to painful stimulation. Moreover, Rampil et al. *(65)* determined that the MAC of isoflurane in rats initially intact ($1.30 \pm 0.25\%$) was unchanged following aspirated decerebration ($1.26 \pm 0.14\%$). These results demonstrate that the movement response to noxious stimulus does not depend upon forebrain structures.

Conversely, memory formation and recollection are aspects of the hypnotic state. For example, a composite of the relationships between the EEG Bispectral Index (described in the section on Bispectral Analysis and the BIS) and the probability of explicit and implicit recall (and unconscious

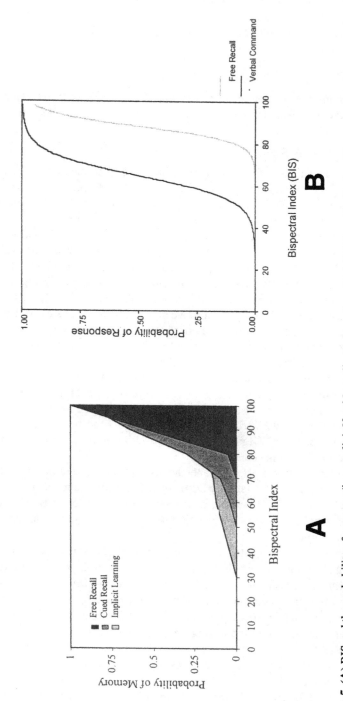

Fig. 5. (A) BIS and the probability of memory (i.e., explicit [frank] recall, cued recall, and implicit learning [i.e., auditory processing]). Lower BIS scores are associated with a lower probability of memory formation and/or recall. (B) BIS and the probabilities of explicit recall and response to verbal command. There is a range of consciousness (e.g., BIS between 70 and 80) where patients are likely to respond to verbal command, but unlikely to form memory that will be explicitly recalled. (Figure 5A is a composite of information gleaned from research that evaluated BIS and memory function (*66–69*). Figure 5 B is adapted from [ref. *66*]).

101

learning) *(66–69)* is shown in Fig. 5A. In order to consolidate memory for explicit recall, patients generally need to be at a level of consciousness that is higher than the minimum consciousness level needed to elicit response to a verbal command (Fig. 5B). Thus the current data supports the hypothesis that anesthetic-induced changes in EEG activity generally reflects changes in the hypnotic, not analgesic, state of the subject.

Modern EEG Monitoring Methods and Limitations

This section will summarize current EEG derived measures, including the Bispectral Index (BIS), entropy, complexity, fractal dimension, and auditory evoked potentials (AEPs), as measures of hypnotic state.

Bispectral Analysis and the BIS

Fourier Analysis of an EEG segment estimates the magnitude and phase of each sinusoidal component for all frequencies. (Magnitude is the absolute value of amplitude. Phase is the fraction of a period time shift relative to the start of the EEG segment.) Power spectral analysis evaluates power information (i.e., the square of the magnitude), but ignores phase information. Power analysis quantifies information about individual components, ignoring information about other components. In contrast, Bispectral Analysis examines the first order nonlinear relationships among the components within the EEG *(70)*. It quantifies the phase coupling (i.e., bicoherence), power coupling (i.e., real triple product), and the effects of phase cancellation on power coupling (i.e., bispectrum.)

Mathematically, the product of a pair of sinusoids of frequencies f1 and f2 produces four sinusoids: two at the frequencies of the original pair, and two at the sum (f1 + f2) and difference frequencies of the original pair. An analysis of the power and phase relationships between three frequency triplets (f1, f2, f1 + f2) will identify whether the component at the sum frequency (f1 + f2) exists from a nonlinear interaction (i.e., multiplication) between the original pair (at frequencies f1 and f2) or whether the component exists independently of the original pair. Bispectral analysis quantifies these relationships among all sets of frequency triplets of the form (f1, f2, f1 + f2) within the EEG. The display of the bispectral metrics (e.g., bispectrum) requires a three dimensional plot: the vertical axis displays the bispectral value above a triangular domain of possible base frequency pairs (f1, f2). Figure 6 shows the change in the EEG, power spectrum and bispectrum for three clinical states of a subject undergoing propofol anesthesia.

The BIS is the first measure of the effect of anesthetics on the brain that has been approved by the Food and Drug Administration. As of January 2001, over 2.5 million anesthetic cases have utilized BIS monitoring, and the use of BIS has been described in over 500 scientific abstracts and manuscripts. Recent review articles describe the development *(70,71)*, clinical validation *(72,73)*, and utility *(74–76)* of the technology.

The Bispectral Index, derived substantially from bispectral EEG descriptors, monitors the hypnotic state of patients during sedation and anesthesia. BIS was developed by combining EEG descriptors that correlated with clinical assessments of consciousness level (*see* Table 1) and were common to a variety of anesthetic agents (i.e., combinations of propofol, midazolam, isoflurane, methohexital, nitrous oxide, and opioids.) The EEG descriptors that comprise BIS are shown in Table 2. An example of the change in these descriptors with increasing propofol anesthesia is tabulated in Fig. 6.

BIS is a composite EEG metric scaled from 100 (wide awake) to 0 (no cortical activity). BIS decreases monotonically with increasing level of hypnotic drug across the full range of hypnotic states, independently of agent (with the exception of the dissociative agent ketamine *[77]*), and is not significantly effected by analgesics. Subjects maintained below 70 have a very low probability of explicit recall (Figs. 5A, B); likewise, subjects with BIS maintained below 60 have a very low probability of responding to verbal command (i.e., being conscious.) (Fig. 5B). In a multicenter study, comparing patients managed using BIS vs standard practice, patients monitored with BIS used less

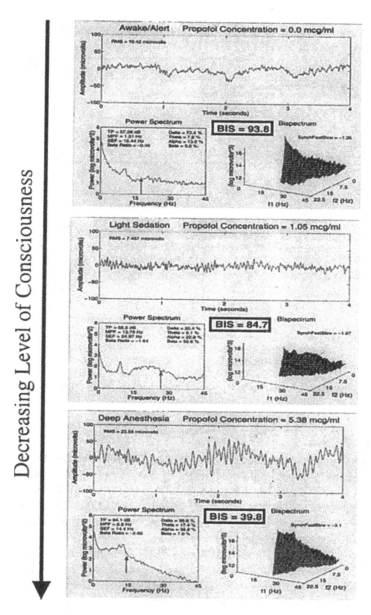

Fig. 6. Changes with increasing sedation in the EEG signal, Power Spectrum, Bispectrum, and components of the BIS (Figure adapted from Rampil *[71]*).

hypnotic agent, woke up faster, were eligible for discharge sooner, and had better recovery scores *(78)*. The use of BIS monitoring to titrate the hypnotic component of anesthesia has been demonstrated to reduce direct and indirect costs, improve post-operative recovery, and monitor for the risk of awareness. When used in conjunction with traditional clinical signs, this additional information allows clinicians to titrate their anesthetic agents to achieve the optimal level of anesthetic through appropriate drug selection and individual agent titration. Recent review articles detail the clinical application of BIS monitoring during anesthesia *(5,79)*.

Table 1
Sedation Level Score assigned using the Modified Observer's Assessment of Sedation Scale

Clinical sedation assessment	Score
Immediate response to name spoken in normal tone.	5
Lethargic response to name spoken in normal tone.	4
Responds only after name is called repeatedly or loudly.	3
Responds only after mild prodding or shaking.	2
Does not respond after mild prodding or shaking.	1

Table 2
Components of the BIS

Name	Description
Beta Ratio	$Log(P_{30-47}/P_{11-20})$
SyncFastSlow	$Log(B_{0.5-47}/B_{40-47})$
QuaziSuppression	
Suppression Ratio	Measures of suppressed EEG within the preceding minute

P_{x-y} is the sum of the spectral power within x and y Hz. B_{x-y} is the sum of the Bispectrum in the area subtended from frequency x to y on both axes. The domain of the bispectrum is triangular due to symmetry conditions and a limit on the highest frequency in the EEG (i.e., half the sampling rate).

Recent Developments

Alternate nonlinear analysis methods, such as entropy, complexity, and fractal dimension, have been employed to quantify structure and predictability within the EEG. Initial work in evaluating these metrics as measures of anesthetic effect has recently been reported. The underlying motivation for the application of these methods stems from the observation that the EEG appears to be a random, desynchronized, high frequency signal in awake states but becomes a predictable, synchronous signal in hypnotically deep states (e.g., delta patterns.)

Entropy quantifies the degree of regularity in the EEG. Estimates of entropy include: Approximate Entropy (ApEn) *(80)*, Shannon Entropy *(81)*, and Spectral Entropy *(82)*. ApEn quantifies the predictability of subsequent EEG given the recent history of EEG. Sleigh and Donnovan evaluated ApEn, BIS and SEF95 at intraoperative endpoints in patients undergoing isoflurane/N20 anesthesia *(83)*. Although ApEn correlated with hypnotic changes, its ability to differentiate awake/sleep states was worse than SEF95, and both were worse than BIS. Bruhn et al., evaluated the Desflurane dose-response relationship of ApEn, BIS, SEF95 and MF *(84)*. ApEn decreased (i.e., regularity increased) continuously with increasing endtidal desflurane concentration. The predictive probability (P_k) of ApEn to predict desflurane concentration (0.86 ± 0.06) was similar to that of BIS and SEF95, but significantly better than MF. (The possible range of P_k is between 0 and 1, where 1 indicates perfect prediction. A fair coin toss has a P_k of 0.5 for predicting the toss outcome *[85]*). Shannon Entropy quantifies the skewness of the amplitude sequences observed within the EEG. Bruhn et al., recently repeated his previous analysis employing Shannon, rather than ApEn and found similar results in predicting desflurane concentration *(86)*.

Complexity is also a measure of regularity, or repeatability, within the EEG. Ziv-Lempel complexity yields the number of distinct patterns within an EEG segment that must be copied to reproduce the EEG segment. The fewer the patterns, the lower the complexity, and the greater the possible data compression. Using a convenience sample of 27 vascular surgery patients undergoing isoflurane, sevoflurane, desflurane, or propofol general anesthesia, Roy and Zhang retrospectively determined a 93% accuracy in predicting sedation level assessed using the Observer's Assessment of Alertness/ Sedation Scale *(87)*.

Fractal dimension quantifies the number of (non-integer, or fractional) dimensions needed to represent the character of the EEG signal *(88)*. A signal that is completely repeatable would require fewer dimensions (i.e., degrees of freedom) to represent the state of the system compared with a signal that is random. In a pilot study of 17 subjects undergoing sevoflurane anesthesia, Widman et al., found that the correlation dimension decreased with increasing sevoflurane, even during burst-suppression patterns *(89)*.

In a comparison of all these methods, Viertio-Oja et al., evaluated Spectral Entropy, ApEn, complexity, fractal dimension and BIS at sedation assessments using the OAAS scale for 150 patients undergoing general anesthesia using propofol, sevoflurane and N2O. They report that all the metrics decreased with decreasing level of consciousness. Spectral Entropy performed best of the entropy and complexity measures, and similar to BIS *(90)*.

Auditory Evoked Potentials

The electrical signature generated in the EEG in response to an auditory stimulus (e.g., a click), is the Auditory Evoked Potential (AEP). Typically, the responses to a rapid sequence of clicks are averaged over time to bring out the small potential buried within the background, spontaneous EEG. The mid-latency AEP (i.e., MLAEP, 20–80 ms after stimulus) shows graded change with increasing dose of hypnotic agents, but shows little change with opioid analgesics. Because most auditory processing ceases with unconsciousness, features extracted from AEPS have been evaluated as potential indicators of hypnotic level *(91–95)*.

Dutton et al. *(96)*, evaluated MLAEP features as predictors of response to verbal command during desflurane and propofol anesthesia. Increasing anesthesia decreased the power of the 40 Hz component, and increased latencies and decreased amplitudes of the primary peaks in the MLAEP (i.e., Na, Pa, and Nb peaks). The power of the 40 Hz component best predicted wakefulness ($P_k = 0.96$) compared to linear combinations of amplitudes and latencies of Na, Pa, and Nb peaks.

Iselin-Chaves, et al. *(97)*, evaluated MLAEP features for predicting loss of consciousness, and for correlating sedation scores with propofol concentration during propofol or propofol and alfentanil anesthesia. MLAEP features (i.e., amplitude and latencies of Pa and Nb peaks) correlated significantly with sedation score ($p < 0.0001$) and were unaffected by the addition of the alfentanil analgesic. Pa and Nb peak latencies predicted loss of consciousness better than peak amplitudes. Mantzaridis and Kenny *(98)* have derived an index from the MLAEP incorporating both amplitude and frequency content called the auditory evoked potential index (AEPidx). AEPidx was comparable to Nb peak latencies in distinguishing consciousness and unconsciousness.

The A-line® Monitor (Danmeter, Denmark) is an emerging MLAEP-based technology. The A-line ARX Index (AAI) employs autoregressive modeling of the AEP signature. This processing requires fewer AEP observations to extract AEP features, thereby increasing its responsiveness to changes in patient state. Initial reports of the AAI indicate that it distinguishes well between consciousness and unconsciousness during propofol anesthesia *(99)*, and correlates with expired sevoflurane concentration *(100)*.

Comparison of Spontaneous and Auditory Evoked EEGs as Hypnotic Measures

Two studies compared the performance of hypnotic measures derived from evoked and spontaneous EEG. Iselin-Chaves et al. *(97)*, reported that BIS correlated significantly better with sedation score and propofol concentration than did MLAEP features ($p < 0.05$). Likewise, BIS predicted loss of consciousness ($P_k = 0.95$) at least as well as what was predicted by Pa and Nb peak latencies, and significantly better than predictions based on Pa and Nb peak amplitudes. Mantzaridis and Kenny *(98)* reported that the AEPidx performed better than BIS in detecting return of consciousness following sedation *(101)*. However, Doi et al. *(102,103)*, demonstrated that BIS correlated better than AEPidx with propofol concentration during emergence from anesthesia. Thus, MLAEP derivatives are good indicators of the transition between consciousness and unconsciousness. But because they have limited dynamic range once subjects are unconscious, MLAEP derivatives do not correlate as well with levels of sedation as do derivatives of spontaneous EEG.

Ultimately, for MLAEP-based indices to become clinically more applicable, future research will need to evaluate whether the relationship between MLAEP-based indices and sedation level is independent of anesthetic agent (or agent combinations), monotonic with agent concentration, and equivalent across a wide variety of patient populations. Other than the obvious exception of the hearing impaired patient, MLAEP-based indices may prove to be suitable indicators of the conscious/unconscious state.

SUMMARY AND CONCLUSION

In summary, we have endeavored to put together a comprehensive picture of anesthetic effects on EEG activity. At the cellular and synaptic level we postulate, via the EPITIDE theory of anesthetic action on patterned brain activity, that anesthetic-induced EEG slowing, burst suppression and isoelectric activity can be accounted for (at least in part) owing to a concentration dependent recruitment of enhanced phasic inhibition, followed by enhanced tonic inhibition, followed by depressed excitation.

Anesthetic induced changes in EEG activity primarily reflect changes in the hypnotic state of the patient. Computerized interpretation of EEG signals provides a tool to manage the hypnotic component of the patient's anesthesia. Although various modalities may prove to be useful for monitoring patient anesthesia, to date only BIS monitoring has been extensively validated in controlled, randomized trials as well as in routine clinical practice. The use of BIS monitoring to titrate the hypnotic component of anesthesia has been demonstrated to reduce costs, improve postoperative recovery, and monitor for the risk of intraoperative awareness.

APPENDIX

Mechanisms of EEG Generation

EEG Physics and Physiology

EEG recordings are thought to monitor electrical activity from hundreds of thousands to millions of neocortical neurons located directly below the skull surface. The prevailing view is that EEG activity represents time varying extracellular potentials that arise from synchronized dendritic currents in large populations of similarly aligned pyramidal neurons *(104)*. At the single neuron level, two main factors contribute to EEG signals recorded at the skull surface; (1) current source magnitude, and (2) current source distance from the EEG recording electrode. Current source magnitude depends on the number of ions which cross a unit area of membrane in a given time period. When ion channels open, many ions flow across a small area of cell membrane in a short period of time, (provided that there is sufficient permeability and electromotive driving force for these ions). This results in a transient and focal separation of charge extracellularly. It is this brief separation of charge that creates well-localized electric dipole moments outside of the neuronal membrane. When many such electric dipole moments are synchronously generated and aligned, these signals summate and are recorded as EEG activity at the skull surface.

In individual neurons, current flows via both active and passive current sources. Conduits for active neuronal current sources include synaptic and voltage activated ion channels, whereas open and "leak" channels provide the permeability for passive current sources. When ligand or voltage activated ion channels open, well-localized currents actively and rapidly sink into neurons creating large focal electric dipole moments. To complete the circuit, current passively sources out to the extracellular space across the membrane resistance, including "leak" channels in dendritic and somatic membranes. These passive currents also give rise to electric dipole moments. However, since ions returning to the current source can pass almost anywhere along the membrane surface, they generally pass over a much larger neuronal membrane area than what they entered through. Therefore, electric dipole moments associated with passive current sources tend to be significantly smaller than those associated with active current sources. Thus, one would predict that scalp recorded EEG activity likely reflects summated activity of active rather than passive current sources.

This is not the whole story however. Physics tells us that electric dipole moment voltage (V) is proportional to one over radius (r) squared: $V \simeq 1/r^2$. As a result of this relationship, scalp recorded EEG signals not only depend on current source magnitudes, but also on the distance that a current source is from the EEG recording electrode. This suggests that active current sources in superficial neocortical layers make the most significant contributions to scalp monitored EEG activity. However, deep layer activity, such as that represented by corticocortical synapse activation in layer 5, is also likely to be represented in scalp recorded EEG signals. In this case, current that actively sinks into neurons in deep cortical layers passively sources out from these neurons in superficial cortical layers. Under these circumstances, the close proximity of passive current sources to EEG recording electrodes would result in EEG signals that reflect passive superficial current sources, rather than deep active current sources. To summarize, scalp recorded EEG activity represents the instantaneous summated activity of multiple electric dipole moments generated by active and passive current sources located throughout the cortical axis, with the most significant contributions coming from current sources located in superficial cortical layers.

Once again, however, this is not the whole story. There are at least three other factors that complicate EEG signal interpretation. The first is that human neocortex is not a planar sheet, instead it is series of ridges (gyri) and invaginations (sulci). This structure materially influences scalp recorded EEG signals by imposing physical constraints on the alignment (and by extension summation or cancellation) of cortically generated electric dipoles. The second factor relates to how EEG signals propagate through cortical matter. Specifically, the proportionality constant ($\simeq$) in the equation ($V \simeq 1/r^2$), is dependent on the dielectric constant of the neuronal tissue (and skull) located between an electric dipole moment and the EEG recording electrode, and this dielectric constant is large and activity dependent. The third factor has to do with how EEG signals are recorded. While it is clear that there is significant heterogeneity in signals generated in different neocortical areas *(105)*, these spatial differences tend to be "blurred out" in typical human EEG recordings that use only a small number of electrodes to measure "gross" brain activity. For a more detailed and quantitative explanation of EEG generation and recording, and its many nuances, the reader is referred to (ref. *1*).

EEG Anatomy and Pharmacology

As described above, scalp recorded EEG signals (such as those monitored during surgical anesthesia), primarily reflect synchronous neuronal activity from the neocortex. At the gross structural level, neocortical synchrony may result from either intrinsic or extrinsic influences. Early studies seeking to address the autonomous nature of neocortical EEG activity yielded conflicting results. Some subcortical regions appeared important for neocortical EEG activity *(106,107)*, while others did not *(108,109)*. In 1949, isolated neocortex was shown to generate rhythmic electrical activity in the 5–12 Hz (theta/alpha) frequency range *(110)*. This result proved that neocortex possesses intrinsic neuronal circuitry capable of sustaining EEG oscillations similar to those observed in intact brains.

More recent studies using intracellular and single unit recordings from various brain regions have yielded a wealth of information regarding the interplay and autonomy of individual cortical structures involved in the generation of different EEG rhythms. For example: theta oscillations appear to critically depend upon ponto-septo-hippocampal structures *(36,111–116)*; delta activity and sleep spindles appear to require cortico-thalamo-cortical feedback loops *(47,117–123)* and neocortical slow oscillations appear to be generated within the neocortex itself *(124–126)*. In addition, the advent of induced rhythmical neuronal oscillations in brain slices *(30,127–134)*, and the ability to perform whole cell recordings in vivo *(135,136)*, have afforded neuroscientists an opportunity to study specific ionic currents that may contribute to synchronous rhythmical EEG activity. Studies using these in vivo and in vitro preparations have demonstrated that different cortical structures sustain synchronous oscillatory activity via a variety of mechanisms *(33,46,122,126,131,132,137–141)*.

ACKNOWLEDGMENTS

The authors would like to acknowledge the kind assistance provided by Frances Monroe and Dr. Bruce MacIver in preparing this chapter.

REFERENCES

1. Nunez, P. L. (1995) Neocortical Dynamics and Human EEG Rhythms. Chapter 1, Oxford University Press, New York.
2. Clark, D. L. and Rosner, B. S. (1973) Neurophysiologic effects of general anesthetics. I. The electroencephalogram and sensory evoked responses in man. *Anesthesiology* **38,** 564–582.
3. Stanski, D. R. (1994) Monitoring depth of anesthesia. In: Miller, R. D., (ed.), *Anesthesia*, Churchill Livingstone, New York, pp. 1127–1159.
4. Bovill, J. G., Sebel, P. S., Wauquier, A., Rog, P., and Schuyt, H. C. (1983) Influence of high-dose alfentanil anaesthesia on the electroencephalogram: correlation with plasma concentrations. *Brit. J. Anaesth.* **55 Suppl. 2,** 199S–209S.
5. Black, S., Mahla, M. E., and Cucchiara, R. F. (2000) Neurologic Monitoring, In: Miller, R. D. (ed.), *Anesthesia*, Churchill Livingstone, New York, pp. 1324–1350.
6. Winters, W. D. (1982) A review of the continuum of drug-induced states of excitation and depresssion. *Prog. Drug Res.* **26,** 225–258.
7. Levy, W. J. (1986) Power spectrum correlates of changes in consciousness during anesthetic induction with enflurane. *Anesthesiology* **64,** 688–693.
8. Reddy, R. V., Moorthy, S. S., Mattice, T., Dierdorf, S. F., and Deitch, R. D., Jr. (1992) An electroencephalographic comparison of effects of propofol and methohexital. *Electroencephalogr. Clin. Neurophysiol.* **83,** 162–168.
9. Tomoda, K., Shingu, K., Osawa, M., Murakawa, M., and Mori, K. (1993) Comparison of CNS effects of propofol and thiopentone in cats. *Brit. J. Anaesth.* **71,** 383–387.
10. Thomsen, C. E. and Prior, P. F. (1996) Quantitative EEG in assessment of anaesthetic depth: comparative study of methodology. *Brit. J. Anaesth.* **77,** 172–178.
11. Stanski, D. R., Hudson, R. J., Homer, T. D., Saidman, L. J., and Meathe, E. (1984) Pharmacodynamic modeling of thiopental anesthesia. *J. Pharmacokinet. Biopharm.* **12,** 223–240.
12. Gustafsson, L. L., Ebling, W. F., Osaki, E., and Stanski, D. R. (1996) Quantitation of depth of thiopental anesthesia in the rat. *Anesthesiology* **84,** 415–427.
13. MacIver, M. B., Mandema, J. W., Stanski, D. R., and Bland, B. H. (1996) Thiopental uncouples hippocampal and cortical synchronized electroencephalographic activity. *Anesthesiology* **84,** 1411–1424.
14. Ebling, W. F., Danhof, M., and Stanski, D. R. (1991) Pharmacodynamic characterization of the electroencephalographic effects of thiopental in rats. *J. Pharmacokinet. Biopharm.* **19,** 123–143.
15. Buhrer, M., Maitre, P. O., Hung, O. R., Ebling, W. F., Shafer, S. L., and Stanski, D. R. (1992) Thiopental pharmacodynamics. I. Defining the pseudo-steady-state serum concentration-EEG effect relationship. *Anesthesiology* **77,** 226–236.
16. Nicoll, R. A., Eccles, J. C., Oshima, T., and Rubia, F. (1975) Prolongation of hippocampal inhibitory postsynaptic potentials by barbiturates. *Nature* **258,** 625–627.
17. Barker, J. L. and Mathers, D. A. (1981) GABA receptors and the depressant action of pentobarbital. *TINS* **4,** 10–13.
18. Jones, M. V. and Harrison, N. L. (1993) Effects of volatile anesthetics on the kinetics of inhibitory postsynaptic currents in cultured rat hippocampal neurons. *J. Neurophysiol.* **70,** 1339–1349.
19. Lukatch, H. S. and MacIver, M. B. (1997) Voltage-clamp analysis of halothane effects on GABA(A fast) and GABA(A slow) inhibitory currents. *Brain Res.* **765,** 108–112.
20. MacIver, M. B., Amagasu, S. M., Mikulec, A. A., and Monroe, F. A. (1996) Riluzole anesthesia: use-dependent block of presynaptic glutamate fibers. *Anesthesiology* **85,** 626–634.
21. Nicoll, R. A. and Madison, D. V. (1982) General anesthetics hyperpolarize neurons in the vertebrate central nervous system. *Science* **217,** 1055–1057.
22. MacIver, M. B. and Kendig, J. J. (1991) Anesthetic effects on resting membrane potential are voltage-dependent and agent-specific. *Anesthesiology* **74,** 83–88.
23. Mody, I., Tanelian, D. L., and MacIver, M. B. (1991) Halothane enhances tonic neuronal inhibition by elevating intracellular calcium. *Brain Res.* **538,** 319–323.
24. Larsen, M., Grøndahl, T. O., Haugstad, T. S., and Langmoen, I. A. (1994) The effect of the volatile anesthetic isoflurane on Ca^{2+}-dependent glutamate release from rat cerebral cortex. *Brain Res.* **663,** 335–337.
25. Carlen, P. L., Gurevich, N., Davies, M. F., Blaxter, T. J., and O'Beirne, M. (1985) Enhanced neuronal K+ conductance: a possible common mechanism for sedative-hypnotic drug action. *Can. J. Physiol. Pharmacol.* **63,** 831–837.

26. Franks, N. P. and Lieb, W. R. (1988) Volatile general anaesthetics activate a novel neuronal K+ current. *Nature* **333**, 662–664.
27. Pinsker, M. C. (1986) Anesthesia: a pragmatic construct. *Anesth. Analg.* **65**, 819–820.
28. Kissin, I. (1993) General anesthetic action: an obsolete notion? *Anesth. Analg.* **76**, 215–218.
29. Amzica, F. and Steriade, M. (1998) Electrophysiological correlates of sleep delta waves. *Electroencephalogr. Clin. Neurophysiol.* **107**, 69–83.
30. Lukatch, H. S. and MacIver, M. B. (1996) Synaptic mechanisms of thiopental-induced alterations in synchronized cortical activity. *Anesthesiology* **84**, 1425–1434.
31. MacIver, M. B., Tanelian, D. L., and Mody, I. (1991) Two mechanisms for anesthetic-induced enhancement of GABAA-mediated neuronal inhibition. *Ann. N. Y. Acad. Sci.* **625**, 91–96.
32. Tanelian, D. L., Kosek, P., Mody, I., and MacIver, M. B. (1993) The role of the GABAA receptor/chloride channel complex in anesthesia. *Anesthesiology* **78**, 757–776.
33. Whittington, M. A., Traub, R. D., and Jefferys, J. G. (1995) Erosion of inhibition contributes to the progression of low magnesium bursts in rat hippocampal slices. *J. Physiol. (Lond.)* **486**, 723–734.
34. Jefferys, J. G., Traub, R. D., and Whittington, M. A. (1996) Neuronal networks for induced "40 Hz" rhythms. *Trends Neurosci.* **19**, 202–208.
35. Sannita, W. G. (2000) Stimulus-specific oscillatory responses of the brain: a time/frequency-related coding process. *Clin. Neurophysiol.* **111**, 565–583.
36 Bland, B. H. (1986) The physiology and pharmacology of hippocampal formation theta rhythms. *Prog. Neurobiol.* **26**, 1–54.
37. Lopes da Silva, F. (1991) Neural mechanisms underlying brain waves: from neural membranes to networks. *Electroencephalogr. Clin. Neurophysiol.* **79**, 81–93.
38. Mori, K. (1973) Excitation and depression of CNS electrical activities induced by general anesthetics. In: Miyasaki, M., Iwatsuki, K., and Fujita, M., (eds.), *Proceedings of the 5th World Congress of Anaesthesiology*, Excerpta Medica, Amsterdam, pp. 40–53.
39. Steriade, M., Amzica, F., and Contreras, D. (1994) Cortical and thalamic cellular correlates of electroencephalographic burst-suppression. *Electroencephalogr. Clin. Neurophysiol.* **90**, 1–16.
40. Schulz, D. W. and Macdonald, R. L. (1981) Barbiturate enhancement of GABA-mediated inhibition and activation of chloride ion conductance: correlation with anticonvulsant and anesthetic actions. *Brain Res.* **209**, 177–188.
41. Sato, M., Austin, G. M., and Yai, H. (1967) Increase in permeability of the postsynaptic membrane to potassium produced by "nembutal". *Nature* **215**, 1506–1508.
42. Berg-Johnsen, J. and Langmoen, I. A. (1990) Mechanisms concerned in the direct effect of isoflurane on rat hippocampal and human neocortical neurons. *Brain Res.* **507**, 28–34.
43. Yost, C. S., Gray, A. T., Winegar, B. D., and Leonoudakis, D. (1998) Baseline K+ channels as targets of general anesthetics: studies of the action of volatile anesthetics on TOK1. *Toxicol. Lett.* **100–101**, 293–300.
44. Hille, B. (1992) Classical biophysics of the squid giant axon, Na and K channels of axons, calcium channels, Sinauer Associates Inc., Sunderland, MA.
45. Llinás, R., and Jahnsen, H. (1982) Electrophysiology of mammalian thalamic neurones in vitro. *Nature* **297**, 406–408.
46. Llinás, R. and Yarom, Y. (1986) Oscillatory properties of guinea-pig inferior olivary neurones and their pharmacological modulation: an in vitro study. *J. Physiol. (Lond.)* **376**, 163–182.
47. Steriade, M., Gloor, P., Llinás, R. R., Lopes de Silva, F. H., and Mesulam, M. M. (1990) Report of IFCN Committee on Basic Mechanisms. Basic mechanisms of cerebral rhythmic activities. *Electroencephalogr. Clin. Neurophysiol.* **76**, 481–508.
48. Swank, R. L. (1949) Synchronization of spontaneous electrical activity of cerebrum by barbiturate narcosis. *J. Neurophysiol.* **12**, 161–172.
49. Henry, C. E. and Scoville, W. B. (1952) Supression-burst activity from isolated cerebral cortex in man. *Electroencephalogr. Clin. Neurophysiol.* **4**, 1–22.
50. Richards, C. D. and White, A. E. (1975) The actions of volatile anaesthetics on synaptic transmission in the dentate gyrus. *J. Physiol. (Lond.)* **252**, 241–257.
51. Richards, C. D., Russell, W. J., and Smaje, J. C. (1975) The action of ether and methoxyflurane on synaptic transmission in isolated preparations of the mammalian cortex. *J. Physiol. (Lond.)* **248**, 121–142.
52. Berg-Johnsen, J. and Langmoen, I. A. (1992) The effect of isoflurane on excitatory synaptic transmission in the rat hippocampus. *Acta Anaesthesiol. Scand.* **36**, 350–355.
53. Gage, P. W. and Robertson, B. (1985) Prolongation of inhibitory postsynaptic currents by pentobarbitone, halothane and ketamine in CA1 pyramidal cells in rat hippocampus. *Brit. J. Pharmacol.* **85**, 675–681.
54. Barker, J. L. (1975) Selective depression of postsynaptic excitation by general anesthetics. In: Fink, B. R. (ed.), Molecular Mechanisms of Anesthesia, Progress in Anesthesiology, Raven Press, New York, pp. 135–153.
55. Anis, N. A., Berry, S. C., Burton, N. R., and Lodge, D. (1983) The dissociative anaesthetics, ketamine and phencyclidine, selectively reduce excitation of central mammalian neurones by *N*-methyl-aspartate. *Brit. J. Pharmacol.* **79**, 565–575.
56. Kullmann, D. M., Martin, R. L., and Redman, S. J. (1989) Reduction by general anaesthetics of group Ia excitatory postsynaptic potentials and currents in the cat spinal cord. *J. Physiol. (Lond.)* **412**, 277–296.
57. Kissin, I., Mason, J. O. D. and Bradley, E. L., Jr. (1987) Pentobarbital and thiopental anesthetic interactions with midazolam. *Anesthesiology* **67**, 26–31.
58. MacIver, M. B. and Roth, S. H. (1988) Inhalation anaesthetics exhibit pathway-specific and differential actions on hippocampal synaptic responses in vitro. *Brit. J. Anaesth.* **60**, 680–691.

59. MacIver, M. B., Tauck, D. L., and Kendig, J. J. (1989) General anaesthetic modification of synaptic facilitation and long-term potentiation in hippocampus. *Brit. J. Anaesth.* **62,** 301–310.
60. Struys, M., Versichelen, L., Mortier, E., et al. (1998) Comparison of spontaneous frontal EMG, EEG power spectrum and bispectral index to monitor propofol drug effect and emergence. *Acta Anaesthesiol. Scand.* **42,** 628–636.
61. Gibbs, F. A., Gibbs, E. L., and Lennox, W. G. (1937) Effect on the electroencephalogram of certain drugs which influence nervous activity. *Arch. Intern. Med.* **60,** 154–166.
62. Sebel, P. S., Lang, E., Rampil, I. J., et al. (1997) A multicenter study of bispectral electroencephalogram analysis for monitoring anesthetic effect. *Anesth. Analg.* **84,** 891–899.
63. Flaishon, R., Windsor, A., Sigl, J., and Sebel, P. S. (1997) Recovery of consciousness after thiopental or propofol. Bispectral index and isolated forearm technique. *Anesthesiology* **86,** 613–619.
64. Antognini, J. F. and Schwartz, K. (1993) Exaggerated anesthetic requirements in the preferentially anesthetized brain. *Anesthesiology* **79,** 1244–1249.
65. Rampil, I. J., Mason, P., and Singh, H. (1993) Anesthetic potency (MAC) is independent of forebrain structures in the rat. *Anesthesiology* **78,** 707–712.
66. Glass, P. S., Bloom, M., Kearse, L., Rosow, C., Sebel, P., and Manberg, P. (1997) Bispectral analysis measures sedation and memory effects of propofol, midazolam, isoflurane, and alfentanil in healthy volunteers. *Anesthesiology* **86,** 836–847.
67. Liu, J., Singh, H., and White, P. F. (1997) Electroencephalographic bispectral index correlates with intraoperative recall and depth of propofol-induced sedation. *Anesth. Analg.* **84,** 185–189.
68. Leslie, K., Sessler, D. I., Schroeder, M., and Walters, K. (1995) Propofol blood concentration and the Bispectral Index predict suppression of learning during propofol/epidural anesthesia in volunteers. *Anesth. Analg.* **81,** 1269–1274.
69. Lubke, G. H., Kerssens, C., Phaf, H., and Sebel, P. S. (1999) Dependence of explicit and implicit memory on hypnotic state in trauma patients. *Anesthesiology* **90,** 670–680.
70. Sigl, J. C. and Chamoun, N. G. (1994) An introduction to bispectral analysis for the electroencephalogram. *J. Clin. Monit.* **10,** 392–404.
71. Rampil, I. J. (1998) A primer for EEG signal processing in anesthesia. *Anesthesiology* **89,** 980–1002.
72. Johansen, J. W. and Sebel, P. S. (2000) Development and clinical application of EEG bispectrum monitoring. *Anesthesiology* **93,** 1336–1344.
73. Johansen, J. W. (2000) Monitoring pharmacologic effects of anesthesia. *Current Anesthesiology Reports* **2,** 369–376.
74. Kissin, I. (2000) Depth of anesthesia and bispectral index monitoring. *Anesth. Analg.* **90,** 1114–1117.
75. Schneider, G., and Sebel, P. S. (1997) Monitoring depth of anaesthesia. *Eur. J. Anaesthesiol. Suppl.* **15,** 21–28.
76. Rosow, C. E. and Manberg, P. J. (1998) Bispectral Index Monitoring. In: Hines, R. and Bowdle, T. A. (eds.), *Annual of Anesthetic Pharmacology: Anesthesiology Clinics of North America,* W. B. Saunders, Philadelphia, pp. 89–107.
77. Sakai, T., Singh, H., Mi, W. D., Kudo, T., and Matsuki, A. (1999) The effect of ketamine on clinical endpoints of hypnosis and EEG variables during propofol infusion. *Acta Anaesthesiol. Scand.* **43,** 212–216.
78. Gan, T. J., Glass, P. S., Windsor, A., et al. (1997) Bispectral index monitoring allows faster emergence and improved recovery from propofol, alfentanil, and nitrous oxide anesthesia. BIS Utility Study Group. *Anesthesiology* **87,** 808–815.
79. Bloom, M. J. (2001) Electroencephalography and monitoring of anesthetic depth. In: Lake, C. L., Hines, R. L., and Blitt, C. D. (eds.), *Clinical Monitoring: Practical Applications for Anesthesia and Critical Care,* WB Saunders Company, New York, pp. 92–101.
80. Pincus, S. M., Gladstone, I. M., and Ehrenkranz, R. A. (1991) A regularity statistic for medical data analysis. *J. Clin. Monit.* **7,** 335–345.
81. Shannon, C. and Weaver, W. (1964) The Mathematical Theory of Communication, University of Illinois Press, Urbana.
82. Rezek, I. A. and Roberts, S. J. (1998) Stochastic complexity measures for physiological signal analysis. *IEEE Trans. Biomed. Eng.* **45,** 1186–1191.
83. Sleigh, J. W. and Donovan, J. (1999) Comparison of bispectral index, 95% spectral edge frequency and approximate entropy of the EEG, with changes in heart rate variability during induction of general anaesthesia. *Brit. J. Anaesth.* **82,** 666–671.
84. Bruhn, J., Röpcke, H., and Hoeft, A. (2000) Approximate entropy as an electroencephalographic measure of anesthetic drug effect during desflurane anesthesia. *Anesthesiology* **92,** 715–726.
85. Smith, W. D., Dutton, R. C., and Smith, N. T. (1996) Measuring the performance of anesthetic depth indicators. *Anesthesiology* **84,** 38–51.
86. Bruhn, J., Lehmann, L. E., Roepcke, H., Bouillin, T. W., and Hoeft, A. (2000) Shannon entropy applied to measurement of the EEG effects of desflurane. *Anesthesiology* **93,** A265.
87. Roy, R. J. and Zhang, X. S. (2000) Evaluation of EEG complexity measure for depth of anesthesia estimation. *Anesthesiology* **93,** A1367.
88. Pritchard, W. S. and Duke, D. W. (1995) Measuring "chaos" in the brain: a tutorial review of EEG dimension estimation. *Brain Cogn.* **27,** 353–397.
89. Widman, G., Schreiber, T., Rehberg, B., Hoeft, A., and Elger, C. E. (2000) Quantification of Depth of Anesthesia by Nonlinear Time Series Analysis of Brain Electrical Activity. *Phys. Rev. E. Stat. Phys. Plasmas. Fluids. Relat. Interdiscip. Topics* **62,** 4898–4903.
90. Viertio-Oja, H., Sarkela, M., Talja, P., Tolvansen-Laakso, H., and Yli-Hankala, A. (2000) Entropy of the EEG signal is a robust index for depth of hypnosis. *Anesthesiology* **93,** A1369.
91. Pockett, S. (1999) Anesthesia and the electrophysiology of auditory consciousness. *Conscious. Cogn.* **8,** 45–61.
92. Capitanio, L., Jensen, E. W., Filligoi, G. C., et al. (1997) On-line analysis of AEP and EEG for monitoring depth of anaesthesia. *Methods Inf. Med.* **36,** 311–314.

93. Ghoneim, M. M., Block, R. I., Dhanaraj, V. J., Todd, M. M., Choi, W. W., and Brown, C. K. (2000) Auditory evoked responses and learning and awareness during general anesthesia. *Acta Anaesthesiol. Scand.* **44,** 133–143.

94. Thornton, C. and Sharpe, R. M. (1998) Evoked responses in anaesthesia. *Brit. J. Anaesth.* **81,** 771–781.

95. Drummond, J. C. (2000) Monitoring depth of anesthesia: with emphasis on the application of the bispectral index and the middle latency auditory evoked response to the prevention of recall. *Anesthesiology* **93,** 876–882.

96. Dutton, R. C., Smith, W. D., Rampil, I. J., Chortkoff, B. S., and Eger, E. I., 2nd (1999) Forty-hertz midlatency auditory evoked potential activity predicts wakeful response during desflurane and propofol anesthesia in volunteers. *Anesthesiology* **91,** 1209–1220.

97. Iselin-Chaves, I. A., El Moalem, H. E., Gan, T. J., Ginsberg, B., and Glass, P. S. (2000) Changes in the auditory evoked potentials and the bispectral index following propofol or propofol and alfentanil. *Anesthesiology* **92,** 1300–1310.

98. Mantzaridis, H. and Kenny, G. N. (1997) Auditory evoked potential index: a quantitative measure of changes in auditory evoked potentials during general anaesthesia. *Anaesthesia* **52,** 1030–1036.

99. Jensen, E. W., Litvan, H., Caminal, P., Campos, J. M., and Villar-Landeira, J. (2000) Comparison of the BIS and the auditory evoked potentials index (AAI) during propofol anesthesia for cardiac surgery. *Anesthesiology* **93,** A1370.

100. Alpiger, S., Helbo-Hansen, H. S., and Jensen, E. W. (2000) Effect of sevoflurane on the middle latency auditory evoked potentials measured by a fast extracting montor. *Anesthesiology* **93,** A261.

101. Gajraj, R. J., Doi, M., Mantzaridis, H., and Kenny, G. N. (1998) Analysis of the EEG bispectrum, auditory evoked potentials and the EEG power spectrum during repeated transitions from consciousness to unconsciousness. *Brit. J. Anaesth.* **80,** 46–52.

102. Doi, M., Gajraj, R. J., Mantzaridis, H., and Kenny, G. N. (1997) Relationship between calculated blood concentration of propofol and electrophysiological variables during emergence from anaesthesia: comparison of bispectral index, spectral edge frequency, median frequency and auditory evoked potential index. *Brit. J. Anaesth.* **78,** 180–184.

103. Gajraj, R. J., Doi, M., Mantzaridis, H., and Kenny, G. N. (1999) Comparison of bispectral EEG analysis and auditory evoked potentials for monitoring depth of anaesthesia during propofol anaesthesia. *Brit. J. Anaesth.* **82,** 672–678.

104. Martin, J. H. (1991) The collective electrical behavior of cortical neurons: the electroencephalogram and the mechanisms of epilepsy. In: Kandel, E. R., Schwartz, J. H., and Jessell, T. M. (eds.), *Principles of Neural Science*, Elsevier, New York, pp. 777–791.

105. Gevins, A. (1998) The future of electroencephalography in assessing neurocognitive functioning. *Electroencephalogr. Clin. Neurophysiol.* **106,** 165–172.

106. Morison, R. S., Finley, K. H., and Lothrop, G. N. (1943) Spontaneous electrical activity of the thalamus and other forebrain structures. *J. Neurophysiol.* **6,** 243–254.

107. Bremer, F. (1949) Considerations sur l'origine et la nature des ondes cerebrales. *Electroencephalogr. Clin. Neurophysiol.* **1,** 177–193.

108. Morison, R. S., Dempsey, E. W., and Morison, B. R. (1941) On the propagation of certain cortical potentials. *Amer. J. Physiol.* **131,** 744–751.

109. Kennard, M. (1943) Effects on EEG of chronic lessions of basal ganglia, thalamus and hypothalamus of monkeys. *J. Neurophysiol.* **6,** 405–415.

110. Kristiansen, K. and Courtois, G. (1949) Rhythmic electrical activity from isolated cerebral cortex. *Electroencephalogr. Clin. Neurophysiol.* **1,** 265–272.

111. Fujita, Y. and Sato, T. (1964) Intracellular recordings from hippocampal pyramidal cells in rabbit during theta rhythm activity. *J. Neurophysiol.* **27,** 1011–1025.

112. Bland, B. H. and Vanderwolf, C. H. (1972) Electrical stimulation of the hippocampal formation: behavioral and bioelectrical effects. *Brain Res.* **43,** 89–106.

113. Vanderwolf, C. H. (1975) Neocortical and hippocampal activation relation to behavior: effects of atropine, eserine, phenothiazines, and amphetamine. *J. Comp. Physiol. Psychol.* **88,** 300–323.

114. Fox, S. E., Wolfson, S., and Ranck, J. B., Jr. (1986) Hippocampal theta rhythm and the firing of neurons in walking and urethane anesthetized rats. *Exp. Brain. Res.* **62,** 495–508.

115. Bland, B. H. and Colom, L. V. (1993) Extrinsic and intrinsic properties underlying oscillation and synchrony in limbic cortex. *Prog. Neurobiol.* **41,** 157–208.

116. Oddie, S. D., Bland, B. H., Colom, L. V., and Vertes, R. P. (1994) The midline posterior hypothalamic region comprises a critical part of the ascending brainstem hippocampal synchronizing pathway. *Hippocampus* **4,** 454–473.

117. Rappelsberger, P., Pockberger, H., and Petsche, H. (1982) The contribution of the cortical layers to the generation of the EEG: field potential and current source density analyses in the rabbit's visual cortex. *Electroencephalogr. Clin. Neurophysiol.* **53,** 254–269.

118. Petsche, H., Pockberger, H., and Rappelsberger, P. (1984) On the search for the sources of the electroencephalogram. *Neuroscience* **11,** 1–27.

119. Steriade, M., Dossi, R. C., and Nunez, A. (1991) Network modulation of a slow intrinsic oscillation of cat thalamocortical neurons implicated in sleep delta waves: cortically induced synchronization and brainstem cholinergic suppression. *J. Neurosci.* **11,** 3200–3217.

120. Nunez, A., Amzica, F., and Steriade, M. (1992) Intrinsic and synaptically generated delta (1–4 Hz) rhythms in dorsal lateral geniculate neurons and their modulation by light-induced fast (30–70 Hz) events. *Neuroscience* **51,** 269–284.

121. Leung, L. S. and Yim, C. Y. (1993) Rhythmic delta-frequency activities in the nucleus accumbens of anesthetized and freely moving rats. *Can. J. Physiol. Pharmacol.* **71,** 311–320.

122. Steriade, M., McCormick, D. A., and Sejnowski, T. J. (1993) Thalamocortical oscillations in the sleeping and aroused brain. *Science* **262,** 679–685.

123. Destexhe, A., Contreras, D., and Steriade, M. (1998) Mechanisms underlying the synchronizing action of corticotha-lamic feedback through inhibition of thalamic relay cells. *J. Neurophysiol.* **79,** 999–1016.
124. Steriade, M., Nunez, A., and Amzica, F. (1993) A novel slow (< 1 Hz) oscillation of neocortical neurons in vivo: depolarizing and hyperpolarizing components. *J. Neurosci.* **13,** 3252–3265.
125. Amzica, F. and Steriade, M. (1995) Short- and long-range neuronal synchronization of the slow (< 1 Hz) cortical oscillation. *J. Neurophysiol.* **73,** 20–38.
126. Contreras, D. and Steriade, M. (1995) Cellular basis of EEG slow rhythms: a study of dynamic corticothalamic rela-tionships. *J. Neurosci.* **15,** 604–622.
127. MacIver, M. B., Harris, D. P., Konopacki, J., Roth, S. H., and Bland, B. H. (1986) Carbachol induced rhythmical slow wave activity recorded from dentate granule neurons in vitro. *Proc. West. Pharmacol. Soc.* **29,** 159–161.
128. Konopacki, J., MacIver, M. B., Bland, B. H., and Roth, S. H. (1987) Carbachol-induced EEG 'theta' activity in hippoc-ampal brain slices. *Brain Res.* **405,** 196–198.
129. MacVicar, B. A. and Tse, F. W. (1989) Local neuronal circuitry underlying cholinergic rhythmical slow activity in CA3 area of rat hippocampal slices. *J. Physiol. (Lond.)* **417,** 197–212.
130. Tell, F. and Jean, A. (1993) Ionic basis for endogenous rhythmic patterns induced by activation of N-methyl-D-aspar-tate receptors in neurons of the rat nucleus tractus solitarii. *J. Neurophysiol.* **70,** 2379–2390.
131. Huguenard, J. R. and Prince, D. A. (1994) Intrathalamic rhythmicity studied in vitro: nominal T-current modulation causes robust antioscillatory effects. *J. Neurosci.* **14,** 5485–5502.
132. Bal, T., von Krosigk, M., and McCormick, D. A. (1995) Synaptic and membrane mechanisms underlying synchronized oscillations in the ferret lateral geniculate nucleus in vitro. *J. Physiol. (Lond.)* **483,** 641–663.
133. Kim, U., Bal, T., and McCormick, D. A. (1995) Spindle waves are propagating synchronized oscillations in the ferret LGNd in vitro. *J. Neurophysiol.* **74,** 1301–1323.
134. Taylor, G. W., Merlin, L. R., and Wong, R. K. (1995) Synchronized oscillations in hippocampal CA3 neurons induced by metabotropic glutamate receptor activation. *J. Neurosci.* **15,** 8039–8052.
135. Metherate, R., and Ashe, J. H. (1993) Ionic flux contributions to neocortical slow waves and nucleus basalis-mediated activation: whole-cell recordings in vivo. *J. Neurosci.* **13,** 5312–5323.
136. Richter, D. W., Pierrefiche, O., Lalley, P. M., and Polder, H. R. (1996) Voltage-clamp analysis of neurons within deep layers of the brain. *J. Neurosci. Meth.* **67,** 121–123.
137. Núñez, A., García-Austt, E., and Buño, W. (1990) Synaptic contributions to theta rhythm genesis in rat CA1-CA3 hippocampal pyramidal neurons in vivo. *Brain Res.* **533,** 176–179.
138. Metherate, R., Cox, C. L., and Ashe, J. H. (1992) Cellular bases of neocortical activation: modulation of neural oscilla-tions by the nucleus basalis and endogenous acetylcholine. *J. Neurosci.* **12,** 4701–4711.
139. Soltesz, I. and Deschênes, M. (1993) Low- and high-frequency membrane potential oscillations during theta activity in CA1 and CA3 pyramidal neurons of the rat hippocampus under ketamine-xylazine anesthesia. *J. Neurophysiol.* **70,** 97–116.
140. Whittington, M. A., Traub, R. D., and Jefferys, J. G. (1995) Synchronized oscillations in interneuron networks driven by metabotropic glutamate receptor activation. *Nature* **373,** 612–615.
141. Flint, A. C. and Connors, B. W. (1996) Two types of network oscillations in neocortex mediated by distinct glutamate receptor subtypes and neuronal populations. *J. Neurophysiol.* **75,** 951–957.
142. Stanski, D. R. (1991) Pharmacodynamic modeling of thiopental depth of anesthesia. In: D'Argenio, (ed.), Advanced Methods of Pharmacokinetic and Pharmacodynamic Systems Analysis, Plenum Press, New York, pp. 79–85.
143. Gray, C. M. and Singer, W. (1989) Stimulus-specific neuronal oscillations in orientation columns of cat visual cortex. *Proc. Natl. Acad. Sci. USA* **86,** 1698–1702.
144. Steriade, M. (1997) Synchronized activities of coupled oscillators in the cerebral cortex and thalamus at different levels of vigilance. *Cereb. Cortex* **7,** 583–604.

7

Cerebral Mechanisms of Analgesia and Anesthesia in Humans Elucidated by In Vivo Brain Imaging

Ferenc Gyulai and Leonard Firestone

INTRODUCTION

Although general anesthetics and opioids have been extensively used in human medicine, the neural mechanisms involved in their mechanism of action remains largely unresolved.

For example, opioids have been shown to exert their analgesic effects at the peripheral (1,2) and central terminals of primary nociceptive afferents both in animals and humans (3). Since the human pain experience, consisting of interacting discriminative, affective-motivational, and cognitive components, is most likely generated in the forebrain (4), the effect of opioids in these structures appears to be of higher importance. Owing to the nature of these behavioral components, however, instead of animal models, human pain studies are required where the effect of analgesics could examined on noninvasively gauged neuronal function and associated behavioral responses in a parallel fashion.

Similarly, abundant in vitro and animal model data support that the postsynaptic gamma aminobutyric acid receptor type A (GABA$_A$-R) is an important target for general anesthetics (reviewed in Tanelian et al. [5] and Franks and Lieb [6]). The involvement of GABA in anesthesia is suggested by in vivo studies showing that GABA-agonists that penetrate the blood-brain barrier can obtund rats (7). In vitro animal studies have shown that volatile anesthetics enhance GABA binding at clinically relevant concentrations (8). Isoflurane, enflurane and halothane enhance GABA-gated Cl$^-$ currents in vitro, in a concentration-dependent manner, at therapeutically relevant concentrations (9), and the potentiation of GABA-mediated Cl$^-$ currents highly correlates with their anesthetizing potency (10). The volatile anesthetic-activated Cl$^-$ current can be blocked by bicuculline and picrotoxin, indicating that the current is mediated by GABA$_A$-Rs (11,12). As demonstrated by receptor binding studies, an increase in the affinity of the binding site for GABA appears to be a mechanism for the augmentation of GABA evoked Cl$^-$ currents by volatile agents (13,14). Halothane at clinically relevant concentrations stimulates Cl$^-$ flux (15) and at the same concentrations increase GABA$_A$-R affinity for muscimol (16). Likewise, isoflurane, halothane, and enflurane potentiate benzodiazepine binding in a concentration- and chloride-dependent fashion by increasing the affinity of the binding site for its ligand (17). Although such studies provide strong support for the GABA$_A$-R hypothesis of anesthetic action, direct evidence from living organisms is lacking, especially under the clinically most relevant circumstances—in the living human brain.

Recent advances in in vivo imaging techniques, such as positron emission tomography (PET) and functional magnetic resonance imaging (fMRI), provide a unique opportunity to map neuronal function both at the receptor and network levels in humans. This chapter focuses on PET and fMRI methodologies available for human experiments reviewing previous studies. In addition, novel

From: *Contemporary Clinical Neuroscience: Neural Mechanisms of Anesthesia*
Edited by: Joseph F. Antognini et al. © Humana Press Inc., Totowa, NJ

experimental approaches using currently available PET and fMRI techniques are discussed that could have the potential to image drug action from the molecular to the network level.

PET METHODOLOGY

PET is based on the measurement of positron-emitting radionuclide concentration in various areas of the body by detecting the collision of positrons and electrons resulting in the emission of two gamma rays simultaneously at the opposite directions (*positron annihilation*). Depending upon the tracer used neuronal function can be assessed either by probing metabolism or receptor availability.

Measuring Neuronal Metabolism

Regional Cerebral Metabolic Rate (rCMR)

Neuronal metabolism can be measured by PET both directly or indirectly by measuring regional cerebral blood flow (rCBF). Quantitative imaging of cerebral metabolism by PET *(18,19)* is based on the modified principles of the autoradiography technique developed by Sokoloff et al. *(20)*. Regional CMR_{glu} is measured using the positron labeled tracer ^{18}F-deoxyglucose (^{18}F-DG), with a halflife of 110 min, which is taken up by neurons as a function of their activity *(18)*. Once inside the cell, ^{18}F-DG becomes metabolically trapped, since it cannot be metabolized by glycolisis. Consequently, the amount of intracellularly accumulated ^{18}F-DG is an accurate reflection of neuronal activity *(19)*. The tracer kinetic model used in this approach assumes 3 compartments: (1) plasma compartment; (2) brain tissue compartment containing glucose and ^{18}F-DG, and (3) compartment for the metabolic products of glucose and ^{18}F-DG. In this model the metabolic product of ^{18}F-DG (as well as glucose) is trapped in compartment #3, and its concentration is directly related to $rCMR_{glu}$. The relationship between the PET-measured brain tissue concentration of ^{18}F-DG and $rCMR_{glu}$ is described by differential equations that can be solved for $rCMR_{glu}$ *(21,18)*.

Regional Cerebral Blood Flow (rCBF)

The underlying principle of measuring rCBF as an index of neuronal metabolism is that synaptic activity generates increases in rCBF. The mechanism of coupling of rCBF and rCMR is still an area of active investigation. The degree of coupling may vary among brain regions and under different experimental circumstances, but it is reliably present in the normal brain *(22)*. Regional CBF is measured by PET using a tracer, such as [^{15}O]water (halflife: 2 min) or [^{15}O]carbon dioxide ($C^{15}O_2$), that freely diffuses across the blood brain barrier, i.e., their uptake in brain tissue is determied by blood flow not diffusion rate. The technique uses the modification of the Kety-Schmidt method *(23)* in which the flow-dependent rate of accumulation or disappearance of a diffusible tracer from the brain is used to measure rCBF at the capillary level. The tracer kinetic model used in this approach assumes 2 compartments: (1) plasma compartment; and (2) brain tissue compartment. The relationship between the PET-measured radiotracer concentration in the brain tissue and rCBF is described by differential equations that can be solved for rCBF *(24,25)*.

Receptor Imaging

Determination of Regional Cerebral Receptor Density

PET can probe the properties of receptors noninvasively in humans by measuring the concentration of radiolabelled receptor-specific ligands in the brain. Instead of quantifying receptor density (B_{max}) and apparent affinity (K_d) separately, a combined binding variable termed distribution volume (DV), the sum of the ratio of these variables (B_{max}/K_d) and nonreceptor specific binding is estimated *(26)*. The advantage of this approach is the ability to estimate DV by a single tracer injection, while estimating B_{max} and K_d requires two or three separate injections with proportionally more scanning time and radioactive exposure. With the provision that B_{max} is not changing under the experimental circumstances, the DV variable can be used as an index of apparent affinity alone.

Similarly to rCBF or rCMR$_{glu}$ measurements, DV is obtained by fitting the PET measured radiotracer concentration brain curve to the curve described by the differential equations of the employed tracer kinetic model. Mostly 2 compartment models are employed: (1) plasma compartment; and (2) brain tissue compartment incorporating both receptor and non-receptor binding sites. To eliminate the nonreceptor component the obtained DV values are normalized to the DV value of a brain area that is essentially devoid of the receptor in question *(26)*.

Displacement Experiment

If a radiolabeled receptor ligand is co-administered with an unlabeled drug, such as an opioid, that is known to bind to the same receptor, the unlabeled drug will compete with the radioligand resulting in its displacement. Because the degree of this displacement is linearly related to the drug's receptor occupancy, by measuring the binding (DV) of a radioligand in the absence and presence of a competing medication, it is possible to derive the percentage of receptors that are occupied by the unlabeled drug:

$$\text{Receptor occupancy (\%)} = 100 \cdot \frac{(DV_{\text{NO DRUG}} - DV_{\text{DRUG}})}{DV_{\text{NO DRUG}}}$$

where DV$_{\text{NO DRUG}}$ and DV$_{\text{DRUG}}$ are the distribution volumes of the radioligand in the absence and presence of the unlabeled, competing drug, respectively *(27)*.

FUNCTIONAL MRI METHODOLOGY

Blood Oxygenation Level-Dependent (BOLD) Effect

Functional MRI uses deoxyhemoglobin as an endogenous contrast agent. Under physiological circumstances, neuronal activation leads to an increase in rCBF. In contrast, neuronal oxidative metabolism does not increase as much as rCBF leading to increases in the oxyhemoglobin-deoxyhemoglobin ratio in the activated brain region. While the ferrous ion in deoxyhemoglobin has a strong magnetic moment, that in oxyhemoglobin possesses no magnetic moment. Consequently, with an increased ratio of oxyhemoglobin, the magnetic field is less disturbed in areas around activated neurons, producing higher signal intensity in T2* (apparent relaxation time)-weighted MRI, a phenomenon called BOLD effect *(28)*. Such signal intensity changes are detected over time, with intervals between hundreds of milliseconds to several seconds depending on the length of repetition time (TR), a fast scanning technique called echo planar imaging *(29)*. Signal intensity starts increasing immediately following neuronal activation, peaking at several seconds after onset, then returning to the baseline in several seconds after neuronal activation ends. Due to this hemodynamic delay the temporal resolution of fMRI is 6–10 s. The relationship between the amplitude of the detected signal and rCBF change is linear within a certain range. Because the BOLD signal requires intact rCBF-metabolism coupling, and the signal is qualitative in nature, using fMRI to elucidate drug action in the brain is still to some extent problematic.

Experimental Design

Block Design

To achieve sufficient statistical power, conventional fMRI studies have been using a "block" paradigm, where the various experimental conditions are repeatedly alternated multiple times during imaging. The most significant disadvantage of this design is that it does not allow the studying of drug action since the repeated presence and absence of the drug condition cannot be achieved.

Event-Related Design

The relatively new, event-related fMRI allows one to avoid the repetition of experimental conditions *(30)*. BOLD signal changes during experimental conditions of 0.5–5 s are detected using the fast scanning technique with TR less than 2 s. This experimental design has been successfully used to elucidate cerebral sites of drug action *(31,32)*.

CEREBRAL SUBSTRATES OF PAIN PERCEPTION, OPIOID AND NITROUS OXIDE ANALGESIA REVEALED BY PET AND FMRI

Brain Regions Activated by Pain Alone

To map the sites of opioid action in the living human brain, first the cerebral substrates of pain perception must be identified. Pain is a conscious experience consisting of discriminative, affective-motivational, and cognitive aspects that are integrated into sensation of pain. These components are each mediated via distinct forebrain areas *(4)*. Animal experiments and observations in humans indicate that pain responsive neurons in the primary somatosensory cortex and ventral posterolateral thalamus, parts of the lateral pain system, have small, contralateral receptive fields *(33)*. This, coupled with human observations showing that lesions of the somatosensory cortex decrease the discriminative aspects of nociception *(34)*, indicates that the lateral pain system is responsible for the spatial localizing and discriminative aspects of pain perception. Another important nociceptive pathway, the medial pain system, is via the medial thalamic nuclei to the anterior cingulate cortex *(35)*. Clinical observations of chronic pain patients following resection of the anterior cingulate cortex indicate that this pathway is responsible for the affective-motivational aspects of pain *(36)*.

Although the above observations had been suggestive of the significant contribution of forebrain areas to the human pain experience, the first experimental evidence came in 1991. Talbot et al. reported activation in the primary and secondary somatosensory cortices, medial thalamus, and anterior cingulate cortex in healthy human volunteers in response to peripheral noxious stimulation using noninvasive O^{15}-water PET methodology. The findings were confirmed and extended by other investigators showing additional responsive areas in the prefrontal cortex, supplementary motor area, and cerebellum *(37–42)*.

Functional MRI have been performed trying to exploit the higher spatial and temporal resolution of the technique. Painful electrical stimulation of the median nerve was shown to activate the contralateral primary somatosensory and anterior cingulate cortices *(43)*. In addition to these areas, other studies found electrical stimulation related activation in the bilateral insular and secondary somatosensory cortices as well *(44)*.

Nociceptive thermal stimulation was shown to evoke activation in the prefrontal, motor, supplementary motor, primary, and secondary somatosensory cortices, in addition to the anterior, posterior cingulate, thalamus, insula, and cerebellum *(45)*.

Using event-related fMRI to correlate BOLD signal intensity changes and subjective ratings of pain activation was shown in secondary somatosensory cortex, anterior cingulate, insular cortex, and thalamus *(46)*.

As illustration of the potential of fMRI to study drug action in humans, accupuncture needle manipulation was shown to decrease activity in the nucleus accumbens, amygdala, hypothalamus, ventral tegmental area, and anterior cingulate cortex in contrast to the increased activity in the somatosensory cortex *(47)*.

Brain Regions Activated by Opioids and Nitrous Oxide

The first attempt to map the cerebral sites of opioid analgesia was reported by Jones et al. *(48)* in one patient suffering from cancer pain in the left jaw. Following a bolus injection of 10 mg of morphine, resulting in complete pain relief, O^{15}-water PET revealed increased rCBF in the prefrontal cortex, anterior cingulate, caudate, and putamen bilaterally and contralaterally in the insular and prefrontal cortices.

To map the cerebral sites of fentanyl's mechanism of action in a statistically meaningful manner, we used O^{15}-water PET in healthy human volunteers *(49)*. Furthermore, in a separate set of experiments, the neural networks mediating the effect of low concentration (20%) of nitrous oxide, were also mapped using PET *(50)*.

Significant rCBF increase was observed in the anterior cingulate (area 25/32), prefrontal cortices (area 8/10), and caudate nuclei, but not in the somatosensory cortical areas following a 1.5 µg/kg intravenous bolus of fentanyl. A significant decrease of rCBF in the left prefrontal (area 11), right temporal cortices (area 39), and cerebellum was also revealed. Inhalation of 20% nitrous oxide was associated with enhanced rCBF in the anterior cingulate cortex (area 24) and decreased rCBF in the hippocampus, posterior cingulate (areas 23, 29), and secondary visual cortices (areas 18, 19).

Modification of Pain-Induced Cerebral Activation by fentanyl and Nitrous Oxide

Since opioids have been shown to evoke neuronal inhibition, fentanyl analgesia was expected to be associated with suppression of pain-evoked local cerebral activation. The observation that nitrous oxide induces met-enkephalin and β-endorphin release in the rat *(51)* and in humans indicates that at least some of nitrous oxide's antinociceptive effect is naloxone reversible *(52)*. This lead to the hypothesis that some of its cerebral targets are shared with those of fentanyl. To test this hypothesis, the effect of fentanyl and nitrous oxide was studied on pain-evoked rCBF changes in healthy volunteers *(53,54)*.

Heat pain to left volar forearm was associated with increased rCBF in the anterior cingulate cortex, ipsilateral thalamus, ipsilateral inferior frontal cortex, and contralateral supplementary motor area, and decreased rCBF in the ipsilateral peristriate cortex (Fig. 1) as previously reported *(37–39)*.

Following the bolus injection of fentanyl, in the presence of pain, rCBF increased in the anterior cingulate and contralateral motor cortices (Fig. 2), and decreased in the bilateral thalamus and ipsilateral posterior cingulate cortex. The rCBF decreases and increases did not overlap in the anterior cingulate cortex. An augmentation of pain-related rCBF increase was also observed in the supplementary motor area and ipsilateral inferior frontal cortex significantly (Fig. 2).

Nitrous oxide abolished all pain-related cerebral responses, and was associated with increased rCBF in the contralateral infralimbic (area 25), and orbitofrontal (areas 10, 11) cortices (Fig. 3). Both fentanyl and nitrous oxide administration was associated with antinociception indicated by the significantly decreased VAS scores.

In contrast to our hypothesis based on the inhibitory effect of fentanyl and nitrous oxide on the cellular level, the presented data show that on the network level these agents exert their analgesic effect via augmentation of pain-evoked cerebral responses in certain areas, as well as both activation and inhibition in other brain regions that are unresponsive to pain stimulation alone. Furthermore, the cerebral substrates of the antinociceptive effect of the two agents do not overlap *(53,54)*.

CEREBRAL TARGETS OF GENERAL ANESTHETICS ELUCIDATED BY PET

Mapping Cerebral Metabolism During General Anesthesia

Although multiple in vitro and animal experiments examined the molecular targets of general anesthetics, their net neurophysiologic effect and the relevance of these influences have not been addressed in the living human brain.

In a series of rCMR$_{glu}$ PET experiments Alkire et al. have shown that propofol, isoflurane, and halothane, titrated to unconsciousness, significantly depress global brain metabolism in humans. Although each examined brain region showed a significant decrease in the presence of the examined anesthetics, no regional heterogenity was could be identified *(55–57)*.

Mapping the Molecular Targets of General Anesthetics

Abundant in vitro and animal model data support that the postsynaptic GABA$_A$-receptor (GABA$_A$-R) is an important target for general anesthetics, but the relevance of these models is untested in humans. Because benzodiazepines (BDZs) have also been shown to act via a specific

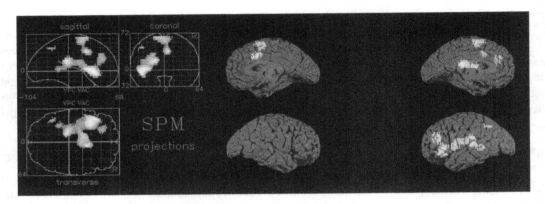

Fig. 1. *Left* Statistical parametric maps of significantly enhanced pain-induced neuronal activity ($p < 0.01$) displayed on sagittal, coronal, and transverse projections of the brain as lighter shades of gray, with the lightest gray indicating the greatest degree of activation. The z score maps were generated from the t scores obtained by averaging images across subjects for each experimental condition and comparing these averages using a t test. R = right hemisphere; VPC = vertical plane through the posterior commissure; VAC = vertical line through the anterior commissure. *Right* Activated areas superimposed upon topographic cortical rendering. (From Adler et al., *(53)*; courtesy of Lippincott Williams and Wilkins.)

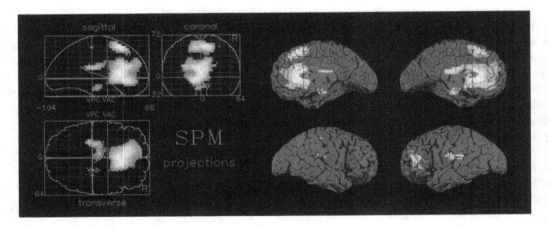

Fig. 2. *Left* Statistical parametric maps of significantly enhanced pain-induced neuronal activity in the presence of fentanyl ($p < 0.01$) displayed on sagittal, coronal, and transverse projections of the brain as lighter shades of gray, with the lightest gray indicating the greatest degree of activation. R = right hemisphere; VPC = vertical plane through the posterior commissure; VAC = vertical line through the anterior commissure. *Right* Activated areas superimposed upon topographic cortical rendering. (From Firestone et al., *(49)*; courtesy of Lippincott Williams and Wilkins.)

GABA$_A$-R site, they provide sensitive probes for the GABA$_A$-R. Availability of the ^{11}C-labeled BDZ ligand, flumazenil (FMZ), allowed us to quantitatively test in humans, whether the volatile anesthetic isoflurane affects GABA$_A$-Rs in vivo in a dose-dependent manner. ^{11}C-FMZ PET scans were obtained in 12 healthy subjects during awake (CONTROL condition) and anesthetized with either 1.0 (1.0 MAC ISOFLURANE group; $n = 7$), or 1.5 MAC (1.5 MAC ISOFLURANE group; $n = 5$) isoflurane (ISOFLURANE conditions). Regions of interest included areas of high, intermediate, and low GABA$_A$/benzodiazepine site density. It was found that DV$_{RATIO}$ increased significantly in each examined region during the ISOFLURANE conditions compared to CONTROL in a dose dependent

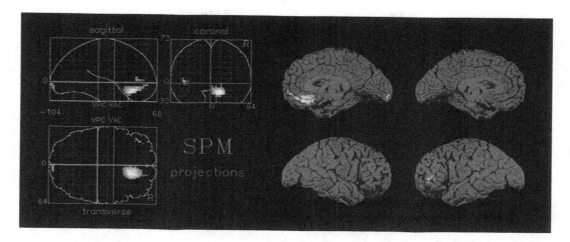

Fig. 3. *Left* Statistical parametric maps of significantly enhanced pain-induced neuronal activity in the presence of nitrous oxide ($p < 0.01$) displayed on sagittal, coronal, and transverse projections of the brain as lighter shades of gray, with the lightest gray indicating the greatest degree of activation. R = right hemisphere; VPC = vertical plane through the posterior commissure; VAC = vertical line through the anterior commissure. *Right* Activated areas superimposed upon topographic cortical rendering. (From Gyulai et al., *(54)*; courtesy of Lippincott Williams and Wilkins.)

manner (Fig. 4) indicating that the conformational change of the $GABA_A$-R is involved in isoflurane's mechanism of action in the living human brain *(58)*.

FUTURE DIRECTIONS

Analgesics

The studies discussed here clearly demonstrate that elucidating the effect of analgesics in the human brain via mapping rCBF or rCMR changes is a powerful technique, but the detected signal provides only limited information about the entire pathway mediating the analgesic response. Opioids bind to neuronal receptors located on cell bodies, which in turn lead to metabolic changes at the level of presynaptic axon terminals *(59)* of the same cells and possibly others downstream to the opioid binding neurons. It follows that by mapping metabolic changes, only the distal end of the pathway is revealed.

Combining currently available PET methodologies, it is possible to map the entire pathway of opioid action from receptor binding to neuronal activity change in the same individual. As shown for triazolam *(60)* and haloperidol *(61)*, by measuring opioid radioligand displacement, such as [^{11}C]buprenorphine *(62)* and [^{11}C]carfentanyl *(63)*, the degree of receptor occupancy of different opioid doses together with regional neuronal activity changes could be measured. Correlation analysis of these two parameters could identify pathways in their entirety through which opioids exert their analgesic effect in the human brain.

General Anesthetics

Although the demonstration of a conformational change at the $GABA_A$-R indicates the involvement of this receptor in anesthetics mechanisms in the living human brain, the relevance of this enhancement of receptor function in terms of its translation into an enhancement of inhibitory synaptic transmission, remains unexplored. This is owing to the limitations of previously employed techniques that did not allow for the maintenance of functional integrity of the nervous system required for the reliable assessment of the relationship between effects of anesthetics on $GABA_A$-R function

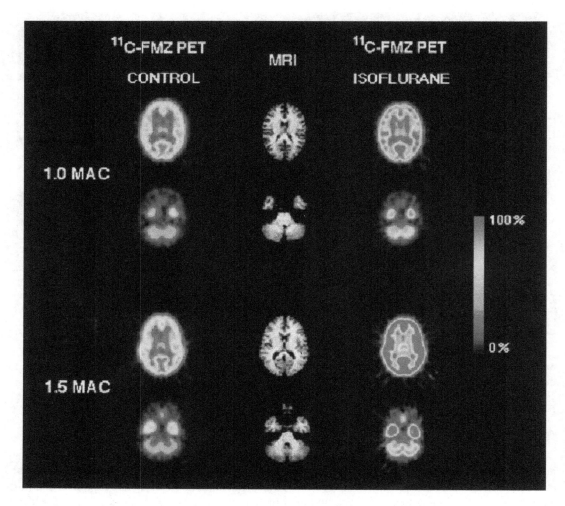

Fig. 4. Summed PET (summed over 20–80 after ^{11}C-flumazenil injection) of ^{11}C-FMZ distribution in two representative volunteers during awake (CONTROL) and when anesthetized (ISOFLURANE) with 1.0 *upper row*; subject 1) and 1.5 MAC isoflurane (*lower row*; subject 1). The plane of both PET and the corresponding MR scans is 4 cm (*upper row*) and 2 cm (*lower row*) superior to the canthomeatal line and show the frontal, temporal and occipital cortical areas, as well as the thalamus. The color scale is shown with red corresponding to 2.7 μCi/ mL brain tissue.

and processes downstream to the receptor. The combination of receptor imaging with ligands such as ^{11}C-FMZ, with metabolic imaging via ^{18}F-deoxyglucose by seeking correlation between direct anesthetic effects on receptors and postsynaptic mechanisms, such as rCMR$_{glu}$, offers the assessment of the translation of receptor effects into inhibition. This unique approach has the potential to shed light on how drug effects are translated into altered brain function in humans.

New Imaging Methodologies—fMRI for Studying Drug Action

Despite the obvious paucity of published results, the potential of fMRI in studying drug action in humans is undeniable. As an early illustration of this, cocaine-related brain activity changes were demonstrated in the prefrontal, temporal cortices, caudate nucleus, basal forebrain, and thalamus *(64)*.

Furthermore, the observed BOLD signal changes were also correlated with drug-induced behavioral responses. Similar studies, focusing on other agents, such as nicotine, shortly followed *(31)*.

Elucidation of anesthetic action in the human brain using fMRI have also begun. For example, isoflurane was shown to decrease and abolish tactile and pain stimulus-related BOLD signal intensity in the primary somatosensory cortex, caudate nucleus, and thalamus at 0.7 and 1.3 vol % concentrations, respectively *(65)*. Similar studies, with careful control experiments to ensure the intactness of cerebral blood flow/metabolism coupling, are needed to further identify the sites of anesthetic action in the human brain. Functional MRI also lends itself to more advanced experimental strategies that have not been exploited yet. One of the major advantages of fMRI is the lack of radioactivity dosimetry constraints allowing the acquisition of scans during multiple experimental conditions. Taking advantage of this unique attribute of the technique a series of scans could be obtained at varying drug concentrations in order to identify BOLD signal intensity drug dose relationships in various brain regions. Integrated experimental findings derived from human studies using the discussed fMRI and PET methodologies have the potential to yield hitherto unobtainable insights into the mechanism of analgesic and anesthetic action under the most clinically relevant circumstance—the intact, living human brain.

REFERENCES

1. Ferreira, S. H. and Nakamura, M. (1979) Prostaglandin hyperalgesia: the peripheral analgesic activity of morphine, enkephalins and opioid antagonists. *Prostaglandins* **18**, 191–200.
2. Joshi, G. P., McCarrol, S., O'Brien, T., and Lenane, P. (1993) Intraarticular analgesia following knee arthroscopy. *Anesth. Analg.* **76**, 333–336.
3. Yaksh, T. L. (1997) Pharmacology and mechanisms of opioid analgesic activity. *Acta. Anaesthesiol. Scand.* **41**, 94–111.
4. Melzack, R. and Casey, K. L. (1968) Sensory, motivational, and central control determinants of pain, The Skin Senses A New Conceptual Model. Edited by Kenshalo, D. Springfield, IL Charles C. Thomas, pp. 423–439.
5. Tanelian, D. L., Kosek, P., Mody, I., and MacIver, M. B. (1993) The role of the GABA$_A$ receptor/chloride channel complex in anesthesia. *Anesthesiology* **78**, 757–776.
6. Franks, N. P. and Lieb, W. R. (1994) Molecular and cellular mechanisms of general anaesthesia. *Nature* **367**, 607–614.
7. Cheng, S. C. and Brunner, E. A. (1985) Inducing anesthesia with a GABA analog, THIP. *Anesthesiology* **63**, 147–151.
8. Cheng, S. C. and Brunner, E. A. (1984) Anesthetic effects on GABA binding. *Anesthesiology* **61**, A326.
9. Jones, M. V., Brooks, P. A., and Harrison, N. L. (1992) Enhancement of γ-aminobutyric acid-activated Cl⁻ currents in cultured rat hippocampal neurones by three volatile anesthetics. *J. Physiol.* **449**, 279–293.
10. Zimmerman, S. A., Jones, M. V., and Harrison, N. L, (1994) Potentiation of gamma-aminobutyric acid A receptor Cl⁻ current correlates with in vivo anesthetic potency. *J. Pharmacol. Exp. Ther.* **270**, 987–991.
11. Hales, T. G., Jones, M. V., and Harrison, N. L. (1992) Evidence for subunit dependent direct activation of the GABA$_A$ receptor by isoflurane. *Anesthesiology* **77**, A698.
12. Yang, J. S. J., Isenberg, K. E., and Zorumski, C. F. (1992) Volatile anesthetics gate a chloride current in postnatal rat hippocampal neurons. *FASEB J.* **6**, 914–918.
13. Wakamori, M., Ikemoto, Y., and Akaike, N. (1991) Effects of two volatile anesthetics and a volatile convulsant on the excitatory and inhibitory amino acid responses in dissociated CNS neurons of the rat. *J. Neurophysiol.* **66**, 2014–2021.
14. Lin, L. H., Chen, L. L., Zirrolli, J. A., and Harris, R. A, (1992) General anesthetics potentiate γ-aminobutyric acid$_A$ receptors expressed by Xenopus oocytes: lack of involvement of intracellular calcium. *J. Pharmacol. Exp. Ther.* **263**, 569–578.
15. Longoni, B. and Olsen, R. W. (1992) Studies on themechanism of interaction of anesthetics with GABA$_A$ receptors. *Adv. Biochem. Psychopharmacol.* **47**, 365–378.
16. Longoni, B., Demontis, G. C., and Olsen, R. W. (1993) Enhancement of GABA$_A$ receptor function and binding by the volatile anesthetic halothane. *J. Pharmacol. Exp. Ther.* **266**, 153–159.
17. Harris, B., Wong, G., and Skolnick, P. (1992) Volatile anesthetics and barbiturates exhibit neurochemical similarities at GABA$_A$ receptors. *Anesthesiology* **77**, A697.
18. Phelps, M. E., Huang, S. C., Hoffman, E. J., Selin, C., Sokoloff, L., and Kuhl, D. E. (1979) Tomographic measurement of local cerebral glucose metabolic rate in humans with (F-18) 2-fluoro-2-deoxy-D-glucose: Validation of method. *Ann. Neurol.* **6**, 371–388.
19. Huang, S. C., Phelps, M. E., Hoffman, E. J., Sideris, K., Selin, C. J., and Kuhl, D. E. (1980) Noninvasive determination of local cerebral metabolic rate of glucose in man. *Am. J. Physiol.* **238**, E69–E82.
20. Sokoloff, L., Reivich, M., Kennedy, C., et al. (1977) The [¹⁴C]deoxyglucose method for the measurement of local cerebral glucose utilization: Theory, procedure, and normal values in the conscious and anesthetized albino rat. *J. Neurochem.* **28**, 897–916.

21. Reivich, M., Alavi, A., Wolf, A., et al. (1985) Glucose metabolic rate kinetic model parameter determination in humans: the lumped constants and rate constants for [^{18}F]fluorodeoxyglucose and [^{11}C]deoxyglucose. *J. Cereb. Blood Flow Metab.* **5**, 179–192.

22. Mraovitch, S., Calando, Y., Pinard, E., Pearce, W. J., and Seylaz, J. (1992) Differential cerebrovascular and metabolic responses in specific neural systems elicited from the centromedian-parafascicular complex. *Neuroscience* **49**, 451–466.

23. Kety, S. S. and Schmidt, C. F. (1948) The nitrous oxide method for quantitative determination of cerebral blood flow in man; theory, procedure and normal values. *J. Clin. Invest.* **27**, 476–483.

24. Herscovitch, P., Markham, J., and Raichle, M. E. (1983) Brain blood flow measured with intravenous H$_2$^{15}O. I. Theory and error analysis. *J. Nucl. Med.* **14**, 782–789.

25. Quarles, R., Mintun, M., Larson, K., Markham, J., MacLeod, A., and Raichle, M. (1993) Measurement of regional cerebral blood flow with positron emission tomography: a comparison of [^{15}O] water to [^{11}C] butanol with distributed-parameter and compartmental models. *J. Cereb. Blood Flow Metab.* **13**, 733–747.

26. Koeppe, R. A., Holthoff, V. A., Frey, K. A., Kilbourn, M. R., and Kuhl, D. E. (1991) Compartmental analysis of [^{11}C]flumazenil kinetics for the estimation of ligand transport rate and receptor distribution using positron emission tomography. *J. Cereb. Blood Flow Metab.* **11**, 735–744.

27. Farde, L., Nordstrom, A.-L., Wiesel, F.-A., Pauli, S., Halldin, C., and Sedvall, G. (1992) Positron emission tomographic analysis of central D1 and D2 dopamine receptor occupancy in patients treated with classical neuroleptics and clozapine. *Arch. Gen. Psychiatry* **49**, 538–544.

28. Ogawa, S., Lee, T. M., Kay, A. R., and Tank, D. W. (1990) Brain magnetic resonance imaging with contrast dependent on blood oxygenation. *Proc. Natl. Acad. Sci. USA* **87**, 9868–9872.

29. Mansfield, P. (1977) Multi-planar image formation using NMR spin echos. *J. Phys. C.* **10**, L55–L58.

30. Buckner, R. L., Bandettini, P. A., O'Craven, K. M., et al. (1996) Detection of cortical activation during averaged single trials of a cognitive task using functional magnetic resonance imaging. *Proc. Natl. Acad. Sci. USA* **93**, 14,878–14,883.

31. Stein, E. A., Risinger, R., and Bloom, A. S. (1999) Functional MRI in pharmacology, Functional MRI. Moonen, C. T. W. and Bandettini, P. A. (eds.). Berlin, Springer pp. 525–538.

32. Leslie, R. A. and James, M. F. (2000) Pharmacological magnetic resonance imaging: a new application for functional MRI. *Trends Pharmacol. Sci.* **21**, 314–318.

33. Kenshalo, D. R., Jr. and Isensee, O. (1983) Responses of primate SI cortical neurons to noxious stimuli. *J. Neurophysiol.* **50**, 1479–1496.

34. Greenspan, J. D. and Winfield, J. A. (1992) Reversible pain and tactile deficits associated with a cerebral tumor compressing the posterior insula and parietal operculum. *Pain* **58**, 29–39.

35. Sikes, R. W. and Vogt, B. A. (1992) Nociceptive neurons in area 24b of rabbit anterior cingulate cortex. *J. Neurophysiol.* **68**, 1720–1732.

36. Corkin, S. (1980) A prospective study of cingulotomy, The Psychosurgery Debate: Scientific, Legal, and Ethical Perspectives. Valenstein, E. S. (ed.). San Francisco: Freeman, pp. 164–204.

37. Jones, A. K. P., Brown, W. D., Friston, K. J., Qi, L. Y., and Frackowiak, R. S. (1991a) Cortical and subcortical localization of response to pain in man using positron emission tomography. *Proc. R. Soc. Lond. B.* **244**, 39–44.

38. Coghill, R. C., Talbot, J. D., Evans, A. C., et al. (1994) Distributed processing of pain and vibration by the human brain. *J. Neurosci.* **14**, 4095–4108.

39. Talbot, J. D., Marrett, S., Evans, A. C., Meyer, E., Bushnell, M. C., and Duncan, G. H. (1991) Multiple representations of pain in human cerebral cortex. *Science* **251**, 1355–1358.

40. Casey, K. L., Minoshima, S., Berger, K. L., Koeppe, R. A., Morrow, T. J., and Frey, K. A. (1994) Positron emission tomographic analysis of cerebral structures activated specifically by repetitive noxious heat stimuli. *J. Neurophysiol.* **71**, 802–807.

41. Svensson, P., Minishima, S., Beydoun, A., Morrow, T. J. and Casey, K. L. (1997) Cerebral processing of acute skin and muscle pain in humans. *J. Neurophysiol* **78**, 450–460.

42. Derbyshire, S. W. G., Jones, A. K. P., Gyulai, F., Clark, S., Townsend, D., and Firestone, L. L. (1997) Pain processing during three levels of noxious stimulation produces differential patterns of central activity. *Pain* **73**, 431–445.

43. Davis, K. D., Wood, M. L., Crawley, A. P., and Mikulis, D. J. (1995) fMRI of human somatosensory and cingulate cortex during painful electrical nerve stimulation. *Neuroreport* **7**, 321–325.

44. Oshiro, Y., Fuijita, N., Tanaka, H., Hirabuki, N., Nakamura, H., and Yoshiya, I. (1998) Functional mapping of pain-related activation with echo-planar MRI: significance of the SII-insular region. *Neuroreport* **9**, 2285–2289.

45. Becerra, L. R., Breiter, H. C., Stojanovic, M., et al. (1999) Human brain activation under controlled thermal stimulation and habituation to noxious heat: an fMRI study. *Magn. Reson. Med.* **41**, 1044–1057.

46. Davis, K. D., Kwan, C. L., Crawley, A. P., and Mikulis, D. J. (1998) Event-related fMRI of pain: entering a new era in imaging pain. *Neuroreport* **9**, 3019–3023.

47. Hui, K. K., Liu, J., Makris, N., et al. (2000) Acupuncture modulates the limbic system and subcortical gray structures of the human brain: evidence from fMRI studies in normal subjects. *Hum. Brain Mapp.* **9**, 13–25.

48. Jones, A. K. P., Friston, K. J., Qi, L. Y., et al. (1991b) Sites of action of morphine in the brain. *Lancet* **338**, 825.

49. Firestone, L. L., Gyulai, F., Mintun, M., Adler, L. J., Urso, K., and Winter, P. (1996) Human brain activity response to fentanyl imaged by positron emission tomography. *Anesth. Analg.* **82**, 1247–1251.

50. Gyulai, F., Firestone, L. L., Mintun, M., and Winter, P. (1996) In Vivo Imaging of human limbic responses to nitrous oxide inhalation. *Anesth. Analg.* **83**, 291–298.

51. Zuniga, J. R., Joseph, S. A., and Knigge, K. M. (1987) The effects of nitrous oxide on the central endogenous pro-opiomelanocortin system in the rat. *Brain Res.* **420,** 57–65.
52. Chapman, C. R. and Benidetti, C. (1979) Nitrous oxide effects on cerebral evoked potential to pain: Partial reversal with a narcotic antagonist. *Anesthesiology* **51,** 135–138.
53. Adler, L. J., Gyulai, F. E., Diehl, D. J., Mintun, M. A., Winter, P. M., and Firestone, L. L. (1997) Regional brain activity changes associated with fentanyl analgesia elucidated by positron emission tomography. *Anesth. Analg.* **84,** 120–126.
54. Gyulai, F. E., Firestone, L. L., Mintun, M. A., and Winter, P. M. (1997a) In vivo imaging of nitrous oxide-induced changes in cerebral activation during noxious heat stimuli. *Anesthesiology* **86,** 538–548.
55. Alkire, M. T., Haier, R. J., Barker. S. J., Shah, N. K., Wu, J. C., and Kao, Y. J. (1995) Cerebral metabolism during propofol anesthesia in humans studied with positron emission tomography. *Anesthesiology* **82,** 393–407.
56. Alkire, M. T., Haier, R. J., Shah, N. K., and Anderson, C. T. (1997) Positron emission tomography study of regional cerebral metabolism in humans during isoflurane anesthesia. *Anesthesiology* **86,** 549–557.
57. Alkire, M. T., Pomfrett, C. J. D., Haie, R. J., et al. (1999) Functional brain imaging during anesthesia in humans. *Anesthesiology* **90,** 701–709.
58. Gyulai, F., Firestone, L., Mintun, M., Price, J., and Winter, P. (1997b) Dose-dependent effects of isoflurane on GABA$_A$ receptor conformation in vivo in humans. *Anesthesiology* **87,** A612.
59. Schwartz, W. J., Smith, C. B., Davidsen, L., et al. (1979) Metabolic mapping of functional activity in the hypothalamo-neurohypophysial system of the rat. *Science* **205,** 723–725.
60. Bottlaender, M., Brouillet, E., Varastet, M., et al. (1994) In vivo high intrinsic efficacy of triazolam: a positron emission tomography study in nonhuman primates. *J. Neurochem.* **61,** 1102–1111.
61. Kapur, S., Remington, G., Jones, C., Wilson, A., DaSilva, J., Houle, S., and Zipursky, R. (1996) High levels of dopamine D$_2$ receptor occupancy with low-dose haloperidol treatment: a PET study. *Am. J. Psychiatry* **153,** 948–950.
62. Galynker, I., Schlyer, D. J., Dewey, S. L., et al. (1996) Opioid receptor imaging and displacement studies with [6-O-[^{11}C]methyl]buprenorphine in baboon brain. *Nucl. Med. Biol.* **23,** 325–331.
63. Frost, J. J., Douglass, K. H., Mayberg, H. S., et al. (1989) Multicompartmental analysis of [^{11}C]-carfentanyl binding to opiate receptors in humans measured by positron emission tomography. *J. Cereb. Blood Flow Metab.* **9,** 398–409.
64. Breiter, H. C., Gollub, R. L., Weisskoff, R. M., et al. (1997) Acute effects of cocaine on human brain activity and emotion. *Neuron* **19,** 591–611.
65. Antognini, J. F., Buonocore, M. H., Disbrow, E. A., and Carstens, E. (1997) Isoflurane anesthesia blunts cerebral responses to noxious and innocuous stimuli: a fMRI study. *Life Sci.* **61,** L349–L354.

Anthony Angel

INTRODUCTION

An inspection of the chapter headings in this book indicates that the action of anesthetic agents, in the whole animal, gives a diverse spectrum of system perturbations. An anesthetized patient shows a change in level of consciousness (*see* Chapter 2), cannot lay down either short- or long-term memory traces (*see* Chapter 3), shows no volitional movements, no gravitational corrective movements, attenuated protective reflexes (*see* Chapter 4), and cannot see, hear, feel, taste or smell. Additionally, there are usually changes in cardiovascular and respiratory performance (except with Xenon *[1,2]* or urethane in animals *[3]*) and an inability to control core temperature. The dose of anesthetic needed to achieve either of the two widely accepted anesthetic endpoints (i.e., loss of righting reflex or withdrawal reflex) varies with age in mammals (*see*, for example, ref. *4*) in that the dose required to anesthetize neonates is higher than that for adult animals. A phenomenon possibly related to central nervous system maturation and development. At the molecular level, anesthetic agents have been shown to interact with ion channels to either enhance or depress channel currents to their specific agonist neurotransmitters (*see* Chapters 16–20). These changes, which are clear-cut for specific ion channels expressed in Xenopus oocytes, are much more difficult to interpret in, or translate to, the whole animal.

The study of anesthetic effects in the whole animal is complicated by the absence of a simple structure/activity relationship that holds for all other bioactive chemicals. Molecules that show anesthetic properties, vary from very simple (e.g., Nitrogen, Xenon) to complex steroids (e.g., Alphadalone and Alphaxalone). Although superficially, the action of anesthetic agents can be "antagonized" by convulsant chemicals, the only effective "antagonist" (using the word antagonist to denote reversal of effect) is to increase the ambient pressure to very high levels (ca. 100 atm or 10 Mpa). This is obviously not classical competitive antagonism at a specific receptor site with a specific chemical agent, but a simple physico-chemical barrier to a theoretical interaction between an anesthetic agent and a putative hydrophobic receptor site. However, since behaviorally, the effect of anesthetic agents can be reversed by high pressure, it allows an experimental tool to tease apart anesthetic effects *per se* as opposed to possible side effects.

This chapter will deal with only one aspect of anesthetic effects, that is the disruption of sensory experience seen with all anesthetic agents and indeed, the phenomenon which has given them their name i.e., without aesthetic sensation. Sensory information in the near (touch), remote (heat sound and light), or the internal (kinaesthetic) environment is transduced by specialized peripheral receptors and transmitted to the nervous system, ultimately to the cerebral cortex, along well-defined sensory pathways. In the somatosensory system, there are two well-defined pathways; that for touch ascends in the dorsal column-medial lemniscal system and that for thermal sensations plus "slow" and "fast" pain in the anterolateral system. Touch and thermal sensations are ultimately routed to the soma-

From: *Contemporary Clinical Neuroscience:* Neural Mechanisms of Anesthesia
Edited by: Joseph F. Antognini et al. © Humana Press Inc., Totowa, NJ

tosensory cortex via the thalamus as a well defined but distorted map of body space–in man the sensory homunculus. (Pain information is routed elsewhere in the nervous system. This is evident from the work of Penfield *(5)* whose patients never reported painful sensations to electrical stimulation of the cerebral mantle, and to the experience of neurosurgeons who can position electrodes for stereotaxic surgery without evoking pain.) For brevity and clarity, this Chapter will only deal with the somatosensory system although all the sensory systems show roughly the same properties.

The peripheral receptors have small (distal structures—below the wrist and ankle), intermediate (from wrist to elbow or ankle to knee), or large (proximal structures–neck and shoulder or leg and trunk) receptive fields. Separate sensory modalities (touch, pressure, hair movement, claw movement, hot and cold) are subserved by different receptor types and the information is processed initially in a parallel fashion (along distinct and separate pathways), then serially processed in the cerebral cortex to give the resultant sensation i.e.; touched with a warm, smooth object. The process of integrating the parallel delivered information is not well understood in the sensory system, but is apparently achieved in a manner analogous to that shown by simple, complex and hypercomplex cells in the visual system. The somatosensory system can be interrogated in the anesthetized animal in two separate ways.

- Because the periphery projects to a specific cortical area, the stimulation of a peripheral nerve, e.g., at the wrist, will be conveyed to the forepaw or hand area of the primary somatosensory cortex at which site a population of cortical cells will be activated. Placing electrodes on the exposed cortical surface, one at the center of the forepaw projection area (active electrode), and one remote from this site (reference electrode), allows the currents generated by this population of cortical cells to be summed between the two electrodes and recorded as a cerebral cortical evoked response. It can be shown that cerebral evoked responses are related to the intensity of peripheral stimulation. The resultant sensation can be related to the sensory stimulation *(6)* and hence the evoked response can be used in animal models as an indication of sensation, or more particularly as a change in sensation. In the lissencephalic (smooth) cortex of the rat, and the consequent simple geometric relationship between the recording electrodes and resultant current flow from the activated cells, the evoked cortical response is relatively simple and easily interpreted (*see* Anesthetic Effects on Evoked Cerebral Responses).

- In addition, all short latency activity evoked by peripheral electrical stimulation of group A fibers or directly applied mechanical stimulation is abolished by section of the dorsal columns and is unaffected by transection of the dorsolateral columns (spinocervical path) or anterolateral columns (spinothalamic path *[7]*). In this fast pathway, afferent information from the periphery ascends in the ipsilateral dorsal columns to synapses on cells in the dorsal column nuclei. The output fibers from these cells cross to the opposite side and ascend to the contralateral ventrobasal thalamus. Cells at this site give rise to the thalamo-cortical radiation fibers that terminate mainly in cortical layer IV, with a small subset going also to cortical layer VI. Thus, the pathway can be interrogated by recording the extracellular current from single cells in the dorsal column nuclei, the ventrobasal thalamus and layers IV–VI of the cerebral cortex.

As the afferent information ascends to the cerebral cortex, it is subjected to a variety of tonic and phasic modulations. This is clearly seen in the cerebral evoked responses which, whatever the basal anesthetic used, are not constant, but vary in latency and conformation on a response-to-response basis.

ANATOMY OF THE THALAMUS

The thalamic nuclei, situated on either side of the third ventricle, can be considered as composed of a paired rod-shaped mass of cells (*see* Fig. 1) whose function is to transmit and modify information from sensory inputs.

- Visual information is transmitted by the lateral geniculate nuclei to the primary visual cortex.
- Auditory information passes via the medial geniculate nuclei to the primary auditory cortex.
- Somatosensory information is passed via the ventrobasal complex: ventroposteromedial nuclei (from face) and ventroposterolateral nuclei (rest of body) to the primary somatosensory cortex.
- Sensory (kinaesthetic and proprioceptive) and motor information from the cerebellum is passed to the primary motor cortical area via the ventrolateral nuclei and from the basal ganglia via the ventral anterior nuclei to the premotor cortex.

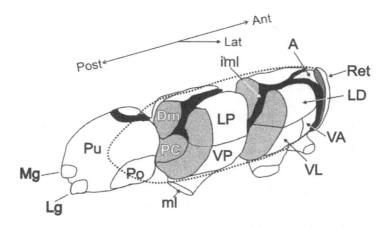

Fig. 1. A schematic diagram of the right thalamic nuclei. Anterior Nuclei, **A**; Dorsomedial nucleus, **Dm**; Internal medullary lamina (which separates the thalamic nuclei into anterior, medial and lateral parts), **iml**; Lateral dorsal nucleus, **LD**; Lateral geniculate nucleus, **Lg**; Lateral Posterior nucleus, **LP**; Medial geniculate nucleus, **Mg**; Medial lemniscus, **ml**; Parafasicular/Centrum medianum complex, **PC**; Posterior group of nuclei, **Po**; Pulvinar, **Pu**; Thalamic reticular nucleus–shown mainly dotted, **Ret**; Ventral anterior nucleus, **VA**; Ventral lateral nucleus, **VL**; Ventroposterolateral and ventroposteromedial nuclei (ventrobasal nuclei), **VP**.

- The lateral nuclei (posterior and dorsal) receive inputs from the medial and lateral geniculate nuclei, as well as from the ventrobasal nuclei and project to the parietal cortex, posterior to the somatosensory cortex.
- The pulvinar projects to wide areas of the temporal, parietal and occipital cortical areas.
- The dorsal medial nuclei relay information from the amygdaloid nucleus and project to the prefrontal cortex.
- The anterior nuclei project to the cingulate gyri.
- The thalamic reticular nucleus covers the dorsolateral, lateral and ventrolateral sides of the thalamic mass and is interconnected with the thalamic nuclei.
- Unlike the other thalamic nuclei the thalamic reticular nucleus does not send any fibers directly to the cerebral cortex.

Figure 2 shows the interrelationships between the thalamic somatosensory relay nucleus, the thalamic reticular nucleus, and the primary somatosensory cortex. A similar arrangement is seen for the auditory, visual, and motor relay paths. The fibers ascending from the dorsal column nuclei end on the thalamic relay cells employing glutamate as their neurotransmitter to excite both AMPA and NMDA receptors. AMPA receptors will give a fast, short-lived excitation and NMDA receptors a slower, longer-lasting excitation. The majority of cells in the rat ventroposterolateral (VPL) nucleus are excited from small receptive fields on the glabrous surface of the paws responding mainly to touch or pressure *(8)*. The output axons from these VPL cells form the cortico-thalamic fibers that project to the primary somatosensory cortex forming three overlapping projections from the touch, pressure, and hair sensitive inputs. In the face area, from the ventroposteromedial nucleus, the projection is mainly to cortical barrels each innervated by one vibrissa *(9)*. As the cortico-thalamic fibers pass through the thalamic reticular nucleus, they give off branches that excite the thalamic reticular cells. In the rat, they also give branches to a different (behaviorally) subset of cells that are interspersed with the thalamic reticular nucleus on the lateral border of the VPL nucleus. These thalamic reticular and boundary cells project back onto the VPL cells from which they receive their input. Cortical cells in layer VI, and possibly layer V, of the primary somatosensory cortex send a return projection to both the VPL cells from which they receive their input and to the thalamic reticular and boundary cells connected to the same VPL cells. Behaviorally, the thalamic reticular cells show

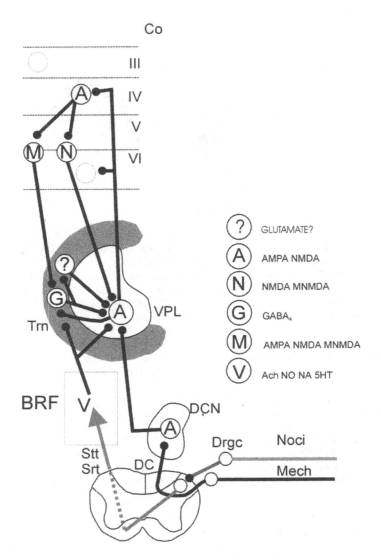

Fig. 2. A schematic diagram of the somatosensory pathway from the forepaw. The letters within the diagrammatic cells (circles) or brain stem box represent the various neurotransmitters released by the terminating fibers. Synaptic connections are represented by small circles. (For further details *see* text). Thalamic reticular cells are labeled **G**, boundary cells are labeled **?**; Brain stem reticular formation, **BRF**; Primary Somatosensory Cortex layer III to VI, **Co**; Dorsal columns, **DC**; Dorsal column nucleus (Cuneate), **DCN**; Dorsal root ganglion cell, **Drgc**; Mechanoceptive input, **Mech**; Thermal and nociceptive input, **Noci**; Spinoreticular path, **Srt**; Spinothalamic path, **Stt**; Thalamic reticular nucleus (shaded), **Trn**; Ventroposterolateral nucleus, **VPL**.

spontaneous activity that is slowed by nociceptive inputs from anywhere on the body surface. The boundary cells also show spontaneous activity, but are excited by nociceptive inputs from anywhere on the body surface. Because there are very few short-axoned interneurons in VPL, the main modulation of thalamic relay cell activity will be given by a series of somatotopically arranged feedback circuits:

- A direct inhibitory feedback from the thalamic reticular cells mediated by GABA$_A$ receptors.
- A direct excitatory, possibly glutamatergic, feedback from the thalamic border cells.

- A direct cortico-thalamic feedback, mainly from cells in cortical layer VI, mediated by both NMDA and metabotropic NMDA receptors which can act directly on thalamic relay cells and also modulate the effect of thalamic reticular GABA inhibition.
- An indirect cortico-thalamic-reticulo-thalamic feedback with the receptor types involved being glutamatergic AMPA, NMDA, and metabotropic NMDA synapses on the thalamic reticular cells.

(For further detailed information about the anatomy and neurochemistry of the thalamic nuclei *see* refs. *11–18*). In addition, the thalamic relay nuclei receive collaterals of fibers passing from the brain stem reticular formation to forebrain sites from the noradrenergic projection arising in the locus coeruleus, the serotonergic (5-hydroxytryptaminergic) projection from the midline raphé nuclei, and a cholinergic projection from the upper brain stem. These projections innervate all of the thalamic nuclei but are particularly dense in the ventral lateral geniculate nuclei and the anterior nuclei. Although usually described as separate specific neurotransmitter systems, it must be remembered that they are functionally interrelated. There are also various glutamatergic and peptidergic projections from other brain-stem sites. The bulk of the ascending reticular activating system also sends projections to the thalamic nuclei via the midbrain reticular system. A possible role for nitric oxide has been put forward also as a method of modulating thalamic relay cell activity *(15)*.

EFFECT OF ANESTHETIC AGENTS ON SENSORY TRANSMISSION

The currents generated by electrical stimulation of a peripheral nerve recorded at the center of the appropriate primary somatosensory cortical receiving area will be superimposed on any spontaneous electrocortical activity and show a moment-to-moment variation. The individual signals will thus show two components: (a) a response related to the stimulus and (b) biological noise. To estimate the activity of the population of cortical cells responding to the sensory stimulus, it is necessary to average a series of consecutive responses. This gives essentially, the sum of all the signals that are time-locked to the stimulus, in direct proportion to the number of signals averaged; whereas, there will be a reduction in the biological noise which, because it occurs at random with respect to the stimulus, it will sum in proportion to the square root of the number averaged. Thus, the average response to 64 stimuli will have its noise component reduced to one eighth. Such averaged evoked cortical responses appear as a wave of positivity interrupted by a series of negative waves or inflections (*see* Fig. 3). From such responses, it is possible to measure the latency of the response (Fig. 3A L), which is the time from the stimulus to the start of the cortical response, the amplitude of the initial positive wave (Fig. 3A Pi), and the amplitude of the initial negative wave (Fig. 3A Ni).

- The latency represents the total time of transmission through the sensory pathway, both peripheral and central, to the sensory cortex.
- The Pi, measured from the baseline to the peak of the initial positive wave, represents the summed excitatory postsynaptic potentials in the cortical cells, and is an index of the size of the thalamo-cortical volley *(19)*.
- The Ni, measured from the peak of the initial positive wave to the trough of the initial negative wave represents the summed action potentials of cortical cells, and is an index of the cortical response to its input *(19)*.

Anesthetic Effects on Evoked Cerebral Responses

To investigate the effects of anesthetics, animals were anesthetized with urethane (ethyl carbamate; 1.25 g/kg), the long acting barbiturate Inactin (sodium thiobutabarbital; 172 mg/kg), or halothane (2-bromo-2-chloro-1,1,1,trifluoroethane; 1.3% in oxygen), and anesthetic depth increased using a variety of anesthetic agents. Earlier work *(20)* had shown that the changes seen as anesthetic depth was increased, was identical if the animal was anesthetized with a single anesthetic agent throughout the experiment, or if the anesthetics were superimposed upon a baseline of urethane. Additionally, in a limited series of experiments, the same changes were seen if animals with implanted cortical electrodes were taken from the unanesthetized to the deeply anesthetized state. By analyzing the effects

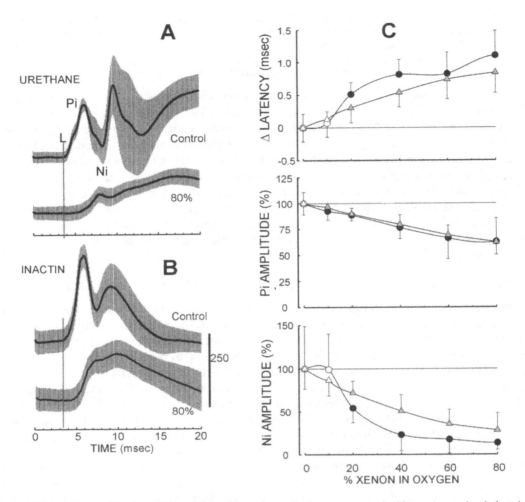

Fig. 3. The effects of the group 1 anesthetic Xenon on cortical responses evoked by supramaximal electrical stimulation at the wrist at a rate of one/s. The averaged responses in **(A)** and **(B)** are to 100 consecutive stimuli, and show the average responses (thick lines) ± SD (fine vertical lines) from an animal anesthetized with urethane (1.25 g/kg [**A**]) and from an animal anesthetized with Inactin, (172 mg/kg [**B**]). (Both anesthetics were given without any premedication. At these doses the animals showed no responses to noxious stimulation of the hindpaw, nor did they show any response to the surgery). The starting latencies are indicated by the vertical lines (labeled **L** in [**A**]) and the initial positive wave and initial negative wave are labeled **Pi** and **Ni** respectively. The averaged effects on the latency and amplitudes of **Pi** and **Ni** of increasing Urethane inspired concentrations of Xenon in Oxygen (*abscissa*) from 12 animals anesthetized with Urethane (*circles*), and 14 animals anesthetized with Inactin (*triangles*) are shown in **(C)**.

The latency results are expressed as change in latency from the starting value with the animal breathing Oxygen alone, and the amplitudes of the initial positive and negative waves are expressed as a percentage change from the starting values. Each point represents the mean, and the bars represent the SD. Filled symbols indicate that the data is statistically significantly different from starting levels ($p < 0.05$). There was no statistically significant difference between the response curves obtained for either basal anesthetic.

of increasing anesthetic depth, and quantifying the three parameters of the evoked response (L, Pi, and Ni), anesthetic agents can be sorted into three basic groups. A fourth group can be defined, somewhat artificially, to isolate those anesthetic agents with specific neurotransmitter agonist or antagonist activity.

All anesthetic agents used gave a dose-dependent increase in the latency of the responses. In the first group of anesthetic agents, (which include urethane, alfentanil, althesin, pentobarbitone, hexabarbitone, thiopentone, inactin, ketamine, trichloroethylene, halothane, forane, enflurane, methoxyflurane, diethyl ether, ethyl vinyl ether, cyclopropane and Xenon), the amplitudes of both the initial positive and initial negative waves showed a dose-dependent decrease as anesthetic depth was increased. For urethane and Halothane, these changes could be reversed by high ambient pressure *(21)*. Figure 3 shows these effects for Xenon applied on either a basal level of urethane or Inactin. There was no statistically significant difference on the changes in the three parameters measured with either anesthetic, as Xenon concentration was increased from 10 to 80%.

In the second group (Etomidate and Propofol; Fig. 4A), the amplitude of the initial positive wave was unaffected as anesthetic depth was increased, but the amplitude of the initial negative wave was decreased in a dose-dependent manner.

In the third group (the benzodiazepines Librium and Midazolam; Fig. 4B). the amplitude of the initial positive wave showed a small dose-dependent decrease, whereas that of the initial negative wave was either unaltered, or actually increased in some experiments as anesthetic depth was increased.

The fourth group (Fig. 4C and D) was separated from the other three, since specific drugs were used to modify noradrenergic, cholinergic, or serotonergic (5-hydroxytryptaminergic) transmission. All the drugs used (*see* ref. *22* for full details), if they displayed any ability to alter the cerebral evoked responses, they gave the same changes as those seen to the first group of anesthetics, or behaved as logical first group "anti-anesthetics," in that they decreased the latency and increased the amplitudes of the initial positive and negative waves. For all the α_2-adrenoreceptor agonists, the most potent of which were Clonidine and Medetomidine, there was a biphasic effect. At low doses, they decreased, slightly but significantly, the anesthetic level, and acted only as anesthetics at high doses. If one assumes that the number of presynaptic adrenergic autoreceptors is smaller than the postsynaptic population, then proportionally more presynaptic receptors could be blocked at low doses. This would mean that the release of endogenous noradrenaline would be decreased at agonist low doses, and hence, decrease anesthetic levels. At a higher dose, the majority of postsynaptic receptors would be activated to reveal the anesthetic effect. The effects of medetomidine were identical in animals anesthetized with Inactin.

The differential effects of the anesthetic agents seen can be summarized as:

- All anesthetic agents delay the transmission of the signal somewhere along the pathway.
- Group 1 and 4 anesthetics decrease the cortical inflow and diminish the cortical cellular response.
- Group 2 anesthetics decrease the cortical cellular response to a virtually unchanged cortical input.
- Group 3 anesthetics slightly decrease the cortical inflow, but the cortical cellular response appears to be enhanced.

The Thalamus as a Potential Site of Anesthetic Action

For a definitive answer of what happens to the sensory input, it is necessary to interrogate the pathway by recording from single cells in the dorsal column nuclei, the ventrobasal thalamus, and in the various cortical layers. Peripheral nerve fibers can be excluded since no effects of anesthetic are seen on nerve fibers until lethal levels of anesthetic are administered. Cells were recorded using extracellular microelectrodes to determine if either their latency or probability of response was altered.

When recording from single cells in the cuneate nucleus, regardless of which basal anesthetic was used, the cells followed each peripheral stimulus, provided that it was supramaximal, with at least one impulse per stimulus, and the responses showed little, or no, variation except in the longer latency discharges (Fig. 5A CUN). For cells in the thalamic relay nucleus, however, a completely different picture was observed. The responses of the cells varied from moment–to–moment in both latency and probability (Fig. 5A VPL). This variability cannot be related to spontaneous discharge rendering them partially refractory to some stimuli because (a), the majority of cells encountered had small receptive fields on the glabrous surface of the forepaw and (b), these cells show little spontaneous

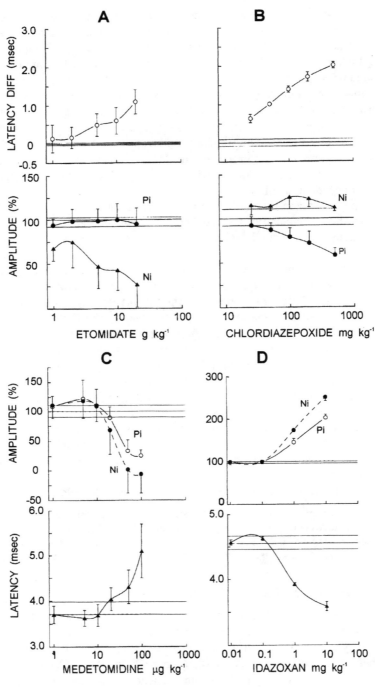

Fig. 4. The effects of the group 2 anesthetic Etomidate (**A**), the group 3 anesthetic Chlordiazepoxide (**B**), and the group 4 chemicals, Medetomidine an adrenoceptor α_2-agonist, which acts as an anesthetic at doses >10 µg/kg (**C**), and Idazoxan an adrenoceptor α_2-antagonist that acts as an antianesthetic at doses >100 µg/kg (**D**). The results, which are expressed in the same way as in Fig. 3, are from five animals for each graph, and the chemicals were superimposed upon a basal anesthetic of urethane (1.25 g/kg). Each point on the graphs represents the mean, the vertical bars represent the SEM. The horizontal lines through the graphs represent the starting level of latency ± SEM. The (*upper*) and (*lower*) lines in the amplitude graphs represent the SEM for **Pi** and **Ni**, respectively.

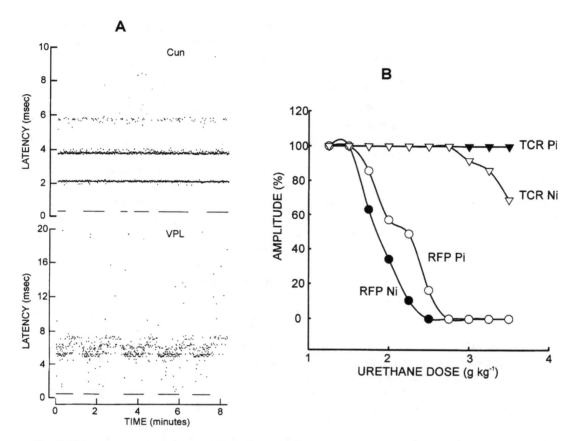

Fig. 5. 500 consecutive responses from a single cuneate neuron (**A**), and 500 consecutive responses from a single ventrobasal thalamic neuron to supramaximal electrical stimulation applied at the wrist, at a rate of 1/s, from two different animals anesthetized with Urethane (1.25 g/kg). The responses of the cells are shown as a dot raster display. If the cell gave an all-or-none action potential to the stimulus, this was converted electronically into a dot and drawn at the latency of its occurrence (Ordinate). The stimuli caused the display to advance to the right and hence, the abscissa shows the timing of the response series. The horizontal lines indicate periods of low voltage high frequency electrocortical activity (**B**).

Graphs of the initial positive and initial negative waves (**Pi** and **Ni**) measured from averaged responses (*N* = 64 1/s) to electrical stimulation at the wrist (**RFP**), or delivered via a microelectrode to the thalamo-cortical radiation fibers (**TCR**) in an animal anesthetized with urethane (1.25 g/kg). The graph shows the effect of increasing levels of urethane anesthesia (abscissa), and the results are expressed as percentage of the starting values for each parameter (**C**).

activity. Cells in the thalamic relay nucleus fail to respond, on average, to one stimulus in five. Thus, they are not very secure synaptically. Another reason that the ventrobasal thalamus could be a target for anesthetic action can be essayed from a comparison of cortical responses evoked by stimulation of the forepaw, to those evoked by stimulation of thalamo-cortical axons via a microelectrode. Stimulation of the thalamo-cortical radiation fibers gives a complex cortical response consisting of an initial positive wave caused by antidromic activation of the cortical cells in layers V and VI, followed by a second positive wave caused by excitation of cells in cortical layers IV–VI by thalamo-cortical afferents. These two positive waves are followed by a negative wave given by the firing of the cortical cells both anti- and orthodromically. In comparing the positive waves to pre- and postthalamic stimulation, the responses representing the summed excitatory postsynaptic currents to prethalamic stimulation show a dose dependent decrease in their amplitudes whereas, those to postthalamic stimulation do not (compare RFP Pi and TCR Pi in Fig. 5B). The cellular cortical responses recorded to postthalamic stimulation are also resistant to anesthetic action (compare RFP Ni and TCR Ni in Fig. 5B). Thus, one can surmise the reduction in cortical responsiveness seen to increasing anesthesia for the group 1 anesthetics takes place at a subcortical level.

Anesthetic Effects on Relay Cells Along the Somatosensory Pathway

For a direct comparison of the behavior of the different cells along the pathway, a restriction must be included in the experimental paradigm. Cells in the cuneate nucleus must be monosynaptically activated by the stimulus. The ventrobasal thalamic relay cells must be monosynaptically activated by the cuneo-thalamic input, and cortical cells, in cortical layers IV and VI, must be monosynaptically activated by the thalamo-cortical input. This means, effectively, that the cells at each locus must have latencies of discharge that are consistent for monosynaptic activation.

For group 1 anesthetics, no cells in the cuneate nucleus showed any decrement in their activity as anesthetic depth was increased, provided that the peripheral stimulus was supramaximal. In complete contrast, all cells recorded from in the thalamic relay nucleus showed a dose-related increase in their latency of discharge, and a dose-related decrease in their probability of response. The same effect was observed in cortical cells in layers IV and VI. From the behavior of the cortical responses to pre- and post-thalamic stimulation, it would seem that these cells merely mirror the decreased thalamic input as anesthetic depth is increased. However, cells recorded from cortical layer V appeared to be more susceptible to anesthetic action. Their dose response curve was shifted to the left compared to cortical layer IV and VI cells. *See* Fig. 6C for summary of the effects of increasing levels of urethane anesthesia on cells at each level of the somatosensory pathway. Identical changes were observed with all the other group 1 anesthetic agents. In addition, the effect of Xenon on somatosensory cells was identical in a comparison made between animals with a basal anesthetic of urethane or Inactin. Similar effects have been reported for isoflurane to "natural" stimulation in the rat, as responses recorded from presumed trigemino-thalamic fibers showed a lesser sensitivity than thalamic trigeminal relay cells as anesthetic depth was increased *(23)*.

For group 2 anesthetics (Etomidate and Propofol), again, there were no changes in the response of cuneate cells as anesthetic depth was increased. In contrast to the action of group 1 anesthetics, they had no effect on the probability of thalamic relay cell responses until very high dose-levels were reached. There was, however, a small increase in response latency at low doses (Fig. 6A, VPL). Cells in cortical layers IV and VI showed a dose-dependant decrease in probability and latency of response (Fig. 6A, Co IV). *See* Fig. 6B for the effects of Etomidate on animals anesthetized with urethane. Again, cells in cortical layer V appear to be more anesthetic susceptible as their dose response curve is shifted to the left.

The benzodiazepines (group 3) again showed no effect on cuneate cell discharge. Cells in the thalamic relay nucleus and all cortical layers had a decreased probability of response and an increased latency of response. The increase in latency depends upon the dose administered, but the reduction in probability is achieved at small doses (<20 mg/kg, for Midazolam). *See* Fig. 7A for an example of a single thalamic relay cell from an animal with a basal anesthetic of urethane to increasing doses of Midazolam. In the control condition, it responded with a bimodal latency distribution of 4.60 and 5.75 ms. After Midazolam, it showed a unimodal latency distribution at modal latencies of 5.80, 5.95, and 6.00 ms for doses of Midazolam of 10, 20, and 40 mg/kg, respectively, with response probabilities of 75.9, 76.3, and 82.3% (compared to the starting level of 100%). Thus, the effect of this group of anesthetic agents appears to be one of stabilization of the cells' response. However, it should be noted that superimposing a low dose of chlordiazepoxide or Midazolam onto a basal level of urethane anesthesia does give a marked change in electrocortical activity. The pattern of HVLF activity changes to one of cortical spindling.

The group 4 anesthetics again show no effect on dorsal column nuclei cells (Fig. 7C). Cholinergic muscarinic antagonists showed an effect on ventrobasal thalamic cells, similar to the group 1 anesthetic agents. However, the anesthetic effect of cholinergic drugs was always modest even at very

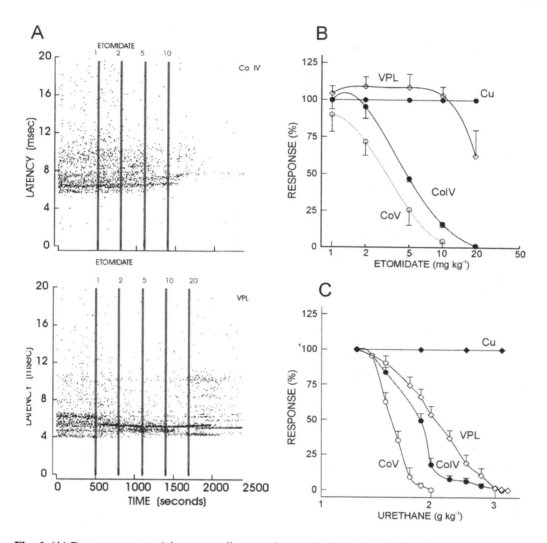

Fig. 6. (A) Dot raster sequential response diagrams from a single cortical cell from layer IV (**Co IV**) and a single thalamic relay cell (**VPL**) recorded from 2 different animals with a basal anesthetic of urethane (1.25 g/kg). Increasing doses of Etomidate were administered by intraperitoneal injection at the vertical lines to give a cumulative dose of Etomidate as shown on the vertical lines (dose as mg/kg). **(B)** and **(C)** Compares the effect of increasing anesthetic depth with Etomidate **(B)** 5 cells from each of the sites recorded from: the cuneate nucleus **Cu**, thalamic relay nucleus **VPL**, Cortical layer IV **CoIV** and cortical layer V **CoV** to supramaximal percutaneous electrical stimulation applied at the wrist at a rate of 1/s) and urethane **(C)** for 35 cuneate cells, 30 thalamic relay cells, 40 cells from cortical layers IV and VI and 4 cells from cortical layer V). Each point on the graph shows the mean probability of response referred to a starting level of 100% for each cell ± SEM (ordinate) versus the increased dose of anesthetic administered (abscissa).

high concentrations. The effect of the α_2-adrenoreceptor agonist drugs are, however, specific. They delay thalamic transmission but markedly prolong the discharge of the cells so that the total number of nerve impulses produced after the administration of these drugs means, the probability of response actually rises, after such chemicals at anesthetic doses between 200 and 300% of starting values. Clearly, this is anomalous. If one considers that the effect of α_2-adrenoreceptor antagonist drugs is to give an overall decrease in anesthetic depth, then it is apparent that the nervous system does not act on the number of impulses evoked per stimulus but, the pattern of such cell discharge must also be of

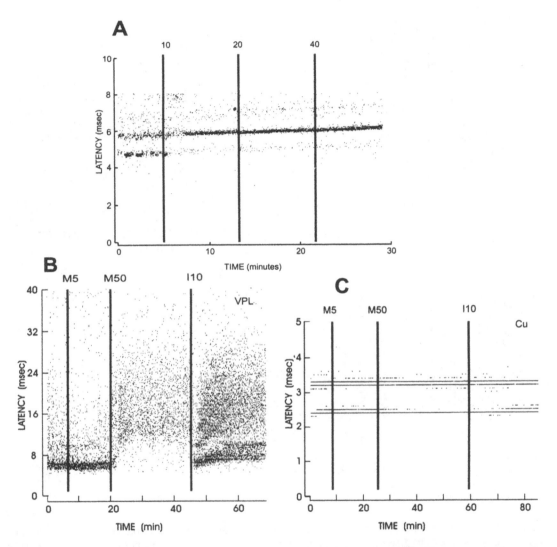

Fig. 7. The effect on a single thalamic relay cell, as a sequential dot raster display from an animal anesthe-tized with urethane (1.25 g/kg) of intraperitoneal injections of Midazolam of 10, 20, and 40 mg/kg (vertical lines) to supramaximal percutaneous electrical stimulation at the wrist at a rate of 1/s (**A**).

The effects of subanesthetic (5 μg/kg M5) and anesthetic doses (50 of μg/kg M50) of the adrenoceptor α_2-agonist Medetomidine, and to the adrenoceptor α_2-antagonist Idazoxan (10 mg/kg I10) from a thalamic relay cell (**VPL**), and a cuneate nucleus cell (**Cu**) from two different animals anesthetized with Urethane (**B** and **C**).

importance together with the timing of the discharge. The effect of Medetomidine (a potent α_2-adrenoreceptor agonist) superimposed on a basal level of urethane anesthesia. Fig. 7C for a single cuneate cell upon which Medetomidine and the α_2-adrenoreceptor antagonist Idazoxan shows little effect, and for a thalamic relay cell (Fig. 7B) on which the effect of the larger dose of Medetomidine is obvious, as is the transient reversal of its effect by Idazoxan. Cells in cortical layers IV and VI mirror the effect seen at the thalamic level, and cells in layer V show, paradoxically, little effect. Again, the same effects are seen in animals anesthetized with Inactin.

Possible Mechanism of Thalamic Modulation

In microelectrode penetrations lateral to the thalamic relay nuclei, cells that are entirely different to thalamic relay cells are encountered. These cells are always spontaneously active, are not influenced, at short latency, by gentle stimulation of the integument i.e., touch, gentle pressure, and hair movement, but do show a change in their activity to noxious stimulation i.e., cutting, pinching or heating the skin. Their "receptive fields" usually extend over the entire body surface. Stimulation of the contralateral body half usually exerts a greater effect than stimulation applied to the ipsilateral body half *(10)*. Two types of such cell are found: those that decrease their frequency of discharge to a noxious stimulus, and those that increase their frequency of discharge after such a stimulus *(10)*. These latter can be easily distinguished from cells responding to hair displacement in the thalamic relay nucleus, which occasionally have their discharge frequency increased by a noxious stimulus, because they never respond, at short latency, to group A nerve stimulation applied at the wrist. Several behavioral correlations show that these cells are probably involved in a modulatory role for the transmission of thalamic sensory information:

- The time course of their discharge after a train of electrical stimuli sufficiently intense to activate group A and group C nerve fibers is exactly the same as that of the increase in thalamic relay cell excitability, after such stimuli *(10)*. As one type always increases their frequency of discharge, it can be postulated that they act as excitatory interneurons, whereas, the other type act as inhibitory interneurons.
- They are found in the anatomical confines of the thalamic reticular nucleus and its boundary zone with the thalamic relay nuclei *(10)*. Cells of opposite type are usually found intermingled with each other, and occasionally, both types of cell can be recorded from the same microelectrode, albeit with different recorded voltages. Because the microelectrodes used (glass micropipets with a tip diameter of 1–2 μm, filled with isotonic sodium acetate and impedances of 10–20 MΩ), extracellular records from single cells usually appear from the background noise and disappear into the background noise for vertical electrode movements of, on average, 80 μm. This implies a close anatomical positioning for the two types of cells encountered.
- The inhibitory neurons are excited by cortical stimulation, and the excitatory neurons are inhibited by such stimuli. In urethane anesthetized rats, the same changes are observed after stimulation of the pyramidal tract, at the level of the pyramidal decussation. Because such stimulation only discharges cells in cortical layer V, then this would point to the cortical cells that control these thalamic cells located in part in this layer *(24)*. This is contrary to the findings of most workers *(see* ref. *18)*, who find retrogradely labeled cells only in cortical layer VI after thalamic injections of horseradish peroxidase.
- After cortical ablation, the excitatory cells show an increase in their spontaneous activity, and the inhibitory cells show a decrease. The cells in the thalamic relay nuclei show a large increase in their probability of response and a decrease in their latency to peripheral stimulation, after cortical ablation *(24)*.
- Both types of cells show long-term changes in their discharge frequencies at stimulation voltages that excite thalamic relay cells. The presumed inhibitory cells show an increased frequency of discharge that peaks at 100 ms and lasts for approx 500 ms after a peripheral stimulus. The presumed excitatory cells show a decrease in their frequency with a similar time course *(24)*.

A similar distribution of two types of spontaneously active cells in the cerebral cortex again either sped up or slowed down by noxious stimulation has been seen. In the cortex, however, each group can be subdivided into two categories: (a) those which, in addition, respond at short latency to gentle peripheral stimulation, and (b), those which only respond, at long latency, to noxious stimuli. Thus these two subsets of cortical cells could be responsible for phasic and tonic modulation of thalamic sensory transmission. Interestingly, these cells appear to be monosynaptically linked to the thalamic reticular cells in such a way that cortical excitatory cells excite thalamic excitatory cells and inhibit thalamic inhibitory cells. Whereas, the reverse is seen for cortical inhibitory cells, which excite thalamic inhibitory cells and inhibit thalamic excitatory cells *(25)*. Thus, behaviorally, one has subsets of thalamo-cortical and cortico-thalamic cells that could be considered as prime candidates for the anatomical modulation circuits already identified *(see* Fig. 2).

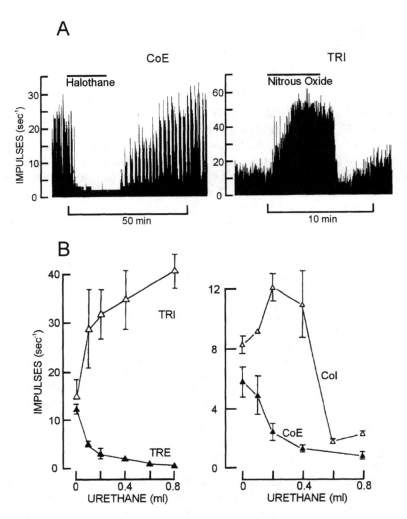

Fig. 8. (A) A representative example of a single cortical presumed excitatory cell to inspiring 1.3% Halothane in oxygen (**CoE**), and a thalamic reticular presumed inhibitory cell (**TRI**) to inspiring 80% nitrous oxide in oxygen from two different animals anesthetized at a basal level with urethane (1.25 g/kg). The graphs (**B**) below show the mean effect of increasing depth of urethane anesthesia (expressed as mL of urethane added intraperitoneally (abscissa) from a basal level of 1.25 g/kg, to a final level of 2.25 g/kg) from thalamic reticular cells of both types (inhibitory, **TRI** $N = 6$ and excitatory **TRE** $N = 6$), 8 cortical excitatory cells (**CoE**), and 4 cortical inhibitory cells (**CoI**). Each point on the graphs represents the mean and the vertical bars ± SD.

In the medullary reticular formation, two types of cell are found which, like those in the thalamus, respond only to noxious peripheral stimulation with extensive "receptive fields."

If the thalamic and cortical cells are involved in the decrease in thalamic transmission seen after administration of anesthetic agents, then logically, those cells which are presumed to be inhibitory should have their frequency of discharge increased, and the excitatory cells should have their frequency of discharge decreased as anesthetic depth increases. This is what is seen for all the group 1 anesthetic agents used (*see* Fig. 8). The thalamic cells behave in the predicted manner, as do the cortical excitatory cells, but the cortical inhibitory cells appear to deviate from the theoretical prediction. However, this can possibly be explained (*see* Changes in Somatosensory Transmission).

OSCILLATIONS IN A PRESUMED STEADY STATE OF ANESTHETIC DEPTH

Changes in Electrocortical Activity

One of the peculiar facets of anesthetized animals is that, with a constant concentration of anesthetic, they show spontaneous and abrupt changes between electrocortical activity of high voltage low frequency (HVLF) and low voltage high frequency (LVHF). So far, this phenomenon has been observed with urethane *(26)* and Inactin, which are extremely slowly metabolized anesthetics, and also in animals inspiring a constant concentration of Halothane. This occurs with a cycle time of 95.8 s (± 4.1 s SEM; $N = 224$) for animals anesthetized with urethane (1.25 g/kg); 116.9 s (± 10.7 s SEM, $N = 11$) for animals anesthetized with Inactin (172 mg/kg); and 117.7 s (± 37.3 s SEM, $N = 6$) for animals breathing 1.3% Halothane.

These changes (*see* Fig. 9A) are:

- Always abrupt and occur between two discrete levels of activity.
- Occur whether the animals are maintained on oxygen or air.
- Occur whether the periphery is being stimulated at an intensity sufficient to activate group A β fibers (tactile input), as well as group A δ fibers (thermal and sharp pain nociceptive input).
- Stimulation of group A and group C fibers always gives a change in electrocortical activity from a pattern of HVLF to LVHF. However, the concept that the fluctuations are owing to a form of pain "breakthrough" is rendered less tenable since these fluctuations are not abolished with morphine.
- Such fluctuations are at the same frequency for any one animal, and are seen throughout the duration of the experimental observational period, usually 12 h—from 1600–0400 h GMT.
- These fluctuations can be recorded at all depths of anesthesia. Figure 9A shows the electrocorticographic activity in an animal anesthetized at two depths with urethane (1.25 and 2.0 g/kg^{-1}). At the latter depth, the electrocorticographic changes observed are of a difference in the frequency of electrocortical spindling activity since at this latter depth of anesthesia, the electrocorticogram is composed of periods of silence interspersed with bursts of rhythmic activity. The changes observed at deeper depths of anesthesia are just as abrupt as at the basal level of anesthesia, but can only be seen when the periphery is not being stimulated. At deeper depths of anesthesia, each peripheral stimulus evokes a cortical spindle or spindle-like cortical response that obscures any change in spindle frequency.
- The proportion of time spent in the LVHF state is also fairly constant from animal to animal (41% ± 3.2% (SEM); $N = 37$; mean observation time 3 h for each animal).

Theoretically, any waveform can be described as a sum of a series of sine waves. Hence, any waveform can be mathematically expressed as a series of sine waves of known amplitude, and phase derived from the original data using a Fast Fourier Transform. The frequency content of the electrocorticographic activity can be conveniently split into four frequency bands (delta: δ 0.5–3.5 Hz, theta: θ 4–7 Hz, alpha: α 8–13 Hz and beta: β 14–30 Hz). *See* Fig. 9B for comparison of the power content of these bands in the unanesthetized, HVLF, LVHF, and "spindling" states. The data from Fig. 9B show that the variation between the HVLF and LVHF states represents a shift of electrocortical activity towards the unanesthetized state, whereas the activity during spindling activity represents a shift to a state between that of the HVLF and LVHF states. Another way of expressing the fluctuations in the basal level is to describe the electrocorticogram shifting from synchronized (HVLF) to desynchronized (LVHF) activity. Analysis of the frequency content of the electrocortical activity shows that the animals at the basal level of anesthesia are oscillating between two depths of anesthesia: one light (LVHF) and one deeper (HVLF), as judged by the changes observed in the spectral power in these two states and changes in the ability of the somatosensory pathway to transmit sensory information in the two states (*see* Changes in Somatosensory Transmission). It must be pointed out that these changes in state are not accompanied by any changes in skeletomotor activity. The changes in electrocortical activity are, however, always accompanied by changes in respiratory activity that are equally dramatic (that for respiratory frequency in Fig. 9A is from 163–174 breaths/min in the basal state, and from 88–79 breaths/min in the spindling state). These respiratory changes

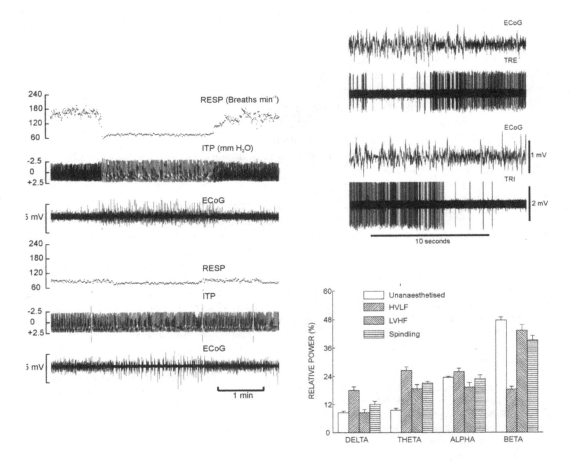

Fig. 9. Each record triplet shows, the instantaneous respiratory frequency (RESP), intratracheal pressure (ITP), and electrocorticographic activity (EcoG). The top record shows a spontaneous change from LVHF to HVLF to LVHF electrocortical activity in a rat anesthetized with urethane (1.25 g/kg) whilst the forepaw was being stimulated at a rate of 1/s. The bottom record shows a spontaneous change, seen as a change in rate of spindling activity, in the same animal after the depth of urethane anesthesia had been increased to 2.0 g/kg; without peripheral stimulation (**A**). The change in spontaneous activity from a single thalamic boundary cell (TRE), and a single thalamic reticular cell (TRI) both recorded from the same rat anesthetized with urethane (1.25 g/kg). The cells were both found in the same microelectrode penetration within 100 μm of each other (**B**). The distribution of the relative powers of the delta, theta, alpha, and beta frequency bands determined in 6 animals taken from the unanesthetized state, and during periods of HVLF, LVHF (1.25 g/kg urethane) and spindling activity (2.0 g/kg). The vertical bars show the mean, and the vertical lines the SD (**C**).

follow those in cortical activity. Taking the time of electrocortical change, as zero then changes in respiratory frequency, commence at +2.72 s (± 1.5 SD; N = 224). Changes in inspiratory effort, seen as an increase in the negative intratracheal pressure on inspiration, occur some 2 s later. The abruptness and timing of the respiratory changes would appear to preclude any influence of blood-gas chemistry on the genesis of these changes. There are also changes in heart rate that increase in the shift from HVLF to LVHF activity, but take a much longer time to start and are not developed fully until 20–30 s later. There are no, or very slight, changes in blood pressure.

Changes in Somatosensory Transmission

When comparing the responses of cells from thalamic and cortical sites to peripheral stimulation, marked changes are seen between HVLF and LVHF states. Cortical responses occur with an earlier latency and increased amplitudes of the initial positive and negative waves (Fig. 10A and C from 31 animals anesthetized with urethane). These data show a decrease in latency of −0.47 ms, an increase in initial positive wave to 110%, and an increase in initial negative wave to 439% from their starting values. The latency changes and increase in Ni were statistically significantly different ($p < 0.01$). With a mean starting latency of 4.11 ms, the latency decrease represents a large change in excitability in the somatosensory pathway. Similar changes were observed in animals anesthetized with Halothane and Inactin. From the dose-response curves for these anesthetics, it is possible to estimate how much of the anesthetic is functionally ignored in the anesthetic depth "switches," amounting to approx 20% of the circulating anesthetic.

Most cells in the dorsal column nuclei show no change in either latency of response or probability of response when the cortical activity shows a change from HVLF to LVHF. Any change seen in cuneate cells is, paradoxically, a slight increase in latency with no change in probability of response (*see* Fig. 10 in ref. *23*). When the responses of cells in the thalamic relay nuclei and all layers of the cortex are examined, all show the same changes i.e., a decrease in the earliest latency at which they respond, and a large increase in response probability (*see* Figs. 5 VPL and 10B,D). Similar changes occurred in animals anesthetized with Inactin or Halothane. In concert with these changes in somatosensory neurons, spontaneously active cells in the thalamic reticular nucleus (inhibitory) and boundary (excitatory) cells, and the excitatory and inhibitory cortical cells, also exhibit changes in their discharge frequencies. Changes in mean frequency of discharge of thalamic boundary cells from 6.9 ± 0.7 to 20.0 ± 1.9 impulses/s (mean ± SEM $N = 43$) and thalamic reticular cells from 38.8 ± 4.3 to 20.1 ± 3.0 impulses/s ($N = 17$) are seen as the cortical activity changes from HVLF to LVHF. These changes in frequency are accompanied by changes in discharge pattern. At low frequencies, the cells discharge irregularly, whereas at high frequencies they show a regular pattern of discharge *(23)*. However, cells in the thalamic reticular nucleus, boundary cells, and spontaneously active cortical cells do not always precede the HVLF to LVHF change. For those cortical cells and boundary cells which speed up in discharge, the frequency change occurs at –0.02 s ± 0.64 s (Cortical excitatory cells mean ± SD; $N = 48$), +0.02 s ± 2.4 (thalamic boundary cells, $N = 17$), taking the change in electrocortical activity as time zero. So far, the only cells that have been found to unequivocally change their frequency of discharge before the electrocortical switch in activity are located in the dorsal part of the medullary dorsal reticular nucleus –0.37 s ± 0.29 ($N = 24$). These cells are functionally in the caudal part of the reticular activating system.

Changes are also observed in cortical evoked responses; thalamic, and cortical cells, but not dorsal column nuclei cells, when their responses are compared in periods of electrocortical silence and spindling activity (*see* Fig. 10B Si and Sp). To collect these data, stimuli were delivered by a manual trigger during periods of electrocortical silence, and 150 ms after the start of a cortical spindle. These changes reflect those seen in the spontaneous changes in electrocortical activity at basal levels of anesthesia in that, for the thalamic relay cells, they are intermediate between those seen in HVLF and LVHF activity. The changes seen in the evoked cortical responses are totally different and would suggest a much greater change in cortical cell activity during a spindle than after a spontaneous desynchronization. This phenomenon requires further experimentation. Nonetheless, the change in cortical inhibitory cells seen as anesthetic depth is increased, is reflected in this intermediate state. This would seem to emphasize the fact that the central nervous system does not appear to interpret a change in frequency of discharge of cells, but rather the more important changes in pattern of discharge. What the graphs for the changes in mean frequency of discharge of thalamic reticular and boundary cells for increasing anesthetic depth do not show is that as the cortex starts spindling activ-

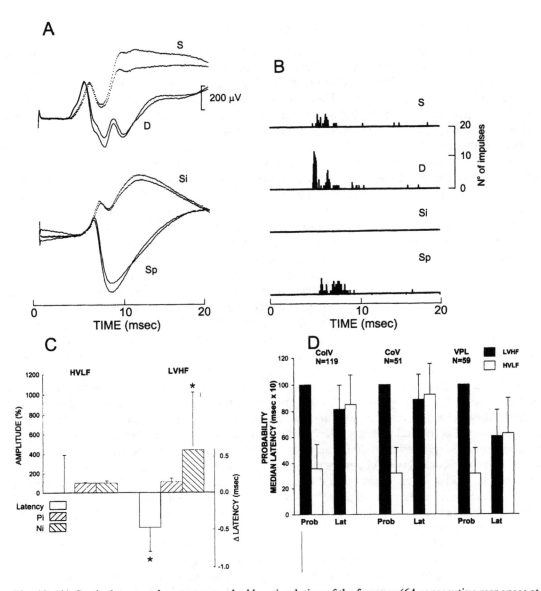

Fig. 10. (A) Cortical averaged responses evoked by stimulation of the forepaw (64 consecutive responses at 1/s) from a rat anesthetized with urethane (1.25 g/kg) obtained during periods of electrocortical **HVLF** (**S**) and **LVHF** activity (**D**) and from periods of spindling (**Sp**) and silent (**Si**) cortical activity after the depth of anesthesia was increased to 2.0 g/kg. **(B)** A series of poststimulus histograms obtained from a single thalamic relay cell to percutaneous electrical stimulation applied at the wrist obtained during the same periods of electrocortical activity. Each histogram shows the responses to 100 consecutive stimuli. **(C)** The average changes from 31 animals anesthetized with urethane (1.25 g/kg) seen in latency and amplitudes of **Pi** and **Ni** during periods of **HVLF** and **LVHF** electrocortical activity. The bars show the mean change the vertical lines the **SD**. **(D)** The mean changes in probability of response and latency in cells in the somatosensory pathway **VPL** thalamic relay cells, **CoIV** and **CoV** from cells in somatosensory cortex layers IV and V. For each cell the starting probability was scaled to 100 for periods of **LVHF** electrocortical activity.

ity, the discharge of both types of cell is modulated following a cortical spindle such that boundary cells (possibly excitatory cells) are momentarily sped up, and thalamic reticular cells (inhibitory) are momentarily slowed down.

THE THALAMIC NUCLEI AS RHYTHM GENERATORS

It is obvious that the central nervous system is capable of generating fixed rhythms of activity. Respiration occurs in fit humans at a rate of 13 breaths/min in the resting state throughout their adult life span. The cortex generates a 10 Hz predominant rhythm when human beings are in a relaxed awake state with their eyes closed, which immediately changes to a predominant 20–30 Hz rhythm if they open their eyes. That it is possible to artificially generate a rhythmic cortical response is seen best in animals anesthetized with barbiturates, after a peripheral stimulus. The same phenomenon is also observed in animals anesthetized with other anesthetics but not with such prominence, longevity, or regularity, with the possible exception of animals anesthetized with a xylazine/ketamine mixture. Figure 11A shows a series of averaged evoked responses taken from a rat anesthetized with the long lasting barbiturate Inactin, after percutaneous electrical stimulation of the forepaw nerves at the wrist. After the initial evoked response, there follows a series of waves at constant frequency, in this example, with an interval of 59 ms i.e., a frequency of approx 17 Hz. This is not solely a cortical phenomenon, as can be shown by the fact that recordings from single thalamic relay cells also show the same behavior (Fig. 11B). This phenomenon can occur as a consequence of activity in the thalamo-cortico-reticulo-thalamic feedback circuitry, as documented above and can be shown by the following observations:

- Examination of the somatosensory pathway to pairs of peripheral stimuli in the anesthetized rat shows that cortical responses are reduced in amplitude and increased in latency for up to 500 ms after the first stimulus of a pair, and that no responses are seen to the second stimulus of a pair, at intervals of 10–40 ms *(28)*. A hyper-excitability is occasionally observed in anesthetized rats at intervals between 80–150 ms, always in animals anesthetized with barbiturates, and in 50% of animals anesthetized with urethane. The same is observed in unanesthetized animals and in man *(19)*.
- In man, the same phenomenon is seen psychophysically. If you ask a human how many stimuli they feel of pairs at intervals of 10–40 ms, they say that they have only been stimulated once. At intervals of 50–80 ms, they give confused replies, and only definitely report two stimuli with intervals greater than 100 ms. At intervals of separation of around 100 ms, some subjects complain about the intensity of the second stimulus (data from class experiments on the Hoffman reflex in Sheffield).
- That this is primarily a thalamic phenomenon can be shown by the fact that the cortical responses to two stimuli delivered to the thalamocortical radiation fibers show a completely different behavior. The responses to the second pair of stimuli are unaltered with separations greater than 10 ms *(27)*.
- Intracellular recordings from cat thalamic relay cells show that after an initial excitation, there is a prolonged period of hyperpolarization lasting for approx 100 ms, followed by a phenomenon the authors describe as "postinhibitory rebound" *(28–30)*.
- This hyperpolarization is generated principally by $GABA_A$ receptors, because it is blocked by bicuculline *(31–32)*.
- There are very few short-axoned neurons in the rat ventrobasal thalamus itself *(33)*, so it would seem unlikely that the general phenomenon of long-lasting thalamic transmission decreases after a peripheral stimulus could be generated by local inhibitory interneurons within the ventrobasal thalamus.
- Rhythmic thalamic activity at approx 10 Hz is not seen if the thalamic nucleus under study is disconnected from its relevant thalamic reticular nucleus projection site *(34)*.
- Recordings from local interneurons in the ferret lateral geniculate nucleus do not show behavior consistent with producing the rhythmic inhibition *(35)*.
- That the spindling activity is generated by the complex thalamo-cortico-reticulo-thalamic feedback loop has been shown to be extremely probable by the work of Steriade *(36)* and his collaborators. Recording from pairs of cells, one reticular, the other thalamic relay, it has been shown that after each thalamic reticular discharge, there is an inhibitory postsynaptic potential in the relay cell. Moreover, the synaptic linkage between the thalamic reticular neurons and thalamic relay neurons is secure.
- The same circuit can generate other rhythms of cortical activity, across the entire spectrum, if the phasing and discharge pattern of the neurons is modified *(see* Chapters 6 and 7 in ref. *18)*.

However, the rhythmic activity seen in the cortex may not solely be caused by subcortical generators. It must be remembered that even in slabs of cortex neurologically isolated from any subcortical input, rhythmic activity can still be evoked by direct stimulation of the cortical surface *(37)*.

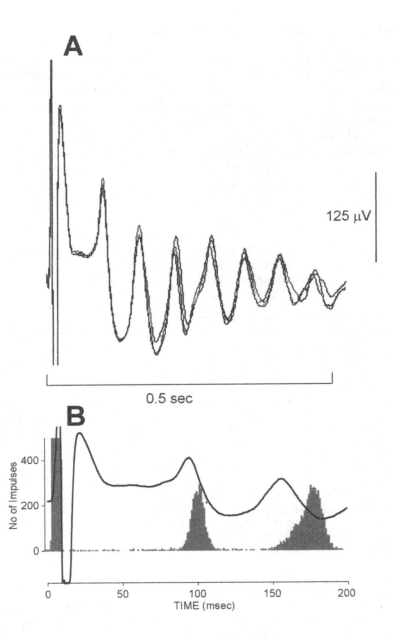

Fig. 11. (A) A series of averaged cortical response to percutaneous electrical stimulation applied at the wrist at a rate of 1/s in a rat anesthetized with Inactin (172 mg/kg). Each average is 64 consecutive peripheral stimuli and there are three consecutive averages superimposed. **(B)** Shows a single average or 100 consecutive peripheral stimuli superimposed upon the poststimulus histogram of a single thalamic relay cell to show the regularity of the cellular response.

CONCLUDING REMARKS

The data presented in this chapter show that the action of the vast majority of anesthetics used to produce "general anesthesia" on the sensory transmission of information is to activate a system (summarized in Fig. 2), to suppress the transfer of this information through the thalamic relay nuclei. In a poorly understood way, the nervous system, even when deeply anesthetized, modulates its anesthetic depth in a cyclical fashion. This is apparently accomplished by modulating the same thalamic reticular-thalamic relay-sensory cortical feedback loop. Present evidence suggests that this cyclical variation is generated in, or at least led by, a part of the caudal reticular formation, which has been implicated in general arousal behavior (38). Finally, this same feedback loop can be used to explain the fast rhythms shown by the spontaneous electrical activity recorded from the cerebral cortex.

Careful perusal of this book will show that there are a variety of ways of addressing the problem of how anesthetics exert their effects. Part of the problem of research into anesthetic action is the vast array of effects they produce on the various body systems (cardiovascular, respiratory, etc.) and on various nervous processes in the whole animal. Another problem is the tendency to interpret the results obtained on a specific action of an anesthetic in a fairly global sense, as if the aspect of anesthetic action under study can be extended and amplified to encompass the whole action of the anesthetic. Considerable difficulties can arise as a result of such imaginative, or speculative interpretation. For example from the data advanced in this particular chapter, one could simplistically state that because the effect of anesthetics is to severely impede the access of information from the sensory paths to the cerebral mantle, then the relevant information to lay down short-term memories is absent. This may be partially true but proving that this would account, by itself, for memory loss would be difficult and would ignore the effects of anesthetics on the higher brain parts involved in memory. Various interactions between anesthetics and specific receptor activated ionophores have been shown. For example, Xenon has been shown to be a potent antagonist at glutamate receptors expressed in *Xenopus* oocytes (39). Any attempt to transfer this observation to the genesis of sensory loss seen in the anesthetic state immediately creates problems. The activation of thalamic relay cells is initially by AMPA receptors, and the expected later activation by the NMDA receptor would be wiped out by the powerful reticular inhibition exerted on the thalamic relay cells. Thus, one cannot explain sensory blockade at this important site given by Xenon to be mediated by its effect on NMDA receptors. Furthermore, reference to Fig. 2 shows that if Xenon is indeed acting to block NMDA transmission, then the system that is activated by Xenon to impede sensory transmission should, in theory, be turned off by this anesthetic. In practice, Xenon, like all the other group 1 anesthetics, turns the system on. Barbiturates, Alphaxalone, and Halothane all have been shown to have a potentiating any effect for GABA on both native and recombinant $GABA_A$ receptors as have Etomidate and Propofol (40). The question thus arises of how the first three of these anesthetics block thalamic relay cell activity and leave cortical neurons in layer IV unaffected, and the latter two anesthetics only exert great effect on the cortical cells? Perhaps there are subtle differences in receptor constitution at the thalamus and cortex. At the moment, there is insufficient information both in the whole animal and isolated receptor research to answer such questions and explain the obvious anomalies. Those who showed the effects of anesthetics on the various *Xenopus* oocyte expressed receptors would claim that they have found the answer to anesthetic action. However, in the whole animal, the nervous system is not so uncomplicated. Each cell will have a variety of receptors to different neurotransmitters on its surface, whose actions will, moreover, be modulated by a whole variety of other chemicals. Another possible explanation for the inability to apply the results seen with isolated receptors is that these actions appear not to be reversed by high pressures (41), which would in turn imply that they are very interesting effects of anesthetics on receptors, but may have nothing to do with the genesis of the anesthetic state. Clearly, a great deal of caution should be exercised when translating the effects seen in reductionist models to the whole animal. On the other hand, it is possible to extract a particular anesthetic/receptor interaction to explain, or partially explain, a single feature of anesthetic action. The effect of pentobarbitone, shown to potentiate the action of the inhibitory transmitter glycine (41), on spinal motoneurons, may partly explain the effects of anesthetics on spinal motoneurons. Glycine plays an important role on the feedback inhibition of spinal motoneurons (42). It could certainly explain the ability of pentobarbitone to reduce the convulsive activity of strychnine.

One other very important aspect of the action of anesthetics remains to be explored. This is their differential effect on nervous pathways. Anesthetics block monosynaptic stretch reflexes at doses that leave protective polysynaptic withdrawal reflexes unaffected *(43)*. Normally, the stretch reflex is very powerful and very difficult to suppress, but it is extremely susceptible to anesthetic action. It has been shown that the monosynaptic activation of dorsal column sensory relay cells is unaffected by anesthetic agents. These observations would seem to indicate that another aspect of anesthetic action could be owing to the organization of a particular system or pathway, i.e., whether a potent excitatory input can be turned off by the anesthetic or the converse, whether a potent inhibitory input can be turned on by the anesthetic and finally, the synaptic security of a particular path. There are many questions that remain to be answered about the mechanism of action of anesthetic agents.

REFERENCES

1. Marx, T., Froeba, G., Wagner, D., Baeder, S., Goertz, A., and Georgieff, M. (1997) Effects on haemodynamics and catecholamine release of xenon anesthesia compared with total i.v. anesthesia in the pig. *Brit. J. Anesth.* **78,** 326–327.
2. Reyle-Hahn, M. and Rossaint, R. (2000) Xenon–a new anesthetic gas. *Anesthetist* **49,** 869–874.
3. DeWildt, D. J., Hillen, F. C., Rauws, A. G., and Sangster, B. (1983) Etomidate-anesthesia, with and without fentanyl, compared with urethane anesthesia in the rat. *Brit. J. Pharmacol.* **79,** 461–469.
4. Ledez, K. M. and Lerman, J (1987) The minimum alveolar concentration (MAC) of isoflurane in preterm neonates. *Anesthesiology* **59,** 421–424.
5. Penfield, W. and Rasmussen, T. (1950) The Cerebral Cortex of Man: A Clinical Study of Localization of Function. New York, Macmillan.
6. Stevens, S. S. (1961) The psychophysics of sensory function. (Rosenblith, W. A. ed, Sensory Communication, MIT Press and John Wiley & Sons, New York.
7. Angel, A., Berridge, D., and Unwin, J. (1973) The effect of anesthetic agents on primary evoked cortical responses. *Brit. J. Anesth.* **71,** 148–163.
8. Angel, A. and Clarke, K. A. C. (1975) An analysis of the representation of the forelimb in the ventrobasal thalamic complex of the albino rat. *J. Physiol.* **249,** 399–423.
9. Woolsey, T. A. and Van der Loos, H. (1970) The structural organization of layer IV in the somatosensory region (S 1) of mouse cerebral cortex. The description of a cortical field composed of discrete cytoarchitectonic units. *Brain Res.* **17,** 205–242.
10. Angel, A. (1964) The effect of peripheral stimulation on units located in the thalamic reticular nuclei. *J. Physiol.* **171,** 42–60.
11. Salt, T. E. and Turner, J. P. (1996) Antagonism of the presumed presynaptic action of L-AP4 on GABAergic transmission in the ventrobasal thalamus by the novel mGluR antagonist MPPG. *Neuropharmacology* **35,** 239–241.
12. Salt, T. E. and Eaton, S. A. (1996) Functions of ionotropic and metabotropic glutamate receptors in sensory transmission in the mammalian thalamus. *Prog. Neurobiol.* **48,** 55–72.
13. Eaton, S. A. and Salt, T. E. (1996) Role of *N*-methyl-D-aspartate and metabotropic glutamate receptors in corticothalamic excitatory postsynaptic potentials in vivo. *Neuroscience* **73,** 1–5.
14. Salt, T. T., Eaton, S. A., and Turner, J. P. (1996) Characterization of the metabotropic glutamate receptors (mGluRs) which modulate GABA-mediated inhibition in the ventrobasal thalamus. *Neurochem. International* **29,** 317–322.
15. Shaw, P. J. and Salt, T. E. (1997) Modulation of sensory and excitatory amino acid responses by nitric oxide donors and glutathione in the ventrobasal thalamus of the rat. *Eur. J. Neurosci.* **9,** 1507–1513.
16. Turner, J. P. and Salt, T. E. (1999) Group III metabotropic glutamate receptors control corticothalamic synaptic transmission in the rat thalamus in vitro. *J. Physiol.* **519,** 481–491.
17. Salt, T. E., Turner, J. P., and Kingston, A. E. (1999) Evaluation of agonists and antagonists acting at group I metabotropic glutamate receptors in the thalamus in vivo. *Neuropharmacol.* **38,** 1505–1510
18. Steriade, M., Jones, E. G., and McCormick, D. A. (eds.) (1997) Thalamus. Volume 1 Organisation and Function. Elsevier Science.
19. Angel, A. (1969) The central control of sensory transmission and its possible relation to reaction time. *Acta Psychologica* **30,** 339–357. N
20. Angel, A., Berridge, D. A., and Unwin, J. (1973) The effects of anesthetic agents on primary evoked cortical responses. *Brit. J. Anesth.* **45,** 824–836
21. Angel, A., Gratton, D. A., Halsey, M. J., and Wardley-Smith, B. (1980) Pressure reversal of the effect of urethane on the evoked cerebral cortical responses in the rat. *Brit. J. Pharmacol.* **70,** 241–247.
22. Angel, A. (1993) Central neuronal pathways and anesthesia. *Brit. J. Anesth.* **71,** 148–163.
23. Detsch, O., Vahle-Hinz, C., Kochs, E., Siemers, M., and Bromm, B. (1999) Isoflurane induces dose-dependent changes of thalamic somatosensory information transfer. *Brain Res.* **829,** 77–89.
24. Angel, A. (1991) The G. L. Brown Lecture. Adventures in anesthesia. *Exper. Physiology* **76,** 1–38.
25. Angel, A. (1983) The functional interrelations between the somatosensory cortex and the thalamic reticular nucleus. Macchi, G., Rustioni, A., and Spreafico, R., eds. Somatosensory Integration in the Thalamus. Elsevier, Amsterdam, pp. 221–239.

26. Angel, A., Dodd, J., and Gray, J. D. (1976) Fluctuating anesthetic state in the rat anesthetized with urethane. *J. Physiol.* **259,** 11P, 12P.

27. Angel, A. (1967) Cortical responses to paired stimuli applied peripherally and at sites along the somatosensory pathway. *J. Physiol.* **191,** 427–448.

28. Andersen, P. and Eccles, J. C. (1962) Inhibitory phasing of neuronal discharges. *Nature* **196,** 645–647.

29. Andersen, P. and Sears, T. A. (1964) The role of inhibition in the phasing of spontaneous thalamo-cortical discharge. *J. Physiol.* **173,** 459–480.

30. Andersen, P., Brooks, C. M., Eccles, J. C., and Sears, T. A. (1964) The ventro-basal nucleus of the thalamus: types of cells, their responses and their functional organisation. *J. Physiol.* **174,** 370–399.

31. Salt, T. E. (1986) Mediation of thalamic sensory input by NMDA and non-NMDA receptors. *Nature* **322,** 263–265.

32. Lee, S. M., Friedberg, M. H., and Ebner, F. F. (1994) The role of GABA-mediated inhibition in the rat ventro-posterior medial thalamus. II. Differential effects of GABA$_A$ and GABA$_B$ receptor antagonists on responses of VPM neurons. *J. Neurophysiol.* **71,** 1716–1726.

33. Scheibel, M. E. and Scheibel, A. B. (1966) Patterns of organization in specific and nonspecific thalamic fields. In The Thalamus.Purpura D. P. and Yahr, M. D., eds., New York, Columbia Univ. Press pp. 13–46.

34. Steriade, M., Dechênes, M., Domich, L., and Mulle, C. (1985) Abolition of spindle oscillations in thalamic neurons disconnected from nucleus reticularis thalami. *J. Neurophysiol.* **54,** 1472–1497.

35. Bal, T., von Krosigk, M., and McCormick, D. A. (1995) Synaptic and membrane mechanisms underlying synchronized oscillations in the ferret LGNd in vitro. *J. Physiol.* **483,** 641–663.

36. Steriade, M., Jones, E. G., and Llinás, R. R., eds. (1990) *Thalamic Oscillations and Signalling.* Wiley-Interscience, New York.

37. Burns, B. D. (1958) *The Mammalian Cerebral Cortex.* Edward Arnold Ltd, London.

38. Moruzzi, G. and Magoun, H. W. (1949) Brain stem reticular formation and activation of the EEG. *Electroencephal. Clini. Neurophysiol.* **1,** 455–473.

39. Franks N. P., Dickinson R., de Sousa S. L. M., Hall A. C., and Lieb W. R. (1998) How does xenon produce anesthesia? *Nature* **396,** 324–324.

40. Lambert, J. L., Belelli, D., Shepherd, S., Muntoni, A.-L., Pistis, M., and Peters, J. A. (1998) The GABA$_A$ receptor: an important locus for intravenous anesthetic action. In (Smith, E. B. and Daniels, S., eds.) Gases in Medicine 8th BOC Priestley Conference. Royal Society of Chemistry. pp. 121–137.

41. Daniels, S. (1998) Interaction between general anesthesia and high pressure. In (Smith, E. B. and Daniels, S., eds.) Gases in Medicine 8th BOC Priestley Conference. Royal Society of Chemistry. pp. 225–233.

42. Bradley, K., Easton, D. M., and Eccles, J. C. (1953) An investigation of primary or direct inhibition. *J. Physiol.* **122,** 474–488.

43. DeJong, R. H., Robles, R., Corbiu, R. W., and Nace, R. A. (1968) Effect of inhalational anesthetics on monosynaptic transmission in the spinal cord. *J. Pharmacol. Exper. Therapeutics* **162,** 326–330.

9

The Hippocampus

M. Bruce MacIver

INTRODUCTION

The hippocampus has been used for studies of anesthetic mechanisms of action for at least twenty years, and has been better studied than any other brain region in this regard. This is because hippocampal cortex is anatomically quite simple, and it is relatively easy to access this brain region in vivo. It is especially well suited for brain slice experiments because several important synaptic connections can be preserved in thin sections. Much has been learned about how various anesthetics alter hippocampal function, and much of this appears to be generalizable to other brain areas.

Overview of the Limbic System and Hippocampal Cortex

The hippocampus is a major component of the mammalian brain limbic system that also includes the dentate gyrus, cingulate cortex, hypothalamus (especially the mammillary bodies), amygdala, and portions of the anterior thalamus. These major structures are interconnected by reciprocal fiber bundles travelling in the fornix, mammillothalamic tract, and stria terminalis. The limbic system has been functionally associated with emotional aspects of behavior related to survival, visceral responses associated with these emotions, and with brain mechanisms for memory. In recent years, the preeminent role of the hippocampus relating to learning and memory has become well established.

Functions of the Hippocampus

The hippocampus is essential for most types of learning and memory in the mammalian brain. Bilateral lesions of the hippocampus result in an inability to learn new information, although memories stored prior to the lesion remain intact. All major forms of declarative memory are disrupted following hippocampal damage (1,2), but some forms of fear conditioning and pure movement related (motor skill) learning are not disrupted. The hippocampus receives sensory inputs from all modalities (olfaction, vision, auditory and somatosensory systems), and outputs from the hippocampus reach widespread regions of neocortex and brainstem centers. Hippocampal neurons respond to noxious (pain) stimuli and are activated during flight-or-fight behavioral responses. In addition, there is good evidence linking voluntary movement initiation to the hippocampal cortex (3), and a strong case has been made for a sensory/motor integration function for this brain area (4,5).

Anesthetic Effects on Hippocampus

General anesthetics produce several important effects, such as block of recall (amnesia), block of pain sensations, and block of movement that could come about, at least in part, through actions at the level of the hippocampus. The hippocampus is clearly effected by anesthetics, and some of the earliest studies of anesthetic actions in the mammalian brain demonstrated a marked alteration of synaptic

From: *Contemporary Clinical Neuroscience:* Neural Mechanisms of Anesthesia
Edited by: Joseph F. Antognini et al. © Humana Press Inc., Totowa, NJ

responses recorded in vivo during anesthesia *(6,7)*. Recent studies of anesthetic effects on EEG responses recorded with microelectrodes in the hippocampus clearly demonstrate that hippocampal electrical activity maps to behavioral responses in a concentration dependent manner *(8,9)* (*see* Chapter 9, *10*). In addition, numerous studies have shown that hippocampal neurons in brain slices are profoundly effected by clinically relevant concentrations of anesthetics (*see* Anesthetic Actions...). It is likely that some important features of the multicomponent state known as anesthesia come about via actions at the hippocampal level.

ANATOMY OF HIPPOCAMPAL CORTEX

Perhaps the most important reason that the hippocampus has been studied in such detail is the relatively simple anatomy of this brain region. The hippocampus is comprised of archicortex, distinguished by a single layer of pyramidal neuron cell bodies separating two layers of synaptic/dendritic zones. Input fibers and output pathways to and from the hippocampus have been well characterized and appear to project in a planar manner, forming a highly laminar structure. The input fibers, synapses, cell bodies and output fibers for a given lamina of hippocampal cortex occur in a plane of a few hundred microns which is perpendicular to the long axis of the hippocampus (Fig. 1). This anatomy is ideally suited to preserve important anatomical connections in 300–500 μ thick slices of hippocampal cortex. Compared to neocortex with multiple pyramidal cell body layers and complex intracolumnar synaptic zones, the hippocampal cortex affords an opportunity to understand synaptic physiology in a fairly straightforward system.

Major Input Pathways to the Hippocampus

The hippocampal formation receives afferent inputs from several sources. Noradrenergic, serotonergic, and dopaminergic fibers diffusely innervate hippocampal neurons and arrive via the fimbria from locus ceruleus, median raphe nuclei, and substantia nigra, respectively. Other brain stem and hypothalamic nuclei provide peptidergic inputs that also appear to diffusely innervate the hippocampus. GABAergic and cholinergic fibers from the septum, via the fimbria, innervate pyramidal neurons in a stratified manner—medial septal inputs synapse on proximal dendrites and lateral septal inputs synapse on distal dendrites. Septal GABAergic fibers appear to innervate hippocampal inhibitory interneurons preferentially. A major glutamatergic input from entorhinal cortex comes into the hippocampus via the perforant path, which strongly innervates dentate gyrus granule neurons, but also appears to synapse with distal dendrites of pyramidal neurons. Glutamatergic inputs from the contralateral hippocampus and other cortical areas, including most regions of neocortex, innervate pyramidal neuron basal and apical dendrites (Fig. 2). These latter glutamatergic systems appear to provide the major excitatory drive to hippocampal neurons, and together with septal inputs are thought to provide the most important, behaviorally relevant inputs.

Trisynaptic Pathway of the Hippocampal Formation

The hippocampal slice preparation preserves a three synapse system that has been well characterized anatomically, physiologically, and pharmacologically. The synapses making up this trisynaptic circuit are distinguished by their high degree of plasticity. They are able to change the gain or strength of the synaptic connection based on the level of activity (frequency) through the circuit. Low frequency action potential discharge activity (0.1–3 Hz) leads to a long lasting decrease in synaptic strength (Long Term Depression; LTD). High frequency activity (8–100 Hz) leads to an increase in synaptic strength (Long Term Potentiation; LTP). This ability to change synaptic strength over long time periods (hours to days) is thought to reflect the plasticity which underlies learning and memory in the hippocampus *(11)*. While other cortical and subcortical synapses also appear to exhibit plasticity, none have been as well studied as the hippocampal trisynaptic circuit.

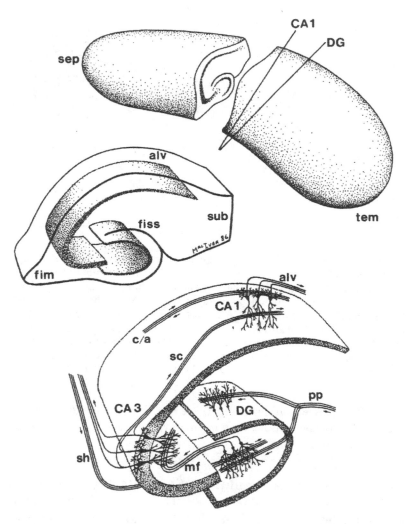

Fig. 1. Diagram of a hippocampus isolated from the right side of a rat brain, straightened and laid flat to facilitate cutting slices perpendicular to the long axis (**sep**–septal and **temp**–temporal ends). Hippocampal neurons form two sheets of cells that look like interlocking Cs when cut in cross section (middle, **fim**–fimbria, **alv** –alveus, **fiss**–hippocampal fissure, and **sub**–subiculum). Input and output connections for the hippocampal trisynaptic pathway are shown: **pp**–perforant path inputs to **DG** (dentate granule) neurons; **mf**–mossy fibers from **DG** to **CA 3** neurons; **sc**–schaffer-collateral fibers from **CA 3**–**CA 1** neurons. Septohippocampal (**sh**) fibers travelling in the fimbria are also shown together with commissural/associational (**c/a**) fibers and **CA 1** neuron output axons travelling in the alveus. The optimal plane of section for preserving **sc** to **CA 1** connections, or **pp** to **DG** connections, are shown at the top. Used with permission from MacIver and Roth, *Brit. J. Anaesth.* 1988 *(52)*.

Dentate Gyrus

As mentioned in the previous section on Pathways to the Hippocampus, the major input to dentate gyrus granule neurons is the perforant path fibers originating in entorhinal cortex. These fibers excite granule neurons by releasing glutamate to activate mainly AMPA/kaninate receptors on granule neuron dendrites in stratum moleculare (Fig. 2). Perforant path fibers also excite local GABAergic inter-

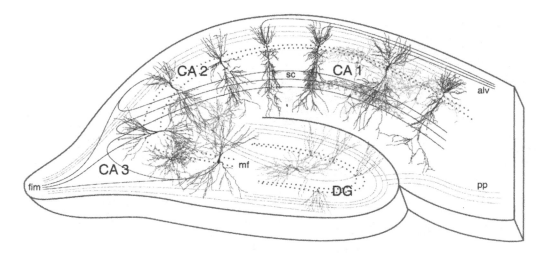

Fig. 2. Diagram of a hippocampal slice showing glutamate mediated excitatory pathways (**pp**, **mf**, and **sc** inputs) to **DG** and **CA** neurons, as well as representative GABAergic inhibitory interneurons (gray cells). Abbreviations are the same as in Fig. 1. The relatively simple anatomy in a hippocampal slice has facilitated electrophysiological studies of anesthetic effects on these neurons. Most studies have investigated effects on **CA 1** pyramidal cell excitability and the **sc** to **CA 1** neuron synapses, but **pp** inputs to **DG** neurons and basal dendritic inputs to **CA 1** neurons have also been shown to be depressed by anesthetics. Only a few studies have investigated anesthetic effects on inhibitory interneurons, due to the sparse distribution of these cells. Glutamate mediated excitatory synapses are made by **sc** fibers onto both **CA 1** and interneuron dendrites. Interneurons make GABA mediated synapses onto dendrites and cell bodies of pyramidal neurons.

neurons in stratum moleculare which appear to provide feed forward inhibition to the granule neurons. Axons from the dentate granule neurons form the mossy fiber pathway that innervates CA 2–CA 4 pyramidal neurons of the hippocampus.

CA 4–CA 2 Pyramidal Cortex

Mossy fibers synapse onto apical dendrites of the CA 2–CA 4 pyramidal neurons (Fig. 2) and provide excitation via mainly AMPA/kaninate receptors. The mossy fibers are distinguished by the abundance of opiate peptides (including enkephalin), which appear to be coreleased with glutamate from their nerve terminals. They, together with hippocampal inhibitory interneurons, are also distinguished from other synapses in showing a high level of cannabinoid receptors on their nerve terminals, which appear to play a role in a unique form of synaptic plasticity termed Depolarization Induced Suppression (DIS; *[12,13]*). When the postsynaptic CA 2 to CA 4 neurons are sufficiently depolarized, they appear to release anandamide from their dendrites, which crosses back over to the presynaptic terminals to transiently inhibit the release of glutamate or GABA. Relatively little is known about the CA 2 and CA 4 pyramidal neurons, however, CA 3 cells have been well characterized. The CA 3 neuron axons provide local excitatory inputs to adjacent CA 3 cells, and also leave the hippocampus via the fimbria/fornix to innervate the mammillary bodies of the hypothalamus. CA 3 axon branches form the Schaffer-collateral pathway that provides a major excitatory input to CA 1 pyramidal neurons within the same hippocampal lamina.

CA 1 Pyramidal Cortex

Schaffer-collateral fibers release glutamate from their nerve terminals to excite CA 1 neuron dendrites in the stratum radiatum (Fig. 2). This excitation occurs via mainly AMPA/kainate receptors, but NMDA receptors also contribute to postsynaptic responses and are known to play an important role in both LTD and LTP forms of plasticity at the Schaffer-collateral to CA 1 neuron synapse.

Schaffer-collateral fibers also excite local GABAergic interneurons in stratum lacunosum moleculare and stratum radiatum which, in turn, provide feed forward inhibition to CA 1 neurons; analogous to the mossy fiber - interneuron—granule cell inhibition seen in the dentate gyrus *(14,15)*. Anesthetic effects have been studied most extensively on the Schaffer-collateral to CA 1 neuron synapses, however, some interesting differences in effect were evident for other synapses onto CA 1 neurons, and for effects on perforant path to granule neuron synapses. Only a few studies have looked at anesthetic effects on hippocampal interneurons.

Major Output Pathways from Hippocampal Cortex

Their are two main outputs from the hippocampus; CA 3 neurons send their axons to other limbic structures via the fimbria/fornix, and CA 1 neurons send their axons to other cortical regions via the alveus and fornix. In addition, each hippocampus is connected to it's contralateral conterpart via the anterior and posterior hippocampal commissural pathways. Most of the axons travelling in the fornix terminate in the mammillary body with a smaller portion ending in the ventromedial hypothalamic nucleus. Smaller numbers of fibers also project to the anterior nucleus of the thalamus and to the septal area and anterior region of the hypothalamus. Thus, efferent output from the hippocampus can reach virtually all regions of the brain through divergent relays through the thalamus, hypothalamus, septum, and other limbic cortical areas.

PHYSIOLOGY OF HIPPOCAMPAL SYNAPTIC CIRCUITS

Hippocampal circuit function has been extensively studied, and the synaptic physiology of this brain region is among the best characterized of any CNS circuitry in the mammalian brain. The vast majority (>80%) of synapses in the hippocampus use the amino acid neurotransmitters glutamate and GABA *(16)*. These neurotransmitters are used primarily for fast synaptic transmission of afferent inputs (including sensory information), for associational information for reciprocal hippocampal connections, and connections to and from other cortical areas. Glutamate is used for excitatory synaptic transmission; GABA is the primary inhibitory transmitter in the hippocampus. Relatively little is known about other neurotransmitters in the hippocampus, but nerve terminals releasing catecholamines, indolamines, peptides, acetylcholine, adenosine and ATP have been described, and many of these transmitters have been shown to modulate hippocampal pyramidal cells and local inhibitory interneurons. This chapter will focus on the physiology of glutamate and GABA synapses, because glutamate is used by all three excitatory synapses of the hippocampal trisynaptic circuit and GABA is used by all of the local inhibitory interneurons within the hippocampus. In addition, anesthetics have been shown to produce strong effects at both amino acid mediated synapse types.

Glutamate-Mediated Synapses

There appear to be at least two types of glutamate synapses in the hippocampus, distinguished by their ability to support pre vs postsynaptic plasticity, and by their sensitivity to receptor antagonists. Mossy fiber glutamate synapses from dentate granule neurons to CA 3 pyramidal neurons appear to support a form of plasticity that involves an increased release of glutamate from presynaptic nerve terminals to produce LTP *(17)*. At the mossy fiber synapse, LTP is not blocked by NMDA (N-methyl-D-aspartate) preferring receptor antagonists. In contrast, Schaffer-collateral fiber glutamate synapses from CA 3–CA 1 neurons exhibit a form of LTP that appears to involve a strengthening of postsynaptic responses, which is blocked by NMDA receptor antagonists *(11)*. In addition, some glutamate mediated synaptic responses can be exclusively mediated by NMDA receptors, while the vast majority appear to be mediated largely by AMPA (amino-3-hydroxy-5-methyl-4-isoxazolepropionic acid) and kainate (KA) receptors *(18)*. There is also good evidence that glutamate released from nerve terminals can also activate receptors that are not associated with the postsynaptic density (extrasynaptic receptors).

AMPA/Kainate Receptors

Most of the excitatory postsynaptic currents (EPSCs) observed at synapses within the hippocampal trisynaptic circuit utilize glutamate receptors of the AMPA/kainate variety. All three synapses can be blocked by the AMPA receptor antagonist, CNQX. Cloning experiments reveal the existence of over nine genes encoding AMPA and KA receptor subunits (19–21). AMPA-preferring receptors consist of homo and heteromeric combinations of the subunits GluR1–4. The KA-preferring receptors consist of subunits GluR5–6 and KA1–2. GluR7 is a KA-preferring receptor, based on binding experiments. AMPA-preferring receptors respond to both AMPA and KA. The homomeric GluR6 receptor is activated by KA but not by AMPA. Heteromeric receptors containing GluR6 and KA2 are activated by both AMPA and KA (22–24). These subunits form ligand-gated channels with a high conductance for cations, especially sodium, and produce depolarizing responses when activated by synaptically released glutamate. These receptor/channels exhibit fast kinetics with rise times of <1–2 ms, and decay times of a few milliseconds to <50 ms in duration. EPSCs resulting from activation of these channels result in excitatory postsynaptic potentials (EPSPs) of several mV in amplitude, which typically last for 10–20 ms. These EPSPs can routinely evoke action potential discharge in the postsynaptic cell when they exceed 5–10 mV in amplitude. At the Schaffer-collateral to CA 1 neuron synapse, these receptor/channels appear to increase in number during LTP and decrease during LTD. Thus, most of the plasticity seen at this synapse appears to result from a regulation of the insertion or removal of AMPA/kainate receptors from the postsynaptic membrane (11,18).

NMDA Receptors

A second type of ligand gated glutamate receptor/channel is commonly observed at some hippocampal synapses and known to play a critical role in synaptic plasticity. These NMDA channels are formed from pentomeres made up of proteins encoded by two subunit families of genes: NR1 consisting of eight alternatively spliced variants (25,26) and, NR2, which contains four homologous subunits (NR2A, NR2B, NR2C, and NR2D). The NR2D subunit exhibits two possible splice isoforms (NR2D-1 and NR2D-2) (27–29). They can be specifically blocked by several NMDA receptor antagonists, including ketamine, MK801 and APV. In addition to being gated by glutamate, NMDA channels are also voltage dependent. At normal resting membrane potentials of −50 to −70 mV, the channels are blocked by Mg ions that bind to the pore and plug the channel. Depolarization of the membrane to nearly 0 mV relieves this channel block by removing Mg ions, allowing sodium, potassium, and most importantly, calcium ions to flow through the channel. This voltage dependent block limits NMDA gated channel function to synapses, which are active at the same time that postsynaptic neurons are strongly depolarized by action potential discharge.

Synaptic plasticity at Schaffer-collateral to CA 1 neuron synapses requires NMDA channel activation, since both LTP and LTD can be blocked by NMDA receptor antagonists.

Metabotropic NMDA Receptors

Glutamate activates a number G protein coupled receptors, known as metabotropic glutamate (mGlu) receptors, which appear to act as regulators of synaptic transmission. These receptors consist of two domains: an extracellular domain to which agonists bind, and a transmembrane heptahelix region involved in G protein activation. Eight different mGlu receptor genes have been identified and classified into three groups (30). Group I (mGlu1 and mGlu5 receptors); are coupled to the activation of phospholipase C; group II (mGlu2 and mGlu3 receptors) and group III (mGlu4, mGlu6, mGlu7, and mGlu8 receptors) are negatively coupled to adenylyl cyclase. Many of these receptors exist in different forms generated by alternative splicing (31) and can be located on presynaptic nerve terminals or postsynaptically. Metabotropic NMDA receptors are thought to play important roles in synaptic plasticity and the growth and maintenance of hippocampal synaptic connections.

GABA-Mediated Synapses

Synapses that release the amino acid transmitter GABA (gamma-aminobutyric acid) are as prevalent in hippocampus as glutamate mediated synapses, and play equally important, albeit opposite, roles. GABA is used as the primary inhibitory neurotransmitter for fast synapses between hippocampal interneurons and pyramidal cells, and for important septal GABAergic inputs to hippocampal interneurons. There are many types of GABA receptors located both at synapses (pre- and postsynaptic), as well as at extrasynaptic sites on both pyramidal and interneurons.

GABA$_A$ Receptors (Slow and Fast) and Chloride Channels

The GABA$_A$ receptor is a ligand gated chloride ion channel comprised of a family of subunits (alpha1–6, beta1–4, gamma1–3, delta, epsilon, and rho1–3) that form pentameric complexes (32–34). The proposed stoichiometry of GABA$_A$ receptors is: two alpha subunits, two beta subunits, and one gamma, or one epsilon, or one rho subunit (34). There appear to be at least three distinct types of GABA$_A$ receptors expressed in hippocampal neurons, and more are likely to be discovered. The first type of receptor is associated with GABA$_{Aslow}$ synapses that are observed in pyramidal neurons following electrical stimulation of afferents that synapse on dendrites (14,35). A second type comprise the GABA$_{Afast}$ receptors which are associated with synapses located on pyramidal neuron cell bodies and axons (35). A third type of receptor has been observed, which does not associate at synapses and this type has been termed extrasynaptic (36). All three receptors form picrotoxin sensitive chloride channels. GABA$_A$ receptors mediate important forms of synaptic inhibition in hippocampal and other cortical circuits and have been well established as targets for anticonvulsant, sedative, and anesthetic drugs.

GABA$_B$ Receptors, G-proteins, and Potassium Channels

GABA$_B$ receptors do not include a channel, but consist of a single protein with seven hydrophobic transmembrane domains, which operate in cooperation with trimeric G proteins through an inhibition of adenylate cyclase. On binding GABA, the activated receptor couples to the alpha subunit of an associated G protein. If this is a GI protein, it inhibits adenylate cyclase and opens a K$^+$ channel (probably via beta subunits). The K$^+$ channel opening leads to neuronal membrane hyperpolarization. If the GABA$_B$ receptor couples to a GO protein, it retards the opening of Ca^{2+} channels, probably via its beta subunits. GABA$_B$ receptors are often located presynaptically on nerve terminals, where they retard the opening of Ca^{2+} channels, so depolarization-induced release of glutamate or GABA from nerve terminals may be depressed.

Cholinergic Synapses and other Neurotransmitters

The most important ascending input to hippocampal neurons uses acetylcholine as an excitatory neurotransmitter and comes from neurons in the septal area of the limbic system (37). These cholinergic synapses mediate both fast and slow membrane currents via both nicotinic and muscarinic receptors on pyramidal cells and inhibitory interneurons. Nicotinic receptors belong to a ligand gated superfamily analogous to the GABA$_A$ receptor family of pentomeric subunits. Muscarinic receptors are G protein linked, similar to GABA$_B$ receptors. A number of other ascending neurotransmitter systems innervate the hippocampus and produce profound modulatory effects on both pyramidal cells and, especially, on inhibitory interneurons; these include: catecholamines, indolamines, and peptide transmitters. These transmitter systems have been poorly characterized in hippocampus, but they offer a potentially fruitful avenue for future research, especially regarding anesthetic effects on neuromodulatory transmitters.

The Theta Rhythm and other EEG Activity

The ascending cholinergic system is known to be essential for coordinating and synchronizing pyramidal neuron discharge activity, as lesions of the septal area and/or muscarinic receptor antagonists produce a profound block of theta rhythms in the hippocampus (38). Theta rhythms are the largest amplitude and among the best characterized EEG signals generated by the mammalian brain. They are thought to be important for learning and memory functions, as well as for sensory/motor integration within the hippocampus and other cortical areas. Theta rhythms are known to be blocked by most general anesthetics, and this could contribute to the loss of recall produced during anesthesia. The hippocampus also generates delta slow wave rhythms (especially during sleep) as well as a miriad of other EEG rhythms covering the full EEG frequency spectrum. Recent attention has focused on high frequency (40–100 Hz) EEG signals which appear to correlate to the processing of sensory information and involve synchronization of GABAergic inhibitory interneurons (15). Studying anesthetic effects on these hippocampal EEG signals could provide a way to link behavioral responses observed in vivo, during anesthesia, with the cellular and synaptic effects observed on pyramidal and interneurons (9).

ANESTHETIC ACTIONS ON HIPPOCAMPAL NEURONS AND SYNAPTIC RESPONSES

Anesthetics Alter Hippocampal EEG Responses In Vivo

It has long been known that anesthetics disrupt the normal EEG signals recorded using microelectrodes from the hippocampus (39,40). General anesthetics produce a concentration dependent continuum of effects on hippocampal EEG signals that are similar to effects produced in other cortical areas, and also similar across species (8,41). At low concentrations that produce ataxia and sedation, anesthetics increase the amplitude of hippocampal EEG rhythms, especially in the delta and theta frequency ranges. Higher concentrations, associated with loss of recall and loss of righting reflex, depress theta frequency responses, but delta activity continues to increase; similar to the EEG patterns observed during deep sleep. Moderate anesthesia, associated with loss of tail pinch and the corneal responses in rats, occurs during burst suppression EEG activity recorded from both the hippocampus and neocortex. At the even higher anesthetic concentrations used for induction to block the gag reflex during intubation, anesthetics produce isoelectric EEG responses (9). Thus, the hippocampus appears to be profoundly affected by anesthetics over the entire clinically relevant concentration ranges used during anesthesia.

Anesthetics Alter Evoked Potentials In Vivo

In contrast to EEG analysis of anesthetic effects, studies looking at synaptically evoked hippocampal recordings in vivo have provided a mixed view of results. The earliest study of anesthetic effects on hippocampal neurons indicated that excitatory EPSP responses were depressed, and that GABA mediated IPSPs were prolonged during anesthesia (6). Subsequent studies have confirmed this EPSP depression (7) or have suggested that the dominant effect is to enhance GABA mediated inhibition (42). Differences in results can readily be explained by differences in anesthetics studied and by whether the effects were observed in already anesthetized vs freely moving subjects. It was evident from all three studies that synaptic responses in the hippocampus were altered during anesthesia, but a detailed study using chronically implanted, freely moving animals would be particularly useful for future research.

Anesthetics Depress Neuronal Excitability

By far, the most detailed studies of anesthetic effects on hippocampal neurons have come from investigations using the in vitro hippocampal slice preparation. Several independent laboratories have studied general anesthetics on many important synaptic and cellular responses. A common theme has emerged for the cellular actions produced by volatile, barbiturate, and propofol anesthetics. All of these agents block synaptically evoked discharge activity of CA 1 pyramidal cells and dentate granule neurons, but the mechanisms producing the block can differ considerably for volatile vs IV anesthetics. Agent specific effects have been observed for actions on excitatory and inhibitory synapses and for changes in postsynaptic excitability. For most anesthetics, multiple sites of action combine in additive or synergistic ways to depress transmission, but other agents appear to act at only one or two sites.

Effects on Resting Membrane Potential

One of the earliest studies using hippocampal brain slices to investigate anesthetic effects found that some agents could hyperpolarize CA 1 neurons *(43)*. This hyperpolarization was observed in the presence of tetrodotoxin, so it was not owing to a generalized depression of synaptic transmission. It appeared to result from a direct effect on the cell membrane, since it was associated with an increase in membrane conductance. Several studies have provided evidence for anesthetic-induced increases in potassium *(44,45)* and chloride *(46,47)* currents in hippocampal neurons, which could account for this hyperpolarization.

Effects on Membrane Resistance

IV agents like propofol can produce marked increases in chloride currents *(36)* of hippocampal neurons. For volatile anesthetics, relatively small hyperpolarizations are produced *(48)* and appear to be both agent selective and dependent on normal resting membrane potentials *(49)*. Cells with more depolarized resting potentials exhibited a greater degree of anesthetic-induced hyperpolariztion. This is consistent with anesthetic-induced increases in potassium or chloride currents, since the reversal potentials for these ions are near the resting potentials of these cells.

Effects on Action Potential Discharge

The shunting effect of a decrease in membrane resistance produced by anesthetics results in a decrease in action potential discharge of hippocampal neurons. This has been observed as decreased discharge frequencies *(44)* and as an increase in discharge thresholds *(50)* for hippocampal neurons. In general, neurons are still capable of firing action potentials in response to depolarizing current injection (Fig. 3), and there do not appear to be strong anesthetic effects on spike amplitude, rise time, or decay kinetics for most agents *(48,51)*.

Effects on Antidromic Discharge

Consistent with a minimal effect on action potential discharge, anesthetics do not appear to effect antidromic spike responses recorded from the pyramidal or granule neuron cell body layers following stimulation of their axons *(52,53)* until high concentrations are achieved, 5–10 fold higher than needed to block synaptically driven discharge.

Anesthetics Depress Excitatory Synaptic Transmission

For hippocampal neurons in brain slices, the most sensitive response measure for anesthetics is synaptically evoked discharge *(48,52–54)*. The ability to fire an action potential following stimulation of afferent synaptic inputs appears to be severely depressed or even blocked by anesthetic concentrations within the clinical range. Although the concentrations which depress synaptic excitation correlate well with clinical levels *(55)*, the mechanisms leading to this depression appear to be somewhat different for each anesthetic studied *(47,49,51–53)*.

Effects on Evoked Population Spike Discharge

Population spikes can be recorded from each of the three main neuron groups in the hippocampal trisynaptic pathway, and represent the summed discharge of large numbers of cells that fire synchronously in response to activation of synaptic inputs to these neurons. Population spikes provide a

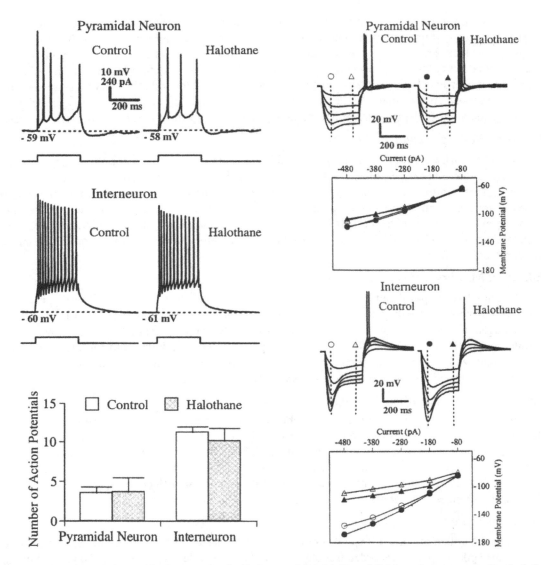

Fig. 3. Anesthetics do not block postsynaptic discharge of CA 1 cells or inhibitory interneurons. On the left, action potential discharges in response to direct depolarizing current injections are shown. Halothane at a concentration of 1 MAC only mildly depressed discharge in the neurons shown. These effects were not statistically significant when compared across all 18 pyramidal neurons studied (*lower bar graph*) or for 13 interneurons studied. On the right, representative membrane voltage responses to hyperpolarizing current injections are shown. 1 MAC concentrations of halothane had little effect on resting membrane potential or membrane resistance for the neurons studied. Figures were used with permission from Nishikawa and MacIver, *J. Neurosci.* 2000 *(48)*.

global measure of circuit function. The amplitude of the response provides a measure of the number of cells that are synaptically activated. Any anesthetic effect on excitatory or inhibitory synaptic inputs will be detected as a change in amplitude of the response. Most agents produce a monotonic, concentration dependent depression of population spike amplitudes *(52,56)*, although some agents like pentobarbital can increase spike amplitudes at low concentrations and block at clinically relevant levels *(53)*. There is a good correlation between the anesthetic concentrations needed to block population spike responses and their clinically effective concentrations for barbiturates, volatile anesthetics, propofol, and even for experimental anesthetics like riluzole *(55,57)*.

Effects on Glutamate-Mediated Synapses

Anesthetic-induced population spike block appears to result, at least in part, from a depression of glutamate-mediated excitatory synaptic transmission. Most agents depress EPSP responses recorded from hippocampal neurons (Fig. 4) and for some, like ketamine and xenon, this can be the dominant effect *(58,59)* leading to population spike block. The mechanisms underlying EPSP depression appear to involve both pre- and postsynaptic sites, but vary among different classes of anesthetics.

PRESYNAPTIC ACTIONS

Volatile anesthetics like halothane appear to act presynaptically to depress the amount of glutamate that is released from nerve terminals. EPSP amplitudes are depressed by anesthetic concentrations that do not alter postsynaptic responses to exogenously applied glutamate *(54,60,61)*. In addition, EPSP depression is accompanied by an increase in paired pulse facilitation, a hallmark for presynaptic actions *(62,63)*. Neither the EPSP depression, nor the increase in facilitation produced by volatile anesthetics is altered in the presence of GABA receptor antagonists or chloride channel blockers, indicating that a direct depressant effect occurs on glutamate nerve terminals *(62,64)*. Studies using synaptomsomes have suggested that glutamate release may be depressed by effects on action potential propagation into nerve terminals *(65)*. At least 15% of the ESPS depression produced by halothane appears to come about by a depression of action potential conduction in presynaptic nerve endings; measured as a depression of fiber volley amplitudes *(60,66)*. The remaining depression could involve depression of calcium channels in presynaptic terminals *(67)*, or effects on proteins associated with vesicular release *(62)*.

POSTSYNAPTIC ACTIONS

It remains to be determined whether anesthetic actions on postsynaptic glutamate receptor mediated responses contribute to the depression of synaptic excitation. Several studies suggest that postsynaptic actions appear to play a role *(58,64,68)*, while others argue for mostly presynaptic effects *(61–63)*. An elegant recent study indicates that although anesthetics can directly depress GluR2 receptors, this effect contributes little to synaptic depression or anesthesia, because effective concentrations for tail pinch responses were not altered in mice expressing mutant GluR2 receptors that were insensitive to anesthetic *(69)*. Postsynaptic actions, in contrast, appeared to play a greater role for isoflurane effects on NMDA-mediated synaptic responses compared to AMPA/kainate, (including GluR2) mediated responses *(64)*.

Comparison of Effects on NMDA vs AMPA Synapses

It is clear that anesthetic effects on postsynaptic NMDA receptors do play an important role for some anesthetics like ketamine *(70,71)*. There is also good evidence that propofol *(72)* and isoflurane (Fig. 5) *(64)* can have selective depressant effects on NMDA receptors compared to AMPA receptor-mediated transmission. Halothane, in contrast, did not appear to have preferential effects on NMDA-mediated responses *(64)*. Further studies will be needed to determine whether other anesthetics also have selective effects on NMDA receptors. It appears likely that this effect will exhibit a high degree of agent selectivity.

Anesthetics Enhance Inhibitory Synaptic Transmission

It has long been recognized that anesthetics enhance synaptic inhibition by prolonging the decay times of IPSCs in hippocampal neurons *(6,73,74)*. Enhanced synaptic inhibition would contribute to the CNS depression produced by anesthetics, but it remains to be determined the extent of this contribution. At this time, it is also unknown whether a single mechanism action is involved, but recent findings indicate that several actions combine to enhance inhibition for some anesthetics.

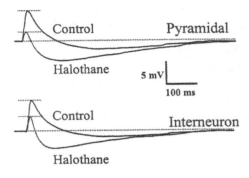

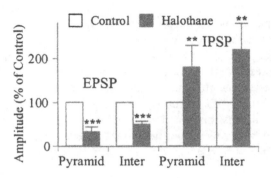

Fig. 4. Anesthetics produce a profound depression of glutamate mediated synaptic responses recorded from CA 1 pyramidal cells and inhibitory interneurons. Halothane at 1 MAC depressed EPSP responses by 50% in both types of neurons averaged across six cells of each type (*bar graph at bottom*). This anesthetic also increased GABA mediated inhibitory synaptic responses in both types of cell. IPSP amplitudes were increased by about 200% in these cells. Used with permission from Nishikawa and MacIver, *J. Neurosci.* 2000 *(48)*.

Effects on Paired Pulse Inhibition

Paired pulse inhibition provides a sensitive measure of anesthetic effects on GABA-mediated inhibition of hippocampal neurons, both in vivo *(42)* and in brain slices *(53,75)*. Paired pulse inhibition appears when two stimulus pulses are delivered with an interpulse interval that is short enough to allow inhibitory synaptic currents generated by the first pulse to depress discharge in response to the second stimulus pulse; between 20–150 ms intervals in hippocampal circuits. Enhanced paired pulse inhibition appears to be a particularly important action for barbiturate anesthetics and propofol, but less important for volatile agents and riluzole *(57)*. This effect would be especially important for determining the discharge frequencies of tonically or rhythmically active neurons. Prolonged paired pulse inhibition has been implicated in the slowing of EEG signals to delta frequencies produced by anesthetics like thiopental *(76)*.

Effects on GABA$_A$-Mediated Synapses

Enhanced paired pulse inhibition produced by anesthetics could come about by several mechanisms. A likely mechanism would simply be that the prolongation of IPSCs provides an increased shunting of second pulse responses. It is interesting, though, that both halothane and thiopental prolong IPSCs to a similar degree, yet only thiopental produces a consistent increase in paired pulse inhibition. It is likely that other mechanisms, including presynaptic effects at GABA nerve terminals also contribute.

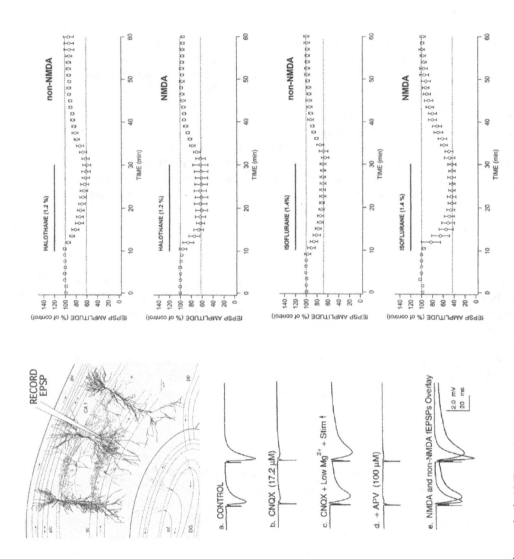

Fig. 5. Anesthetics depress both AMPA and NMDA receptor mediated EPSP responses recorded from the dendritic fields of CA 1 neurons (*upper left*). AMPA receptor dependent EPSPs can be blocked with the receptor antagonist CNQX and NMDA receptor responses are blocked with the antagonist APV (*lower left recordings*). Anesthetic effects on pharmacologically isolated AMPA (non-NMDA) and NMDA EPSPs were agent selective. Halothane depressed both types of glutamate mediated EPSP to a similar degree (*top right*). Isoflurane, in contrast, produced a greater depression of NMDA EPSPs compared to AMPA receptor mediated responses (*bottom right*). Both agents were applied at their equivalent 1 MAC concentrations, and each point represents the mean ± SD for 5 separate experiments. Used with permission from Nishikawa and MacIver, Anesthesiology 2000 (*64*).

161

PRESYNAPTIC ACTIONS

GABA nerve terminals experience feed back inhibition of release via $GABA_B$ receptors located on the terminal membrane. These receptors respond to released GABA and appear to downregulate further release, thus limiting paired pulse inhibition under normal conditions (77,78). It is possible that anesthetics enhance paired pulse inhibition by depressing this feedback system, but this effect was not observed for volatile agents at CA 1 neuron synapses (75). It is also possible that anesthetics have a direct effect to enhance the release of GABA from nerve terminals. Such an effect has been observed for halothane (79,80), midazolam, and propofol (36) and was evident as an increase in the frequency of IPSCs recorded from hippocampal neurons. For halothane, this increase in frequency appeared to result from an anesthetic-induced release of calcium from internal stores in the GABA nerve terminal leading to a greater release probability for vesicles (79,81).

POSTSYNAPTIC ACTIONS

There is now ample evidence that the prolongation of IPSCs involves direct anesthetic actions on postsynaptic $GABA_A$ receptors (74), *see also* Chapters 6, 15, 16, and 20 in this book). The prolongation can be reduced by lowering calcium concentrations in postsynaptic neurons using the chelator BAPTA (46), and elevated calcium concentrations modulate membrane patch clamp responses to pulses of exogenously applied GABA (35). In addition, anesthetic effects on $GABA_A$ receptors persist in membrane patches and occur too quickly to involve second messenger systems (82). Instead, they appear to result from a direct anesthetic-induced slowing in the dissociation of GABA from the receptor (83).

INTERNEURON ACTIONS

Little is known about the effects produced by anesthetics on GABAergic interneurons, but a few studies have indicated that a generalized depression occurs, comparable to effects seen on excitatory pyramidal neurons. Volatile anesthetics have been shown to depress glutamate synaptic inputs to interneurons (84). This effect appears to result from presynaptic depression of transmitter release, similar to effects in CA 1 pyramidal neurons (48,63). Volatile agents have also been shown to enhance GABA-mediated inhibition for synapses made between interneurons (47). The combined effects at glutamate and GABA synapses can account for a majority of the depressant effects on interneurons (48), and demonstrates that the inhibitory components of CA 1 neuronal circuitry are effectively removed at the same time that the pyramidal neurons are depressed.

Combined Effects at GABA and Glutamate Synapses

It appears that most anesthetics that have been studied in hippocampal brain slices depress glutamate mediated excitatory synapses and enhance GABA-mediated inhibitory synapses over the same concentration ranges that are used clinically. Combined effects on both types of synapses summate with direct depressant effects on membrane excitability to render neurons silent during anesthesia produced by halothane, nitrous oxide, thiopental, pentobarbital, and isoflurane (55,85). A few anesthetics like ketamine and xenon appear to act exclusively to depress synaptic excitation, with little effect on GABA inhibitory synapses (59,86). At least one agent, propofol, appears to act mostly at $GABA_A$ receptors, since most of the propofol-induced depression can be reversed by the $GABA_A$ receptor antagonist, bicuculline, with little residual depression seen at glutamate synapses (36,58,68).

Pathway Specific and Anesthetic Selective Effects

Concentration-response analysis of anesthetic effects on three synaptic pathways in hippocampal slices indicate that effects can differ considerably. Barbiturates produce biphasic effects (enhancement at low concentrations and depression at clinical levels) on two inputs to CA 1 neurons, but only depression at inputs to dentate granule neurons (53). Similar concentration effect differences are apparent for volatile anesthetic effects *(52)* at hippocampal synapses. These pathway specific differences in effect are not surprising in light of the multitude of GABA and glutamate receptor subtypes and their heterogeneous distribution at different synapses. Future research will no doubt reveal even greater degrees of selectivity, reflecting differential anesthetic sensitivities for receptors with unique subunit compositions.

Anesthetics Block Long-Term Potentiation of Synapses

Anesthetic-induced depression of hippocampal neurons could play a role in the loss of recall that occurs during anesthesia. Volatile anesthetics block LTP at hippocampal synapses *(87)*, consistent with the idea that LTP provides a synaptic locus for learning ant memory in the hippocampus. Recent studies have also shown that anesthetics block the other major form of hippocampal synaptic plasticity, LTD *(88)*. Preliminary studies suggest that actions at glutamate nerve terminals *(89)* and/or at GABA synapses *(88)* can account for the anesthetic-induced block of synaptic plasticity.

CONCLUSIONS

Anesthetics Depress Hippocampal Synaptic Circuits

There is now ample evidence from both in vivo and brain slice studies to indicate that anesthetic effects on hippocampal neurons contribute to the CNS depression that underlies anesthesia. It is likely that effects observed on hippocampal synapses also occur in other brain areas, especially cortical regions; although subtle differences in effect will likely been seen to depend on the specific subunit pharmacology that exists at each particular synapse or group of synapses. It is already apparent that anesthetics can act on three distinct GABA$_A$ receptors expressed in hippocampal CA 1 pyramidal neurons alone *(36,90)*, and more GABA$_A$ receptors will likely be found on other hippocampal neurons. Similarly, effects on glutamate mediated synapses indicate that anesthetics can have selective effects on responses mediated by NMDA and non-NMDA receptors *(64)*. Regardless of the particular mechanisms associated with a given anesthetic, the block of hippocampal population spike responses correlates very well with clinical concentrations for several classes of volatile and intravenous anesthetics *(55)*. In coming years, the use of hippocampal slice preparations will further increase our understanding of anesthetic sites and mechanisms of action.

Multiple Sites of Anesthetic Action

One of the most interesting findings to emerge from anesthetic research using hippocampal neurons is that anesthetics can depress population spikes via several actions occurring at the cellular and synaptic level; and the particular profile of actions can differ for each anesthetic. Early unitary theories of anesthetic action predicted a single effect at a common site would explain the CNS depression produced by all anesthetics. It is now evident that multiple sites of action are involved. For example, halothane appears to depress CA 1 neuron population spikes by at least five effects that combine to depress excitatory transmission and enhance inhibitory synaptic inputs. Halothane depresses action potential conduction in presynaptic glutamatergic nerve fibers. This anesthetic also depresses glutamate release from nerve terminals through a separate mechanism, and may blunt postsynaptic excitation by shunting dendritic currents. Halothane also acts on GABAergic nerve terminals to increase the release of this inhibitory transmitter, an effect opposite to that seen a glutamate synapses. Clear postsynaptic effects on GABA$_{Aslow}$ and GABA$_{Afast}$ types of receptors are observed, which result in a decrease in postsynaptic membrane resistance and would contribute to membrane hyperpolarization of CA 1 neurons. These five effects appear to account for most of the population spike depression produced by halothane, but additional effects on postsynaptic potassium and calcium currents in CA 1 neurons have been reported and can readily account for the reminder of depressant actions.

Other anesthetics, including volatile agents share a similar pattern of effects on CA 1 neurons, but appear to differ in the degree of effect seen at each site. For some agents, like propofol and xenon, fewer sites of action appear to be involved, but even for these anesthetics, effects at GABA or glutamate synapses play a major role in population spike depression, and both produce effects that correlate with their clinical potencies. Taken together, results from studies using hippocampal neurons support a Multisite Agent Selective (MAS) hypothesis for anesthetic mechanisms of action. No single effect can account for the depression produced by most anesthetics, and differing sites of action or degrees of effect are apparent for different agents. The MAS hypothesis predicts that even more sites of action will become apparent when anesthetic effects on other transmitter systems in the hippocampus are studied. For example, cholinergic synapses are known to play as important a role as glutamate synapses for controlling hippocampal neuron excitability, yet anesthetic effects on septal-hippocampal inputs remain to be determined. The same is true for catecholamine, indolamine, and peptidergic transmitter systems within the hippocampus. It is likely that both pre- and postsynaptic sites of action will provide anesthetic targets on these important ascending pathways. The MAS hypothesis provides a better paradigm than a unitary theory for future studies directed at the development of safer and more effective anesthetics that target discrete sites at CNS synapses.

Relationship to Clinical/Behavioral Effects of Anesthetics

Anesthesia encompasses a number of interrelated CNS effects, some of which may critically involve the hippocampus. The loss of consciousness and block of recall produced by anesthetics almost certainly involves hippocampal and cortical circuit depression. It is possible that depressed sensory perception and even the block of purposeful movement produced by anesthetics could include actions on hippocampal function, although effects at the spinal cord level undoubtedly contribute as much or more to these components of anesthesia. Future studies of anesthetic actions in the hippocampus will likely provide insights into the normal function and physiology of this important brain area. In addition to providing a more detailed understanding of the synaptic and cellular basis of anesthesia.

REFERENCES

1. Milner, B., Squire, L. R., and Kandel, E. R. (1998) Cognitive neuroscience and the study of memory. *Neuron* **20,** 445–468.
2. Bannerman, D. M., Yee, B. K., Good, M. A., Heupel, M. J., Iversen, S. D., and Rawlins, J. N. (1999) Double dissociation of function within the hippocampus: a comparison of dorsal, ventral, and complete hippocampal cytotoxic lesions. *Behavioral Neuroscience* **113,** 1170–1188.
3. Vanderwolf, C. H. (1998) Brain, behavior, and mind: what do we know and what can we know? *Neurosci. Biobehav. Rev.* **22,** 125–142.
4. Bland, B. H. and Colom, L. V. (1993) Extrinsic and intrinsic properties underlying oscillation and synchrony in limbic cortex. *Prog. Neurobiol.* **41,** 157–208.
5. Oddie, S. D. and Bland, B. H. (1998) Hippocampal formation theta activity and movement selection. *Neurosci. Biobehav. Rev.* **22,** 221–231.
6. Nicoll, R. A., Eccles, J. C., Oshima, T., and Rubia, F. (1975) Prolongation of hippocampal inhibitory postsynaptic potentials by barbiturates. *Nature* **258,** 625–627.
7. Leung, L. S. (1981) Differential effects of pentobarbital and ether on the synaptic transmission of the hippocampal CA1 region in the rat. *Electroencephalogr. Clin. Neurophysiol.* **51,** 291–305.
8. Tomoda, K., Shingu, K., Osawa, M., Murakawa, M., and Mori, K. (1993) Comparison of CNS effects of propofol and thiopentone in cats. *Brit. J. Anaesth.* **71,** 383–387.
9. MacIver, M. B., Mandema, J. W., Stanski, D. R., and Bland, B. H. (1996) Thiopental uncouples hippocampal and cortical synchronized electroencephalographic activity. *Anesthesiology* **84,** 1411–1424.
10. Lukatch, H. S. and Greenwald, S. (2002) Chapter 6. Cerebral Cortex–Anesthetic action on the electroencephalogram: Cellular and synaptic mechanisms and clinical monitoring, in Neural Nechanisms of Anesthesia, (Antognini, J., ed.) Humana Press Inc., Totowa, NJ.
11. Malenka, R. C. and Nicoll, R. A. (1999) Long-term potentiation—a decade of progress? *Science* **285,** 1870–1874.
12. Ameri, A., Wilhelm, A., and Simmet, T. (1999) Effects of the endogeneous cannabinoid, anandamide, on neuronal activity in rat hippocampal slices. *Brit. J. Pharmacol.* **126,** 1831–1839.
13. Wilson, R. I. and Nicoll, R. A. (2001) Endogenous cannabinoids mediate retrograde signalling at hippocampal synapses. *Nature* **410,** 588–592.

14. Pearce, R. A. (1993) Physiological evidence for two distinct GABAA responses in rat hippocampus. *Neuron* **10,** 189–200.
15. Banks, M. I., White, J. A., and Pearce, R. A. (2000) Interactions between distinct GABA(A) circuits in hippocampus. *Neuron* **25,** 449–457.
16. Shepherd, G. M. (1994) Neurobiology, Third Oxford University Press, New York, pp. 28–66.
17. Mellor, J. and Nicoll, R. A. (2001) Hippocampal mossy fiber LTP is independent of postsynaptic calcium. *Nat. Neurosci.* **4,** 125–126.
18. Montgomery, J. M., Pavlidis, P., and Madison, D. V. (2001) Pair recordings reveal all-silent synaptic connections and the postsynaptic expression of long-term potentiation. *Neuron* **29,** 691–701.
19. Seeburg, P. H. (1993) The TINS/TiPS Lecture. The molecular biology of mammalian glutamate receptor channels. *Trends Neurosci.* **16,** 359–365.
20. Hollmann, M., and Heinemann, S. (1994) Cloned glutamate receptors. *Annu. Rev. Neurosci.* **17,** 31–108.
21. Nakanishi, S. and Masu, M. (1994) Molecular diversity and functions of glutamate receptors. *Annu. Rev. Biophys. Biomol. Struct.* **23,** 319–348.
22. Sommer, B., Keinanen, K., Verdoorn, T. A., et al. (1990) Flip and flop: a cell-specific functional switch in glutamate-operated channels of the CNS. *Science* **249,** 1580–1585.
23. Egebjerg, J., Bettler, B., Hermans-Borgmeyer, I., and Heinemann, S. (1991) Cloning of a cDNA for a glutamate receptor subunit activated by kainate but not AMPA. *Nature* **351,** 745–748.
24. Herb, A., Burnashev, N., Werner, P., Sakmann, B., Wisden, W., and Seeburg, P. H. (1992) The KA-2 subunit of excitatory amino acid receptors shows widespread expression in brain and forms ion channels with distantly related subunits. *Neuron* **8,** 775–785.
25. Sugihara, H., Moriyoshi, K., Ishii, T., Masu, M., and Nakanishi, S. (1992) Structures and properties of seven isoforms of the NMDA receptor generated by alternative splicing. *Biochem. Biophys. Res. Commun.* **185,** 826–832.
26. Hollmann, M., Boulter, J., Maron, C., et al. (1993) Zinc potentiates agonist-induced currents at certain splice variants of the NMDA receptor. *Neuron* **10,** 943–954.
27. Monyer, H., Sprengel, R., Schoepfer, R., et al. (1992) Heteromeric NMDA receptors: molecular and functional distinction of subtypes. *Science* **256,** 1217–1221.
28. Nakanishi, S. (1992) Molecular diversity of glutamate receptors and implications for brain function. *Science* **258,** 597–603.
29. Ishii, T., Moriyoshi, K., Sugihara, H., Sakurada, K., Kadotani, H., Yokoi, M., Akazawa, C., Shigemoto, R., Mizuno, N., Masu, M., and et al. (1993) Molecular characterization of the family of the N-methyl-D-aspartate receptor subunits. *J. Biol. Chem.* **268,** 2836–2843.
30. Conn, P. J. and Pin, J. P. (1997) Pharmacology and functions of metabotropic glutamate receptors. *Annu. Rev. Pharmacol. Toxicol.* **37,** 205–237.
31. Pin, J. P., De Colle, C., Bessis, A. S., and Acher, F. (1999) New perspectives for the development of selective metabotropic glutamate receptor ligands. *Eur. J. Pharmacol.* **375,** 277–294.
32. Amin, J. and Weiss, D. S. (1996) Insights into the activation mechanism of rho1 GABA receptors obtained by coexpression of wild type and activation-impaired subunits. *Proc. R. Soc. Lond. B. Biol. Sci.* **263,** 273–282.
33. Carlson, B. X., Engblom, A. C., Kristiansen, U., Schousboe, A., and Olsen, R. W. (2000) A single glycine residue at the entrance to the first membrane-spanning domain of the gamma-aminobutyric acid type A receptor beta(2) subunit affects allosteric sensitivity to GABA and anesthetics. *Mol. Pharmacol.* **57,** 474–484.
34. Tretter, V., Ehya, N., Fuchs, K., and Sieghart, W. (1997) Stoichiometry and assembly of a recombinant GABAA receptor subtype. *J. Neurosci.* **17,** 2728–2737.
35. Banks, M. I. and Pearce, R. A. (2000) Kinetic differences between synaptic and extrasynaptic GABA(A) receptors in CA1 pyramidal cells. *J. Neurosci.* **20,** 937–948.
36. Bai, D., Zhu, G., Pennefather, P., Jackson, M. F., MacDonald, J. F., and Orser, B. A. (2001) Distinct functional and pharmacological properties of tonic and quantal inhibitory postsynaptic currents mediated by gamma-aminobutyric acid(A) receptors in hippocampal neurons. *Mol. Pharmacol.* **59,** 814–824.
37. Bland, B. H., Oddie, S. D., and Colom, L. V. (1999) Mechanisms of neural synchrony in the septohippocampal pathways underlying hippocampal theta generation. *J Neurosci.* **19,** 3223–3237.
38. Bland, B. H. and Oddie, S. D. (1998) Anatomical, electrophysiological and pharmacological studies of ascending brainstem hippocampal synchronizing pathways. *Neurosci. Biobehav. Rev.* **22,** 259–273.
39. Gray, J. A. and Ball, G. G. (1970) Frequency-specific relation between hippocampal theta rhythm, behavior, and amobarbital action. *Science* **168,** 1246–1248.
40. Kramis, R., Vanderwolf, C. H., and Bland, B. H. (1975) Two types of hippocampal rhythmical slow activity in both the rabbit and the rat: relations to behavior and effects of atropine, diethyl ether, urethane, and pentobarbital. *Exp. Neurol.* **49,** 58–85.
41. Stanski, D. R. and Watkins, W. D. (1982) Drug Disposition in Anesthesia, Grune & Stratton, New York, pp. 72–96.
42. Pearce, R. A., Stringer, J. L., and Lothman, E. W. (1989) Effect of volatile anesthetics on synaptic transmission in the rat hippocampus. *Anesthesiology* **71,** 591–598.
43. Nicoll, R. A. and Madison, D. V. (1982) General anesthetics hyperpolarize neurons in the vertebrate central nervous system. *Science* **217,** 1055–1057.
44. Carlen, P. L., Gurevich, N., Davies, M. F., Blaxter, T. J., and O'Beirne, M. (1985) Enhanced neuronal K+ conductance: a possible common mechanism for sedative-hypnotic drug action. *Can. J. Physiol. Pharmacol.* **63,** 831–837.
45. Ries, C. R. and Puil, E. (1999) Ionic mechanism of isoflurane's actions on thalamocortical neurons. *J. Neurophysiol.* **81,** 1802–1809.

46. Mody, I., Tanelian, D. L., and MacIver, M. B. (1991) Halothane enhances tonic neuronal inhibition by elevating intracellular calcium. *Brain Res.* **538**, 319–323.
47. Nishikawa, K. and MacIver, M. B. (2001) Agent-selective effects of volatile anesthetics on $GABA_A$ receptor- mediated synaptic inhibition in hippocampal interneurons. *Anesthesiology* **94**, 340–347.
48. Nishikawa, K. and MacIver, M. B. (2000) Membrane and synaptic actions of halothane on rat hippocampal pyramidal neurons and inhibitory interneurons. *J. Neurosci.* **20**, 5915–5923.
49. MacIver, M. B. and Kendig, J. J. (1991) Anesthetic effects on resting membrane potential are voltage-dependent and agent-specific. *Anesthesiology* **74**, 83–88.
50. Langmoen, I. A. (1983) Some mechanisms controlling hippocampal pyramidal cells. *Prog. Brain Res.* **58**, 61–69.
51. MacIver, M. B. and Kendig, J. J. (1989) Enflurane-induced burst discharge of hippocampal CA1 neurones is blocked by the NMDA receptor antagonist APV. *Brit. J. Anaesth.* **63**, 296–305.
52. MacIver, M. B. and Roth, S. H. (1988) Inhalation anaesthetics exhibit pathway-specific and differential actions on hippocampal synaptic responses in vitro. *Brit. J. Anaesth.* **60**, 680–691.
53. MacIver, M. B. and Roth, S. H. (1987) Barbiturate effects on hippocampal excitatory synaptic responses are selective and pathway specific. *Can. J. Physiol. Pharmacol.* **65**, 385–394.
54. Richards, C. D. and White, A. E. (1975) The actions of volatile anaesthetics on synaptic transmission in the dentate gyrus. *J. Physiol.* **252**, 241–257.
55. MacIver, M. B. (1997) General anesthetic actions on transmission at glutamate and GABA synapses, in Anesthesia: Biological Foundations, (Biebuyck, J. F., Lynch III, C., Maze, M., Saidman, L. J., Yaksh, T. L., and Zapol, W. M., eds.) Lippincott-Raven Publishers, New York, pp. 277–286.
56. Hagan, C. E., Pearce, R. A., Trudell, J. R., and MacIver, M. B. (1998) Concentration measures of volatile anesthetics in the aqueous phase using calcium sensitive electrodes. *J. Neurosci. Methods* **81**, 177–184.
57. MacIver, M. B., Amagasu, S. M., Mikulec, A. A., and Monroe, F. A. (1996) Riluzole anesthesia: use-dependent block of presynaptic glutamate fibers. *Anesthesiology* **85**, 626–634.
58. Wakasugi, M., Hirota, K., Roth, S. H., and Ito, Y. (1999) The effects of general anesthetics on excitatory and inhibitory synaptic transmission in area CA1 of the rat hippocampus in vitro. *Anesthesia and Analgesia* **88**, 676–680.
59. de Sousa, S. L., Dickinson, R., Lieb, W. R., and Franks, N. P. (2000) Contrasting synaptic actions of the inhalational general anesthetics isoflurane and xenon. *Anesthesiology* **92**, 1055–1066.
60. Richards, C. D. and Smaje, J. C. (1976) Anaesthetics depress the sensitivity of cortical neurones to L-glutamate. *Brit. J. Pharmacol.* **58**, 347–357.
61. Perouansky, M., Kirson, E. D., and Yaari, Y. (1998) Mechanism of action of volatile anesthetics: effects of halothane on glutamate receptors in vitro. *Toxicol. Lett.* **100–101**, 65–69.
62. MacIver, M. B., Mikulec, A. A., Amagasu, S. M., and Monroe, F. A. (1996) Volatile anesthetics depress glutamate transmission via presynaptic actions. *Anesthesiology* **85**, 823–834.
63. Kirson, E. D., Yaari, Y., and Perouansky, M. (1998) Presynaptic and postsynaptic actions of halothane at glutamatergic synapses in the mouse hippocampus. *Brit. J. Pharmacol.* **124**, 1607–1614.
64. Nishikawa, K. and MacIver, M. B. (2000) Excitatory synaptic transmission mediated by NMDA receptors is more sensitive to isoflurane than are non-NMDA receptor mediated responses. *Anesthesiology* **92**, 228–236.
65. Ratnakumari, L. and Hemmings, H. C., Jr. (1998) Inhibition of presynaptic sodium channels by halothane. *Anesthesiology* **88**, 1043–1054.
66. Mikulec, A. A., Pittson, S., Amagasu, S. M., Monroe, F. A., and MacIver, M. B. (1998) Halothane depresses action potential conduction in hippocampal axons. *Brain Res.* **796**, 231–238.
67. Study, R. E. (1994) Isoflurane inhibits multiple voltage-gated calcium currents in hippocampal pyramidal neurons. *Anesthesiology* **81**, 104–116.
68. Hirota, K., Roth, S. H., Fujimura, J., Masuda, A., and Ito, Y. (1998) GABAergic mechanisms in the action of general anesthetics. *Toxicol. Lett.* **100-101**, 203–207.
69. Joo, D. T., Xiong, Z., MacDonald, J. F., Jia, Z., Roder, J., Sonner, J., and Orser, B. A. (1999) Blockade of glutamate receptors and barbiturate anesthesia: increased sensitivity to pentobarbital-induced anesthesia despite reduced inhibition of AMPA receptors in GluR2 null mutant mice. *Anesthesiology* **91**, 1329–1341.
70. Orser, B. A., Pennefather, P. S., and MacDonald, J. F. (1997) Multiple mechanisms of ketamine blockade of N-methyl-D-aspartate receptors. *Anesthesiology* **86**, 903–917.
71. Duchen, M. R., Burton, N. R., and Biscoe, T. J. (1985) An intracellular study of the interactions of N-methyl-DL-aspartate with ketamine in the mouse hippocampal slice. *Brain Res.* **342**, 149–153.
72. Orser, B. A., Bertlik, M., Wang, L. Y., and MacDonald, J. F. (1995) Inhibition by propofol (2,6 di-isopropylphenol) of the N-methyl-D-aspartate subtype of glutamate receptor in cultured hippocampal neurones. *Brit. J. Pharmacol.* **116**, 1761–1768.
73. Nicoll, R. A. (1972) The effects of anaesthetics on synaptic excitation and inhibition in the olfactory bulb. *J. Physiol.* **223**, 803–814.
74. Tanelian, D. L., Kosek, P., Mody, I., and MacIver, M. B. (1993) The role of the GABAA receptor/chloride channel complex in anesthesia. *Anesthesiology* **78**, 757–776.
75. Pearce, R. A. (1996) Volatile anaesthetic enhancement of paired-pulse depression investigated in the rat hippocampus in vitro. *J. Physiol.* **492**, 823–840.
76. Lukatch, H. S. and MacIver, M. B. (1996) Synaptic mechanisms of thiopental-induced alterations in synchronized cortical activity. *Anesthesiology* **84**, 1425–1434.

77. Otis, T. S. and Mody, I. (1992) Modulation of decay kinetics and frequency of GABAA receptor mediated spontaneous inhibitory postsynaptic currents in hippocampal neurons. *Neuroscience* **49**, 13–32.
78. Otis, T. S. and Mody, I. (1992) Differential activation of GABAA and GABAB receptors by spontaneously released transmitter. *J. Neurophysiol.* **67**, 227–235.
79. Doze, V. A., Monroe, F. A., and MacIver, M. B. (1997) Halothane enhances presynaptic GABA release by increasing internal calcium. *Anesthesiology* **87**, A626.
80. Banks, M. I. and Pearce, R. A. (1999) Dual actions of volatile anesthetics on GABA(A) IPSCs: dissociation of blocking and prolonging effects. *Anesthesiology* **90**, 120–134.
81. Doze, V. A. and MacIver, M. B. (1998) Halothane acts on ryanodine sensitive calcium release channels to enhance GABA release. *Anesthesiology* **89**, A722.
82. Li, X., Czajkowski, C., and Pearce, R. A. (2000) Rapid and direct modulation of GABAA receptors by halothane. *Anesthesiology* **92**, 1366–1375.
83. Li, X. and Pearce, R. A. (2000) Effects of halothane on GABA(A) receptor kinetics: evidence for slowed agonist unbinding. *J. Neurosci.* **20**, 899–907.
84. Perouansky, M., Kirson, E. D., and Yaari, Y. (1996) Halothane blocks synaptic excitation of inhibitory interneurons. *Anesthesiology* **85**, 1431–1438; discussion 29A.
85. Mennerick, S., Jevtovic-Todorovic, V., Todorovic, S. M., Shen, W., Olney, J. W., and Zorumski, C. F. (1998) Effect of nitrous oxide on excitatory and inhibitory synaptic transmission in hippocampal cultures. *J. Neurosci.* **18**, 9716–9726.
86. Yamakura, T., Chavez-Noriega, L. E., and Harris, R. A. (2000) Subunit-dependent inhibition of human neuronal nicotinic acetylcholine receptors and other ligand gated ion channels by dissociative anesthetics ketamine and dizocilpine. *Anesthesiology* **92**, 1144–1153.
87. MacIver, M. B., Tauck, D. L., and Kendig, J. J. (1989) General anaesthetic modification of synaptic facilitation and long-term potentiation in hippocampus. *Brit. J. Anaesth.* **62**, 301–310.
88. Simon, W., Hapfelmeier, G., Kochs, E., Zieglgänsberger, W., and Rammes, G. (2001) Isoflurane Blocks Synaptic Plasticity in the Mouse Hippocampus. *Anesthesiology* **94**, 1058–1065.
89. Anderson, R. J., Hornung, B., Pittson, S., Monroe, F. A., and MacIver, M. B. (2000) Low concentrations of isoflurane block long term potentiation of hippocampal neuron synapses. *Anesthesiology* **93**, A776.
90. Lukatch, H. S. and MacIver, M. B. (1997) Voltage-clamp analysis of halothane effects on GABA(A fast) and GABA(A slow) inhibitory currents. *Brain Res.* **765**, 108–112.

10

Anesthetic Effects on the Reticular Formation, Brainstem and Central Nervous System Arousal

Joseph F. Antognini and Earl Carstens

INTRODUCTION

The reticular formation (RF) and brainstem are critically involved in normal neurological processes, such as nociception and consciousness. The RF is often called an "activating system" because of its ability to increase "arousal," presumably by activation of subcortical and cortical structures. Furthermore, numerous sites in the brainstem are involved in descending modulation of nociception. Thus, it is likely that anesthetics exert some of their effects via actions at the RF and brainstem. This chapter will describe the anatomy, physiology, and neurochemistry of the RF and brainstem, anesthetic effects at these sites, and how these actions might contribute to anesthesia. In addition, we discuss how these actions might affect the "arousal" state of the brain, and thereby affect clinically important goals such as amnesia and unconsciousness. We also discuss the use of auditory evoked potentials as a method of monitoring depth of anesthesia.

ANATOMY AND PHYSIOLOGY

The RF is a loose group of cells that is longitudinally spread throughout the hindbrain and midbrain including the thalamus. Individual cells in the RF may send axons caudally as far as the upper cervical cord and rostrally into the thalamus (1). The RF is to the brainstem and midbrain what the interneuronal network is to the spinal cord, although the RF is more extensive. Since the 19th century, neuroscientists have postulated that the RF governed the arousal state of the animal. In anesthetized animals, electrical stimulation of the RF was associated with EEG desynchronization (2). This change from a sleep-like EEG to an "awake" EEG was taken as proof that the RF was intimately involved with arousal. It is speculative whether electrical stimulation of the RF and its subsequent EEG activation is similar to what occurs naturally. That is, just because the EEG assumes an "awake" pattern does not mean that the functional state of the brain is shifting towards consciousness. Several investigators found that cortical and thalamic neurons had enhanced responses to stimuli during RF stimulation that resulted in increased arousal (3–5).

The RF is not functionally and structurally diffuse. It has discrete nuclei with discrete neurochemical profiles. A major neuronal group is the locus ceruleus that uses norepinephrine as its primary neurotransmitter. The brainstem raphe contains neurons rich in serotonin. These cells project to distant parts of the central nervous system (CNS), including the forebrain. Other cell groups rely upon acetylcholine as a neurotransmitter. The cells include those in the laterodorsal tegmental nucleus and the pedunculopontine nucleus. These cells also project to, among other sites, the forebrain, and are thought to be involved in regulation of sleep and consciousness. RF cells involved in sensory and

From: *Contemporary Clinical Neuroscience:* Neural Mechanisms of Anesthesia
Edited by: Joseph F. Antognini et al. © Humana Press Inc., Totowa, NJ

motor systems rely heavily upon glutamate and GABA for neurotransmission *(6)*. The RF receives sensory information from the spinoreticular tract that originates mostly from the deep dorsal horn and the ventral horn, although all parts of the dorsal and ventral horns probably contribute to some extent. Noxious stimuli clearly result in transmission of impulses to the RF via this pathway (Fig. 1) *(7,8)*.

The RF has other functions aside from arousal. Muscle tone depends in part on pontine and medullary neurons *(6)*. The RF also controls breathing and the cardiovascular system. Reticulospinal neurons are involved in nociception. In this regard, the reticular spinal neurons send axons to the dorsal horn of the spinal cord, where nociceptive information is modulated *(7)*. Several brainstem sites likely are involved in the action of anesthetics. These sites include the periaqueductal gray (PAG), rostroventral medulla (RVM), and locus coerelus (LC). These sites are part of the system that modulates nociception via descending fibers.

The role of midbrain RF neurons in control of consciousness is stressed in a report by Steriade et al., who found that discharge rates were correlated with waking and active sleep *(9)*. For example, activity of midbrain RF neurons during waking and active sleep was twice that during synchronized sleep. Furthermore, increased activity proceeded EEG desynchronization and behavioral changes (e.g., going from sleep to awaking) by 10–15 s.

The PAG can have profound influences on nociception. In fact, in Reynolds' original report of the role of the PAG in nociception he described surgical procedures being performed in awake rats that had had PAG stimulation *(10)*. Following that report, Hosobuchi et al. described pain relief in humans that received PAG stimulation *(11)*. Roizen et al. reported a 25% reduction in halothane minimum alveolar concentration (MAC) in humans that had PAG stimulation via electrodes implanted to treat chronic pain *(12)*. These results clearly indicate that the PAG can influence anesthetic requirements, but it is unclear whether any anesthetic actually exerts its effect at the PAG. For example, Rampil and colleagues reported that isoflurane MAC was unchanged after precollicular decerebration and spinal cord transection *(13,14)*. Taken in isolation, these studies suggest that no supraspinal site is important to the ability of isoflurane to suppress movement. However, because the spinal cord is capable of complex movements (*see* Chapter 11), it is possible that in the absence of supraspinal influences MAC is unchanged, but that in the normal animal, supraspinal sites might none the less influence anesthetic requirements.

Some have speculated that RF pathology might be associated with diverse disorders such as schizophrenia, REM behavior disorder, and narcolepsy. Although these claims remain to be substantiated, it is clear that the RF is intimately involved in many normal neurophysiological functions, and RF dysfunction might lead to diverse neurological pathophysiology *(15)*.

The medulla oblongata is critically involved in control of consciousness as well as the cardiopulmonary system. The solitary tract of the medulla is involved in the sleep cycle. For example, it "deactivates" the RF, thereby inhibiting normal states of consciousness. In addition, thalamocortical loops and spindle-production are altered as the result of neurophysiological processes in the medulla *(16)*.

Further evidence of the role of the brainstem in cortical function is the finding that fast oscillations (20–40 Hz) in thalamocortical systems are potentiated by cholinergic nuclei located in the mesopontine area *(17)*. This presumably occurs as a consequence of cholinergic input onto muscarinic receptors in the thalamus.

In a series of studies, Fields and colleagues described groups of cells in the nucleus raphe magnus (NRM) whose activities appeared to correlate with movement resulting from noxious stimulation *(18,19)*. OFF cells were defined as cells that decreased their firing rate immediately preceding initiation of a withdrawal reflex. ON cells on the other hand, increased their firing rate prior to the withdrawal. Activity in REGULAR cells increased only slightly in response to noxious stimulation, whereas activity of NEUTRAL cells did not change. These authors concluded that ON/OFF cells are involved in the initiation of movement that occurs during noxious stimulation. Leung and Mason determined that changes in ON and OFF-cell activity occurred after the initial movement. They con-

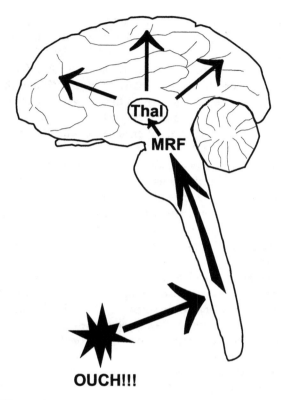

Fig. 1. Noxious stimulation results in impulse transmission to the spinal cord, which leads to impulse propagation rostrally to the midbrain reticular formation (MRF) and thalamus (Thal), and finally to cerebral cortex. Spinothalamic neurons send axons directly to the thalamus.

cluded that these cells might therefore be involved in not only the initiation of movement, but also the propagation of movement *(20,21)*.

ANESTHETIC EFFECTS IN BRAINSTEM AND RETICULAR FORMATION

Although anesthetics are distributed throughout the entire CNS, this does not imply that the anesthetic state results from equally diffuse actions. As pointed out in Chapter 11 , anesthetic action in the spinal cord accounts for the immobility-producing effects of isoflurane. Interestingly, discrete localized injections of barbiturates can lead to altered neurophysiological functions. Hayashi et al. found that injection of pentobarbital into the medulla of dogs lowered intracranial pressure and altered the EEG *(22)*. These ketamine-anesthetized dogs had experimentally-induced elevated intracranial pressure. The EEG changed from an "activated" pattern to a synchronized pattern (e.g., to low frequency, high amplitude). Devor and Zalkind *(23)* found that pentobarbital injected into the mesopontine tegmentum bilaterally produced unconsciousness.

Shimoji and Bickford *(24)* examined the effects of various anesthetics (halothane, ether, N_2O, and thiopental) on mesencephalic reticular neurons. The spontaneous activity of most neurons was depressed by these anesthetics, (compared to the awake state) but a few neurons were excited (e.g., increased spontaneous activity). This was particularly true upon exposure to 75% N_2O, where four of ten neurons had increased activity. In a separate report, Shimoji and colleagues investigated excitatory and inhibitory responses of MRF neurons *(25)*. They found halothane, ether, and isoflurane suppressed excitation responses, although N_2O did not have a consistent depressive effect. Thiopental and thiamylal potentiated inhibitory response while halothane, ether, and isoflurane had variable effects. In fact, at "light" levels of anesthesia, the inhalation anesthetics were more likely to block inhibitory responses. In a companion paper, Shimoji, and Bickford found that various anesthetics depressed MRF neuronal responses to peripheral electrical stimulation *(26)*.

Goodman and Mann *(27)* recorded multiunit activity in the RF and thalamus of cats. During drowsiness and slow wave sleep, neuronal activity in the RF was depressed, although it returned to waking levels during paradoxical sleep. Anesthetics, such as halothane and barbiturates, depressed activity progressively. However, at light levels of anesthesia with ether or barbiturates, RF and thalamic neurons had increased activity *(27)*.

The possible role of brainstem sites in anesthetic action is underscored by the results of Roizen et al. *(28)*. These investigators produced lesions of the locus coeruleus, nucleus raphe dorsalis, and ventral bundle. Lesions at each of these sites decreased halothane MAC $\approx$30%. In addition, locus coeruleus lesions decreased cortical norepinephrine content by 75%, whereas lesions of the nucleus raphe dorsalis resulted in a similar decrease in cortical serotonin. These rats, in general, appeared to function normally while awake *(28)*. Thus, these data suggest that discrete brain stem sites might be involved in anesthetic action.

Further evidence of the possible role of supraspinal sites in anesthetic-induced immobility can be found in our study of differential anesthetic (isoflurane) delivery. When isoflurane concentration was preferentially decreased in the torso (and hence spinal cord), the isoflurane concentration in the head required to stop movement increased 140% *(29)*. Despite the conclusion that the spinal cord is the major site where isoflurane produces immobility, we were nonetheless able to produce immobility via a supraspinal action, albeit at a high isoflurane concentration.

Leung and Mason *(30)* examined the effect of isoflurane on activity of ON- and OFF cells in rats. Isoflurane was administered at concentrations less than (low), equal to (medium), or exceeding (high) the concentration required to block movement in response to supramaximal stimulation. ON- and OFF cells were variably affected at the low and medium isoflurane concentrations, but were inhibited at the high isoflurane concentration. A similar observation was made with regard to NEUTRAL cells. REGULAR cells were not affected at any isoflurane concentration studied, so the depressant effect on the ON- and OFF cells was specific *(30)*. The authors concluded that isoflurane did not exert part of its immobilizing effect via action at cells in the NRM. However, a limited number of cells were studied. Although cells were initially classified according to responses to noxious stimulation, isoflurane effects on spontaneous activity were examined, as opposed to responses to noxious stimuli. Thus, more work is required before these cells can be discarded as sites of anesthetic action.

The brainstem and other subcortical areas are not only involved in descending analgesia, but also motor control. For example the mesencephalic locomotor region (MLR) is located in the mesopontine area and contributes substantially to locomotion. This site has been exploited experimentally in studies where a decerebrate animal is made to walk via stimulation of the MLR, which thereby causes locomotion *(31)*. The MLR is connected to central pattern generators in the spinal cord. This group of interneurons (excitatory and inhibitory) propagate movement by alternating excitation and inhibition of motoneurons. The thalamus also contains an area that when stimulated leads to locomotion. In essence, these supraspinal sites "tell" the requisite circuitry in the spinal cord to carry out the actual complex series of movements *(32)*. The complexity of this system can be observed when at lesser levels of MLR stimulation, an animal walks on a treadmill with alternating movements of the extremities, while at greater levels of MLR stimulation, the pattern changes to a gallop where the hind limbs move in concert but opposite to the forelimbs *(33)*.

It is interesting to note that the spinal cord is relatively more resistant to halothane's metabolic depressant effect compared to the brain. Crosby and Atlas *(34)* found that 1 MAC Halothane depressed glucose utilization 12–35% in various sections of the spinal cord, but it decreased utilization in various cerebral structures by 45–70%. These data parallel the greater anesthetic sensitivity of memory and consciousness (processes that occur in the brain) as compared to the anesthetic sensitivity of the movement response (a process that occurs primarily in the spinal cord).

Not all anesthetics depress RF activity. Tamásy et al. *(35)* compared ketamine and pentobarbital and determined that while pentobarbital markedly decreased multi-unit activity in the RF, ketamine increased it. Furthermore, responses to various stimuli (auditory, visual, tactile, noxious) were profoundly depressed by pentobarbital. Responses to tactile and noxious stimuli were preserved during ketamine anesthesia.

In addition to depression, anesthetics may cause dishabituation of RF neurons. In brief, RF neurons habituate to stimuli, and halothane, N_2O, and thiopental interfere with this process *(24–26)*. This led the authors to conclude that anesthetics might exert some of their effect by inactivation of facilitation as well as inhibition. Nonetheless, the most significant finding of the study of Shimoji et al. *(24)* is the 50–75% reduction of spontaneous activity. Their conclusions regarding habituation are based on comparison to the reduced spontaneous activity, making it difficult to interpret their data.

Alkire and colleagues examined regional cerebral metabolism during halothane, isoflurane, and propofol anesthesia *(36–39)*. The midbrain, like all structures examined, decreased its metabolic rate for glucose. During propofol anesthesia, however, the midbrain was less affected as compared to other structures. The reasons for these findings are unknown.

Anesthesia requirements may also be altered by injection of carbachol into the pontine reticular nucleus *(40,41)*. Ishizawa et al. determined that carbachol decreased MAC nearly 50% when injected into the pontine reticular nucleus, and this was reversed by atropine, a nonselective muscarinic antagonist. Mecamylamine, a nicotinic antagonist, did not reverse the MAC decline, suggesting that the anesthetic-sparing effect of carbachol is modulated via muscarinic receptors. Interestingly, mecamylamine did reverse the antinociceptive effect of carbachol, indicating that the effect on MAC was not likely due to an analgesic effect. In rats, systemic physostigmine decreased halothane MAC. However, the EEG shifted towards a waking pattern. Zucker, however *(42)* determined that systemic physostigmine increased MAC. These discrepant results are unexplained. It is interesting to reconcile the anesthetic-sparing effect of physostigmine with its activating effect on the EEG. Because physostigmine appears to partially reverse the hypnotic effect of propofol and volatile anesthetics *(43,44)*, it seems possible that drugs that modulate the cholinergic system might alter anesthesia in divergent ways.

BRAINSTEM AUDITORY EVOKED POTENTIALS

Midlatency auditory evoked potentials (AEPs) have been used as a tool to measure depth of anesthesia. Brainstem AEPs are recorded in the first 10–12 ms, and represent potentials arising from repetitive auditory stimulation *(45)* (Fig. 2). These are recorded from surface electrodes, and the waveforms are buried in the electroencephalogram, because their amplitudes are smaller than those of electroencephalographic waveforms. By presenting hundreds or thousands of auditory stimuli (via headphones), these waveforms can be collected by a computer, and the "randomness" of the electroencephalogram can be eliminated. The impulses are transmitted via the auditory nerve to the brainstem, where synaptic events contribute to generation of the AEPs. As the impulses travel to the lateral geniculate body, then to the auditory cortex, additional potentials are generated. The AEPs occurring 12–50 ms after the stimulus are termed midlatency AEPs. Because the potentials occurring in this time range are the result of cortical and subcortical auditory processing, there has been some interest in using the midlatency AEPs as a method to measure depth of anesthesia. Usually, there are three peaks in the midlatency AEP, two negative and one positive *(45)*. In general, a number is associated with each peak and signifies the time (in ms) when it occurs. These latencies usually occur at around 15, 28, and 40 ms. Anesthetics depress the midlatency AEP at concentrations associated with onset of unconsciousness. In general, the latencies of these peaks are prolonged, and the amplitudes are depressed. At sufficient anesthetic concentrations, the waveforms are abolished. Thus, there is interest in exploiting this effect in order to measure anesthetic depth.

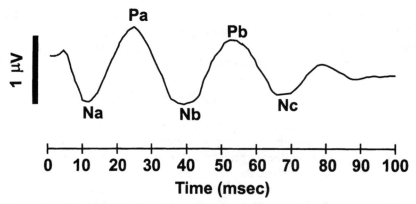

Fig. 2. Midlatency auditory evoked potentials. The various components are shown, including the negative (Na, Nb, Nc) and positive (Pa, Pb) waves. The tracing resembles a sine wave. The cycle (peak-to-peak) is approx 25 ms, which represents 40 Hz.

One interesting aspect of the midlatency AEP is the 40-Hz oscillation *(46,47)*. This represents the frequency activity of the waveforms. For example, the waveforms generally are sinusoidal in shape, and because the first and third peaks are about 25 ms apart, the pattern resembles a 40-Hz oscillation (Fig. 2). Coincidentally, 40-Hz oscillations occur in thalamocortical loops. It is thought that these loops are critical to consciousness, and their interruption can result in unconsciousness. Dutton et al. investigated the effect of desflurane and propofol on 40-Hz oscillations and correlated these effects with consciousness *(46)*. They found that 40-Hz power, as well as latency and amplitude effects, predicted wakefulness.

In isoflurane-anesthetized patients, Newton et al. *(48)* examined the relationship among midlatency AEPs, consciousness, and isoflurane concentration. Increasing the isoflurane concentration from 0.1–0.4 MAC caused progressive depression of the amplitudes and prolongation of the latencies of the AEP waveforms. This occurred in concert with progressive depression of consciousness and memory, as measured by the ability of patients to follow commands and remember words spoken to them. Thornton et al. *(49)* found that surgical stimulation partially reversed the depression of the midlatency AEPs that resulted from halothane anesthesia. These data suggest that at light levels of anesthesia, noxious stimulation, such as a surgical incision, can cause CNS arousal and bring the patient closer to consciousness. These same investigators, in a different study, determined that neuromuscular blockade did not affect midlatency AEPs *(50)*. Interestingly, similar to their prior study *(49)*, they found that the noxious stimulation of laryngoscopy increased Pa amplitude and decreased Nb latency, suggesting that the patients were shifting towards consciousness (although they were clearly not conscious).

Schwender et al. *(51)* further evaluated the utility of the AEPs by testing implicit and explicit memory in patients that had received either flunitrazepam, isoflurane, or propofol during high-dose fentanyl administration for cardiac surgery. No patient had explicit recall, but several had implicit memory. Furthermore, the patients without implicit memory had attenuated or absent AEP waveforms, while those with implicit memory had measurable waveforms, and less prolongation of the Pa latency.

Interestingly, lower esophageal contractility (LEC) was once proposed as a method to monitor depth of anesthesia *(52)*. The esophagus is innervated by the vagus nerve, with its nucleus residing in the brainstem. The peristalsis and contractility of the lower esophagus is affected by anesthesia, presumably by action in the brainstem. Although LEC does decrease in a dose-dependent fashion during anesthesia, there is unfortunately insufficient sensitivity and specificity for LEC to function as an accurate monitor of anesthetic depth. Furthermore, its effectiveness varies with the type of anesthetic used. For example, opiates can alter the tone of the gastro-esophageal sphincter, independent of any anesthetic effect.

ANESTHETIC EFFECTS ON THE BRAIN'S "AROUSAL" STATE

Direct and Indirect Effects on Arousal

In the past, the brain was hypothesized to be the critical site of anesthetic action, insofar as the three anesthetic end-points could occur via a cerebral action of anesthetics. Recent evidence, however, clearly points to the spinal cord as an important site of anesthetic action. In particular, movement occurring as the result of noxious stimulation is strongly affected by anesthetic action in the spinal cord (*14,29*; Chapter 11). These observations are not entirely surprising inasmuch as the spinal cord contains the requisite circuitry to initiate and propagate complex movements (*53,54*). What remains unclear is whether anesthetic effects in the spinal cord might indirectly affect CNS "arousal" and thus amnesia and unconsciousness, two other important clinical goals of general anesthesia (*55*). We have determined that isoflurane and propofol, two diverse anesthetics, can alter cerebral responses to noxious stimuli indirectly via an action in the spinal cord (*56–58*). Relay of nociceptive input through ascending sensory pathways to the MRF, thalamus, and brain can clearly result in cerebral activation, and thus, increased "arousal". Anesthetic depression at the spinal dorsal horn (e.g., spinothalamic cells) could attenuate spinofugal transmission of nociceptive input and thereby diminish "arousal" (Figs. 3 and 4). This would presumably depress consciousness and memory. Noxious stimulation does in fact increase arousal (and, presumably, consciousness and memory), an effect that is blocked during isoflurane inhalation (0.4–0.8%) (*59*). While our prior studies indicate that anesthetic action in the spinal cord can influence arousal, further work is required to determine specific characteristics, such as the anatomic sites and neurotransmitters involved in this process.

Nociception and its Effect on Central Nervous System Arousal

Following activation of peripheral nociceptors by a noxious stimulus, an action potential propagates along the afferent nerve, reaching the nerve terminal in the dorsal horn of the spinal cord and releasing excitatory neurotransmitters such as glutamate, aspartate, and neuropeptides such as Substance P (*60*). The second order neuron may either project to an interneuron, a motorneuron, or it may send an axon up to the thalamus and/or reticular formation (e.g., spinothalamic, spinoreticular, spinomesencephalic neurons). Some of these thalamic and reticular neurons project to the cerebral cortex (Fig. 1). The major neurotransmitters in this process include glutamate, GABA, glycine, and ACh (*61*).

Whether cerebral activation (enhanced arousal) occurs during noxious stimulation clearly depends on sufficient transmission of nociceptive impulses to the brain. The ascending transmission of nociceptive input is modulated by, among other things, the balance of excitation and inhibition resulting from glutamate, GABA, and glycine actions on thalamic and reticular neurons (*61,62*). Diminished release of (or sensitivity to) glutamate, or enhanced release of (or sensitivity to) GABA or glycine would tend to diminish the ascending transmission of the nociceptive impulse to the brain (*63–65*). Cholinergic activity within the thalamus modulates sensory information (*66,67*). In addition, cortical neurons receive cholinergic input from basal forebrain neurons (thalamus and reticular formation) (*68*). The magnocellular nucleus in the forebrain also projects cholinergic fibers to the cerebral cortex (*69*). These various cholinergic inputs modulate arousal, as determined by the behavioral state and the EEG. For example, cortical ACh levels increase with increased arousal and are accompanied by EEG activation (desynchronization) (*70–72*). Thus, the transmission of nociceptive impulses to the brain, and the subsequent result (e.g., increased arousal and EEG activation) is modulated by the glutamatergic, GABAergic, glycinergic, and cholinergic neurotransmitter systems.

The role of various neurotransmitter systems in the production of anesthesia is not completely understood. It is conceivable that different neurotransmitter systems modulate different anesthetic

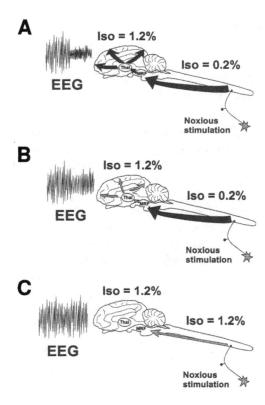

Fig. 3. (A) The anesthetic concentration (isoflurane) in the spinal cord is sufficient to effectively block the ascending transmission of nociceptive impulses to the MRF, thalamus, and brain; no EEG activation occurs. In one scenario **(B)**, decreasing the spinal concentration of anesthesia facilitates ascending transmission of nociceptive impulses, but the sensitivity of the brain is unchanged (as compared to **[A]**). There is minimal EEG activation, owing to the added nociceptive impulses that are transmitted to the brain. In **(C)**, we hypothesize that the brain is more sensitive to the additional nociceptive impulses, and there is marked EEG activation (desynchronization). Thus, we hypothesize that the "arousal" level of the brain is reset by changing the anesthetic concentration in the spinal cord.

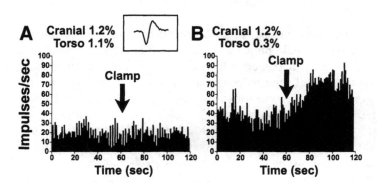

Fig. 4. Peri-stimulus time histograms from a goat anesthetized with isoflurane, in which differential anesthetic delivery was accomplished. Single unit activity was recorded from a neuron in the midbrain reticular formation (action potential shown in inset). **(A)** When the cranial and torso isoflurane was 1.2 and 1.1% respectively, application of a noxious stimulus (clamp) for one minute did not increase the neuron's activity. **(B)** When the torso isoflurane was decreased to 0.3% while maintaining the cranial isoflurane at 1.2%, spontaneous activity was increased, and there was a significant increase in the neuron's activity with application of the clamp. These data indicate that activity in the reticular formation can be affected indirectly by anesthetic action in the spinal cord.

end points *(73)*. Anesthetic-induced immobility may result from action on motoneurons *(74)*, as anesthetics (such as ethanol and enflurane) depress glutamate currents independent of glycine and $GABA_A$ receptors *(75,76)*. Effects on dorsal horn cell responses however depend, at least in part, on $GABA_A$ receptors *(77)*. Also, ACEA-1021, an antagonist at the glycine recognition site of the NMDA receptor, has no effect on consciousness or righting reflex in rats at a dose that decreases halothane MAC by 50% *(78)*. Thus, any knowledge we have regarding neurotransmitters involved in the movement response may not be applicable to our understanding of the neurotransmitters involved in anesthetic-induced unconsciousness or the ascending transmission of nociceptive impulses.

There are at least two experimental methods to investigate the neurotransmitter systems that participate in consciousness and ascending transmission of nociceptive input. Pharmacological manipulation of neurotransmitter systems operant at the spinal cord is one method. For example, direct placement of a glutamate antagonist onto the spinal cord would tend to blunt the effect of glutamate, if it was involved in the transmission of nociceptive impulses. A GABA agonist would enhance the GABAergic system. If these systems were not important, then such pharmacologic manipulation at the spinal level would not significantly affect the EEG activation pattern resulting from noxious stimulation. Administering agonists and antagonists is a powerful use of classical pharmacology to determine what spinal neurotransmitters modulate the EEG blunting effect of anesthetics. Such methods have recently been used to determine what neurotransmitters are involved in anesthetic-induced immobility. Mason et al. *(79)* found that GABA antagonists partially reversed halothane's antinociceptive effect. Likewise, some investigators have reported that picrotoxin, a $GABA_A$ antagonist, increased isoflurane MAC by 40%, indicating that the $GABA_A$ receptor modulates, in part, the immobility caused by isoflurane *(80,81)*.

In addition to pharmacological manipulation, direct measurement of neurotransmitter concentration would aid elucidation of the relative roles of various neurotransmitter systems. For example, how does isoflurane affect glutamate and ACh concentrations in the thalamus and cerebral cortex? Microdialysis is one accepted method to measure in vivo changes in neurotransmitter concentration *(82)*. For example, microdialysis of the cerebral cortex could detect changes in ACh concentration that might be correlated with EEG changes *(83)*. Furthermore, because glutamate is a major excitatory neurotransmitter in the thalamus *(84)*, anesthetic action in the spinal cord could indirectly depress thalamic glutamate concentrations. Most research into anesthetic effects on neurotransmitter physiology has focused on in vitro systems, with less use of in vivo preparations. Thus, little information is available regarding how anesthetic effects at various CNS sites combine to modulate neurotransmitters in the intact animal.

Anesthetics Effects on Transmission of Nociceptive Impulses

Anesthetics might affect nociceptive transmission at multiple sites. Peripheral actions of anesthetics appear to have no significant effect *(85,86)*, or in fact they may excite peripheral nociceptors *(87,88)*. On the other hand, several decades of classical studies have shown that anesthetics depress dorsal horn cellular responses to somatosensory stimuli *(89,90)*. Thus, the dorsal horn is likely to be the first anatomic point at which anesthetics could exert their effect. Because the dorsal horn contains cells with ascending projections (e.g., spinothalamic), as well as cells with connections to reflex motor pathways, action within the dorsal horn could contribute to each of the anesthetic end-points either directly or indirectly. For example, anesthetics could depress spinothalamic responses to noxious stimuli and thereby depress the ascending transmission of nociceptive impulses.

Anesthetics also have effects at numerous brain sites and on numerous neurotransmitter systems. Isoflurane and proprofol decrease metabolic rate within the thalamus and cerebral cortex *(36,91)*. In addition, anesthetics affect ACh release. Shichino et al. *(92)* demonstrated that isoflurane depressed basal ACh concentrations in the cortex. Kurosawa et al. *(93)* determined that noxious mechanical stimuli increased cortical ACh concentrations. This effect was most prominent with hindpaw stimulation. Meuret et al. *(43)* determined that intravenous physostigmine, a centrally acting acetylcholinesterase inhibitor, partially reversed propofol's sedative and EEG effect. Others have found that physostigmine can reverse the effect of other anesthetics, such as halothane *(44)*. Taken together, these data suggest that inhaled (e.g., isoflurane) and intravenous (e.g., propofol) anesthetics exert their effects, at least in part, by action on supraspinal cholinergic systems. It is unclear, however, how anesthetics such as isoflurane affect ACh relative to its effect on the EEG. For example, isoflurane blunts, or completely prevents, the desynchronization response that occurs as the result of noxious stimulation *(94)*. We have observed that isoflurane action in the spinal cord indirectly affects the EEG *(56,57)*. It is unclear what neurotransmitters (such as ACh) are involved in these findings.

The Relationship Among Neurotransmitters, Nociceptive Input, and Understanding Anesthetic Mechanisms

Our understanding of anesthetic mechanisms is intricately dependent upon the neurotransmitter systems that (1) are modulated by anesthetics, and (2) are involved in the transmission of nociceptive impulses. The use of agonists and antagonists at the spinal cord level might elucidate those neurotransmitters that facilitate nociceptive impulse transmission. A facilitatory (or inhibitory) effect of a particular agonist on anesthetic action does not necessarily imply that a neurotransmitter system is a site of anesthetic action. However, determination of neurotransmitter concentrations would be useful as a guide to establishing which neurotransmitters are affected by anesthesia. Furthermore, and perhaps more importantly, knowing which neurotransmitters are pertinent to each anesthetic endpoint could permit clinical modulation *(95)*. For example, if a particular neurotransmitter at the spinal cord level was critically involved in the ascending transmission of nociceptive impulses (which increased brain arousal and thereby facilitate consciousness and memory formation), then intrathecal (or systemic) administration of the appropriate agonist or antagonist could decrease anesthetic requirements for unconsciousness and amnesia.

Studies of anesthetic mechanisms at any level (molecular, cellular, whole body) require a judicious choice of anesthetics to be examined. Isoflurane and propofol are commonly used. First, these drugs are representative of inhalational and intravenous anesthetics. Secondly, isoflurane and propofol are widely used clinically. Third, the hypothesized mechanisms of action of these two drugs have similarities and differences. For example, both isoflurane and propofol appear to act at $GABA_A$ receptors. However, isoflurane has effects on AMPA/Kainate glutamate receptors, while propofol does not *(96)*. We also recognize that these anesthetics, while perhaps not having significant effects on a particular receptor, might have effects on the ligand that binds to that receptor (e.g., decreased neurotransmitter release via a presynaptic action).

COULD SPINAL CORD ACTION OF ANESTHETICS INFLUENCE CONSCIOUSNESS AND MEMORY?

It is convenient to assume that anesthetic action in the brain (and brain alone) results in amnesia and unconsciousness, but that is not necessarily so. Several investigators working with animal models and humans have found that blocking afferent impulses (as occurs with neuroaxial blockade) decreases the amount of sedative drug (such as midazolam) required to achieve a given level of sedation. For example, Hodgson et al. *(97)* determined that epidural lidocaine decreased the amount of sevoflurane required to produce a bispectral (BIS) number of 50 on the processed EEG. They hypothesized that afferent transmission was blocked, which thereby decreased the "arousal" state of the brain. Interestingly, they also observed that epidural blockade decreases sevoflurane MAC assessed rostral to the level of the block *(98)*. Others have found that central neuroaxial blockade decreases midazolam, thiopental, and propofol requirements for sedation *(99,100)*. In rats, spinal bupivacaine decreases the amount of thiopental needed to sedate the animals and prevent responses to noxious simulation *(101)*. Finally, spinal anesthesia itself results in sedation in humans *(102)*. These studies clearly indicate that the elimination of afferent transmission of normal input from the majority of the body decreases the "arousal" of the brain; this would lead to decreased consciousness and presumably (although not necessarily) decreased memory formation.

Anesthetic-induced amnesia is closely correlated with certain EEG parameters (e.g., the BIS number) *(103,104)*. Anything that decreases the "arousal" level in the brain (and thereby results in EEG slowing) would tend to decrease memory formation. Because general anesthetics also decrease afferent transmission, we hypothesize that they would decrease brain "arousal" not only by the obvious direct cerebral effect, but also by an action in the spinal cord, and thereby help to blunt memory formation.

The available evidence suggests that blockade of ascending transmission "resets" the arousal level of the brain, as measured by the EEG activation response. During differential delivery of a low concentration of isoflurane to the torso, goats are much more likely to exhibit spontaneous EEG desynchronization, indicating that the brain's arousal level is increased compared to when the torso isoflurane concentration is greater (authors' unpublished observations). One potential experimental approach to this question would be to examine neurotransmitter levels in the thalamus and cerebral cortex during differential isoflurane delivery, in the absence of noxious stimulation. Also, electrical stimulation of the mesencephalic reticular formation (MRF) can cause EEG desynchronization *(2)*. Electrical stimulation of the MRF during differential anesthetic delivery to brain and torso may prove useful in elucidating the sensitivity of the brain vis-à-vis EEG desynchronization. For example, EEG desynchronization might be more likely to occur at lower torso isoflurane concentrations when the cranial anesthetic concentration remains unchanged (authors' unpublished observations).

SUMMARY

The RF and brainstem play critical roles in consciousness, memory, motor function, nociception, and awareness—all of which are ablated by anesthetics. It is not surprising that, over the decades, researchers have closely examined anesthetic action at these sites. As with other studies, however, conflicting results have been obtained. Nonetheless, continued efforts in these areas should continue to yield fruitful and provocative results.

REFERENCES

1. de Groot, J. (1991) *Reticular Formation. Correlative Neuroanatomy* Appleton-Lange, Norwalk, Connecticut, pp. 179–183.
2. Moruzzi, G. and Magoun, H. W. (1949) Brain stem reticular formation and activation of the EEG. *Electroencephalogr. Clin. Neurophysiol.* **1,** 455–473
3. Bremer, F. and Stoupel, N. (1959) Nouvelles recherches sur la facilitation et inhibition des potentiels evoques corticaux dans l'eveil cerebral. *Arch. Int. Physiol. Biochem.* **67,** 240–275
4. Dumont, S. and Dell, P. (1960) Facilitation reticulare des mecanismes visuels corticaux. *Electroencephalogr. Clin. Neurophysiol.* **12,** 769–796.
5. Munk, M. H., Roelfsema, P. R., Konig, P., Engel, A. K., and Singer, W. (1996) Role of reticular activation in the modulation intracortical synchronization. *Science,* **272,** 271–274
6. Hobson, J. A. (1999) Sleep and Dreaming. In: Fundamental Neuroscience (Zigmond, M. J., Bloom, F. E., Landis, S. C., Roberts, J. L., and Squire, L. R., eds.) Academic Press, San Diego, pp. 1207–1227.
7. Willis, W. D. and Westlund, K. N. (1997) Neuroanatomy of the pain system and of the pathways that modulate pain. *J. Clin. Neurophysiol.* **14,** 2–31.
8. Bowsher, D. (1976) Role of the reticular formation in responses to noxious stimulation. *Pain* **2,** 361–378.
9. Steriade, M., Oakson, G., and Ropert, N. (1982) Firing rates and patterns of midbrain reticular neurons during steady and transitional states of the sleep-waking cycle. *Exp. Brain. Res.* **46,** 37– 51.
10. Reynolds, D. V. (1969) Surgery in the rat during electrical analgesia induced by focal brain stimulation. *Science* **164,** 444–445.
11. Hosobuchi, Y., Adams, J. E., and Linchitz, R. (1977) Pain relief by electrical stimulation of the central gray matter in humans and its reversal by naloxone. *Science* **197,** 183–186.
12. Roizen, M. F., Newfield, P., Eger, E. I., Hosobuchi, Y., Adams, J. E., and Lamb, S. (1985) Reduced anesthetic requirement after electrical stimulation of periaqueductal gray matter. *Anesthesiology* **62,** 120–123.
13. Rampil, I. J., Mason, P., and Singh, H. (1993) Anesthetic potency (MAC) is independent of forebrain structures in the rat. *Anesthesiology* **78,** 707–712.
14. Rampil, I. J. (1994) Anesthetic potency is not altered after hypothermic spinal cord transection in rats. *Anesthesiology* **80,** 606–610.
15. Garcia-Rill, E. (1997) Disorders of the reticular activating system. *Med. Hypotheses* **49,** 379–387.
16. Gottesmann, C. (1999) The neurophysiology of sleep and waking: intracerebral connections, functioning and ascending influences of the medulla oblongata. *Prog. Neurobiol.* **59,** 1–54.

17. Steriade, M., Dossi, R. C., Pare, D., and Oakson, G. (1991) Fast oscillations (20–40 Hz) in thalamocortical systems and their potentiation by mesopontine cholinergic nuclei in the cat. *Proc. Natl. Acad. Sci. USA* **88**, 4396–4400.

18. Fields, H. L., Malick, A., and Burstein, R. (1995) Dorsal horn projection targets of ON and OFF cells in the rostral ventromedial medulla. *J. Neurophysiol.* **74**, 1742–1759.

19. Mason, P. and Fields, H. L. (1989) Axonal trajectories and terminations of on- and off-cells in the cat lower brainstem. *J. Comp. Neurol.*, 288, 185–207.

20. Leung, C. G. and Mason, P. (1998) Physiological survey of medullary raphe and magnocellular reticular neurons in the anesthetized rat. *J. Neurophysiol.* **80**, 1630–1646.

21. Leung, C. G. and Mason, P. (1999) Physiological properties of raphe magnus neurons during sleep and waking. *J. Neurophysiol.* **81**, 584–595.

22. Hayashi, M., Kobayashi, H., Kawano, H., Handa, Y., and Kabuto, M. (1987) The effects of local intraparenchymal pento-barbital on intracranial hypertension following experimental subarachnoid hemorrhage. *Anesthesiology* **66**, 758–765.

23. Devor, M. and Zalkind V. I. (2001) Reversable analgesia, atonia, and loss of consciousness on bilateral intracerebral microinjection of pentobarbital. *Pain* **94**, 101–112.

24. Shimoji, K. and Bickford, R. G. (1971) Differential effects of anesthetics on mesencephalic reticular neurons. I. Spontaneous firing patterns. *Anesthesiology* **35**, 68–75.

25. Shimoji, K., Fujioka, H., Fukazawa, T., Hashiba, M., and Maruyama, Y. (1984) Anesthetics and excitatory/inhibitory responses of midbrain reticular neurons. *Anesthesiology* **61**, 151– 155.

26. Shimoji, K. and Bickford, R. G. (1971) Differential effects of anesthetics on mesencephalic reticular neurons. II. Responses to repetitive somatosensory electrical stimulation. *Anesthesiology* **35**, 76–80.

27. Goodman, S. J. and Mann, P. E. (1967) Reticular and thalamic multiple unit activity during wakefulness, sleep and anesthesia. *Exp. Neurol.* **19**, 11–24.

28. Roizen, M. F., White, P. F., Eger, E. I., and Brownstein,M. (1978) Effects of ablation of serotonin or norepinephrine brain-stem areas on halothane and cyclopropane MACs in rats. *Anesthesiology* **49**, 252–255.

29. Antognini, J. F. and Schwartz, K. (1993) Exaggerated anesthetic requirements in the preferentially anesthetized brain. *Anesthesiology* **79**, 1244–1249.

30. Leung, C. G. and Mason, P. (1995) Effects of isoflurane concentration on the activity of pontomedullary raphe and medial reticular neurons in the rat. *Brain. Res.* **699**, 71–82.

31. Adreani, C. M. and Kaufman, M. P. (1998) Effect of arterial occlusion on responses of group III and IV afferents to dynamic exercise. *J. Appl. Physiol.* **84**, 1827–1833.

32. Grillner, S., Parker D., and Manir A. E. (1998) Vertebrate locomotion-a lamprey perspective. *Ann. NY Acad. Sci.* **860**, 1–18.

33. Mori, S., Sakamoto, T., Ohta, Y., Takakusaki, K., and Matsuyama, K. (1989) Site-specific postural and locomotor changes evoked in awake, freely moving intact cats by stimulating the brainstem. *Brain Res.* **505**, 66–74.

34. Crosby, G. and Atlas, S. (1988) Local spinal cord glucose utilization in conscious and halothane- anaesthetized rats. *Can. J. Anaesth.* **35**, 359–363.

35. Tamásy, V., Korányi, L., and Tekeres, M. (1975) E.E.G. and multiple unit activity during ketamine and barbiturate anaesthesia. *Br. J. Anaesth.* **47**, 1247–1251.

36. Alkire, M. T., Haier, R. J., Barker, S. J., Shah, N. K., Wu, J. C., and Kao, Y. J. (1995) Cerebral metabolism during propofol anesthesia in humans studied with positron emission tomography. *Anesthesiology* **82**, 393–403;

37. Alkire, M. T., Pomfrett, C. J., Haier, R. J., Gianzero, M. V., Chan, C. M., Jacobsen, B. P., and Fallon, J. H. (1999) Functional brain imaging during anesthesia in humans, effects of halothane on global and regional cerebral glucose metabolism. *Anesthesiology* **90**, 701–709.

38. Alkire, M. T. (1998) Quantitative EEG correlations with brain glucose metabolic rate during anesthesia in volunteers. *Anesthesiology* **89**, 323–333.

39. Alkire, M. T., Haier, R. J., Shah, N. K., and Anderson, C. T. (1997) Positron emission tomography study of regional cerebral metabolism in humans during isoflurane anesthesia. *Anesthesiology* **86**, 549–557.

40. Ishizawa, Y., Ma, H. C., Dohi, S., and Shimonaka, H. (2000) Effects of cholinomimetic injection into the brain stem reticular formation on halothane anesthesia and antinociception in rats. *J. Pharmacol. Exper. Thera.* **293**, 845–851.

41. Ishizawa, Y. (2000) Selective blockade of muscarinic receptor subtypes in the brain stem reticular formation in rats: effects on anesthetic requirements. *Brain Res.* **873**, 124–126.

42. Zucker, J. (1991) Central cholinergic depression reduces MAC for isoflurane in rats. *Anesth. Analg.* **72**, 790–795.

43. Meuret, P., Backman, S. B., Bonhomme, V., Plourde, G., and Fiset, P. (2000) Physostigmine reverses propofol-induced unconsciousness and attenuation of the auditory steady state response and bispectral index in human volunteers. *Anesthesiology* **93**, 708–717.

44. Hill, G. E., Stanley, T. H., and Sentker, C. R. (1977) Physostigmine reversal of post-operative somnolence. *Can. Anaesht. Soc. J.* **24**, 707–711

45. Celesia, G. G. and Peachey, N. S. (1999) Auditory evoked potentials. In: Electroencephalography: Basic priciples, clinical applications and related fields. Eds: Niedermeyer, E., Lopes da Silva F. Lippincott, Williams and Williams, Philadelphia, pp. 994–1013.

46. Dutton, R. C., Smith, W. D., Rampil, I. J., Chortkoff, B. S., and Eger, E. I. 2nd. (1999) Forty-hertz midlatency auditory evoked potential activity predicts wakeful response during desflurane and propofol anesthesia in volunteers. *Anesthesiology* **91**, 1209–1220.

47. Plourde, G. (1999) Auditory evoked potentials and 40-Hz oscillations. *Anesthesiology* **91**, 1187–1189.

48. Newton, D. E., Thornton, C., Konieczko, K. M., et al. (1992) Auditory evoked response and awareness: a study in volunteers at sub-MAC concentrations of isoflurane. *Br. J. Anaesth.* **69,** 122–129.

49. Thornton, C., Konieczko, K., Jones, J. G., et al. (1988) Effect of surgical stimulation on the auditory evoked response. *Br. J. Anaesth.* **60,** 372–378.

50. Richmond, C. E., Matson, A., Thornton, C., Dore, C. J., and Newton, D. E. (1996) Effect of neuromuscular block on depth of anaesthesia as measured by the auditory evoked response. *Br. J. Anaesth.* **76,** 446–448.

51. Schwender, D., Faber-Zullig, E., Klasing, S., Poppel, E., and Peter, K. (1994) Motor signs of wakefulness during general anaesthesia with propofol, isoflurane and flunitrazepam/fentanyl and midlatency auditory evoked potentials. *Anaesthesia* **49,** 476–484.

52. Kuni, D. R. and Silvay, G. (1989) Lower esophageal contractility: a technique for measuring depth of anesthesia. *Biomedical Instrumentation and Technology* **23,** 388–395.

53. Sherrington, C. S. (1906) The integrative action of the nervous system. New Haven, Yale University, pp. 44–48.

54. Fukson, O. I., Berkinblit, M. B., and Feldman, A. G. (1980) The spinal frog takes into account the scheme of its body during the wiping reflex. *Science* **209,** 1261–1263.

55. Kendig, J. J. (1993) Spinal cord as a site of anesthetic action. *Anesthesiology* **79,** 1161–1162.

56. Antognini, J. F., Carstens, E., Sudo, M., and Sudo, S. (2000) Isoflurane depresses electroencephalographic and medial thalamic responses to noxious stimulation via an indirect spinal action. *Anesth. Analg.* **91,** 1282–1288

57. Antognini, J. F., Wang, X. W., and Carstens, E. (2000) Isoflurane action in the spinal cord blunts electro-encephalographic and thalamic-reticular formation responses to noxious stimulation in goats. *Anesthesiology* **92,** 559–566.

58. Antognini, J. F., Saadi, J., Wang, X. W., Carstens, E., and Piercy, M. (2001) Propofol action in the spinal cord and brain blunts electroencephalographic responses to noxious stimulation in goats. *Sleep* **24,** 26–31.

59. Munglani, R., Andrade, J., Sapsford, D. J., Baddeley, A., and Jones J. G. (1993) A measure of consciousness and memory during isoflurane administration: the coherent frequency. *Brit. J. Anaesth.* **71,** 633–641.

60. Fürst, S. (1999) Transmitters involved in antinociception in the spinal cord. *Brain Res. Bulletin* **48,** 129–141.

61. McCormick, D. A. (1992) Neurotransmitter actions in the thalamus and cerebral cortex and their role in neuromodulation of thalamocortical activity. *Prog. Neurobiol.* **39,** 337–388.

62. Pollard, M. (2000) Ionotropic glutamate receptor-mediated responses in the rat primary somatosensory cortex evoked by noxious and innocuous stimulation in vivo. *Exp. Brain Res.* **131,** 282–292.

63. Murugaiah, K. D. and Hemmings, H. C., Jr. (1998) Effects of intravenous general anesthetics on [3H]GABA release from rat cortical synaptosomes. *Anesthesiology* **89,** 919–928.

64. Eilers, H., Kindler, C. H., and Bickler P. E. (1999) Different effects of volatile anesthetics and polyhalogenated alkanes on depolarization-evoked glutamate release from cortical brain slices. *Anesth. Analg.* **88,** 1168–1174.

65. Larsen, M. and Langmoen, I. A. (1998) The effect of volatile anaesthetics on synaptic release and uptake of glutamate. *Toxicol. Lett.* **100–101,** 59–64.

66. Rico, B. and Cavada, C. (1998) A population of cholinergic neurons is present in the macaque monkey thalamus. *Eur. J. Neurosci.* **10,** 2346–2352.

67. Williams, J. A., Comisarow, J., Day J., Fibiger H. C., and Reiner, P. B. (1994) State-dependent release of acetylcholine in rat thalamus measured by in vivo microdialysis. *J. Neurosci.* **14,** 5236–5242.

68. Detari, L., Rasmusson, D. D., and Semba, K. (1999) The role of basal forebrain neurons in tonic and phasic activation of the cerebral cortex. *Prog. Neurobiol.* **58,** 249–277.

69. Bigl, V., Woolf, N. J., and Butcher, L. L. (1982) Cholinergic projections from the basal forebrain to frontal, parietal, temporal, occipital, and cingulate cortices: a combined fluorescent tracer and acetylcholinesterase analysis. *Brain Res. Bull.* **8,** 727–749.

70. Celesia, G. G. and Jasper, H. H. (1966) Acetylcholine released from cerebral cortex in relation to state of activation. *Neurology* **16,** 1053–1063.

71. Jones, B. E. (1993) The organization of central cholinergic systems and their functional importance in sleep-waking states. *Prog. Brain Res.* **98,** 61–71.

72. Semba, K. (1991) The cholinergic basal forebrain: a critical role in cortical arousal. In: The basal forebrain: anatomy to function. (Napier, T. C. et al., eds.) pp. 197–218. Plenum, New York

73. Collins, J. G., Kendig, J. J., and Mason P. (1995) Anesthetic actions within the spinal cord: contributions to the state of general anesthesia. *Trends Neurosci.* **18,** 549–553

74. Rampil, I. J. and King B. S. (1996) Volatile anesthetics depress spinal motor neurons. *Anesthesiology* **85,** 129–134.

75. Wang, M. Y., Rampil, I. J., and Kendig, J. J. (1999) Ethanol directly depresses AMPA and NMDA glutamate currents in spinal cord motor neurons independent of actions on $GABA_A$ or glycine receptors. *J. Pharmacol. Exp. Therap.* **290,** 362–367.

76. Cheng, G. and Kendig J. J. (2000) Enflurane directly depresses glutamate AMPA and NMDA currents in mouse spinal cord motor neurons independent of actions on $GABA_A$ or glycine receptors. Anesthesiology **93,** 1075–1084.

77. Ota, K., Yanagidani, T., Kishikawa, K., Yamamori, Y., and Collins, J. G. (1998) Cutaneous responsiveness of lumbar spinal dorsal horn neurons is reduced by general anesthesia, an effect dependent in part on $GABA_A$ mechanisms. *J. Neurophysiol.* **80,** 1383–1390.

78. McFarlane, C., Warner, D. S., Nader, A., and Dexter, F. (1995) Glycine receptor antagonism. Effects of ACEA-1021 on the minimum alveolar concentration for halothane in the rat. *Anesthesiology* **82,** 963–968.

79. Mason, P., Owens, C. A., and Hammond, D. L. (1996) Antagonism of the antinocifensive action of halothane by intrathecal administration of $GABA_A$ receptor antagonists. *Anesthesiology* **84,** 1205–1214.

80. Zhang, Y., Sonner, J., Wu, S., and Eger, E. I. (1999) The increased MAC produced by picrotoxin application to the rat's spinal cord has a ceiling effect: More than GABA$_A$ enhancement mediates MAC. *Anesthesiology* **91**, A321.

81. Zhang, Y., Wu, S., Eger, E. I., and Sonner, J. M. (2001) Neither GABA$_A$ nor strychnine-sensitive glycine receptors are the sole mediators of MAC for isoflurane. *Anesth. Analg.* **92**, 123–127.

82. Lydic, R., Baghdoyan, H. A., and Lorinc, Z. (1991) Microdialyis of cat pons reveals enhanced acetylcholine release during state-dependent respiratory depression. *Am. J. Physiol.* **261**, R766–R770.

83. Marrosu, F., Portas, C., Mascia, M. S., et al. (1995) Microdialysis measurement of cortical and hippocampal acetylcholine release during sleep-wake cycle in freely moving cats. *Brain Res.* **671**, 329–332.

84. Bordi, F. and Ugolini, A. (2000) Involvement of mGluR(5) on acute nociceptive transmission. *Brain Res.* **871**, 223–233.

85. Antognini, J. F. and Kien N. D. (1995) Potency (minimum alveolar anesthetic concentration) of isoflurane is independent of peripheral anesthetic effects. *Anesth. Analg.* **81**, 69–72.

86. Bosnjak, Z. J., Seagard, J. L., Wu, A., and Kampine, J. P. (1982) The effects of halothane on sympathetic gamglionic transmission. *Anesthesiology* **57**, 473–479.

87. MacIver, M. B. and Tanelian, D. L. (1990) Volatile anesthetics excite mammalian nociceptor afferents recorded in vitro. *Anesthesiology* **72**, 1022–1030.

88. Campbell, J. N., Raja, S. N., and Meyer, R. A. (1984) Halothane sensitizes cutaneous nociceptors in monkeys. *J. Neurophysiol.* **52**, 762–770

89. de Jong, R. H. and Wagman, I. H. (1968) Block of afferent impulses in the dorsal horn of monkey. A possible mechanism of anesthesia. *Exp. Neurol.* **20**, 352–358.

90. Namiki, A., Collins, J. G., Kitahata, L. M., Kikuchi, H., Homma, E., and Thalhammer, J. G. (1980) Effects of halothane on spinal neuronal responses to graded noxious heat stimulation in the cat. *Anesthesiology* **53**, 475–480.

91. Fiset, P., Paus, T., Daloze, T., et al. (1999) Brain mechanisms of propofol-induced loss of consciousness in humans: a positron emission tomographic study. *J. Neurosci.* **19**, 5506–5513.

92. Shichino, T., Murakawa, M., Adachi, T., et al. (1997) Effects of isoflurane on in vivo release of acetylcholine in the rat cerebral cortex and striatum. *Acta Anaesthesiol. Scandina.* **41**, 1335–1340.

93. Kurosawa, M., Sato, A., and Sato, Y. (1992) Cutaneous mechanical sensory stimulation increases extracellular acetylcholine release in cerebral cortex in anesthetized rats. *Neurochem. Int.* **21**, 423–427.

94. Antognini, J. F. and Carstens E. (1999) Isoflurane blunts electroencephalographic and thalamic-reticular formation responses to noxious stimulation in goats. *Anesthesiology* **91**, 1770–1779.

95. Saidman, L. J. (1995) Anesthesiology. *JAMA* **273**, 1661–1662.

96. Krasowski, M. D. and Harrison, N. L. (1999) General anaesthetic actions on ligand-gated ion channels. *Cell. Mol. Life Sci.* **55**, 1278–1303.

97. Hodgson, P. S. and Liu, S. S. (2001) Epidural lidocaine decreases sevoflurane requirement for adequate depth of anesthesia as measured by the Bispectral Index monitor. *Anesthesiology* **94**, 799–803.

98. Hodgson, P. S., Liu, S. S., and Gras, T. W. (199) Does epidural anesthesia have general anesthetic effects? *Anesthesiology* **91**, 1687–1692.

99. Tverskoy, M., Shagal, M., Finger, J., and Kissin, I. (1994) Subarachnoid bupivacaine blockade decreases midazolam and thiopental hypnotic requirements. *J. Clin. Anesth.* **6**, 487–490.

100. Tverskoy, M., Fleyshman, G., Bachrak, L., and Ben-Shlomo, I. (1996) Effect of bupivacaine-induced spinal block on the hypnotic requirement of propofol. *Anesthesia* **51**, 652–653.

101. Eappen, S. and Kissin, I. (1998) Effect of subarachnoid bupivacaine block on anesthetic requirements for thiopental in rats. *Anesthesiology* **99**, 1036–1042.

102. Pollock, J. E., Neal, J. M., Liu, S. S., Burkhead, D., and Polissar, N. (2000) Sedation during spinal anesthesia. *Anesthesiology* **93**, 728–734.

103. Glass, P. S., Bloom, M., Kearse, L., Rosow, C., Sebel., P., and Manberg, P. (1997) Bispectral analysis measures sedation and memory effects of propofol, midazolam, isoflurane, and alfentanil in healthy volunteers. *Anesthesiology* **86**, 836–847.

104. Iselin-Chaves, I. A., Flaishon, R., Sebel, P. S., et al. (1998) The effect of the interaction of propofol and alfentanil on recall, loss of consciousness, and the Bispectral Index. *Anesth. Analg.* **87**, 949–955.

11

Anesthesia, the Spinal Cord and Motor Responses to Noxious Stimulation

Joseph F. Antognini and Earl Carstens

INTRODUCTION

The spinal cord has emerged as an important site of anesthetic action. For many decades, studies that examined the effects of anesthetics on spinal cord function had unknown impact, since it was unclear what clinical endpoint might be affected by such action. For example, when an anesthetic depresses spinal dorsal horn neuronal responses to tactile stimulation, what endpoint is achieved? Because the movement response that accompanies noxious stimulation is ablated in large part via a spinal cord action of anesthetics (1–3), there is renewed interest in the effects of anesthetics on the spinal cord.

This chapter will examine the role of the spinal cord in anesthesia. After a brief description of anatomy and neurophysiology, we will discuss the complex neurocircuitry that permits the spinal cord to initiate and propagate complex movements. We will discuss how anesthetics might alter spinal cord processing and how these effects result in each anesthetic goal (amnesia, unconsciousness, immobility). In particular, we will discuss the movement that occurs with noxious stimulation and how anesthetics affect that movement.

ANATOMY AND NEUROPHYSIOLOGY

Embryology

The spinal cord develops from the primitive neural tube. The spinal nerves arise from motor neuroblasts (basal plate) and sensory neuroblasts (neural crest) An axon emerges from the motor neuroblast and eventually enters a muscle. The sensory neuroblast develops axons that either grow proximally into the dorsal horn of the spinal cord, or distally to a peripheral site, such as skin. This process is complete at birth (4).

One unanswered question is how the embryological, fetal, and neonatal development of the nervous system (both structurally and physiologically) affects anesthetic requirements. We know that the minimum alveolar concentration (MAC) in neonates, while higher than MAC for adults, is lower compared to that of infants aged 3–6 months (5,6). Is this difference due to the maturation of the complex neurocircuitry of the spinal cord? Is it related to changes in neurotransmitters in the spinal cord? Is there less descending supraspinal inhibition in neonates as compared to adults (7)? No definitive answers are yet available to these intriguing questions.

From: *Contemporary Clinical Neuroscience:* Neural Mechanisms of Anesthesia
Edited by: Joseph F. Antognini et al. © Humana Press Inc., Totowa, NJ

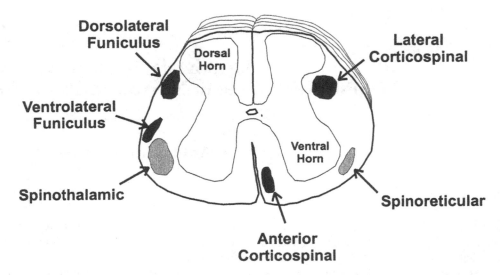

Fig. 1. Diagram of spinal cord anatomy. The dorsal horn contains the second order neurons that receive sensory input from the periphery. The ventral horn contains the motoneurons that send axons out to muscle. Various tracts are shown that transmit impulses to (gray) and from (black) supraspinal structures.

Anatomy

Since the early work of Bell and Magendie the spinal cord is descriptively divided into dorsal and ventral halves (Fig. 1) that have been generally related to sensory and motor function, respectively. Sensory primary afferent nerve fibers transmit impulses from the periphery, and their central branches terminate on second order neurons in the dorsal horn. Primary afferent fibers of mechanoreceptors tend to enter the spinal cord in a medial position in the dorsal root and terminate in deeper laminae (III–VI) of the dorsal horn, while small-diameter afferents from nociceptors and thermoreceptors enter more laterally to terminate in more superficial laminae I–II (8).

Second-order neurons receiving direct synaptic input from primary afferent fibers can be generally categorized according to the following functional classes: some neurons contribute to ascending sensory pathways such as the spinothalamic tract, while others function as interneurons in segmentally-organized reflex pathways. A recent double-label study provides evidence that ascending spinothalamic and spinoreticular tract neurons, and segmental interneurons constitute almost exclusively separate populations (9). Other neurons form part of segmentally-organized circuits, called "central pattern generators" (CPGs), that are involved in generating rhythmic limb movements; it is not known if such neurons receive direct synaptic input from primary afferents. It is also uncertain if neurons involved in reflex pathways also participate in CPG circuits. Another group of "propriospinal" neurons give rise to ascending and/or descending projections to other spinal segments, and are involved in inter-segmental coordination of multi-limb movements, such as locomotion in quadrupeds. It is important to point out that the physiological function of each class of neuron is different (10), and each neuron may be more important to a particular anesthetic endpoint than another neuronal type.

The structure of the motor system is remarkably conserved across species. Even in lamprey, the lowest vertebrate, there is significant supraspinal input into the spinal cord (11). When comparing mice and iguanas, Ryan et al. found that pools of motoneurons representing different muscles were in the same relative positions in both species (12). Given these and other similarities, it is not surprising that many species have similar MAC values (13) (if one assumes that anesthetics act at motoneurons to suppress movement—*see* Chapter 13).

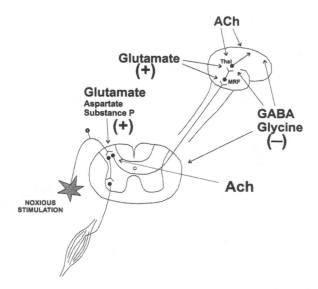

Fig. 2. Peripheral noxious stimulation initiates impulse propagation to the spinal dorsal horn where excitatory neurotransmitters are released, such as glutamate and aspartate; Substance P, a neuropeptide, plays a lesser role in acute pain *(118)*. The impulse may then travel to motoneurons (via interneurons in this example) which initiate movement. The peripheral axon may also synapse on a dorsal horn cell with ascending projections (such as a spinoreticular cell). Again, glutamate is the major excitatory neurotransmitter. The midbrain reticular formation (MRF) cell may synapse on a cell in the medial thalamus, which then projects to cortex, where acetylcholine (ACh) and glutamate modulate cerebral function. GABA and glycine, the major inhibitory neurotransmitters, also modulate cerebral and spinal cord function. This simplified diagram does not include other, more complex pathways.

Neurophysiology

The transmission of impulses from the periphery to the spinal cord and then to the brain depends on synapses, and synaptic transmission occurs via neurotransmitters (NTs) *(14)*. There are several classifications of NTs, including excitatory or inhibitory, amino acids, or peptides. The major excitatory NT is glutamate, while gamma-aminobutyric acid (GABA) and glycine are the major inhibitory NTs *(see* Chapters 16–20). It is very possible that anesthetics exert their effects by actions on NTs, either by decreased release or by altered binding of the NT to receptors.

The spinal cord uses several NTs (Fig. 2). For example, glutamate and aspartate excite post-synaptic cells (e.g., the motoneuron) resulting in movement. Glycine is an important inhibitory NT in the spinal cord. GABA, while present in the spinal cord, appears to be more important in the brain. Normal spinal cord function depends on other NTs such as acetylcholine (ACh). In fact, manipulation of ACh can alter responses to noxious stimulation. Intrathecal neostigmine provides analgesia *(15)*. Substance P is a peptide that is released by small-diameter primary afferents including nociceptors, and thus may be important to pain and withdrawal reflexes evoked by noxious stimuli. However, the importance of the role played by substance P in pain has recently been questioned, based on evidence that knockout mice lacking substance P or the neurokinin-1 (NK-1) receptor to which substance P binds, show fairly normal pain-like behavioral responses to noxious stimulation *(16–18)*. However, substance P may be involved in chronic inflammatory or neuropathic pain, since behavioral measures of chronic pain (e.g., hyperalgesia; allodynia) induced by limb inflammation or nerve injury were significantly reduced in knockout mice or in rats in which spinal NK-1 receptor-expressing neurons were selectively destroyed *(19)*.

The first order neurons in the dorsal horn act as a "spinal gate" *(20)*. Depending on the balance of inhibition and excitation within the spinal cord, excitatory afferent input arising from noxious peripheral stimulation may result in movement, or just in autonomic activation. Inhibitory influences in the spinal cord descend from supraspinal structures such as the rostral ventromedial medulla (RVM) and locus coeruleus *(10)*. These brainstem neurons give rise to descending axons that travel in the dorsolateral funiculus (DLF) and ventrolateral funiculus (VLF) that convey inhibitory signals to the dorsal horn *(10)* *(see* Fig. 3).

SPINAL CORD AS A SITE OF ANESTHETIC ACTION

The Spinal Cord and MAC

Three studies describe the importance of the spinal cord as a site of anesthetic action. In one study *(1)*, the forebrain was removed in rats anesthetized with isoflurane. MAC was determined before and after pre-collicular decerebration *(1)*. There was no significant change in MAC after decerebration, suggesting that structures rostral to the transection (thalamus, cerebral cortex, etc.) were not important sites where isoflurane exerted its effect on movement. In another study, a hypothermic spinal cord transection was performed at the thoracic level, and MAC was determined in both forelimbs and hindlimbs before and after the transection *(2)*. MAC was unchanged below the level of the transection, suggesting that the movement response is generated within the spinal cord in the absence of descending influences, and that isoflurane prevented movement by acting there.

In a study performed in goats, we found that anesthetic action in the spinal cord appeared to be important to the suppression of movement *(3)*. In this model, it is possible to differentially deliver anesthetics to the head (brain) and torso (spinal cord). When isoflurane was delivered throughout the body, MAC was about 1.2%. When we delivered the isoflurane to the cranial circulation (with only 0.2–0.3% in the torso), the isoflurane concentration required in the brain to suppress movement was 2.9% indicating that anesthetic action in the spinal cord was very important in suppressing the movement response.

These three studies *(1–3)* represent two bodies of evidence that are important for several reasons. First, different species (rats, goats) were used. This suggests that these findings might be more easily extrapolated to other species, such as humans. Second, different methods were used. Rampil and colleagues either removed brain tissue or transected the spinal cord *(1,2)*, while we employed differential anesthetic delivery. These techniques provided important clues that the movements elicited by supramaximal noxious stimulation (during anesthesia) can be generated primarily or solely within the spinal cord and brainstem. Because the spinal cord is capable of complex movements, it is not surprising that these complex movements persist despite removal of supraspinal influences. A natural conclusion of the studies by Rampil et al. is that anesthetic action in the brain or brainstem does not play any role in suppression of movement *(1,2)*. However, this conclusion may be too far-reaching. The differential delivery of isoflurane to the brain (albeit at high concentrations) can prevent movement, suggesting that the brain and brainstem are not completely without influence on movement resulting from noxious stimulation applied during anesthesia *(3)*.

The ability of subcortical structures to produce complex movements is best illustrated by the behaviors observed in rats that have had a pre-collicular decerebration. Woods and Lovick *(21,22)* documented normal righting reflexes, grooming, and locomotion in rats with pre-collicular decerebration. Noxious stimuli elicited jumping, vocalization, and head turning towards the stimulus. Not surprisingly, these animals did not respond to visual stimuli, but did so to auditory stimuli. The issue of anesthetic effects on spinally-organized movement patterns is further discussed below *(see* Section on Movement Patterns).

If, as hypothesized, the spinal circuits generating complex movement (i.e., CPGs) are more resistant to anesthesia than supraspinal mechanisms involved in consciousness and memory, then one would expect to see clinical evidence of this possibility. This, in fact, does appear to be the case.

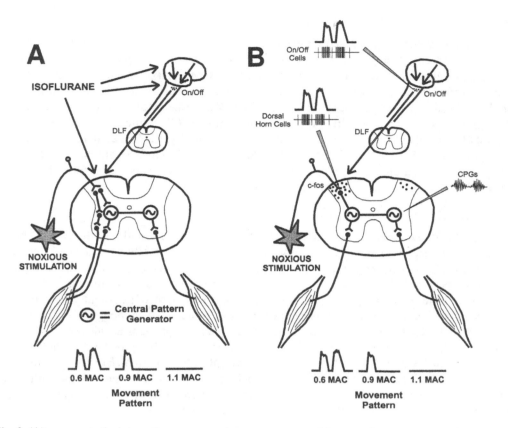

Fig. 3. (A) represents the interaction among various components of the central nervous system in response to noxious stimulation, and how anesthetics such as isoflurane might affect that interaction. A noxious stimulus generates impulses that travel to the dorsal horn and are then transmitted to muscles that initiate a response (movement pattern). CPGs may be involved in the movement response. Movement is also likely to result from participation of "private" reflex pathways that do not necessarily involve CPGs (seen on the left side of the cord; pathway to crossed extensor not shown). Supraspinal influences (ON/OFF cells and possibly higher CNS structures, such as the cerebral cortex and thalamus) modulate the response. These supraspinal sites exert control via the dorsal lateral funiculus (DLF), although other spinal pathways might also be used (e.g., corticospinal tract). CPGs generate rhythmic patterns that govern the movement. Anesthetics might affect the supraspinal and the spinal components. **(B)** represents how different techniques can be used to investigate spinal cord action of anesthetics, especially effects on movement. Single-cell recording of ON/OFF cells and dorsal horn cells, and correlation to the movement, might establish whether ON/OFF cell and dorsal horn cells activities correlate with the movement. Likewise, c-fos studies might determine to what extent anesthetics depress dorsal horn function, particularly in the sub-MAC range. Determining anesthetic effects on CPGs would determine if CPG output is affected in the same clinical range as the movement associated with noxious stimulation. The "private" pathway shown in Fig. 3A has been removed for clarity.

Commonly seen during induction and emergence of anesthesia in patients who have received a predominant or exclusive volatile anesthetic, muscle rigidity can occur. This is often described as clonic in nature, but can resemble shivering. This was investigated by Sessler et al. *(23)*, who found that at low isoflurane concentrations during emergence, clonic muscle activity occurred that was distinctly different from thermoregulatory shivering. They hypothesized that this muscle activity was the result of a pharmacological "decerebration". The loss of descending inhibition might have occurred because the brain was still "asleep", while the spinal cord was "awake". This movement occurs when the patient is still unresponsive and unable to form memories.

Spinal Opiates—Effects on Anesthetic Requirements

Numerous studies have examined the effect of spinal opiates on MAC. As expected, most of the available data strongly suggest that spinal opiates such as morphine, fentanyl, and buprenorphine lower MAC by as much as 50%. This presumably occurs as the result of opiates acting at opiate receptors in the spinal cord to suppress transmission of noxious impulses (*see* Fig. 8C). This effect has been shown in animals (rat, dog) as well as humans *(24–26)*. Drasner et al. *(25)* administered morphine 0.75 mg intrathecally, and found that halothane MAC was 0.46%, while it was 0.81% in a control group that had received a similar morphine dose intramuscularly. Lincina et al. *(27)*, however, in a well-controlled double-blind study determined that intrathecal morphine did not affect halothane MAC. The reasons for the discrepancy between these two studies are unclear. Nonetheless, the bulk of the data indicate that spinal opiates will decrease MAC.

Hyperalgesia and the Spinal Cord

Anesthetics in low doses are associated with hyperalgesia. In a rat study, Archer et al. *(28)* found that thiopental enhanced nociceptive responses at low plasma concentrations associated with drowsiness. Further increases in thiopental concentrations resulted in unconsciousness and unresponsiveness to noxious stimuli. In a similar study, Zhang et al. *(29)* determined that isoflurane, diethyl ether, halothane, and nitrous oxide produced hyperalgesia at low (0.1 MAC) concentrations. Clinically, there is evidence that anesthetics produce hyperalgesia in humans *(30)*, although this is controversial *(31)*. It is unclear what sites of action might be responsible for hyperalgesia. One possibility is sensitization of peripheral nociceptors by halothane *(32)*. Another possibility is that anesthetic action in the brain induces descending facilitation of spinal nociceptive transmission. However, we have found that propofol and thiopental did not enhance the nociceptive responses of spinal dorsal horn neurons via a cerebral action *(33,34)*. Further work is required to determine to what extent, if any, anesthetics cause hyperalgesia, and whether the spinal cord is critically involved.

METHODS TO INVESTIGATE ANESTHETIC ACTION IN THE SPINAL CORD

There are numerous approaches to indirectly and directly examine anesthetic action in the spinal cord, although space limitations permit us to discuss only a few. Some of these methods are discussed in Chapters 12 and 13.

Motoneuron Excitability as Assessed by F-Wave and H-Reflex

Relatively noninvasive electrophysiological tests have been available for many decades to investigate neurological status. It is possible to monitor and determine anesthetic effects on spinal reflexes. Two commonly studied reflexes are the F-wave and the H-reflex *(35,36)*. The F-wave represents the antidromic activation of spinal motoneurons by peripheral motor nerve stimulation, resulting in the generation of recurrent action potentials that are transmitted orthodromically to the muscle. Depolarization of a small number of muscle fibers can be detected using electromyography. Of note, the F-wave does not rely upon a synapse within the spinal cord *(36)*, and is thought to reflect the "excitability" of the motoneuron *(37)*. That is, if a group of motoneurons was more prone to discharge (as might occur if the resting membrane voltage was close to the threshold), then the F-wave would be large. In a series of studies in rats conducted by Rampil and colleagues, anesthetics such as isoflurane, halothane, and N_2O depressed the F-wave at concentrations that produce immobility *(36,38,39)*. Similar studies in humans also have shown that isoflurane *(40,41)* or propofol *(42)* depresses the F-wave at clinically relevant concentrations Furthermore, we reported in the goat that isoflurane depresses the F-wave primarily via a direct spinal action, with little or no supraspinal effect *(43)*. Thiopental, however, produces immobility at concentrations that have minimal effect on the F-wave *(44)*, so any effect on the F-wave cannot be generalized to all anesthetics. Thus, it is possible that some, but not all, anesthetics prevent movement by a direct effect on motoneurons (*see* Chapter 13).

The H-reflex is elicited by peripheral nerve stimulation at a threshold that selectively activates the largest myelinated Ia fibers from muscle spindles. These fibers conduct impulses orthodromically into the spinal cord to synapse directly onto motoneurons (monosynaptic reflex), which in turn project to the homonymous muscle, causing it to contract. Changes in H-reflex threshold are thought to reflect changes in motoneuron excitability. As with the F-wave, anesthetics affect the H-reflex *(35,45)*, providing further evidence in support of a direct action of anesthetics on motoneurons to prevent movement.

Single-unit Recording in the Spinal Cord In Vivo

The spinal cord can also be investigated at the level of single neurons or "units." Single-unit activity can be recorded extracellularly or intracellularly. For extracellular recording, a microelectrode near the neuron can register the extracellular currents generated when the neuron fires an action potential. This method allows one to quantify the number of action potentials fired by a neuron spontaneously or in response to a stimulus. For intracellular recording, the tip of a microelectrode placed inside the neuron's membrane measures the voltage difference between the inside and outside of the cell. This allows one to measure subthreshold changes in the membrane potential as well as action potentials. A variant is whole-cell patch-clamp recording, which is beginning to be done in vivo, and allows recording of ionic currents flowing through the cell's membrane, which is maintained at a constant voltage.

With each technique, the effect of anesthesia on the cell's response to a given stimulus can be recorded. In vivo extracellular single-unit recording methods have been used for several decades to show that anesthetic agents have dose-related depressant actions on nociceptive and non-nociceptive dorsal horn neurons, e.g., halothane and isoflurane *(20,46–51)*; nitrous oxide *(20,52–55)*, thiopental *(100)*, and propofol *(33,56)*, as discussed in more detail in Chapter 12. To date, few if any studies have employed intracellular or patch-clamp techniques in vivo to investigate anesthetic effects on spinal cord neurons. As single-unit recording methods have contributed to our understanding of anesthetic effects on dorsal horn neurons, there are several limitations. Most importantly, only one or a few neurons can be recorded at one time, although techniques to record from multiple single units simultaneously are rapidly improving. It can also be technically difficult to isolate and hold a single neuron long enough to assess anesthetic effects, especially with intracellular or patch-clamp techniques. This is particularly true for single-unit recordings in awake behaving animals; most studies to date have been performed in anesthetized animals. Another problem is that it can be difficult to determine the exact function of a given neuron. The technique of antidromic stimulation can be used to determine whether a neuron projects to supraspinal structures. However, to show that a neuron participates as an interneuron in a local neural circuit is much more difficult, as discussed further below (*see* Organized Movement Patterns).

Spinal Withdrawal Reflexes

In MAC studies, gross, purposeful movement in response to supramaximal stimulation is the measured end-point. Simple withdrawal of a single limb is usually considered negative. Nonetheless, withdrawal reflexes are commonly used to assess pain, and may also provide useful information regarding the spinal action of anesthetic agents. Furthermore, flexion reflexes are normally accompanied by the crossed-extensor reflex, which is adaptive in maintaining body posture *(57)*. Indeed, this alternating pattern may form the basis for the rhythmically alternating limb movements of walking. Currently, the functional relationship between flexion reflexes and locomotor CPGs is poorly understood.

In conscious or lightly anesthetized animals, limb withdrawal can be elicited by noxious cutaneous stimulation. Examples are flexion withdrawal of a hind limb in response to noxious mechanical or thermal stimulation of the paw *(57–60)*, or the rat tail flick reflex in response to noxious thermal stimulation of the tail *(61)*. The magnitude of the withdrawal can be monitored by recording EMG activity from limb flexor muscles, or by tethering the limb to a force transducer. EMG activity provides a relative measure, while limb withdrawal force provides an absolute measure *(62)*. Such methods have been used to show that limb withdrawal reflexes are suppressed by pentobarbital *(63)* and morphine *(64)*.

Recent work indicates that limb withdrawal reflexes do not represent a largely invariant flexion movement of the limb in response to stimulation at spatially diverse sites, as originally suggested by Sherrington *(57)*, and conceptualized by the flexor reflex afferent (FRA) pathway *(65)*. Instead, a "modular" organization of withdrawal reflexes has been proposed, based on the observation of distinct patterns or "local signs" of limb movements elicited by stimulation at different skin sites *(66,67)*. The distinguishing feature is that the stimulated skin surface is moved directly away from the source of stimulation *(68)*, thereby serving to protect the limb and to reduce maladaptive movements toward the stimulus. Such modular reflex organization has recently been shown for withdrawal of the leg in response to noxious stimulation of the plantar or dorsal surface of the foot in humans *(69,70)*. Previous studies of the RIII flexion reflex in humans showed that it is depressed by morphine *(71)*. Such reflex recordings in humans or animals may thus prove to be valuable in assessing anesthetic action.

There are a number of sites along the reflex pathway at which anesthetics could act to reduce movement, as illustrated in Fig. 4. Anesthetic agents could affect properties of cutaneous (or other) tissue (e.g., blood flow), or peripheral nociceptors, influencing the transduction of noxious stimuli into nerve impulses. Halothane may increase the excitability of polymodal nociceptors *(32)*, although studies with isolated limb perfusion indicate that MAC is not affected by a peripheral action of anesthetics studied *(72)*.

A much more likely site of anesthetic action is within the spinal cord, reducing the excitability of interneurons in the reflex pathway. Many previous studies have shown that nociceptive and non-nociceptive dorsal horn neurons are depressed in a dose-related manner by anesthetic agents (*see* Single Unit Recording). If some of these dorsal horn neurons participate as reflex interneurons, then their depression by anesthetics would contribute to reflex suppression. The anesthetic-induced depression might be due to direct hypolarization of the dorsal horn neuron, or to presynaptic inhibition of transmitter release from afferent fibers. In addition, anesthetics might act supraspinally to change the activity in descending modulatory pathways (e.g., increased descending inhibition) to indirectly reduce excitability of the dorsal horn neurons. This possibility is addressed in more detail in section 5. Anesthetics might also reduce excitation of motoneurons by the interneuronal pathway, either by depressing interneuronal input or by directly hyperpolarizing the motoneuron cell body (*see* Chapter 13). There is evidence that barbiturates depress synaptic transmission to motoneurons *(73)*. Although unlikely, anesthetics might block conduction in motor axons. The data from indirect assessment of motoneuron excitability (F-wave, H-reflex; *see* above) suggest that some anesthetics may reduce motoneuronal excitability by one or more of these mechanisms. Finally, anesthetics could theoretically act at the neuromuscular junction or on muscle fibers directly to reduce contraction and thereby depress movement, although there is no evidence for this.

One of the greatest difficulties in determining the site of anesthetic action within the spinal cord is separating the relative roles of the sensory and motor systems. To specify the exact site along the reflex pathway at which anesthetics might act to reduce noxious stimulus-evoked withdrawal reflexes is a technically challenging problem. It is possible to directly or indirectly assess the excitability of motoneurons driving the reflex (*see* Motoneuron Excitability as Assessed by F-wave and H-reflex). However, it is more difficult to assess the effect of anesthetics on premotor interneurons in the reflex pathway. This requires demonstrating a functional, excitatory connection from the interneuron to the motoneuron. One approach is to electrically stimulate within a motoneuron pool and identify interneurons that are antidromically excited. However, this only works for the last-order interneuron, and not for interneurons that are interposed in a multisynaptic chain before the last-order interneuron. Further, this technique does not allow one to determine if the synaptic connection is excitatory or

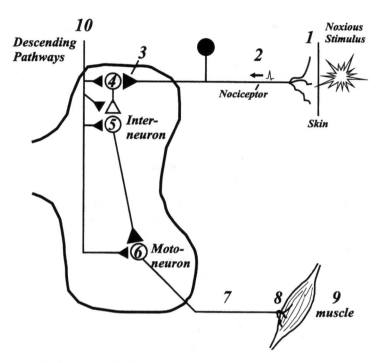

Fig. 4. Sites where anesthetics could influence MAC. **1:** stimulus transduction by nociceptor; **2:** conduction by afferent nerves; **3:** spinal synaptic transmission; **4, 5:** dorsal horn interneurons; **6:** motoneuron; **7:** conduction by motor axon; **8:** neuromuscular junction; **9:** muscle; **10:** descending pathways.

inhibitory. The most powerful technique is spike-triggered averaging *(74)*, but again this can only be applied for last-order interneurons. This method requires that action potentials recorded extracellularly from the putative interneuron be used to synchronize intracellular recordings from a simultaneously recorded motoneuron, so that a monosynaptic EPSP can be shown to occur reliably with each presynaptic action potential. To date, this method has been used successfully to characterize a small number of interneurons *(74,75)* but has not been applied to polysynaptic pathways. Technically more feasible alternatives are indirect, such as simultaneous recordings from dorsal horn cells and motoneurons *(63,76–78)*. In such studies, motoneuronal activity can be measured indirectly using single-fiber electromyography (EMG) or by monitoring the force of withdrawal. These techniques permit the investigator to examine the timing of dorsal horn neuronal responses in relation to motoneuron responses. Furthermore, a high degree of cross-correlation between dorsal horn and motor unit firing would be strong, although not incontrovertible, evidence that they are functionally linked. Carstens and Campbell (63) simultaneously recorded single-unit activity from lumbar wide dynamic range (WDR) dorsal horn neurons, flexor motor units, as well as the force of limb withdrawal, in response to noxious thermal paw stimulation. In most cases, the dorsal horn neuronal response preceded and overlapped that of the single motor unit and reflex withdrawal, suggesting that the neurons participated in driving the reflex even though they never exhibited a 1:1 correspondence in firing with motor units and thus may or may not have been functionally connected. Furthermore, the reflex and motor unit firing were more susceptible than WDR neurons to pentobarbital anesthesia, as well as to descending inhibition evoked by midbrain stimulation. More recently, Morgan *(76)* recorded from WDR and nociceptive-specific dorsal horn neurons during withdrawal reflexes in lightly-anesthetized rats, and found that most units fired prior to the reflex but some were not active until after the initiation of the reflex movement.

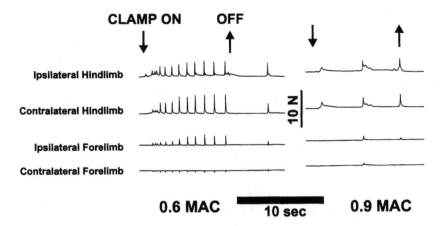

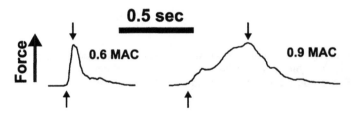

Fig. 5. Raw force tracings from one rat. Each limb was attached to a force transducer. Note the vigorous movement when the clamp was applied at 0.6 MAC of isoflurane (down arrow = clamp on, up arrow = clamp off). At 0.9 MAC, the movement number decreased, but the force of the movements was affected less. The extremity movements were synchronous, and there was no evidence of an alternating pattern. At 1.1 MAC and 1.4 MAC no movement occurred and the tracings are omitted. The data demonstrate that the transition from 0.6–0.9 MAC mainly affected the number of movements, and less so the force of those movements (data not reported from *79*).

Fig. 6. Examples of limb movement at 0.6 and 0.9 MAC isoflurane in an individual rat. The limb was attached to a force transducer. Note that the time to achieve maximal force was prolonged at 0.9 MAC. The arrows indicate the start of movement and the time when the maximal force was achieved (data not reported from *79*).

Organized Movement Patterns

Another approach to investigate the spinal action of anesthetics is to assess their effect on organized movement patterns, because such movement patterns are very likely to be generated by CPGs within the spinal cord. Indeed, most MAC studies use gross purposeful movement in response to a supramaximal stimulus as an end-point. However, few previous studies have attempted to quantify such movements *(79)*.

We have investigated effects of inhaled anesthetics on multi-limb movement patterns *(79)*. Rats were in a prone position with each of the four limbs fully extended and attached to force transducers, as was the snout. A supramaximal mechanical stimulus was applied to one hind paw (or the tail), and the force, speed, and number of limb and head movements were measured at different concentrations of isoflurane or halothane. At sub-MAC concentrations, the movement consisted of a synchronized, flexion-extension pattern in all limbs (Fig. 5). It was surprising that rhythmically alternating limb movements were not observed, possibly because all limbs were in a fully-extended starting position. From 0.6–0.9 MAC, there was a reduction in the number of limb movements but not their force, while at 1.1 MAC the force of movements also decreased. A reanalysis of the data from this study revealed that the time to development of maximal force was also prolonged by isoflurane (Fig. 6, Table 1), as was the time from stimulus onset to initiation of the first movement (1.4 ± 2.3 s

Table 1
Time to Achievement of Maximal Force

	Isoflurane Concentration	
	0.6 MAC	0.9 MAC
Ipsilateral Hindlimb	0.10 ± 0.02 s	0.20 ± 0.10 s*
Contralateral Hindlimb	0.09 ± 0.03 s	0.23 ± 0.13 s*

*$p < 0.05$ compared to 0.6 MAC value; 244 movements were analyzed from 9 rats (data not reported from ref. *79*).

at 0.8–0.9% isoflurane and 7.7 ± 2.0 s at 1.3–1.4% isoflurane [$p < 0.001$]). We also observed that movements sometimes persisted after the noxious stimulus was removed (*see*, e.g., Fig. 3 in ref. *79*). This is perhaps not surprising, given the experience in the operating room when patients sometimes continue to move after the surgeon has ceased stimulation. The neural circuits involved in the movement are presumably still in a heightened state of activity. Dorsal horn neurons often continue to fire after a noxious stimulus is removed (afterdischarge), and thus might promote continuation of the movement *(80)*. Thus, it is not unexpected that movement may continue after a noxious stimulus has been removed with maintained activity in the neural circuitry involved in generating the movement.

Correlation of the parameters of movement (number, force, speed) with the intensity of a noxious stimulus is a valid and accepted method to investigate the neural circuits involved in nociception. For example, in the rodent formalin test, the number of paw flinches induced by subcutaneous injection of formalin is a measured end-point *(81)*. In addition, the force of flexion hind limb withdrawal evoked by graded noxious thermal stimuli in rats correlates well with stimulus intensity *(60)*. Similarly, the intensity of noxious stimulation correlated with the force and latency of an operantly-conditioned bar-press escape response in monkeys *(82)*.

Neuroanatomical Techniques

Electrophysiological techniques, although yielding information regarding dynamic actions, are limited by the ability to study one or perhaps a few cells at any one time. Anatomical techniques, on the other hand, allow the assessment of entire populations of neurons that may contribute to neural circuits underlying behavior.

An anatomical method that is used increasingly to investigate nociceptive neurons is c-fos immunohistochemistry *(83,84)*. Neuronal cellular production of c-fos, a proto-oncogene, is increased after noxious stimulation *(85)*. While a significant amount of c-fos data has been collected using moderately noxious stimulation (e.g., subcutaneous formalin), little work has been performed examining supramaximal stimulation, and the effect of anesthetics. Sun et al. *(86)* found that halothane and N_2O failed to suppress c-fos activation in the lumbar dorsal horn following subcutaneous formalin injection. Another group of investigators *(87)* determined that formalin injection increased c-fos expression in all layers of the dorsal horn, and that N_2O and halothane suppressed c-fos expression in deeper, but not superficial, layers. Such data could yield valuable insight into spinal cord sites that are affected by anesthetics. Recent data indicate that c-fos staining is an appropriate method to investigate anesthetic effects. An NMDA antagonist (MK-801) and opiates both depress c-fos expression *(88,89)*. It has been known for some time that MK-801 and opiates decrease MAC *(90,91)*. These c-fos and MAC studies complement each other and suggest that anesthetic effects on c-fos expression will likely yield data that are directly relevant to anesthetic mechanisms.

Anatomical methods have also been applied to the perplexing problem of tracing multisynaptic reflex pathways in the spinal cord. One approach is retrograde transneuronal labeling. When wheat germ agglutinin conjugated to horseradish peroxidase (WGA-HRP) is injected into a hind limb muscle, it is taken up by motor nerve terminals and transported retrogradely to the motoneuronal cell bodies. Some WGA-HRP escapes from the motoneuron cell body and is taken up by the synaptic terminals of last-order interneurons projecting to those motoneurons. These interneurons can be visualized histochemically, and are located mainly in the intermediate zone and ventral horn with some in the dorsal horn *(75)*. A variant of this method is the use of herpes or pseudorabies viruses, which have the advantage that the tracer "signal" is amplified due to viral replication within each serially, retrogradely infected neuron *(92)*. Injection of pseudorabies virus into hindlimb *(93,9)* or tail muscles *(9)* led to distinct, staged patterns of spinal cell labeling, suggesting that neurons in a multisynaptic chain were serially infected. Several potential reflex pathways were deduced in this manner, including a pathway from the substantia gelatinosa (lamine II) to lamina I to motoneurons *(9)*. This latter pathway is of particular interest since nociceptor afferents terminate in the superficial layers (I and II) of the dorsal horn. A drawback of this method is that the functional nature (i.e., excitatory or inhibitory) of the connections cannot be specified.

MOVEMENT PATTERNS DURING NOXIOUS STIMULATION

Why is the Pattern of Movement Important?

Noxious stimulation initiates a complex set of nocifensive behavioral responses, the collective goal of which is to remove or escape from the source of stimulation. Anesthetics suppress this behavior. Since the introduction of the concept of MAC as a measure of anesthetic potency *(94)*, little work has been performed to objectively describe and quantify the actual type of movement that occurs with supramaximal stimulation, and how anesthetics affect it. A more accurate description of the movement pattern will aid further investigation of the underlying neural circuits and the sites and mechanisms by which anesthetics affect that movement. Thus, before the question of "how" and "where" anesthetics alter movement is addressed, the question of "what" movement is altered must be answered.

Organized Movement Patterns in Response to Noxious Stimulation and Spinal Sites at Which Anesthetics Suppress Movement

The movement that occurs with supramaximal noxious stimulation has been poorly described. In a MAC study, gross, purposeful movement is considered to be a positive response, and usually includes a pawing motion or turning of the head *(13,94)*. The stimulus is usually removed once this movement occurs, although the movement quite often persists for a short period afterwards. Isoflurane and halothane at 0.6–0.9 MAC decreased the number of limb movements elicited by supramaximal mechanical stimulation with little effect on the force of movement, while at the transition from 0.9–1.1 MAC movement force was also reduced *(79)*. What could account for these effects?

Noxious stimulation can initiate complex movements that are generated within the spinal cord. Noxious cutaneous stimulation can elicit flexion withdrawal of the limb, accompanied by extension of the opposite limb, via circuits at the segmental spinal level *(95)*. However, the spinal cord is capable of generating considerably more complex movement patterns. Chronically spinalized cats suspended above a treadmill with the paws in contact can exhibit walking, and as the treadmill speed is increased the alternating pattern seen in each pair of limbs shifts to a synchronized pattern as the gait switches from walk to gallop *(96)*. Frogs with upper cervical cord transections maintain the wiping reflex, which involves extension of the hindlimb to contact the site of a noxious stimulus (such as acid-soaked paper) applied to the forelimb followed by wiping; if the forelimb is moved, the trajectory of the hindlimb movement is "automatically" adjusted to accurately reach the stimulus *(97)*. In brain dead humans, complex movements can occur, including extremity flexion across the chest, sitting up in bed, and turning of the head *(98)*. These movements are possible, in part, because

CPGs within the spinal cord are capable of producing movement patterns such as walking, running, and scratching *(99)*.

Very little work has addressed anesthetic effects on CPGs. A well-accepted model for investigating vertebrate CPGs is the lamprey, a parasitic fish *(100)*. As in all vertebrates, supraspinal structures in the lamprey brain give rise to descending pathways that influence spinal circuits to initiate, maintain, and modulate the speed and pattern of locomotion *(11)*. Sensory information is integrated centrally and when a decision to move is made (excluding peripherally-initiated escape responses), commands are sent down to the spinal CPGs to initiate locomotion. This organizational scheme applies generally to higher vertebrates, in which locomotor centers have been described in the brain stem, where electrical stimulation initiates rhythmic movement patterns *(101)*. Swimming in the lamprey involves alternating contraction of muscles on each side of the body wall. Despite differences between lamprey swimming and mammalian walking, the CPGs involved in generating the rhythmically alternating motor pattern appear to rely on similar types of excitatory and inhibitory interneurons, neurotransmitters (glutamate, glycine), receptors (e.g., AMPA, NMDA), and ion channels *(11)*. These similarities, together with the large size and smaller number of neurons in the CPG of lampreys compared to mammals, have made the lamprey an excellent model to study locomotion and motor behavior.

Yamamura et al. *(102)* investigated the effects of halothane on behavioral responses and synaptic transmission in lamprey. By monitoring escape (darting away) from a noxious electrical stimulus, these authors determined the "MAC" to be 0.32 mM, and "MAC$_{95}$" to be 0.51 mM. These concentrations are quite similar to those required to anesthetize mammals *(103)*. At these halothane concentrations, EPSPs in motoneurons were moderately depressed. In another study, the same authors briefly reported that ketamine, an NMDA antagonist, suppressed fictive locomotion *(102)*. Fictive locomotion is studied by recording the activity of motor axons in ventral roots on both sides of the spinal cord, and can be quantified in terms of frequency, phase-relations, and amplitude. It is possible to assess the effects of anesthetics on these different parameters of movement to determine, for example, if frequency, number of movements, or force (amplitude) are selectively affected at different anesthetic concentrations. If CPG activity ceased at an anesthetic concentration that still permitted nocifensive behavior, one could infer that anesthetic action at CPGs is not likely to be an important part of anesthetic-induced immobility.

In our study of the effects of isoflurane and halothane on multi-limb movement patterns in rats *(79)*, the reduction in movement number at 0.6–0.9 MAC might reflect decreased synaptic drive (e.g., from nociceptive pathways) onto the motoneurons which, however, still elicit strong contraction. The reduction in force observed at the 0.9–1.1 MAC transition might reflect anesthetic effects on the motoneurons or CPGs or both. As discussed in Single Unit Recording, it is well-known that anesthetic agents depress nociceptive dorsal horn neurons, although most earlier studies examined a wide range of anesthetic concentrations *(46,50,51)*. We reason that as the anesthetic concentration increases from 0.6–0.9 MAC, there is a reduction in nociceptive transmission through the dorsal horn, with little change in motoneuron excitability. Indeed, we found that at the 0.9–1.1 MAC transition, nociceptive dorsal horn neuronal responses to a supramaximal noxious stimulus were reduced by only about 15% *(80)* In assessing isoflurane effects on motoneuron excitability using the F-wave *(39)*, there was little or no change in the 0.6–0.8 MAC range, while it was significantly depressed at 0.8–1.2 MAC *(39)*. Collectively, these data suggest that as the concentration of inhaled anesthetics approaches 1 MAC, the reduction in the number of movements elicited by supramaximal stimulation is attributed to depression of nociceptive dorsal horn transmission. As the concentration increases above 1 MAC, the resulting depression of motoneurons contributes to the observed reduction in force of movements. Based on this reasoning, it may be hypothesized that isoflurane and halothane have a relatively greater depressant effect on nociceptive dorsal horn neurons in the 0.6–0.9 than the 0.9–1.1 MAC range, and that dorsal horn activity is correlated with the movement response at low (0.6 MAC) but not high (>0.9 MAC) anesthetic concentrations.

Supraspinal Modulation of Movement Responses to Noxious Stimulation

While the spinal cord is a critical site of anesthetic action to block movement, anesthetic actions in the brain are not insignificant. As noted in the Section on The Spinal Cord and MAC, a sufficiently high concentration of isoflurane delivered differentially to the cranial circulation will block movement in response to supramaximal stimulation *(3)*. Rampil et al. have noted that although MAC was unchanged following spinal cord transection in rats, the movement was not as vigorous as before transection *(2)*; it was not stated whether this was due to a reduced number and/or force of movements. Electrophysiological studies *(see* Differential Delivery below) are consistent with these observations. Using the method of differential delivery of anesethetics in goats, increasing the concentration of cranial isoflurane from 0.3–1.3% (with the spinal concentration held at 0.8%) resulted in a decrease in dorsal horn neuronal responses to noxious stimulation *(49)*. Moreover, spinal cord isoflurane concentrations of 1.3% significantly depressed dorsal horn neuronal responses, thereby potentially "masking" any supraspinal influences. Thus, anesthetic action at supraspinal sites might be important in the sub-MAC range (e.g., 0.6–0.9 MAC), although they might be superceded by spinal actions at concentrations approaching or exceeding 1 MAC. Interestingly, supraspinal modulation does not appear to be important to halothane's reduction of low-threshold receptive field size *(105)* *(see* Chapter 12).

The supraspinal modulation of rhythmic movement patterns by descending pathways is a poorly-understood issue. In quadrupeds, propriospinal connections coordinate the timing and pattern of the rhythmic synchronized movements of the fore- and hind limbs. CPGs involved in generating rhythmic limb movements are under supraspinal control from locomotor centers *(99)*, and spinal nociceptive pathways are modulated by multiple descending pathways *(10)* *(see* Subheading 5.). The relative effects of these various descending pathways in terms of spinal anesthetic actions to block movement are not known. Since spinalization is well known to disinhibit nociceptive dorsal horn neurons *(106)*, it may be hypothesized that high cervical transection of the spinal cord would enhance nociceptive input through the dorsal horn, leading to an increase in the number and/or force of movements evoked by a supramaximal stimulus and thereby increasing MAC. Upper cervical spinalization would block tonic descending facilitatory as well as inhibitory influences. An alternative hypothesis is that this would result in a net disfacilitation of CPGs in the spinal cord, leading to a decreased number of movements in response to noxious stimulation without necessarily affecting the anesthetic concentration at which the movement is abolished (i.e., MAC). Future studies of the effects of upper cervical transection on the parameters of movement following supramaximal stimulation, and effects of anesthetic agents, should contribute to our understanding of the interplay between descending pathways and spinal cord circuitry involved in generating movement.

THE RELATIVE CONTRIBUTIONS OF SPINAL VS SUPRASPINAL ANESTHETIC ACTIONS TO IMMOBILITY IN RESPONSE TO NOXIOUS STIMULATION

Use of Differential Delivery to Investigate Spinal vs Supraspinal Anesthetic Actions

Based on the unique anatomy of goats, it is possible to isolate the cerebral circulation and connect it to a blood oxygenator to selectively deliver anesthetic agents to the brain independent of the rest of the body *(3)*. Use of this technique has shown that anesthetic requirements are several-fold higher for the brain compared to the torso (i.e., spinal) circulation *(3)*. Using this preparation, we showed that when the cerebral concentration of isoflurane was increased from 0.3–1.3%, while holding the isoflurane concentration to the torso constant at 0.8%, there was a depression of the responses of WDR and nociceptive-specific spinal dorsal horn neurons to a supramaximal noxious mechanical stimulus *(48)*. This was particularly evident at supraclinical concentrations of cranial isoflurane (3–8.5%). In contrast, when the concentration of isoflurane delivered to the brain was reduced to

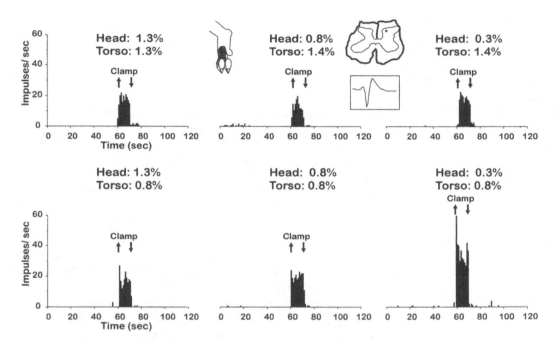

Fig. 7. Individual response of a wide dynamic range cell. These peri-stimulus time histograms (PSTHs, bin width 1 s) show the response to changing cranial and torso isoflurane concentrations. In the top row of PSTHs, torso isoflurane was kept at 1.3–1.4%, and as the cranial isoflurane concentration was decreased, the evoked response was unchanged. In the bottom row of PSTHs, torso (and hence spinal cord) isoflurane was 0.8%, and decreasing cranial isoflurane from 1.3 to 0.3% increased the evoked response. Adapted from ref. *49* with permission.

0.3%, while holding the torso concentration constant at 0.8%, there was a significant facilitation of the dorsal horn neuronal response *(49)*. Therefore, when the direct spinal effect of isoflurane was minimized, high cranial isoflurane depresses, and low cranial isoflurane facilitates nociceptive dorsal horn neuronal responses (Fig. 7). These data indicate that anesthetic action in the brain contributes to depression of spinal nociceptive transmission, although this effect is usually masked by the direct spinal action of the anesthetic. These findings are discussed in On- and Off-Cells in relation to descending antinociceptive pathways.

We have utilized this approach to investigate additional anesthetics. Nitrous oxide had divergent effects on nociceptive spinal neurons when delivered systemically or differentially to the torso *(55)*, a finding that may relate to its low potency. Both propofol *(33)* and thiopental *(34)* significantly depressed nociceptive spinal neurons in a dose-related manner when injected into the torso circulation (with cranial anesthesia maintained by 0.8% isoflurane), while having no effect when delivered to the cranial circulation at comparable plasma concentrations. These results indicate that supraspinal actions of propofol and thiopental at clinically relevant concentrations do not have a significant effect on spinal nociceptive transmission.

Descending Antinociceptive Pathways and Anesthesia

As discussed in the preceding section, inhaled anesthetics such as isoflurane may act supraspinally to partially depress spinal nociceptive transmission indirectly by engaging descending pathways, an effect that may contribute to immobility in response to supramaximal stimulation. A discussion of descending antinociceptive pathways is therefore relevant to mechanisms of anesthetic action.

The major sources of descending inhibitory input to spinal nociceptive dorsal horn neurons arise from serotonergic and noradrenergic cell groups in the rostral ventromedial medulla (RVM), including the raphe nuclei, and locus coeruleus and related nuclei. These pathways are shown in Fig. 8. The panels show schematics of the brain and spinal cord in longitudinal section. Noxious stimuli excite nociceptors that send afferent fibers into the spinal cord to excite dorsal horn neurons via release of glutamate and substance P to act at postsynaptic glutaminergic and NK-1 receptors, respectively. Neurons in RVM, many of which are serotonergic, give rise to descending fibers which travel in the spinal dorsolateral funiculi to terminate in the spinal dorsal horn. The RVM-spinal pathway has a direct inhibitory effect on spinal projection neurons via a 5HT-1a receptor, as well as an indirect inhibitory action via excitation of inhibitory GABA interneurons through a 5HT-3 receptor. The GABA interneuron inhibits the projection cell via a GABA receptor. Descending inhibition of spinal nociceptive neurons can be reduced by administration of drugs that antagonize both 5-HT-1a, 5-HT-3, and GABA receptors *(107–109)*. RVM receives excitatory glutaminergic input from the midbrain periaqueductal gray (PAG). The PAG also excites noradrenergic neurons in locus coeruleus and surrounding cell groups, which give rise to descending projections to the spinal cord (Fig. 8B). These pathways can inhibit nociceptive spinal projection cells directly via an alpha-2 adrenoreceptor, and indirectly by exciting GABA inhibitory interneurons via an alpha-1 receptor. Inhibition of spinal neurons evoked by PAG stimulation is reduced by alpha-1, alpha-2, and GABA antagonists *(110,111)*.

Opiates such as morphine inhibit spinal projection neurons via direct spinal and indirect supraspinal actions (Fig. 8C). They act supraspinally by exciting PAG neurons. The mechanism probably involves direct inhibition of GABA interneurons via a μ-receptor to disinhibit the PAG neurons. The PAG excites the RVM-spinal pathway, which inhibits nociceptive projection neurons directly, as well as indirectly by exciting enkephalinergic inhibitory interneurons. The enkephalinergic interneurons inhibit projection neurons both pre- and postsynaptically via μ-receptors. The analgesic effect of systemically administered morphine is due to a synergistic interaction of its supraspinal and direct spinal effects *(112)*.

ON- and OFF-Cells

Insight into mechanisms of supraspinal modulation of nociceptive transmission came with the discovery of ON- and OFF-cells in the RVM *(113)*. These cells are characterized by their change in firing rate just prior to the occurrence of a nociceptive spinal withdrawal reflex, most commonly the rat's tail flick reflex. OFF-cells fire spontaneously and cease firing just prior to the occurrence of the reflex, while ON-cells are generally silent and only begin to fire just prior to the reflex. Both cell types give rise to descending projections to the spinal cord *(114)*. OFF-cells are thought to have an inhibitory effect on dorsal horn neurons, while ON-cells are thought to have a facilitatory effect. Thus, cessation of activity in the OFF-cell, and increased activity of the ON-cells, produces less inhibition and more excitation of spinal neurons, respectively, thereby permitting spinal nociceptive reflexes to occur.

During morphine analgesia, nociceptive spinal reflexes are depressed. Interestingly, OFF-cells continue firing without cessation even when a noxious stimulus is applied *(115)*. When the opiate antagonist naloxone is given, the reflex occurs again, as does the pause in OFF-cell firing. This indicates that morphine analgesia is partly due to a lack of removal of spinal inhibition by the OFF-cells. Morphine disinhibits OFF-cells, so they continue to fire while ON-cells are inhibited. This shifts the balance of descending influences in favor of inhibition, thereby suppressing the reflex.

Based on the function of ON- and OFF-cells, we propose a model to explain how isoflurane might act in the brain to affect spinal nociceptive reflex transmission. This model requires two important assumptions: (1) the spinal transmission of nociceptive signals depends on a balance of descending inhibition and facilitation, and (2) the descending inhibitory (OFF-cell) pathway is more resistant to inhibition by anesthetic compared to the descending excitatory (ON-cell) pathway. The model is

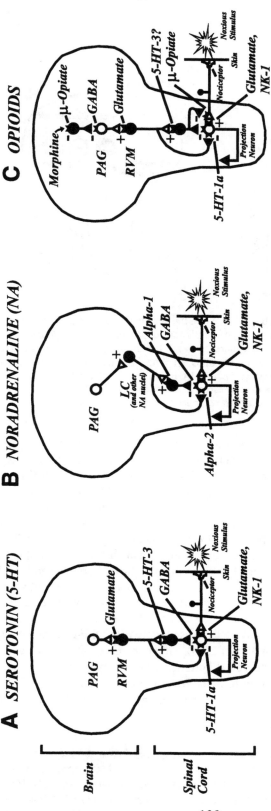

Fig. 8. Descending antinociceptive pathways. **A:** Serotonin (5-HT). descending pathway. Schematic depicts longitudinal section through brain and spinal cord. In this and subsequent figures, + (and open triangle) denotes excitatory and – (filled triangle) denotes inhibitory synapse, respectively. Noxious stimulus normally excites nociceptor in skin. Action potentials are conducted along afferent fiber to spinal cord, with excitatory synapse onto spinal projection neurons. Nociceptor input excites spinal projection neuron via glutamate and NK-1 receptors (receptors indicated by polygons). Descending pathway involves excitatory glutaminergic connection from PAG to RVM. Axons from RVM descend to inhibit projection neuron directly via 5-HT-1a receptor, and indirectly by excitation (through 5-HT-3 receptor) of inhibitory GABAergic interneuron. **B:** Noradrenergic (NA) descending pathway. Descending pathway from PAG excites NA cell groups in locus coeruleus (LC) and adjacent areas of lateral brainstem. Axons of NA neurons descend to inhibit spinal projection neuron directly via alpha-2 receptor, and indirectly by exciting (via alpha-1 receptor) an inhibitory GABAergic interneuron. **C:** Opioidergic descending pathway. Morphine acts at μ-receptor to inhibit GABAergic inhibitory interneuron and thus disinhibit PAG. This activates the serotonergic NRM-spinal pathway to inhibit projection neurons directly (5-HT-1a receptor), and indirectly by activating inhibitory opioidergic interneuron via μ-receptor.

199

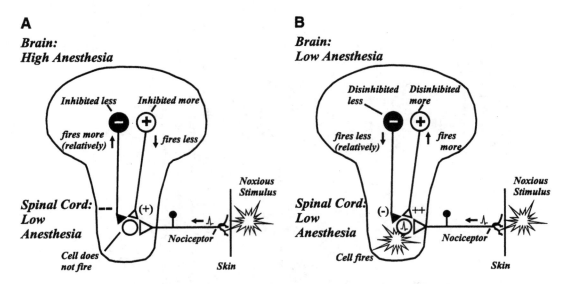

Fig. 9. Model of anesthetic action in the brain. **A:** When the anesthetic concentration to the brain is high, it is proposed that descending inhibitory neurons (OFF-cells) are depressed less than descending facilitatory (ON-cells) by the anesthetic. This leads to a net increase in inhibition in the spinal cord, so that nociceptive spinal neurons do not fire in response to a noxious stimulus. **B:** When the anesthetic concentration to the brain is low, it is proposed that descending inhibitory neurons (OFF-cells) are disinhibited less than descending facilitatory neurons (ON-cells) by withdrawal of anesthetic. This leads to a net increase in excitation in the spinal cord, so that nociceptive spinal neurons fire in response to a noxious stimulus.

shown schematically in Fig. 9. When the anesthetic concentration is high to the brain and low to spinal cord (so that the direct spinal inhibitory action of anesthetic does not mask descending effects), we propose that ON-cells are inhibited more than OFF-cells (Fig. 9A). OFF-cell firing is therefore relatively higher compared to ON-cell firing. Thus, there is a balance favoring inhibition in the spinal cord via the OFF-cell pathway, so that a noxious stimulus is incapable of exciting the dorsal horn neuron. When anesthesia is low to the brain and spinal cord, we propose that ON-cells will be disinhibited more than OFF-cells by withdrawal of the anesthetic (Fig. 9B). Greater disinhibition of ON-cells means that their firing will increase relatively more than OFF-cells. This shifts the balance in favor of descending excitation in the spinal cord, so that the dorsal horn neuron is facilitated and gives a larger response to the noxious stimulus. This scheme is therefore consistent with the actions of ON- and OFF-cells, and also with the observation that anesthesia globally depresses neurons in the brain. Furthermore, the predictions of this model are testable. Indeed, there is limited evidence that the steady-state firing of some ON-cells may be depressed more than OFF-cells at moderate-to-high concentrations of isoflurane ($\approx$ 0.9–1.4 MAC) *(116)*, although more data are needed. Moreover, indirect inhibitory effects of isoflurane on dorsal horn neurons were only observed when the spinal cord isoflurane concentration was relatively low (0.6 MAC) *(49)*. ON- and OFF-cell activity might be therefore be expected to correlate with nociceptive reflex movements in the 0.6–0.9 MAC range.

SUMMARY

Research into mechanisms of anesthesia has rapidly progressed over the last decade. In great part, this has been due to investigation at the cellular and molecular level. Interpretation of these data is difficult, however, in the absence of our understanding of effects on whole animals. Each anesthesia end-point likely occurs as the result of anesthetic action at different sites *(117)*. Thus, we will need to know what CNS sites are involved in order to have an integrated understanding of anesthetic effects.

The spinal cord appears to be a critical site of anesthetic action-the movement response that results from noxious stimulation is abolished by anesthetic action in the spinal cord. It also appears likely that anesthetics affect memory and consciousness in part via an action in the spinal cord (*see* Chapter 10).

REFERENCES

1. Rampil, I. J., Mason, P., and Singh, H. (1993) Anesthetic potency (MAC) is independent of forebrain structures in the rat. *Anesthesiology* **78,** 707–712.
2. Rampil, I. J. (1994) Anesthetic potency is not altered after hypothermic spinal cord transection in rats. *Anesthesiology* **80,** 606–610.
3. Antognini, J. F. and Schwartz, K. (1993) Exaggerated anesthetic requirements in the preferentially anesthetized brain. *Anesthesiology* **79,** 1244–1249.
4. Gilbert, S. G. (1989) Pictorial human embryology. University of Washington Press, Seattle, pp.109–131.
5. Gregory, G. A., Eger, E. I., and Munson E. S. (1969) The relationship between age and halothane requirement in man. *Anesthesiology* **30,** 488–491.
6. LeDez, K. M. and Lerman, J. (1987) The minimum alveolar concentration (MAC) of isoflurane in preterm neonates. *Anesthesiology* **67,** 301–307.
7. Fitzgerald, M. and Jennings, E. (1999) The postnatal development of spinal sensory processing. *Proc. Nat. Acad. Sci. USA* **96,** 7719–7722.
8. Willis, W. D. and Coggeshall, R. E. (1991) Sensory Mechanisms of the Spinal Cord, 2nd Ed., Plenum NY, p. 575.
9. Jasmin, L., Carstens, E., and Basbaum, A.I. (1997) Interneurons presynaptic to rattail flick motoneurons as mapped by transneuronal transport of pseudorabies virus: few have long ascending collaterals. *Neuroscience* **76,** 859–876.
10. Willis, W. D. and Westlund, K. N. (1997) Neuroanatomy of the pain system and of the pathways that modulate pain. *J.Clin.Neurophysiol.* **14,** 2–31.
11. Grillner, S., Parker, D., and Manir, A. E. (1998) Vertebrate locomotion-a lamprey perspective. *Ann. NY Acad. Sci.* **860,** 1–18.
12. Ryan, J. M., Cushman, J., Jordan, B., Samuels, A., Frazer, H., and Baier, C. (1998) Topographic position of forelimb motoneuron pools is conserved in vertebrate evolution. *Brain Behav. Evol.* **51,** 90–99.
13. Quasha, A. L., Eger, E. I., and Tinker, J. H. (1980) Determination and applications of MAC. *Anesthesiology* **53,** 315–334.
14. Furst, S. (1999) Transmitters involved in antinociception in the spinal cord. *Brain Res. Bull.* **48,** 129–141.
15. Lauretti, G. R., Hood, D. D., Eisenach, J. C., and Pfeifer, B. L. (1998) A multi-center study of intrathecal neostigmine for analgesia following vaginal hysterectomy. *Anesthesiology* **89,** 913–918.
16. De Felipe, C., Herrero, J. F., O'Brien, J. A., et al. (1998) Altered nociception, analgesia and aggression in mice lacking the receptor for substance P. *Nature* **392,** 394–397.
17. Cao, Y. Q., Mantyh, P. W., Carlson, E. J., Gillespie, A. M., Epstein, C. J., and Basbaum, A.I. (1998). Primary afferent tachykinins are required to experience moderate to intense pain [see comments]. *Nature* **392(6674),** 390–394.
18. Mantyh, P. W., Rogers, S. D., Honore, P., et al. (1997). Inhibition of hyperalgesia by ablation of lamina I spinal neurons expressing the substance P receptor. *Science* **278(5336),** 275–279.
19. Nichols, M. L., Allen, B. J, Rogers, S. D., et al. (1999) Transmission of chronic nociception by spinal neurons expressing the substance P receptor. *Science* **286(5444),** 1558–1561.
20. de Jong, R. H., Robles, R., and Morikawa, K. I. (1969) Actions of halothane and nitrous oxide on dorsal horn neurons ("The Spinal Gate"). *Anesthesiology* **31,** 205–212.
21. Woods, J. W. (1964) Behavior of chronic decerebrate rats. *J. Neurophysiol.* **27,** 635–644
22. Lovick, T. A. (1972) The behavioural repertoire of precollicular decerebrate rats. *J. Physiol.* **226,** 4P–6P.
23. Sessler, D. I., Israel, D., Pozos, R. S., Pozos, M., and Rubinstein, E. H. (1988) Spontaneous post-anesthetic tremor does not resemble thermoregulatory shivering. *Anesthesiology* **68,** 843–850.
24. Lang, E., Kapila, A., Shlugman, D., Hoke, J. F., Sebel, P. S., and Glass, P. S. (1996) Reduction of isoflurane minimal alveolar concentration by remifentanil. *Anesthesiology* **85,** 721–728.
25. Drasner, K., Bernards, C. M., and Ozanne, G. M. (1988) Intrathecal morphine reduces the minimum alveolar concentration of halothane in humans. *Anesthesiology* **69,** 310–312.
26. Valverde, A., Dyson, D. H., and McDonell, W. N. (1989) Epidural morphine reduces halothane MAC in the dog. *Can. J. Anesth.* **36(6),** 629–632.
27. Licina, M. G., Schubert, A., Tobin, J. E., Nicodemus, H. F., and Spitzer, L. (1991) Intrathecal morphine does not reduce minimum alveolar concentration of halothane in humans: results of a double-blind study. *Anesthesiology* **74,** 660–663.
28. Archer, D. P., Ewen, A., Roth, S. H., and Samanani, N. (1994) Plasma, brain, and spinal cord concentrations of thiopental associated with hyperalgesia in the rat. *Anesthesiology* **80,** 168–176.
29. Zhang, Y., Eger, E. I., 2nd, Dutton, R. C., and Sonner, J. M. (2000) Inhaled anesthetics have hyperalgesic effects at 0.1 minimum alveolar anesthetic concentration *Anesthesia and Analgesia* **91,** 462–466.
30. Petersen-Felix, S., Arendt-Nielsen, L., Bak, P., Fisher, M., and Zbinden, A. M. (1996) Psychophysical and electrophysiological responses to experimental pain may be influenced by sedation: comparison of the effects of a hypnotic (propofol) and an analgesic (alfentanil). *Brit. J. Anaesth.* **77,** 165–171.
31. Wilder-Smith, O. H. G., Kolletzki, M., and Wilder-Smith, C. H. (1995) Sedation with intravenous infusions of propofol or thiopentone. Effects on pain perception. *Anaesthesia* **50,** 218–222.

32. Campbell, J. N., Raja, S. N., and Meyer, R. A. (1984) Halothane sensitizes cutaneous nociceptors in monkeys. *J. Neurophysiol.* **52(4)**, 762–770.
33. Antognini, J. F., Wang, X. W., Piercy, M., and Carstens, E. (2000) Propofol directly depresses lumbar dorsal horn neuronal responses to noxious stimulation in goats. *Canadian J. Anaesth.* **47**, 273–279.
34. Sudo, M., Sudo, S., Chen, X. G., Piercy, M., Carstens, E., and. Antognini, J. F. (2001) Thiopental directly depresses lumbar dorsal horn neuronal responses to noxious mechanical stimulation in goats. *Acta Anaesthesiologica Scandinavica* **45**, 823–839.
35. de Jong, R. H., Hershey, W. N., and Wagman, I. H. (1967) Measurement of a spinal reflex response (H-reflex) during general anesthesia in man. Association between reflex depression and muscular relaxation. *Anesthesiology* **28**, 382–389.
36. Rampil, I. J. and King, B. S. (1996) Volatile anesthetics depress spinal motor neurons. *Anesthesiology* **85**, 129–134.
37. Leis, A. A., Stetkarova, I., Beric, A., and Stokic, D. S. (1996) The relative sensitivity of F wave and H reflex to changes in motoneuronal excitability. *Muscle Nerve* **19**, 1342–1344.
38. Friedman, Y., King, B. S., and Rampil, I. J. (1996) Nitrous oxide depresses spinal F waves in rats. *Anesthesiology* **85**, 135–141.
39. King, B. S. and Rampil, I. J. (1994) Anesthetic depression of spinal motor neurons may contribute to lack of movement in response to noxious stimuli. *Anesthesiology* **81**, 1484–1492.
40. Zhou, H. H., Jin, T. T., Qin, B., and Turndorf, H. (1998) Suppression of spinal cord motoneuron excitability correlates with surgical immobility during isoflurane anesthesia. *Anesthesiology* **88**, 955–961.
41. Zhou, H. H., Mehta, M., and Leis, A. A. (1997) Spinal cord motoneuron exci30tability during isoflurane and nitrous oxide anesthesia. *Anesthesiology* **86**, 302–307.
42. Kakinohana, M., Motonaga, E., Taira, Y., and Okuda, Y. (2000) [The effects of intravenous anesthetics, propofol, fentanyl and ketamine on the excitability of spinal motoneuron in human: an F-wave study] Masui. *Japanese J. Anesthesiol.* **49(6)**, 596–601.
43. Antognini, J. F., Carstens, E., and Buzin, V. (1999) Isoflurane depresses motoneuron excitability by a direct spinal action: an F-wave study. *Anesth. Analg.* **88**, 681–685.
44. Gupta, D. K., King, B., and Rampil, I. J. (2000) The effects of the Thiopental on spinal motor neurons. *Anesth. Analg.* S416.
45. Soriano, S. G., Logigian, E. L., Scott, R. M., Prahl, P. A., and Madsen, J. R. (1995) Nitrous oxide depresses the H-reflex in children with cerebral palsy. *Anesthesia and Analgesia* **80**, 239–241.
46. de Jong, R. H. and Wagman, I. H. (1968) Block of afferent impulses in the dorsal horn of monkey. A possible mechanism of anesthesia. *Exp. Neurology* **20**, 352–358.
47. de Jong R. H., Robles, R., and Heavner, J. E. (1970) Suppression of impulse transmission in the cat's dorsal horn by inhalation anesthetics. *Anesthesiology* **2**, 440–445.
48. Antognini, J. F., Carstens, E., Tabo, E., and Buzin, V. (1998) The effect of differential delivery of isoflurane to head and torso on lumbar dorsal horn activity. *Anesthesiol.* **88**, 1055–1061.
49. Jinks, S., Antognini, J. F., Carstens, E., Buzin, V., and Simons, C. (1999) Isoflurane can indirectly depress lumbar dorsal horn activity in the goat via action within the brain. *Brit. J. Anaesth.* **82**, 244–249.
50. Kitahata, L. M., Ghazi-Saidi, K., Yamashita, M., Kosaka, Y., Bonikos, C., and Taub, A. (1975) The depressant effect of halothane and sodium thiopental on the spontaneous and evoked activity of dorsal horn cells: lamina specificity, time course and dose dependence. *J. Pharmacol. Exp. Therapeutics* **195**, 515–521.
51. Kishikawa, K., Uchida, H., Yamamori, Y., and Collins, J. G. (1995) Low-threshold neuronal activity of spinal dorsal horn neurons increases during REM sleep in cats: comparison with effects of anesthesia. *J. Neurophysiol.* **74**, 763–769.
52. Taub, A., Hoffert, M., and Kitahata, L. M. (1974) Lamina-specific suppression and acceleration of dorsal-horn unit activity by nitrous oxide: a statistical analysis. *Anesthesiology* **40**, 24–31.
53. Utsumi, J., Adachi, T., Miyazaki, Y., et al (1997). The effect of xenon on spinal dorsal horn neurons: a comparison with nitrous oxide, Anesthesia and Analgesia, **84**, 1372–1376.
54. Miyazaki, Y., Adachi, T., Utsumi, J., Shichino, T., and Segawa, H., (1999). Xenon has greater inhibitory effects on spinal dorsal horn neurons than nitrous oxide in spinal cord transected cats, Anesthesia and Analgesia **88**, 893–897.
55. Antognini, J. F., Chen, X. G., Sudo, M., Sudo, S., and Carstens, E. (2001) Variable effects of nitrous oxide at multiple levels of the central nervous system in goats *Vet. Res. Comm.* **25**, 523–538.
56. Uchida, H., Kishikawa, K., and Collins, J. G. (1995) Effect of propofol on spinal dorsal horn neurons. Comparison with lack of ketamine effects. *Anesthesiology* **83(6)**, 1312–1322.
57. Sherrington, C. S. (1910) Flexion-reflex of the limb, crossed extension reflex and reflex stepping and standing. *J. Physiol.* **40**, 28–121.
58. Carstens, E. and Campbell, I. G. (1998) Parametric and pharmacological studies of midbrain suppression of the hindlimb flexion withdrawal reflex in the rat. *Pain* **33**, 201–213.
59. Carstens, E. and Ansley, D. (1993) Hindlimb flexion withdrawal evoked by noxious heat in conscious rats: magnitude measurement of stimulus-response function, suppression by morphine, and habituation. *J. Neurophysiol.* **70**, 621–629.
60. Carstens, E. and Douglass, D. K. (1995) Midbrain suppression of limb withdrawal and tail flick reflexes in the rat: correlates with descending inhibition of sacral spinal neurons. *J. Neurophys.* **73**, 2179–2194.
61. Carstens, E. and Wilson, C. G. (1993) Rattail flick reflex: magnitude measurement of stimulus-response function, suppression by morphine, and habituation. *J. Neurophysiol.* **70**, 630–639.
62. Carstens, E. (1993) Quantitative assessment of nocifensive behavioral responses and the underlying neuronal circuitry. *Der Schmerz* **7**, 204–215.
63. Carstens, E. and Campbell, I. G. (1992) Responses of motor units during the hind limb flexion withdrawal reflex evoked by noxious skin heating: phasic and prolonged suppression by midbrain stimulation and comparison with simultaneously recorded dorsal horn units. *Pain* **48**, 215–226.

64. Carstens, E., Hartung, M., Stelzer, B., and Zimmermann, M. (1990) Suppression of a hindlimb flexion reflex by micro-injection of glutamate or morphine into the periaqueductal gray in the rat. *Pain* **43**, 105–112.
65. Schomburg, E. D. (1990) Spinal sensorimotor systems and their supraspinal control. *Neurosci. Res.* **7**, 265–340.
66. Schouenborg, J. and Kalliomäki, J. (1990) Functional organization of the nociceptive withdrawal reflexes. I. Activation of hindlimb muscles in the rat. *Exper. Brain Res.* **83 (1)**, 67–78.
67. Schouenborg, J., Weng, H. R., and Holmberg, H. (1994) Modular organization of spinal nociceptive reflexes. *News Physiol. Sci.* **9**, 261–265.
68. Schouenborg, J. and Weng, H. R. (1994) Sensorimotor transformation in a spinal motor system. *Exp. Brain Res.* **100(1)**, 170–174.
69. Andersen, O. K., Sonnenborg, F. A., and Arendt-Nielsen, L. (1999) Modular organization of human leg withdrawal reflexes elicited by electrical stimulation of the foot sole. *Muscle and Nerve* **22(11)**, 1520–1530.
70. Sonnenborg, F. A., Andersen, O. K., and Arendt-Nielsen, L. (2000) Modular organization of excitatory and inhibitory reflex receptive fields elicited by electrical stimulation of the foot sole in man. *Clin. Neurophysiol.* **111(12)**, 2160–2169.
71. Willer, J. C. (1985) Studies on pain. Effects of morphine on a spinal nociceptive flexion reflex and related pain sensation in man. *Brain Res.* **331(1)**, 105–114.
72. Antognini J. F. and Kien N. D. (1995) Potency (minimum alveolar anesthetic concentration) of isoflurane is independent of peripheral anesthetic effects. *Anesth. Analg.* **81**, 69–72.
73. Weakly, J. N. (1969) Effect of barbiturates on 'quantal' synaptic transmission in spinal motoneurones. *J. Physiol.* **204(1)**, 63–77.
74. Bras, H., Cavallari, P., Jankowska, E., and Kubin, L. (1989) Morphology of midlumbar interneurones relaying information from group II muscle afferents in the cat spinal cord. *J. Comp. Neurol.* **290**, 1–15
75. Jankowska, E. and Edgley, S. (1993) Interactions between pathways controlling posture and gait at the level of spinal interneurones in the cat. *Progress in Brain Research* **97**, 161–171.
76. Morgan, M. M. (1998) Direct comparison of heat-evoked activity of nociceptive neurons in the dorsal horn with the hindpaw withdrawal reflex in the rat. *J. Neurophysiol.* **79**, 174–80.
77. Schouenborg, J., Weng, H. R., Kalliomäki, J., and Holmberg, H. (1995) A survey of spinal dorsal horn neurones encoding the spatial organization of withdrawal reflexes in the rat. *Exper. Brain Res.* **106(1)**, 19–27.
78. Nishioka, K., Harada, Y., Kitahata, L. M., Tsukahara, S., and Collins J. G. (1995) Role of WDR neurons in a hind limb noxious heat evoked flexion withdrawal reflex. *Life Sci.* **56**, 485–489.
79. Antognini, J. F., Wang, X. W., and Carstens, E. (1999) Quantitative and qualitative effects of isoflurane on movement occurring after noxious stimulation. *Anesthesiology* **91**, 1064–1071.
80. Antognini, J. F. and Carstens, E. (1999). Increasing isoflurane from 0.9 to 1.1 minimum alveolar concentration minimally affects dorsal horn cell responses to noxious stimulation. *Anesthesiology* **90**, 208–214.
81. Wheeler-Aceto, H. and Cowan, A. (1991) Standardization of the rat paw formalin test for the evaluation of analgesics. *Psychopharmacology* **104**, 35–44.
82. Cooper, B. Y. and Vierck, C. J., Jr. (1986) Measurement of pain and morphine hypalgesia in monkeys. *Pain* **26(3)**, 361–392.
83. Harris, J. A. (1998) Using c-fos as a neural marker of pain. *Brain Res. Bull.* **45**, 1–8.
84. Herrera, D. G. and Robertson, H. A. (1996) Activation of c-fos in the brain. *Progr. Neurobiol.* **50**, 83–107.
85. Hunt, S. P., Pini, A., and Evan, G. (1987) Induction of c-fos-like protein in spinal cord neurones following sensory stimulation. *Nature* **328**, 632–634.
86. Sun, W. Z., Shyu, B. C., and Shieh, J. Y. (1996) Nitrous oxide or halothane, or both, fail to suppress c-fos expression in rat spinal cord dorsal horn neurones after subcutaneous formalin. *Br. J. Anaesth.* **76**, 99–105.
87. Hagihira, S., Taenaka, N., and Yoshiya, I. (1997) Inhalational anesthetics suppress expression of c-fos protein evoked by noxious somatic stimulation in the deeper layer of the spinal cord in the rat. *Brain Res.* **751**, 124–130.
88. Zhai, Q. Z. and Traub, R. J. (1999) The NMDA receptor antagonist MK-801 attenuates c-Fos expression in the lumbosacral spinal cord following repetitive noxious and non-noxious colorectal distention. *Pain* **83**, 321–329.
89. Huang, W. and Simpson, R. K. (1999) Intrathecal treatment with MK-801 suppresses thermal nociceptive responses and prevents c-fos immunoreactivity induced in rat lumbar spinal cord neurons. *Neurol. Res.* **21**, 593–598.
90. Scheller, M.S., Zornow, M. H., Fleischer, J. E., Shearman, G. T., and Greber, T. F. (1989) The noncompetitive N-methyl-D-aspartate receptor antagonist, MK-801 profoundly reduces volatile anesthetic requirements in rabbits. *Neuropharmacology* **28**, 677–681.
91. Munson, E. S., Saidman, L. J., and Eger, E. I. (1965) Effect of nitrous oxide and morphine on the minimum anesthetic concentration of fluroxene. *Anesthesiology* **26**, 134–139.
92. Loewy, A. D. (1998) Viruses as transneuronal tracers for defining neural circuits. *Neurosci. Biobehav. Rev.* **22(6)**, 679–684.
93. Rotto-Percelay, D. M., Wheeler, J. G., Osorio, F. A., Platt, K. B., and Loewy, A. D. (1992) Transneuronal labeling of spinal interneurons and sympathetic preganglionic neurons after pseudorabies virus injections in the rat medial gastrocnemius muscle. *Brain Research* **574(1–2)**, 291–306.
94. Eger, E. I., Saidman, L. J., and Brandstater, B. (1965) Minimum alveolar anesthetic concentration: a standard of anesthetic potency. *Anesthesiology* **26**, 756–763.
95. Gordon, J. (1991) Spinal mechanisms of motor coordination. In: Principles of Neuroscience, 3rd Ed. (Kandel, E., Schwartz, and Jessel, eds.) Elsevier, NewYork. pp. 581–607.
96. Pearson, K. (1976) The control of walking. *Scien. Amer.* **235**, 72–86.
97. Fukson, O. I., Berkinblit, M. B., and Feldman, A. G. (1980) The spinal frog takes into account the scheme of its body during the wiping reflex. *Science* **209**, 1261–1263.
98. Christie, J. M., O'Lenic, T. D., and Cane, R. D. (1996) Head turning in brain death. *J. Clin. Anesth.* **8**, 141–143.

99. Grillner, S. and Wallen, P. (1985) Central pattern generators for locomotion, with special reference to vertebrates. *Ann. Rev. Neurosci.* **8,** 233–2361.

100. Sigvardt, K. A. and Williams, T. L. (1996) Effects of local oscillator frequency on intersegmental coordination in the lamprey locomotor CPG: Theory and experiment. *J. Neurophysiol.* **76,** 4094–4103.

101. Grillner, S. and Shik, M. L. (1973) On the descending control of lumborsacral spinal cord from the "mesencephalic locomotor region". *Acta Physiol. Scand.* **87,** 320–333.

102. Yamamura, T., Stevens, W. C., Okamura, A., Harada, K., and Kemmotsu, O. (1993) Correlative study of behavior and synaptic events during halothane anesthesia in the lampry. *Anesth. Analg.* **76,** 342–347.

103. Franks, N. P., and Lieb, W. R. (1996) Temperature dependence of the potency of volatile general anesthetics. Implications for in vitro experiments. *Anesthesiology* **84,** 716–720.

104. Yamamura, T., Harada, K., Okamura, A., and Kemmotsu, O. (1990) Is the site of action of ketamine anesthesia the N-methyl-D-aspartate receptor? *Anesthesiology* **72,** 704–710.

105. Yamamori, Y., Kishikawa, K., and Collins, J. G. (1995) Halothane effects on low-threshold receptive field size of rat spinal dorsal horn neurons appear to be independent of supraspinal modulatory systems. *Brain Res.* **702,** 162–168.

106. Handwerker, H. O., Iggo, A., and Zimmermann, M. (1975) Segmental and supraspinal actions on dorsal horn neurons responding to noxious and non-noxious skin stimuli. *Pain* **1,** 147–165.

107. Lin, Q., Peng, Y. B., and Willis, W. D. (1996a) Antinociception and inhibition from the periaqueductal gray are mediated in part by spinal 5-hydroxytryptamine (1A) receptors. *J. Pharmacol. Exp. Ther.* **276,** 958–967.

108. Lin, Q., Peng, Y. B., and Willis, W. D. (1996b) Role of GABA receptor subtypes in inhibition of primate spinothalamic tract neurons: difference between spinal and periaqueductal gray inhibition. *J. Neurophysiol.* **75,** 109–123.

109. Peng, Y. B., Lin, Q., and Willis, W. D. (1996a) The role of 5-HT3 receptors in periaqueductal gray-induced inhibition of nociceptive dorsal horn neurons in rats. *J. Pharmacol. Exp. Ther.* **276,** 116–124.

110. Peng, Y. B., Lin, Q., and Willis, W. D. (1996b) Effects of GABA and glycine receptor antagonists on the activity and PAG-induced inhibition of rat dorsal horn neurons. *Brain Res.* **736,** 189–201.

111. Peng, Y. B., Lin, Q., and Willis, W. D. (1996c.) Involvement of alpha-2 adrenoceptors in the periaqueductal gray-induced inhibition of dorsal horn cell activity in rats. *J. Pharmacol. Exp. Ther.* **278,** 125–135.

112. Yeung, J. C. and Rudy, T. A. (1980) Multiplicative interaction between narcotic agonisms expressed at spinal and supraspinal sites of antinociceptive action as revealed by concurrent intrathecal intracerebroventricular injections of morphine. *J. Pharmacol. Exp. Ther.* **215,** 633–642.

113. Fields, H. L., Heinricher, M. M., and Mason, P. (1991) Neurotransmitters in nociceptive modulatory circuits. *Ann. Rev. Neurosci.* **14,** 219–245.

114. Fields, H. L., Malick, A., and Burstein, R. (1995) Dorsal horn projection targets of ON and OFF cells in the rostral ventromedial medulla. *J.Neurophysiol.* **74,** 1742–1759.

115. Heinricher, M. M., Morgan, M. M., and Fields, H. L. (1992) Direct and indirect actions of morphine on medullary neurons that modulate nociception. *Neuroscience* **48,** 533–543.

116. Leung, C. G. and Mason, P. (1995) Effects of isoflurane concentration on the activity of pontomedullary raphe and medial reticular neurons in the rat. *Brain Research* **699,** 71–82.

117. Eger, E. I., Koblin, D. D., Harris, R. A., et al. (1997) Hypothesis: inhaled anesthetics produce immobility and amnesia by different mechanisms at different sites. *Anesth. Analg.* **84,** 915–918.

118. Mantyh, P., Rogers, S. D., Honore, P., et al. (1997) Inhibition of hyperalgesia by ablation of lamina I spinal neurons expressing the substance P receptor. *Science* **278,** 275–279.

12

Spinal Cord–Dorsal Horn

J. G. Collins

INTRODUCTION

Although the scientific method is designed to test hypotheses rather than to discover a scientific truth, it is easy to fall into the trap of assuming that we finally understand how a biological system operates (the truth). In an effort to avoid that trap, this chapter begins with several statements about assumptions that underlie most of the work to which references will be made.

The first assumption is that the number of action potentials produced by a neuron encodes information. It is widely assumed that the firing frequency of a neuron conveys a message and, therefore, a change in that frequency will change or perhaps destroy the message. While there is much support for frequency coding, we should not assume that the number of action potentials or even the presence or absence of an action potential is the only way that a neuron transmits information. A recent review *(1)* highlights likely biochemical means of neuronal information handling independent of voltage signals. Without exception, the work discussed in this chapter is focused on changes in voltage-dependent signals. Future scientists are likely to view our current understanding of neuronal information transmission in a very different way.

The second assumption is that general anesthetics alter information flow by actions at synapses, rather than by actions on axons. Although that assumption is supported by early studies of general anesthetics *(2,3)*, the implications for this chapter could be significant. Much of the electrophysiology upon which this chapter is based is derived from extracellular recordings of activity assumed to be generated in or near cell bodies. We assume that if an action potential is recorded near a cell body of a neuron in the spinal dorsal horn, that action potential has survived an anesthetic effect and will be transmitted to the terminals of the cell's axon to participate in the passage of information at the next synapse. However, it is likely that axonal branching points have a greater sensitivity to signal alteration than is currently appreciated *(4)*. It is, therefore, possible that changes seen at the cell body may not accurately reflect what reaches the next synapse.

The third assumption is that experiments conducted in an animal model with associated interventions to allow for the experiment (anesthesia, surgery, decerebration, etc.) accurately reflect the human condition when a general anesthetic is used in a clinical setting. However, preparation of the animal for the experiment may alter the system under study. It was reported that the degree of surgical preparation of an animal altered spinal neuronal sensitivity to general anesthetics *(5)*. The animal models in use today, of necessity, include uncontrolled variables that may confound our interpretation of anesthetic effects at the level of the spinal cord.

Recognizing both the limitations of the above assumptions as well as the likely limits of our current knowledge, it is still possible to propose reasonable hypotheses about the importance of anesthetic actions on spinal dorsal horn neurons. The history of studies of anesthetic effects is bracketed

From: *Contemporary Clinical Neuroscience:* Neural Mechanisms of Anesthesia
Edited by: Joseph F. Antognini et al. © Humana Press Inc., Totowa, NJ

by reports that suggest possible physiological significance of anesthetic actions on the spinal dorsal horn. Wall *(6)* and deJong *(7)* proposed that general anesthetic actions at the level of the spinal dorsal horn may contribute to anesthesia. Most recently, Antognini and colleagues *(8)* reported that isoflurane acts in the spinal cord to blunt transmission of noxious inputs to the thalamus and cerebral cortex, and thus might indirectly contribute to anesthetic end points such as amnesia and unconsciousness. To better understand how this could happen, we will first consider the anatomy and physiology of the spinal dorsal horn. This chapter does not provide an exhaustive catalog of all published studies of aesthetic effects on spinal dorsal horn neurons. Rather, it contains selected references that support the author's view of our current state of understanding of the implications of general anesthetic depression of spinal dorsal horn neurons.

SPINAL DORSAL HORN ANATOMY AND PHYSIOLOGY

It is widely assumed that general anesthetic disruption of information transmission within the spinal dorsal horn contributes to general anesthesia. Dubner and Bennett *(9)* described the spinal dorsal horn and its homolog, the trigeminal system, as consisting of three major components: (1) central terminals of primary afferents; (2) output and intrinsic neurons; (3) terminals of extrinsic neurons that modulate activity of other neurons.

That verbal image is reproduced in Fig. 1, revealing the potentially important role the spinal dorsal horn plays in the handling of information about both the outside world and the interior status of the animal. If general anesthetics have important actions at synapses, then the spinal dorsal horn is where both the first synapse between many primary afferents and the central nervous system occurs, as well as the site where modulatory systems exist to influence those synapses.

In the early 1950s, Rexed described a laminar organization of the cell bodies within the spinal cord *(10,11)* based upon cytoarchitectonic detail. The spinal dorsal horn is composed of Rexed laminae 1–6 and for this chapter, the focus will be limited to cell bodies located within those 6 Rexed laminae.

Primary Afferent Input to the Spinal Dorsal Horn

Primary afferents that make an initial synapse within the spinal dorsal horn include fibers of all sizes, from the largest myelinated A-fibers to the smallest unmyelinated C-fibers. Primary afferents that synapse on second order neurons in the spinal dorsal horn are associated with receptors in all tissues of the body, and convey information about cutaneous touch, temperature, pain, visceral sensations, and muscle and joint sensations, including proprioception *(12–19)*. Those anatomical connections provide potential sites of action for general anesthetics that could result in changes in the central processing of information about all these sensations. However, not all of those sensations are transmitted exclusively through the dorsal horn. As an example, many primary afferents communicating information about light touch travel directly to the dorsal column nuclei by the dorsal column pathways. Anesthetic effects in the dorsal horn would not directly influence those pathways, although the first synapse made within the dorsal column nuclei provides a likely potential site of action for general anesthetics as well.

A consideration of the anatomy and physiology of the output from the dorsal horn will provide a better appreciation of the systems likely to be influenced by anesthetic actions on synapses within the spinal dorsal horn *(14,18,19)*. Table 1 contains a listing of major ascending tracks that derive input from spinal dorsal horn neurons as well as the types of natural stimulation known to activate the spinal dorsal horn neurons that contribute to those specific pathways. These ascending tracts are in addition to the obvious connections to motor output that originate in the spinal dorsal horn. If general anesthetics can reduce or block the response of spinal dorsal horn second order neurons to activation by primary and afferents, then it is reasonable to assume the sensory modalities represented in Table 1 may be disrupted by general anesthetic actions on the spinal dorsal horn.

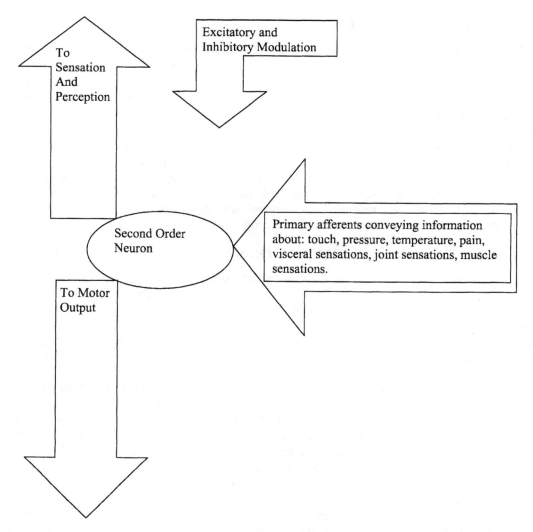

Fig. 1. Outline of Spinal Dorsal Horn Sensory Transmission.

Table 1
Major Ascending Tracts Derived from Spinal Dorsal Horn Neurons

Tract	*Cells of origin activated by:*
Postsynaptic dorsal column pathway	Hair movement, pressure or pinch of the skin or underlying tissue.
Spinocervicothalamic tract	Hair movement, pressure or pinch of the skin or underlying tissue.
Spinothalamic tract	Noxious (heating, cooling, mechanical, chemical) and non-noxious stimulation of skin, viscera, and muscles, proprioceptive stimuli.
Spinomesencephalic tract	Noxious and non-noxious stimulation of skin, joints and muscle.
Spinoreticular tract	Noxious and non-noxious stimulation of skin, joints, periosteum, muscle, tendons, and viscera.

Descending Modulatory Systems

The anatomy and physiology of the spinal dorsal horn contains one additional component that may serve as an important target for general anesthetic actions. As depicted in Fig. 1, in addition to sending information to motor neurons and supraspinal centers, the dorsal horn is a site of modulation by either propriospinal or descending modulatory systems. Modulation of neurons that give rise to the spinothalamic tract is an example of such an action. Willis and Coggeshall *(18)* listed the following sites that could exert either an inhibitory (nucleus raphe magnus, medullary reticular formation, periaquaductal gray and adjacent midbrain reticular formation, regions of the cerebral cortex) or an excitatory (medullary reticular formation, regions of the cerebral cortex) effect on spinal dorsal horn spinothalamic tract neurons. Descending pathways from those supraspinal regions ultimately synapse on spinothalamic tract neurons, and exert both tonic and phasic control of their activity. Anesthetic actions on those modulatory systems, either suprspinally, or within the doral horn, may also be responsible for anesthetic induced changes in behavior.

EFFECTS OF GENERAL ANESTHETICS ON SPINAL DORSAL HORN NEURONS

Neurons of the spinal dorsal horn that respond to activation of the peripheral terminals of primary afferents have been divided into several broad categories. The first category is composed of neurons that respond maximally to low intensity stimuli (usually mechanical). They also respond to high intensity stimuli, but the ceiling of their response is quite low, resulting in no increase in response as the intensity of the stimulus increases. We will refer to those neurons as low threshold (LT) neurons. The second category is made up of neurons that only respond to high intensity stimuli (many modalities). Those neurons do not become activated until the stimulus at the peripheral end of the primary afferent is approaching or has reached a tissue damaging intensity. We will refer to those neurons as high threshold (HT) neurons. The third category encompasses characteristics of the first two. These neurons will respond weakly to low intensity stimuli of many modalities but will have an increasing rate of response as the stimulus intensity increases with a maximum response occurring when stimuli are in the noxious range. We will refer to those neurons as wide dynamic range (WDR) or multi-receptive (MR) neurons. The last category responds to joint and muscle stimulation and will be referred to as proprioceptive neurons.

In spite of the fact that almost 35 yr have passed since initial reports of general anesthetic effects on spinal sensory neurons, there is a relative dearth of information about those anesthetic effects. This can be attributed to an initial recognition that opioids, as well as general anesthetics, could block the response of spinal dorsal horn neurons to peripheral receptive field stimulation *(20–22)*. The resulting focus on spinal opioid analgesia drew researchers away from studies of general anesthetic effects on those systems.

There are, however, some studies that provide insight into general anesthetic actions on the spinal dorsal horn. Initial studies of general anesthetic actions on spinal dorsal horn neurons revealed that depression of neuronal activity was generally seen *(7,23–29)*. In some of the earlier studies, emphasis was placed on either spontaneous activity or drug effects on neurons of a particular Rexed lamina. The laminar focus was owing to the assumption, later proven incorrect, that laminar organization reflected physiological function. That concept was, however, soon replaced by the realization that the response profile of a neuron to natural stimulation of peripheral receptive fields was a better way to define the physiologic function of the neuron. As more emphasis was placed on a neuron's response to natural stimuli, it became apparent that anesthetics could depress responses to both non-noxious and noxious receptive field stimulation e.g., ref. *25.* Later studies confirmed and expanded on these earlier reports. Of relevance to this chapter, we need to know if general anesthetics can depress the four types of neurons that we described above. Recall that one of the classes of neurons, the WDR neuron, responds to both non-noxious and noxious stimuli, a fact that was not appreciated during the earliest anesthetic studies. Although, in early studies, responses to both noxious and non-noxious stimuli were reported to be depressed, it was not always possible to determine the cell type from which recordings were being made.

LT NEURONS

General anesthetics can depress the response of spinal dorsal horn LT neurons to receptive field stimulation. Halothane has been shown to depress the response of LT neurons in an awake cat preparation, as well as in an acute rat preparation *(30,31)*. Not only was the response of the neurons diminished, but the receptive field area on the skin from which responses could be elicited was reduced in size. The effect appeared to be dose dependent and independent of supraspinal modulatory systems. However, Herrero and Headley *(32)* reported that the receptive field size in sheep was increased by halothane, suggesting possible species differences.

WDR Neurons

The responses of WDR neurons to both noxious and non-noxious stimuli have been reported to be depressed by, among other anesthetic agents, xenon *(33)* and halothane *(31,32)* in rats, cats, and sheep. As with LT neurons, both the response of the neurons and the receptive field area from which activity was elicited was decreased, although a reduction in the receptive field area was not seen in sheep *(32)*. Responses of WDR neurons to noxious visceral stimulation (colorectal distention) have also been observed (Collins et al., unpublished observation).

HT Neurons/Proprioceptive Neurons

We are unaware of any systematic studies of general anesthetic effects on HT spinal dorsal horn neurons or proprioceptive neurons. However, limited unpublished work in our laboratory demonstrated halothane depression of HT neurons, and proprioceptive neuronal responses to natural stimulation.

The above brief review of general anesthetic effects paints a very simplistic picture in need of challenging. Do all anesthetics produce similar effects? Do general anesthetics always depress spinal dorsal horn neurons? The answer to both questions is no, as demonstrated by published studies and additional unpublished work from our laboratory. In one of the early studies of anesthetic effects on spinal dorsal horn neurons, Conseiller and colleagues *(27)* reported that ketamine depressed neuronal response to high intensity stimuli, but not responses to low intensity stimuli. However, neuronal types were not described. We repeated those experiments in an intact, awake animal preparation, and reported that anesthetic doses of ketamine did depress the response of WDR neurons to noxious stimuli, but did not alter the response of LT neurons to low threshold receptive field stimulation *(34)*. We have had an opportunity to examine a large number of general anesthetic agents, including halothane, enflurane, isoflurane, nitrous oxide, pentobarbital, propofol, and dexmetatomine, as well as ketamine. In all of those experiments, ketamine is the only general anesthetic which we have found not to depress the response of low threshold neurons to receptive field stimulation. As mentioned previously, halothane did not change the mechanical thresholds to low intensity stimuli in sheep *(32)*, nor did it change the threshold for noxious mechanical stimulation of HT neurons in the sheep. We must therefore conclude that anesthetic effects on spinal dorsal horn neurons are likely to be both drug and species specific, even though our general expectation is that neuronal responses will be depressed.

ARE DEPRESSIVE EFFECTS SIMPLY OWING TO LOSS OF CONSCIOUSNESS?

Although general anesthetics appear, in general, to depress the responses of spinal dorsal horn neurons to receptive field stimulation, we do not know for sure if the effect is the direct result of the drug or simply the result of drug induced sleep. A partial answer was obtained when effects of rapid eye movement (REM) sleep and propofol-induced sleep (anesthesia) were compared in the same animals on the same neurons *(35)*. The greatest sleep induced change in neuronal response to receptive field stimulation was apparent during REM sleep. Unlike motor neurons that are inhibited during REM sleep, spinal dorsal horn neurons demonstrated a greatly increased response. In spite of the fact that spinal dorsal horn neuronal responses to receptive field stimulation were greatly enhanced during REM sleep, when propofol was administered to the animal and the response of the same neuron was examined, the effect was in the opposite direction. Propofol produced profound depression of the neuron response. These opposite effects of REM sleep and propofol-induced sleep in the same neurons suggest that anesthetic depression of spinal dorsal horn neurons is not simply due to drug-induced loss of consciousness.

ANESTHETIC EFFECTS ON MODULATORY SYSTEMS

Figure 1 tells us that anesthetics may not only have a direct effect on the spinal dorsal horn, but may also influence those neurons by altering modulatory systems that impinge on them. In the early anesthetic studies, deJong and colleagues *(25)* reported that nitrous oxide could only depress noxiously-evoked activity in the spinal cord if the animals had an intact spinal cord. (Contrast that with the more recent studies by Antonini and colleagues and Rampil and colleagues *(36–39)* that support a primary spinal role for MAC. Recently, Maze and colleagues have confirmed these early observations and demonstrated that the analgesic effects of nitrous oxide result ultimately from activation of descending noradrenogeric systems capable of depressing the response of spinal dorsal horn neurons to noxious peripheral stimuli *(40)*.

Previously, we reported that pentobarbital unmasked the response of some spinal dorsal horn neurons to noxious peripheral stimuli *(41)*. When the neurons were studied in the awake drug-free animal, they did not respond to the test noxious stimulus. However, when the animal was anesthetized with pentobarbital, they did. This pentobarbital effect appeared to be dose-dependent, and was most apparent with lower doses. This would be in keeping with the clinical suggestion that low doses of barbiturates can increase rather than decrease an individual's response to noxious stimuli. We interpreted our findings to reflect an anesthetic induced disinhibition of tonic modulation resulting in an increased responsivity of neurons to peripheral receptive field stimulation.

Those two studies demonstrated that general anesthetics may influence spinal dorsal horn neurons indirectly by changing modulatory influences on them, as well as by acting directly on to the neurons from primary afferents.

IS IT REALLY THAT SIMPLE?

Figure 2 affords any opportunity to consider the implications of the studies cited above. If general anesthetics depress information transmission by second order neurons, either by a direct pre- or postsynaptic action (Number 1 in Fig. 2), or by actions on propriospinal or descending modulatory systems (Number 2 in Fig. 2) then the impact on sensory and motor output should be predictable. If we focus on pain input from primary afferents and use spinal opioid analgesia as a model for comparison, we would predict that with adequate depression of second order neurons, the sensation and perception of pain is eliminated (Number 3 in Fig. 2), along with the driving force for the reflex withdrawal to a painful stimulus (Number 4 in Fig. 2). While that assumption seems appropriate, there are a series of unanswered questions that must be addressed if we are to truly appreciate the impact of general anesthetics on the spinal dorsal horn.

The first question relates to the degree of depression necessary to completely block information transmission. How much of a change in stimulus-evoked activity is associated with a detectable change in behavior or sensation? This is an unanswered question of relevance to all parts of the

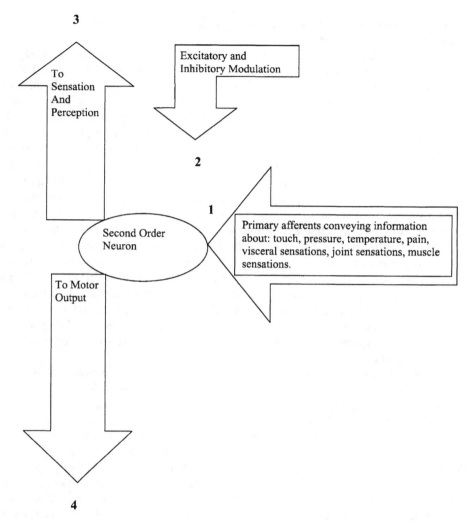

Fig. 2. Impact of anesthetic depression on spinal sensory neurons. Inhibitory influence on information transmission to (**1**) or modulation of (**2**) second order neurons should decrease sensations (**3**) and motor reponses (**4**).

nervous system. Namiki et al *(42)* reported that one MAC of halothane suppressed spinal WDR neuronal response to noxious thermal stimuli by approx 60%, whereas 1.5 MAC reduced the same response by 80%. Both numbers represent a population mean taken from a relatively small number of animals ($n = 12$–13). Can we assume that an 80% reduction in noxiously evoked activity is adequate to block a pain message? This question has yet to be answered.

The challenge we face in understanding the real impact of anesthetic actions on the spinal dorsal horn is perhaps best conveyed by a sequence of studies focused on the importance of the spinal cord in the production of MAC *(36–39)*. It has been assumed that the absence of a withdrawal reflex to a noxious stimulus reflects an adequate depth of anesthesia. In one of the original papers that defined MAC *(43)*, the authors state "We believe that in none of these or the subsequent studies did any dog suffer pain on application of these noxious stimuli." This belief is based on published and unpublished observations in man at similar depths of anesthesia. That assumption, i.e., that lack of a coordinated motor response to a noxious stimulus means an absence of the sensation of pain, although not often stated, has been widely associated with the concept of MAC. If the patient or animal does not move, then they do not feel pain.

If immobility in the presence of a noxious stimulus truly reflects the production of analgesia, then work by Rampil and colleagues *(36,38)* and Antognini and colleagues *(37,39)* should have had a profound effect on our understanding of how general anesthetics produce analgesia. In a series of elegant studies, those two laboratories demonstrated that MAC i.e., immobility in the presence of a noxious stimulus, was mainly, if not exclusively, the result of general anesthetic actions at the level of the spinal cord, with little or no involvement of anesthetic actions at supraspinal sites. If immobility was in fact analgesia, then the production of analgesia is due to mechanisms described by the earlier studies, i.e., depression of spinal dorsal horn neurons. Unfortunately, it does not appear to be that simple. As investigators continue to test hypotheses, Kendig and colleagues *(44)* threw the proverbial monkey wrench into the works. They reported that the inhalation anesthetic enflurane directly depresses the response of spinal motor neurons to simulation by excitatory neurotransmitters. With that report, previous assumptions that immobility was owing to block of pain singling in the spinal cord were formally challenged. In the extreme, the work from Kendig's lab exposed the possibility that the immobility was due exclusively to anesthetic depression of spinal motor neurons, totally unrelated to any anesthetic effects on spinal sensory neurons. In support of that possibility, Paik and colleagues reported that responses of spinal motor neurons to noxious primary afferent stimulation were much more sensitive to suppression by pentobarbital than were the responses of spinal dorsal horn neurons *(45)*. Additional support comes from the report by Carstens and Campbell *(48)* that barbiturate depression of spinal motor neurons was not always accompanied by depression of WDR spinal dorsal horn neurons.

This mounting doubt about the real impact of general anesthetics is compounded by our lack of understanding of spinal dorsal horn physiology and pharmacology. This is reflected in the fact that we still do not have a good appreciation of which spinal sensory neurons may be interacalated in the reflex pathways that cause withdrawal from a noxious stimulus. The interneurons that relay input from primary afferent nociceptors to motor neurons have not been identified. The literature has been focused on WDR neurons as most likely to be involved in passing information about noxious stimuli to spinal motor neurons *(47–50)*. However, Morgan has recently provided data that supports involvement of subsets of both HT and WDR neurons in nociceptive hind limb reflexes *(51,52)*. Morgan showed that only some HT and WDR neurons had response-latencies that were quick enough for them to participate in a noxious reflex that was occurring at the same time that the neuronal activity was being studied. He reported that only 41% of the HT neurons and 55% of the WDR neurons were active before the nociceptive reflex began.

To the best of our knowledge, there are no reports of studies in which it was determined if anesthetics were depressing neurons with short enough latencies to initiate a noxious reflex at the same time that the reflex was being recorded. Positive results of such a study would support, but not prove, a cause and effect relationship between an anesthetic depression of spinal sensory neurons and depression of a noxious reflex. However, negative results would support the hypothesis that anesthetic depression of spinal sensory neurons does not contribute to the depression of noxious reflexes.

We face a similar dearth of information about spinal sensory neurons associated with ascending fiber tracts, and therefore positioned to communicate information rostrally. We know that several ascending fiber tracts associated with information about noxious cutaneous stimuli originate in the spinal dorsal horn *(18)*. However, there is no information about anesthetic effects on cells that are known to transmit information rostrally. To add complexity to this situation, convincing anatomical studies have been published recently that strongly support the hypothesis that separate spinal nociceptive cell populations participate in information transmission for sensory vs motor functions, rather than having a common population of cells sharing those functions *(53)*. It is possible that anesthetic effects on the spinal dorsal horn HT and WDR neurons involved in nociceptive reflexes may be different than anesthetic effects on spinal dorsal horn HT and WDR neurons involved in the rostral transmission of information about noxious stimuli.

CONCLUSION

There is reasonable evidence that general anesthetics are capable of depressing information transmission at the level of the spinal dorsal horn. It is reasonable to hypothesize that the upstream systems (motor output and perception) will receive less information about the stimulus event as a result of that anesthetic action. It is, therefore, likely that future studies will confirm that anesthetic induced immobility in the presence of a noxious stimulus is due, at least in part, to drug actions on spinal dorsal horn neurons. It is also likely that future studies will reveal that anesthetic depression of spinal dorsal horn neurons, by reducing pain signals that reach supraspinally, contributes to reduced pain sensations. Likewise, reductions in information about other sensory modalities may be found to contribute to additional anesthetic actions (e.g. amnesia, loss of consciousness).

ACKNOWLEDGMENT

Work in the author's laboratory has been supported by grants from NIH-NIGMS.

REFERENCES

1. Katz, P. S. and Clemens, S. (2001) Biochemical networks in nervous systems: Expanding neuronal information capacity beyond voltage signals. *Trends Neurosci.* **24,** 18–25.
2. Larrabee, M. G. and Holaday, D. A. (1952) Depression of transmission through sympathetic ganglia during general anesthesia. *J. Pharm. Exp. Ther.* **105,** 400–408.
3. Larrabee, M .G. and Posternack, J. M. (1952) Selective actions of anesthetics on synapses and axons in mammalian sympathetic ganglia. *J. Neurophy.* **15,** 72–114.
4. Waikar, S. S., Thalhammer, J. G., Raymond, S. A., Huang, J. H., Change, D. S., and Strichartz, G. R. (1996) Mechanoreceptive afferents exhibit functionally-specific activity dependent changes in conduction velocity. *Brain Res.* **721,** 91–100.
5. Hartell, N. A. and Headley, P. M. (1991) Preparative surgery enhances the direct spinal actions of three injectable anesthetics in the anesthetized rat. *Pain* **24,** 75–80.
6. Wall, P. D. (1967) The mechanisms of general anesthesia. *Anesthesiology* **28,** 46–53.
7. deJong, R. H. and Wagman, I. H. (1968) Block of afferent impulses in the dorsal horn of monkey. a possible mechanism of anesthesia. *Exp. Neurol.* **20,** 352–358.
8. Antognini, J. F., Carstens, E., Sudo, M., and Sudo, S. (2000) Isoflurane depresses electroencephalographic and medial thalamic responses to noxious stimulation via an indirect spinal action. *Anesth. Analg.* **91,** 1282–1288.
9. Dubner, R. and Bennett, G. S. (1983) Spinal and trigeminal mechanisms of nociception. *Ann. Rev. Neurosci.* **6,** 381–418.
10. Rexed, B. (1952) The cytoarchitectonic organization of the spinal cord in the rat. *J. Comp. Neurol.* **96,** 415–466.
11. Rexed, B. (1954) The cytoarchitectonic organization of the spinal cord in the cat. *J. Comp. Neurol.* **100,** 297–380.
12. Light, A. R. and Perl, E. R. (1979) Spinal termination of functionally identified primary afferent neurons with slowly conducting myelinated fibers. *J. Comp. Neurol.* **186,** 133–150.
13. Cervero, F. and Iggo, A. (1980) The substantiagelatinosa of the spinal cord. A critical review. (1980) *Brain* **103,** 717–772.
14. Brown, A. G. (1981) Organization in the spinal cord: The anatomy and physiology of identified neurons. Springer-Verlag, Berlin.
15. Craig, A. D. and Mense, S. (1983) The distribution of afferent fibers from the gastrocnemius-soleus muscle in the dorsal horn of the cat, as revealed by the transport of horseradish peroxidase. *Neurosci. Lett.* **41,** 233–238.
16. Craig, A. D., Heppelmann, B., and Schaible, H. G. (1988) Projection of the medial and posterior articular nerves of the cat's knee to the spinal cord. *J. Comp. Neurol.* **266,** 279–288.
17. Sugiura, Y., Teruci, N., and Hosoya, Y. (1989) Differences in distribution of central terminals between visceral and somatic unmyelinated primary afferent fibers. *J. Neurophys.* **62,** 834–840.
18. Willis, W. D. and Coggeshall, R. E. (1991) Sensory mechanisms of the spinal cord, 2nd ed. Plenum, New York.
19. Davidoff, R. A. (ed.) (1987) Handbook of the spinal cord. Vol. 2–3. Anatomy and Physiology. New York.
20. Besson, J. M., Wyon-Maillard, M. C., Benoist, J. M., Conseiller, C., and Hamann, K. F. (1973) Effects of phenoperidine on lamina V cells in the cat dorsal horn. *J. Pharm. Exp. Ther.* **187,** 239–245.
21. Calvillo, O., Henry, J. L., and Neuman, R. S. (1974) Effects of morphine and naloxone on dorsal horn neurons in the cat. *Can. J. Physiol. Pharmacol.* **52,** 1207–1211.
22. Kitahata, L. M., Kosaka, Y., Taub, A., Bonikos, K., and Hoffert, M. (1974) Lamina-specific suppression of dorsal horn unit activity by morphine sulfate. *Anesthesiology* **41,** 39–48.
23. Wall, P. D. (1967) The laminar organization of dorsal horn and effects of descending impulses. *J. Physiol.* **188,** 403–423.
24. deJong, R.H., Robles, R., and Morikawa, K. (1969) Actions of halothane and nitrous oxide on dorsal horn neurons ('the spinal gate'). *Anesthesiology* **31,** 205–212.

25. deJong, R. H., Robles, R., and Heavner, J. E. (1970) Suppression of impulse transmission in the cat's dorsal horn by inhalation anesthetics. *Anesthesiology* **32,** 440–445.

26. Kitahata, L. M., Taub, A., and Sato, I. (1971) Lamina-specific suppression and facilitation of dorsal horn unit activity by nitrous oxide and by hyperventilation. *J. Pharmacol. Exp. Ther.* **176,** 101–108.

27. Conseiller, C., Benoist, J. M., Hamann, K. F., Maillard, M. C., and Besson, J. M. (1972) Effects of ketamine (C1581) on cell response to coetaneous stimulations in laminae IV and V in the cat's dorsal horn. *Europ. J. Pharmacol.* **18,** 346–353.

28. Kitahata, L. M., Taub, A., and Yosaka, Y. (1973) Lamina-specific suppression of dorsal horn unit activity by ketamine hydrochloride. *Anesthesiology* **38,** 4–11.

29. Heavner, J. E. and deJong, R. H., (1974) Modulation of dorsal horn throughput by anesthetics., in Pain Advances in Neurol, Vol. 4, (Bonica, J., ed.), Raven Press, New York, pp. 179–185.

30. Yamamori, Y., Kishikawa, K., and Collins, J. G. (1995) Halothane effects on low-threshold receptive field size of rat spinal dorsal horn neurons appear to be independent of supraspinal modulatory systems. *Brain Research* **702,** 162–168.

31. Ota, K., Yanagidani, T., Kishikawa, K., Yamamori, Y., and Collins, J. G. (1998) Cutaneous responsiveness of lumbar spinal dorsal horn neurons is reduced by general anesthesia, An effect dependent in part on GABA$_A$ mechanisms. *J. Neurophysiol.* **80,** 1383–1390.

32. Herrero, J. F. and Headley, P. M. (1995) Cutaneous responsiveness of lumbar spinal neurons in awake and halothane-anesthetized sheep. *J. Neurophysiology* **74,** 1549–1562.

33. Miyazaki, Y., Adache, T., Utsumi, J., Shidino, T., and Segawa, H. (1999) Xenon has greater inhibitory effects on spinal dorsal horn neurons than nitrous oxide in spinal cord transected cats. *Anesth. Analg.* **88,** 893–897.

34. Collins, J. G. (1986) Effects of ketamine on low threshold tactile sensory input are not dependent upon a spinal site of action. *Anesth. Analg.* **65,** 1123–1129.

35. Kishikawa, K., Uchida, H., Yamamori, Y., Collins, and J. G. (1995) Low-threshold neuronal activity of spinal dorsal horn neurons increases during REM sleep in cats: Comparison with effects of anesthesia. *J. Neurophys.* **74,** 743–769.

36. Rampil, I. S., Mason, P., and Singh, H. (1993) Anesthetic potency (MAC) is independent of forebrain structures in the rat. *Anesthesiology* **78,** 707–712.

37. Antognini, J. F. and Schwartz, K. (1993) Exaggerated anesthetic requirements in the preferentially anesthetized brain. *Anesthesiology* **79,** 1244–1249.

38. Rampil, I. J. (1994) Anesthetic potency is not altered after hypothermic spinal cord transection in rats. *Anesthesiology* **80,** 606–610.

39. Antognini, J. F. (1997) The relationship among brain, spinal cord and anesthetic requirements. *Med. Hypotheses* **48,** 83–87.

40. Zhang, C., Davies, M. F., Guo, T.-Z, and Maze, M. (1999) the analgesic action of nitrous oxide is dependent on the release of norepinephrine in the dorsal horn of the spinal cord. *Anesthesiology* **91,** 1401–1407.

41. Collins, J. G. and Ren, K. (1987) WDR response profiles of spinal dorsal horn neurons may be unmasked by barbiturate anesthesia. *Pain* **28,** 369–378.

42. Namiki, A., Collins, J. G., Kitahata, L. M., Kikuchi, H., Homma, E., and Thalhammer, J. G. (1980) Effects of halothane on spinal neuronal responses to graded noxious heat stimulation in the cat. *Anesthesiology* **53,** 475–480.

43. Eger, E. I., II, Saidman, L. J., and Brandstater, B. (1965) Minimum alveolar ansthetic concentration: A standard of anesthetic potency. *Anesthesiology* **26,** 756–763.

44. Cheng, G. and Kendig, J. J. (2000) Enflurane directly depresses glutamate AMPa and NMDA currents in mouse spinal cord motor neurons independent of actions on GABAA or glycine receptors. *Anesthesiology* **93,** 1075–1084.

45. Paik, K. S., Nam, S. C., and Chung, J. M. (1989) Different classes of cat spinal neurons display differential sensitivity to sodium pentobarbital. Neuroscience Research 23107–115.

46. Carstens, E. and Campbell, I. G. (1992) Responses of motor units during the hind limb flexion withdrawal reflex evoked by noxious skin heating: Phasic and prolonged suppression by midbrain stimulation and comparison with simultaneously recorded dorsal horn units. *Pain* **48,** 215–226.

47. Schonenburg, J. and Sjolun, B. H. (1983) Activity evoked by A- and C-afferent fibers in rat dorsal horn neurons and its relation to a flexion reflex. *J. Neurophysiol.* **50,** 1108–1121.

48. Schonenburg, J. and Dickenson, A. (1985) The effects of a distant noxious stimulation on A and C fibre-evoked flexion reflexes and neuronal activity in the dorsal horn of the rat. *Brain Res.* **320,** 23–32.

49. Falinower, S., Willer, J. C., Junien, J. L., and LeBars, D. (1994) A C-fiber reflex modulated by heterotropic noxious somatic stimuli in the rat. *J. Neurophys.* **72,** 194–213.

50. Nishioka, K., Harada, Y., Kitahata, L. M., Tsukahara, S., and Collins, J. G. (1995) Role of WDR neurons in a hind limb noxious neat evoked flexion withdrawal reflex. *Life Sci.* **56,** 485–489.

51. Morgan, M. (1999) Paradoxical inhibition of nociceptive neurons in the dorsal horn of the rat spinal cord during a nociceptive hind limb reflex. *Neuroscience* **88,** 489–498.

52. Morgan, M. (1998) Direct comparison of heat-evoked activity of nociceptive neurons in the dorsal horn with the hindlimb withdrawal reflex in the rat. *J. Neurophys.* **79,** 174–180.

53. Jasmin L, Carstens, E., and Bashaum, A. I. (1997) Interneurons presynaptic to rat tail-flick motorneurons as mapped by transneuronal transport of pseudorabies virus: Few have long ascending collaterals. *Neuroscience* **76,** 859–876.

13
Spinal Cord

Anesthetic Actions on Motor Neurons

Joan J. Kendig

INTRODUCTION

Anesthesia and Immobility

Anesthesia as a Constellation of Endpoints

Recently it has become not only apparent but obvious that anesthesia is a group of endpoints rather than a single state, and that these endpoints have fundamentally different mechanisms. This concept is perhaps most clearly and comprehensively presented in an editorial by Kissin *(1)*, with examples drawn from the entire range of intravenous and inhalation anesthetic agents. It is widely acknowledged that there are mechanistic differences at the molecular level between receptor-specific agents with anesthetic properties, such as benzodiazepines, opioids, and α2 receptor agonists. However even within the class of inhaled agents, there are differences in potency ratios for partial pressures required to reach two different endpoints: loss of righting reflex, and abolition of movement in response to a noxious stimulus *(2,3)*. Different mechanisms are also indicated for amnesia vs immobility; a group of fluorinated compounds which do not cause immobility nevertheless do interfere with learning *(4)*.

Anesthetic endpoints commonly used in experimental studies of mechanism include hypnosis or unconsciousness, which operationally in humans is loss of response to verbal commands; loss of righting reflex in vertebrates; and loss of movement in response to a noxious stimulus (immobility). Analgesia is covered in detail in several chapters in this section. Analgesia, meaning loss of painful sensation before immobility, a loss of consciousness is clearly a property of some agents but may not be of others. In considering analgesic properties with respect to human pain, it is difficult to separate sedation and anxiolysis from analgesia. Animal models of acute pain, measured as tail flick latency, suggest that sub-immobilizing concentrations of inhalation agents are analgesic *(5)*, but at very low concentrations may be hyperalgesic *(6)*. In a model of human experimental pain, isoflurane did not reduce perceived pain intensity *(7)*. In a tail pressure test, barbiturates and propofol reduce the threshold for withdrawal at levels below those which prevent movement altogether; however this may represent hyperreflexia rather than enhanced nociception *(8,9)*.

Immobility as an Anesthetic Endpoint; Importance in Development and Testing of Theories of Anesthesia

Among all the endpoints the most widely accepted for inhalation agents is immobility in response to a noxious stimulus. The development of a standard for anesthetic potency, defined as the minimum alveolar anesthetic concentration (MAC) required to prevent movement in 50% of subjects in response to a standardized noxious stimulus *(10)*, has facilitated the comparison of potency among inhalation

From: *Contemporary Clinical Neuroscience: Neural Mechanisms of Anesthesia*
Edited by: Joseph F. Antognini et al. © Humana Press Inc., Totowa, NJ

agents and served as the gold standard for anesthetic concentrations relevant to proposed mechanisms of anesthesia. It should be emphasized that concentrations associated with immobility are higher than those for other anesthetic endpoints described above. In studies of mechanism, the endpoint should be specified and chosen to be relevant to the functional role of the tissue being studied. For example, in amygdala and hippocampal studies, the relevant concentrations are probably those associated with amnesia rather than immobility.

Since MAC is determined as loss of motor response to a noxious stimulus, in some minds, this anesthetic action has been equated with antinociception or analgesia. However, antinociception and immobility are probably distinct from each other. Not only does reflex threshold increase in human experimental pain while sensation remains unchanged *(7)*, but recent evidence suggests that mouse strains that differ markedly in their responses in pain models *(11)* display only small differences in MAC *(12)*.

For a long time it was automatically assumed that immobility, like some other anesthetic endpoints, is due to anesthetic actions in brain. The seminal studies by Rampil and Antognini described in the Introduction and in Chapter 11, showing that the site of MAC is primarily in spinal cord, induced a profound shift in thinking about anesthesia and contributed to the growing realization that anesthetic endpoints are distinct and site-specific.

Spinal Determinants of MAC

As the studies by Rampil *(13)* show, the ability to mount a withdrawal movement in response to a noxious stimulus and the action of anesthetics on it is independent of supraspinal structures. The anatomy of the spinal components that may contribute to MAC is discussed at length in Chapter 11. There are three elements, as diagrammed in Fig. 1A. These include the central terminations of the sensory primary afferent neurons, interneurons of many types, and the cell bodies and initial axon segments of motor neurons. The peripheral axons of motor neurons distal to the spinal cord probably do not contribute to immobility, nor do actions at the neuromuscular junction *(14)*. Conduction in large diameter myelinated axons like those of motor neurons is not sensitive to anesthetic agents at concentrations relevant to MAC, as many studies have shown. The roles of elements in the dorsal horn are described in Chapter 2. The present chapter will focus on anesthetic actions on motor neurons, with comments on actions mediated by interneurons presynaptic to them. The hypothesis will be presented that direct actions of anesthetic agents, in particular volatile agents, on motor neurons contribute importantly to immobility.

MOTOR NEURONS AS A CELLULAR LOCUS FOR THE IMMOBILIZING ACTIONS OF ANESTHETIC AGENTS

Prologue

This section presents some basic aspects of motor neuron structure, describes some early studies of anesthetic action done before the rich diversity of receptors and ion channels was appreciated, and outlines potential targets for anesthetic action on motor neurons, only a few of which have been investigated.

Motor Neurons as the Final Common Path Before the Initiation of Movement

Inputs to Motor Neurons

The integration of peripheral input by interneurons is described in Chapter 11. Motor neurons receive products of that integration, the output of local circuits that function as the central pattern generators for coordinated movement, propriospinal interneurons that provide intersegmental coordination, descending input from supraspinal motor regions of the central nervous system, and direct excitatory input from peripheral proprioceptors. In their role as integrators that translate all

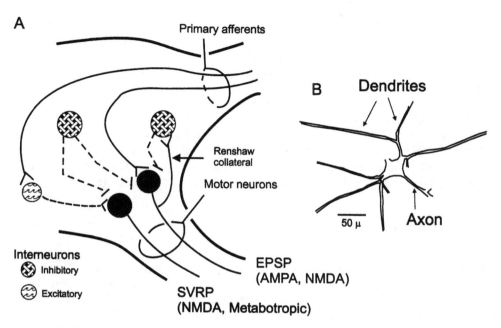

Fig. 1. (A) Simplified diagram of spinal cord connections to motor neurons. Large diameter primary afferent nerves from proprioceptors make direct excitatory synaptic contact with motor neurons to form the anatomic substrate for the monosynaptic reflex excitatory postsynaptic potential (EPSP). The transmitter released from these terminals is glutamate; the receptors mediating it are of both AMPA and NMDA subtypes. Primary afferents from small diameter sensory neurons, including nociceptors, make excitatory synaptic connections with interneurons which in turn, make excitatory synaptic connections to motor neurons; there may be more than one interneuron in this chain. The slow ventral root potential (SVRP) is a depolarization lasting many seconds; the transmitters which mediate it include NMDA and metabotropic receptors of several types, including glutamate and NK. **(B)** Tracing of a motor neuron cell body and its processes taken from a photograph of a cell *in situ*; the cell was fluorescently labeled with DiI injected postmortem into the gastrocnemius muscle of a 6-d-old rat, which traveled retrogradely to the cell body in the spinal cord. The fine dendritic terminals were not visible in the photograph. Identification of one of the processes as the axon is presumptive based on direction of travel. The sum of excitatory and inhibitory inputs to synapses on dendrites and cell body are integrated in the cell body and initiate impulses if they exceed the threshold of the spike initiating zone distal to the axon hillock. A adapted with permission from *(51)*.

these sources into patterned impulse activity leading to release of transmitter at the muscle endplate, the motor neurons serve as the final common path *(15)*, translating central cellular activity to muscle contraction and relaxation. The flexion reflex withdrawal in response to a painful stimulus, the behavioral endpoint for MAC, is a polysynaptic reflex involving sensory afferents, local interneuronal circuits, and motor neurons.

Structure and Properties of Motor Neurons

The structure of motor neurons is appropriate to their role as the final common path converting the sum of inputs into a motor command. A large cell body supports a number of dendritic processes; synaptic connections are made onto both dendrites and cell body (Fig. 1B), although dendritic synaptic boutons are far more numerous than somatic. Excitatory synaptic inputs generate depolarizations that spread electrotonically toward the cell body. As in other cells, some may generate dendritic action potentials, which permit them to travel greater distances than decaying passive events. However because of the cable properties of the large cell body and relatively small diameter dendrites, these do not initiate action potentials in the cell body of the motor neuron. Rather, the sum of depolarizations from all inputs spreads throughout the cell body to the spike initiating zone between the axon hillock and the beginning of the myelinated portion of the axon. A depolarization sufficient to cross the threshold of this specialized region will generate an action potential, which regeneratively travels down the axon to the motor nerve terminal, and retrogradely initiates an action potential in the higher threshold cell body and dendrites.

In this discussion, motor neurons will be treated as a homogeneous population. This is almost certainly an oversimplification, because motor neurons vary in size and position according to the muscles they innervate, flexors vs extensors and proximal vs distal muscles. Motor units differ in properties such as speed of adaptation to a sustained stimulus. In mammals, there is also a separate population of small motor neurons that innervate muscle spindles. The extent to which these populations of motor neurons differ in basic properties and in response to anesthetic agents is uncertain.

Early Studies in Spinal Cord

Basic Neurophysiology

Most early basic neurophysiological studies in vertebrates were done in spinal cord motor neurons, which became the cell type for understanding vertebrate neurophysiology *(16)*. Interpretation of experimental results was facilitated by several advantages of the vertebrate spinal cord. The separation of afferent input from motor output in dorsal and ventral roots permitted a defined input by stimulating a dorsal root; extracellular recording could be done from ventral roots in the knowledge that this reflected responses of motor neurons *(17)*. Following the introduction of microelectrode intracellular recording, the large size of motor neurons made them nearly the only vertebrate neuron that offered advantages comparable to the large axons and cell bodies of crustaceans and mollusks. Functionally, a cell impaled by blind probing could be unambiguously identified as a motor neuron by antidromically activating it via the ventral root.

Anesthetic Actions

Much of the initial knowledge of anesthetic actions was developed by grueling in vivo studies, requiring hours of surgical preparation and painstaking maintenance of the experimental animal. In a landmark series of such studies, Somjen *(18)* demonstrated that ether and thiopental depressed the monosynaptic excitatory postsynaptic potential in all motor neurons, elevated the threshold for impulse initiation in approximately half, and had no consistent effect on resting membrane potential. There were no discernable effects on conduction in the primary afferent nerve terminals *(19)*. The results of his studies led to the hypothesis that these two anesthetics decrease reflex responses predominantly by depressing excitatory synaptic transmission to motor neurons, with an uncertain and variable contribution from increase in threshold. Depression of excitatory synaptic transmission was postulated to be due to postsynaptic changes, although a decrease in excitatory transmitter release could not be ruled out in these experiments *(20)*. With only minor modifications due to the proliferation of receptors and ion channels now known to influence neurons, hypotheses such as these still form the nucleus of the debate concerning anesthetic actions on motor neurons.

Evolution of Neurophysiological Techniques

These difficult in vivo studies were superseded by the development in the early 1970s of the in vitro hippocampal slice preparation, which became the dominant neuronal preparation just in time to participate in and benefit from the development of new knowledge about the multiplicity of neurotransmitters and the complexity of determinants of excitability. Anesthesia related studies in hippocampus are described in Chapter 9. However, almost simultaneously with the growth of hippocampal slice studies, Otsuka and his colleagues developed an in vitro preparation of neonatal rat spinal cord *(21)*, which has been used extensively in studies of anesthetic and analgesic actions. Later, Takahashi and Konnerth showed it was possible to study visually identified motor neurons in spinal cord slices, initially by sharp electrode recording *(22)*, and eventually with whole cell patch clamp *(23,24)*. This preparation is now in widespread use.

Regulation of Excitability in Motor Neurons

Organization of the Section

The section below outlines receptors and ion channels that determine motor neuron excitability, with anesthetic actions where known. Voltage gated channels are covered in detail in Chapter 9, but are briefly included here for the sake of completeness.

Intrinsic Properties

All neurons maintain a resting potential difference between the inside and the outside of the cell membrane. The ultimate cause of this is active ion transport, predominantly of sodium ions from inside to outside the cell and a passive redistribution of potassium ions to the cell interior. However, the more immediate contributor is the selective potassium permeability of voltage-independent (non-gated) ion channels. Increased activity of these channels, by increasing the conductance to potassium, will move the resting potential toward the potassium equilibrium potential and away from the threshold of impulse initiation. In addition, by lowering membrane resistance, these channels will short-circuit excitatory synaptic input and render it less effective. An anesthetic that increased the passive flow of current through such channels would thus reduce excitability. Channels of particular current interest are tandem pore potassium channels. At least some types of this channel have a response to volatile anesthetic agents that would move excitability in this direction *(25,26)*. Halothane and sevoflurane activate a potassium current in hypoglossal motor neurons that has a pH sensitivity similar to that of the TASK-1 tandem pore potassium channel *(27)*.

Some types of sodium channels are sensitive to volatile anesthetic agents at reasonable concentrations *(28)*. A persistent inward sodium current in hypoglossal motor neurons carried through TTX insensitive sodium channels is reduced by halothane *(29)*. Other channels active near the resting potential that will modulate excitability are low voltage activated (LVA) calcium channels. Halothane decreases current through these channels, and thus may modulate excitability through an action on them *(30)*. Motor neurons also exhibit long-lasting depolarizing plateau potentials owing to LVA calcium channels. Some intravenous agents depress plateau potentials and thus decrease excitability *(31)*. In addition, fast transient K channels may be activated under certain conditions, causing a delay in reaching the threshold for impulse initiation. However, isoflurane inhibits such channels *(32)*.

Motor neurons respond to persistent depolarization above threshold by generating a train of action potentials. The frequency and number of impulses in the train are limited by calcium dependent potassium channels; alcohols, ketamine, and a barbiturate reduce current through channels of this type, but volatile anesthetics exert little effect at anesthetically relevant concentrations *(33)*.

Synaptic Inputs

EXCITATORY

Most of the fast ligand-gated excitatory synaptic input to motor neurons is mediated by receptors of the AMPA subtype (GluR1–4). However, at least in the very young rat spinal cord, NMDA receptors provide a greater contribution to the depolarization than is observed in hippocampal cells (Fig. 2A). Although some kainate receptors, particularly GluR5 and KA1, are present on motor neurons *(34)* kainate receptors provide a vanishingly small contribution to excitatory input (Fig. 2B). Motor neurons are themselves cholinergic, but there appears to be little contribution from nicotinic receptors to excitatory input. The response to application of nicotinic agonists is very small (Knape and Kendig, unpublished data). It is not certain whether $5HT_3$ receptors are present on motor neurons.

In addition to fast excitatory transmission, there are slower forms of excitatory transmission mediated by metabotropic (G-protein coupled) receptors of various types. These include serotonin, NK1–3, a1 and α2, dopamine, adenosine, cholinergic muscarine, and metabotropic glutamate

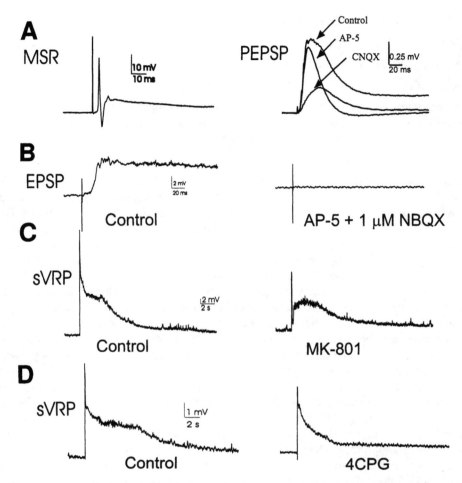

Fig. 2. Responses recorded extracellularly from a lumbar ventral root of isolated neonatal rat spinal cord in response to stimulation of a dorsal root; these represent the synchronous responses of all the excitable motor neurons that send axons out that root. (**A**, *left*) The monosynaptic reflex (MSR) consisting of a compound action potential rising very early on an excitatory postsynaptic potential, the initial phase of which is obliterated by the action potential. Right, the population excitatory postsynaptic potential (PEPSP) can be observed without the compound action potential by offsetting stimulating and recording electrodes by one or more segments. Arrows indicate the AMPA receptor component revealed by blocking the NMDA response with AP-5, and the slower NMDA receptor response revealed when AMPA receptors are blocked by CNQX. (**B**) There is no significant kainate response. When NMDA receptors are blocked by AP-5 and AMPA by a low concentration of NBQX, little or no response remains. In some preparations a few percent of the initial response remains which is sensitive to a kainate antagonist. (**C**) The initial component of the slow ventral root potential (sVRP) is sensitive to another NMDA receptor antagonist, MK-801, leaving a very slow, relatively small response which rises from near baseline. (**D**) The very slow component is depressed by a variety of antagonists at second messenger operated receptors; among the most effective is a glutamate metabotropic receptor antagonist 4CPG.

receptors (Fig. 2C,D). The functional roles of these receptors on motor neurons is not certain, and some may be inhibitory rather than excitatory *(34)*.

INHIBITORY INPUTS

Unlike other parts of the central nervous system the major ionotropic inhibitory transmitter in the spinal cord is glycine, although GABA also contributes. There is evidence that the two ligands of inhibitory chloride channels are co-released at the same synaptic terminals *(35)*. Motor neurons are subject to tonic inhibitory input as evidenced by spontaneous miniature synaptic currents, and also to both feed-forward and feedback inhibition. The feed-forward inhibition permits coordinated movement by enforcing alternate relaxation of flexor and extensor muscles and prevents the exaggerated reflexes characteristic of some central nervous system (CNS) disorders. The feedback inhibition is represented by the classic Renshaw cell, innervated by a collateral branch from the motor neuron axon, in turn forming inhibitory synaptic connections with the motor neuron (Fig. 1). The early component of this inhibition is owing to glycinergic input, the later to GABA. In addition to the fast ligand-gated chloride channels, there are other inhibitory inputs to motor neurons mediated by second messenger-linked receptors including those for $GABA_B$ receptors. There is a vast literature on anesthetic actions on $GABA_A$ and glycine receptors, but little on slower modulatory inhibitory channels. In hippocampus, a volatile anesthetic agent enhances both $GABA_A$ and $GABA_B$ currents *(36)*, but there is no information available about anesthetics and $GABA_B$ receptors in motor neurons.

ANESTHETIC ACTIONS ON MOTOR NEURONS: EXPERIMENTAL STRATEGIES AND THEIR LIMITATIONS

Outline

This section outlines several methods of probing anesthetic actions on motor neurons and describes their advantages and limitations. In each section, recent studies using each method are cited, together with the conclusions that may be drawn from them.

Peripheral to the Spinal Cord

Behavioral Tests

Behavioral tests of motor neuron excitability are common in anesthesia research, including those used to test MAC levels as abolition of movement in response to a supramaximal noxious stimulus, and various tests of pain and analgesia, such as paw withdrawal and tail flick. The advantage of these methods is that they measure the sum of all inputs to the motor neurons in addition to the intrinsic excitability of the motor neurons themselves. The disadvantage with respect to understanding mechanism is the same, in that they cannot separate actions on various components of the circuit. Abolition of movement may be closest in this respect, as it is predominantly a spinal phenomenon with fewer supraspinal components than the others; the tail flick response to a noxious stimulus may be predominantly spinal as well. However, few conclusions about the site of anesthetic action within the spinal cord can be drawn from these studies.

Electromyographic Studies of Reflexes

The H-reflex has similar limitations to behavioral studies, but with the advantage that it can be examined in humans. Evoked by peripheral nerve stimulation, it is a monosynaptic reflex mediated by large-diameter primary afferent sensory nerves, involving all elements in the arc except transduction of the sensory stimulus at sensory afferent peripheral terminals. The measure is electromyographic. H-reflexes are depressed by volatile agents at subanesthetic concentrations *(14,37,38)*, but only at high blood levels of propofol *(39)*. Etomidate and ketamine actually increase H-reflex amplitude *(40,41)*.

The F-wave is a cleaner index of motor neuron excitability. It too is evoked by peripheral nerve stimulation and recorded electromyographically, but represents antidromic invasion of central motor neurons that is sufficiently depolarizing to trigger orthodromic impulses after the absolute refractory period has passed. The F-wave, although a measure of motor neuron excitability, is not restricted to intrinsic excitability, since the motor neurons are subject to tonic excitatory and inhibitory influences. F-waves are depressed by inhalation agents including nitrous oxide at clinically relevant concentrations *(14,42–46)*. Both H- and F-wave depression are correlated with loss of movement in response to a noxious stimulus *(47)*.

Spinal Cord Population Evoked Potentials

Methods, Advantages, and Limitations

The sum of the responses of a population of motor neurons can be recorded from an electrode placed over a ventral root in close proximity to the ventral horn, with stimuli applied to a dorsal root. This can be done in vitro, with intact spinal cords taken from very young rats. Many of the early studies on anesthetic actions cited above employed this method in vivo. In addition to the usual advantages of controlled conditions for in vitro recording, the method has the advantages over H-wave recording of employing a purely sensory volley as opposed to a mixed, and the capability of measuring subthreshold motor neuron responses. However, the circuits are essentially still a black box, with the advantage of revealing everything the entire spinal cord can do. The disadvantage in mechanistic terms is that changes induced by anesthetics cannot be isolated to one element or another. Extracellular recording, by its nature, does not produce meaningful absolute values for the amplitudes of the recorded responses, so changes must be expressed as a percent of control amplitude for each experiment. Furthermore, under most experimental conditions, only relatively fast and large transients can be observed, again giving limited insight into underlying changes in resting potential or membrane resistance in the individual motor neurons. One type of extracellular recording, in which potentials in a ventral root are measured across a very high resistance sucrose gap, partially resolves these limitations, although only average changes can be measured, not absolute values of potentials in individual motor neurons. The method thus obscures variability in the population of motor neurons, and is predominantly influenced by the largest motor neurons in the pool. However, this method was used in a very influential paper that demonstrated frog spinal cord motor neuron hyperpolarization to a broad range of anesthetics, including barbiturates, ether, and α-chloralose *(48)*. The hyperpolarization was not blocked by GABA$_A$ antagonists (glycine antagonists were not employed), and was hypothesized to be caused by an increase in potassium conductance, because parallel experiments on hippocampal neurons showed hyperpolarization accompanied by a conductance increase.

Monosynaptic Reflex and Population Excitatory Postsynaptic Potential

PHYSIOLOGY AND PHARMACOLOGY

Stimulating a lumbar dorsal root and recording from the corresponding ipsilateral ventral root elicits the classic monosynaptic reflex, observed as a compound action potential in the ventral nerve root (Fig. 2A). Thresholds for eliciting this response are so low that little of the underlying excitatory postsynaptic potential can be seen before it is obliterated by the action potential. Offsetting the stimulating and recording electrodes by one or two segments permits a large subthreshold excitatory postsynaptic potential to be recorded without contamination by the compound action potential (Fig. 2A). The fast population excitatory postsynaptic potential in motor neurons is mediated by both AMPA and NMDA receptors; a combination of AMPA-selective and NMDA-selective antagonists nearly completely abolishes it (Fig. 2B). Motor neurons are subject to tonic inhibition via both GABA$_A$ and glycine receptors; application of a GABA$_A$ antagonist bicuculline or a glycine antagonist strychnine elevates the response.

ANESTHETIC SENSITIVITY

The population EPSP and the monosynaptic reflex are sensitive to volatile anesthetic agents including halothane *(49)*, isoflurane *(50)*, enflurane *(51)*, and ethanol *(52)*, at concentrations equivalent to MAC or lower (Fig. 3A,B). Concentrations that inhibit the monosynaptic reflex correlate well with MAC *(53)*. An experimental anesthetic (cyclobutane) depresses the monosynaptic reflex, whereas a related nonimmobilizing compound does not *(54)*. Alcohols depress both the AMPA and NMDA receptor-mediated components of the EPSP *(52)*, but with some apparent selectivity for the NMDA component (Fig. 3D). The monosynaptic reflex is not diminished by barbiturates *(55)*, propofol *(55)*, α$_2$ adrenergic agonists *(50)*, opiates *(56)*, or ketamine *(57,58)*. The population EPSP

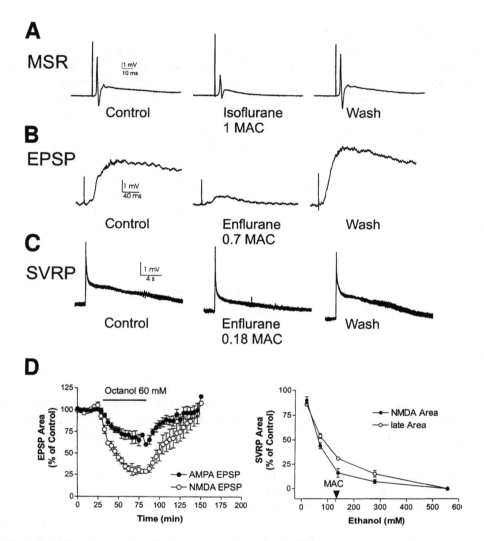

Fig. 3. Anesthetic actions on the population evoked responses shown in Fig. 2. **(A)** Isoflurane depresses the monosynaptic reflex at 1 MAC. **(B)** Enflurane depresses the underlying population EPSP, and this action accounts for at least some of the depression of the monosynaptic reflex if it falls below the threshold for part of the motor neuron population. **(C)** The slow ventral root potential is more sensitive than the monosynaptic reflex. **(D)** Selective anesthetic actions are shown when antagonists are used to block one or another of the components of ventral root responses (*see* Fig. 2 for examples). Left, octanol is more potent in depressing the NMDA component of the EPSP. Right, ethanol displays some selectivity for the NMDA-mediated component of the slow ventral root potential over the slower metabotropic component. Data points in **D** represent averages of 4–6 individual spinal cords; error bars are SEM. **A, D** from rat spinal cord; **B, C** from mouse. Portions of this figure adapted with permission from *(51)*.

has not been examined for these agents, but presumably would be little affected. However, depression of the somewhat slower NMDA receptor-mediated component of the EPSP, which one might expect for ketamine, does not necessarily lead to depression of the monosynaptic reflex, since the latter is triggered very early on the rising phase of the AMPA component. An earlier study in cats suggested that propofol, but not ketamine or a barbiturate, depressed monosynaptic reflexes. However, the propofol results were obtained on a background of barbiturate anesthesia, which might be expected to exert additive effects with propofol *(59)*.

INFORMATION FROM GENETICALLY ENGINEERED MICE

Studies on population evoked ventral root responses in intact cord are limited in the extent to which mechanistic explanations can be derived. However, some progress can be made. We have investigated responses to enflurane in spinal cords from mice that lack the β3 subunit of the $GABA_A$ receptor *(51)*, which behavioral studies showed to have an increased enflurane requirement to prevent movement in response to a noxious stimulus *(60)*. However, ventral root responses in spinal cords from the null mutants did not differ in sensitivity to enflurane from those from wild type animals. The contributions of $GABA_A$ receptors to enflurane actions did change however. Bicuculline significantly attenuated enflurane's depressant actions in cords from wild type mice, but not in mutant cords. The results suggested that EPSP depression results from anesthetic actions on multiple targets in spinal cord, and that the mutation caused an unpredicted shift in the proportions of targets in the mix. $GABA_A$ receptors became less important, but in order to maintain the same sensitivity, other targets must have played a greater role in the mutants than in the wild types. In the same studies, glycine receptors appeared to be upregulated in the mutants. These receptors also contributed slightly to anesthetic actions on the EPSP, but to the same extent in wild type and mutant animals. Thus, some other unidentified receptors took on a greater role in anesthetic depression in the mutant animals. The results are theoretically highly interesting, but illustrate the riskiness of assuming that global knockout mutations will provide simple solutions to the puzzle of anesthetic mechanisms.

The Nociceptive-Related Slow Ventral Root Potential

PHYSIOLOGY AND PHARMACOLOGY

The slow ventral root potential is a complex polysynaptic response that requires small diameter sensory nerve activation for its full expression *(61)*. By this criterion, by its evocation by true noxious stimuli, and by its sensitivity to analgesic agents, it is believed to be related to nociception *(62,63)*. The slow ventral root potential has an early component sensitive to NMDA receptor antagonists, and a late component that appears to be mediated by a variety of metabotropic receptors *(61)* (Fig. 2C,D).

ANESTHETIC SENSITIVITY

The slow ventral root potential is more sensitive to anesthetic agents than the fast EPSP (Fig. 3C,D). The late metabotropic receptor-mediated component is selectively sensitive to α_2 adrenoceptor agonists *(50)* and opioids *(56)*, whereas volatile anesthetic agents *(50)*, ketamine *(57)* midazolam *(64)*, and alcohols *(52)* display some selectivity for the early component (Fig. 3D). It is not certain where the receptors that mediate these anesthetic actions are located. Certainly there are NMDA receptors on motor neurons, and possibly metabotrobic receptors of various types as well. However, it is also probable that at least some of the anesthetic depression of the slow ventral root potential is due to anesthetic actions on interneurons presynaptic to the motor neurons. This question cannot be resolved by studies on intact cord.

Single Motor Neurons

Methodology, Advantages, and Limitations

The disadvantages of extracellular recording are resolved by studies of single motor neurons, most commonly in recent times using patch clamp techniques to record from cell bodies. The method of preparing slices from spinal cord, combined with visualization of cells in the cord via infrared illumination on closed circuit TV and fluorescent labeling, allows identification of large cells in the ventral horn as motor neurons. With a different technique, using antidromic activation via a ventral root, motor neurons can be functionally identified in intact or semi-intact cord.

When motor neurons are stimulated via a dorsal root (or in slices via an electrode placed in the dorsal root entry zone), the changes induced by anesthetics can be directly related to studies of population evoked responses in the intact cord, with greater insights into their mechanistic basis.

Furthermore, by evoking responses in motor neurons directly with glutamate, meanwhile blocking presynaptic impulse activity, it is possible to bypass presynaptic elements and unambiguously identify anesthetic actions on motor neurons themselves. There are also some disadvantages to single cell recording. In intact cord, finding and identifying motor neurons by blind probing is cumbersome, and the yield low. In slice, visual control makes establishing a recording easy, but with much of the connectivity stripped away, important elements may be lost.

Responses Evoked by Electrical Stimulation of a Dorsal Root

METHODS AND ADVANTAGES

Dorsal root-evoked responses are the single neuron counterpart of the population ventral root responses evoked by dorsal root stimulation in the intact cord. Although it is possible in intact cord to examine slow depolarizations that are the counterparts of the population slow ventral root potential, in spinal cord slice any such responses are small because of the diminished input. Most studies have therefore examined relatively fast events that correspond to the short-latency population EPSP. In addition to examining excitatory synaptic transmission, single cell studies using whole cell patch techniques in current clamp mode, or intracellular sharp electrodes can look at changes in threshold and in resting membrane potential. Studies in voltage clamp mode can exclude changes in response owing to resting membrane potential changes, at least in the cell body and proximal dendrites; clamp control in distal dendrites is problematic.

ANESTHETIC ACTIONS

Using intracellular electrodes, Takenoshita and Takahashi *(49)* found that halothane hyperpolarized motor neuron cell membranes in rats by several millivolts while increasing input conductance. Threshold for spike initiation did not change; they concluded that the larger current required for impulse initiation was due to the hyperpolarization and increase in conductance, which they attributed to an increase in potassium permeability. In studies with whole cell patch electrodes, our studies also showed that halothane consistently hyperpolarized motor neurons with a reduction in number of impulses evoked by depolarizing current injections, which could be attributed to the hyperpolarization. However, there was no significant change in input resistance (Cheng and Kendig, unpublished data). Ethanol also decreased the number of impulses evoked by a given level of depolarizing input current, but without changes in resting potential whereas input resistance increased, as did threshold *(65)*. Enflurane also hyperpolarized mouse spinal cord neurons, but again with no significant change in input resistance (Cheng and Kendig, unpublished data). The early studies by Somjen *(18–20)* suggested hyperpolarization was inconsistent for ether and thiopental. Our studies show that hyperpolarization varies among agents, but there is no consistent change in membrane conductance. Thus, reduction in number of impulses in a train and increase in threshold appear to have different causes for different agents, and our laboratory differs from others in finding no decrease in membrane resistance.

As in the intact cord, single cell studies show that volatile anesthetic agents and ethanol depress the fast excitatory postsynaptic potential and the corresponding excitatory postsynaptic current *(49,65–67)* (Fig. 4A). Enflurane and ethanol depress both AMPA and NMDA receptor-mediated components of excitatory postsynaptic potentials and currents *(66,67)*.

Pharmacologically Isolating the Motor Neuron

BLOCKING PRESYNAPTIC IMPULSE ACTIVITY AND EVOKING RESPONSES BY NEUROTRANSMITTER APPLICATION TO THE MOTOR NEURON

When presynaptic impulses are blocked by tetrodotoxin to cut out the presynaptic circuitry, and excitatory potentials and currents are evoked by brief pulses of glutamate, ethanol and enflurane depress glutamate-evoked potentials and currents *(66,67)* (Fig. 4B). This result shows that at least some of the actions of these agents can be attributed to direct actions on the motor neurons themselves, in addition to any effects mediated via presynaptic elements.

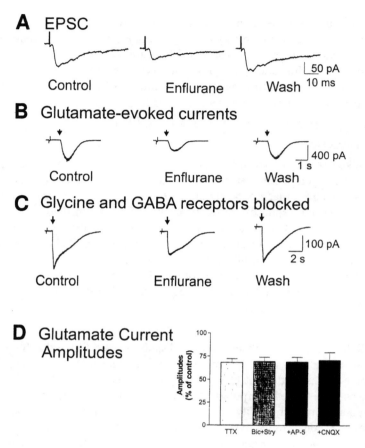

Fig. 4. Enflurane actions on individual motor neurons in mouse spinal cord slice recorded with a patch electrode in whole cell voltage clamp. All enflurane concentrations are approx 1 MAC. **(A)** The excitatory postsynaptic current evoked by stimulation in the dorsal root entry area is depressed by enflurane in a reversible fashion. **(B)** The motor neuron is pharmacologically isolated from presynaptic activity by TTX (300 nM) and responses evoked by pulses of glutamate (5 mM) applied at the time points are indicated by the arrows. Enflurane depresses this response, indicating a direct action of the agent on motor neurons. **(C)** When glycine and GABA$_A$ receptors are blocked by strychnine and bicuculline respectively, enflurane still depresses glutamate-evoked currents indicating that actions on the inhibitory chloride channels are not essential to depressant actions of this agent on motor neurons. **(D)** Glutamate-evoked responses are depressed to the same extent in the untreated preparation (TTX), when inhibitory chloride channels are blocked (Bic+Stry), and when either AMPA (+AP-5) or NMDA (+CNQX) receptors mediate the response. Numbers in **D** are averages of 5–9 individual neurons, error bars are SEM. Figure adapted with permission from *(66)*.

ELIMINATING POSTSYNAPTIC RECEPTORS

It has been a dominant theory that enhancement of activity at GABA$_A$ receptors is an important component, perhaps the only component, of the mechanism of action of a wide variety of anesthetic agents *(68–70)*. Although there has been a recent retreat from the universality of this view *(71)*, it remains pervasive in discussions of molecular mechanisms of anesthesia. For the spinal cord, similar or greater importance is attached to enhancement of glycine receptor mediated inhibition. In order to test whether postsynaptic actions on either or both of these receptors might account for anesthetic depression of glutamate-evoked responses in motor neurons, both receptors were blocked by their respective antagonists. In the presence of either bicuculline, strychnine or both, ethanol and enflurane still depressed both AMPA and NMDA types of glutamate-evoked currents *(66,67)* (Fig. 4C,D).

Application of any of the antagonists, alone or in combination, did not change the sensitivity of glutamate-evoked currents to the anesthetic agents. This result shows that volatile anesthetics can exert depressant actions on spinal motor neurons independent of actions on either of the inhibitory chloride channels, and equally on currents mediated by both major subtypes of glutamate receptors. The result does not, however, demonstrate that these anesthetics act directly on the glutamate receptors, since the depression of currents may be mediated indirectly via an action elsewhere.

DISCUSSION AND CONCLUSIONS

Relative Roles of Anesthetic Actions on Motor Neurons vs Presynaptic Elements

Although the studies outlined in the preceding section show clearly that anesthetics can act directly on motor neurons to depress responses to transmitter and to reduce the probability of impulse generation, the methods of isolating postsynaptic responses preclude assignment of relative sensitivity. Direct application of glutamate does not precisely mimic glutamatergic synaptic transmission. The concentration of glutamate applied does approximate the millimolar concentrations released into the synaptic cleft, but exogenous glutamate also activates extrasynaptic receptors, and the time course of action is different. In spite of these limitations, the results do show that motor neuron responses to glutamate are depressed at the same concentrations of anesthetic that depress circuit-mediated synaptic transmission in intact cord. Thus, in a sense, the question of relative importance is somewhat like the chicken and the egg. If the motor neuron cannot respond, it does not matter whether or not presynaptic input is also reduced, and vice versa.

There is a difference between synaptically evoked responses and glutamate-evoked currents with respect to the contributions of $GABA_A$ and glycine receptors to anesthetic actions. Blockade of these inhibitory chloride channels does not alter the anesthetic sensitivity of motor neurons when the probe is exogenously applied glutamate, but does attenuate anesthetic actions measured as depression of the monosynaptic EPSP. The attenuation is not large, particularly in the case of glycinergic receptors, and clearly the response is still depressed in the presence of antagonists to these receptors. It might be argued that the ability of actions on inhibitory channels to modify glutamate-evoked responses is limited when spontaneous activity is blocked. However, there is considerable tonic release, particularly of glycine, even under these conditions (Cheng and Kendig, [72]), and both bicuculline and strychnine increase the amplitude of glutamate-evoked currents.

Relation Between Studies on Motor Neurons and Movement In Vivo

In view of the role of motor neurons as the final common path that integrates all upstream input into a move/no move decision, anesthetic actions that limit the ability of motor neurons to generate a train of impulses in response to excitatory transmitter are directly relevant to the anesthetic endpoint of immobility in response to a noxious stimulus. Results in vivo are in agreement with a limited role for inhibitory chloride channels in blocking movement; block of these channels by intrathecal application of bicuculline and strychnine increases anesthetic requirement by a maximum of approx 40% (73).

Major Contributors to Depression of Motor Neuron Excitability

As the reports of the studies cited above make clear, there are multiple targets for anesthetic actions both on motor neurons themselves, and on elements presynaptic to them. Anesthetics depress the ability of motor neurons to generate action potentials, by acting on a number of different ion channels that may vary from agent to agent. Some of these may generate a hyperpolarization but this is not universal, and is not a prerequisite for reducing impulse generation for at least some agents. The section above suggests a number of voltage-gated and voltage-independent channels that regulate excitability. It is probable that not all the targets that modulate intrinsic excitability have been identified.

No one would argue that actions of anesthetic agents on $GABA_A$ and glycine receptors are unimportant. However, in particular for volatile agents, they are not the sole or even the major contributors to anesthetic depression of motor neuron excitability. Actions on these receptors may be more important for some intravenous agents including propofol and barbiturates. In fact, there is evidence that enhancement of GABA-mediated responses in spinal cord is more prominent for these agents than for ethanol or isoflurane *(50,52,55,73,74)*.

Actions on glutamate receptors on motor neurons are probably important. For ethanol and enflurane, there is no apparent selective sensitivity for NMDA vs AMPA currents. Selective actions on NMDA vs AMPA currents have been reported for xenon but not isoflurane in another preparation *(71)*. However, the caution still persists that there is as yet no identified site for volatile agents on the glutamate receptor itself, and anesthetic actions on the currents may be indirect. Ketamine, on the other hand, almost certainly exerts its actions, on motor neurons as elsewhere, predominantly as a noncompetitive antagonist at NMDA receptors.

There are large areas to which little attention has been paid that will probably be important in the future. In particular, anesthetic actions on the intracellular metabolic pathways that lead to changes in receptor phosphorylation is an area of research that has hardly been touched. In addition, except in the case of opioids and α_2 adrenoceptor agonists, anesthetic actions on receptors coupled to G-proteins have not been investigated.

REFERENCES

1. Kissin, I. (1993) General anesthetic action: an obsolete notion? *Anesth. Analg.* **76,** 215–218.
2. Deady, J. E., Koblin, D. D., Eger, E. I. D., Heavner, J. E., and D'Aoust, B. (1981) Anesthetic potencies and the unitary theory of narcosis. *Anesth. Analg.* **60,** 380–384.
3. Kissin, I., Morgan, P. L., and Smith, L. R. (1983) Anesthetic potencies of isoflurane, halothane, and diethyl ether for various end points of anesthesia. *Anesthesiology* **58,** 88–92.
4. Eger, E. I., 2nd, Koblin, D. D., Harris, R. A., et al. (1997) Hypothesis: inhaled anesthetics produce immobility and amnesia by different mechanisms at different sites. *Anesth. Analg.* **84,** 915–918.
5. Sonner, J., Li, J., and Eger, E. I., 2nd (1998) Desflurane and nitrous oxide, but not nonimmobilizers, affect nociceptive responses. *Anesth. Analg.* **86,** 629–634.
6. Zhang, Y., Eger, E. I., Dutton, R. C., and Sonner, J. M. (2000) Inhaled anesthetics have hyperalgesic effects at 0.1 minimum alveolar anesthetic concentration. *Anesth. Analg.* **91,** 462–466.
7. Petersen-Felix, S., Arendt-Nielsen, L., Bak, et al. (1995) Analgesic effect in humans of subanaesthetic isoflurane concentrations evaluated by experimentally induced pain. *Brit. J. Anaesth.* **75,** 55–60.
8. Ewen, A., Archer, D. P., Samanani, N., and Roth, S. H. (1995) Hyperalgesia during sedation: effects of barbiturates and propofol in the rat. *Can. J. Anaesth.* **42,** 532–540.
9. Archer, D. P., Samanani N., and Roth S. H. (2000) Pentobarbital induces nocifensive yhyperreflexia, not hyperalgesia in rats. *Can. J. Anaesth.* **47,** 687–692.
10. Eger, E. I., 2nd, Saidman, L. J., and Brandstater, B. (1965) Minimum alveolar anesthetic concentration: a standard of anesthetic potency. *Anesthesiology* **26,** 756–763.
11. Mogil, J. S., Wilson, S. G., Bon, K., et al. (1999) Heritability of nociception I: responses of 11 inbred mouse strains on 12 measures of nociception. *Pain* **80,** 67–82.
12. Sonner, J. M., Gong, D., Li J., Eger E. I., 2nd, and Laster M. J. (1999) Mouse strain modestly influences minimum alveolar anesthetic concentration and convulsivity of inhaled compounds. *Anesth. Analg.* **89,** 1030–1034.
13. Rampil, I. J. (1994) Anesthetic potency is not altered after hypothermic spinal cord transection in rats. *Anesthesiology* **80,** 606–610.
14. Pereon, Y., Bernard, J. M., Nguyen The Tich, S., Genet, R., Petitfaux, F., and Guiheneuc, P. (1999) The effects of desflurane on the nervous system: from spinal cord to muscles. *Anesth. Analg.* **89,** 490–495.
15. Sherrington, C. S. (1906) The Integrative Action of the Nervous System. Yale University Press, New Haven and London.
16. Eccles, J. C. (1957) The Physiology of Nerve Cells. The Johns Hopkins Press, Baltimore, MD.
17. Eccles, J. C. (1946) Synaptic potentials of motor neurons. *J. Neurophysiol.* **9,** 87–120.
18. Somjen, G. G. and Gill, M. (1963) The Mechanism of the blockade of synaptic transmission in the mammalian spinal cord by diethyl ether and by thiopental. *J. Pharmacol. Exper. Ther.* **140,** 19–30.
19. Somjen, G. G. (1963) Effects of ether and thiopental on spinal presynaptic terminals. *J. Pharmacol. Exper. Ther.* **140,** 395–402.
20. Somjen, G. (1967) Effects of anesthetics on the spinal cord of mammals. *Anesthesiology* **28,** 135–143.
21. Otsuka, M. and Konishi, S. (1974) Electrophysiology of mammalian spinal cord in vitro. *Nature* **252,** 733–734.
22. Takahashi, T. (1978) Intracellular recording from visually identified motoneurons in rat spinal cord slices. *Proc. R. Soc. Lond. B. Biol. Sci.* **202,** 417–421.

23. Konnerth, A., Keller, B. U., and Lev-Tov, A. (1990) Patch clamp analysis of excitatory synapses in mammalian spinal cord slices. *Pflugers Arch.* **417,** 285–290.
24. Takahashi, T. (1990) Membrane currents in visually identified motoneurones of neonatal rat spinal cord. *J. Physiol.* **423,** 27–46.
25. Gray, A. T., Winegar, B. D., Leonoudakis, D. J., Forsayeth, J. R., and Yost, C. S. (1998) TOK1 is a volatile anesthetic stimulated K+ channel. *Anesthesiology* **88,** 1076–1084.
26. Yost, C. S., Gray, A. T., Winegar, B. D., and Leonoudakis D. (1998) Baseline K+ channels as targets of general anesthetics: studies of the action of volatile anesthetics on TOK1. *Toxicol. Lett.* **100–101,** 293–300.
27. Sirois, J. E., Lei, Q., Talley, E. M., Lynch, C., and Bayliss, D. A. (2000) The TASK-1 two-pore domain K+ channel is a molecular substrate for neuronal effects of inhalation anesthetics. *J. Neurosci.* **20,** 6347–6354.
28. Scholz, A., Appel, N., and Vogel, W. (1998) Two types of TTX-resistant and one TTX-sensitive Na+ channel in rat dorsal root ganglion neurons and their blockade by halothane. *Eur. J. Neurosci.* **10,** 2547–2556.
29. Sirois, J. E., Pancrazio, J. J., Iii, C. L., and Bayliss, D. A. (1998) Multiple ionic mechanisms mediate inhibition of rat motoneurones by inhalation anaesthetics. *J. Physiol.* **512,** 851–862.
30. Takenoshita, M. and Steinbach J. H. (1991) Halothane blocks low-voltage-activated calcium current in rat sensory neurons. *J. Neurosci.* **11,** 1404–1412.
31. Guertin, P. A. and Hounsgaard, J. (1999) Non-volatile general anaesthetics reduce spinal activity by suppressing plateau potentials. *Neuroscience* **88,** 353–358.
32. Franks, N. P. and Lieb, W. R. (1991) Stereospecific effects of inhalational general anesthetic optical isomers on nerve ion channels. *Science* **254,** 427–430.
33. Dreixler, J. C., Jenkins, A., Cao, Y. J., Roizen, J. D., and Houamed, K. M. (2000) Patch-clamp analysis of anesthetic interactions with recombinant SK2 subtype neuronal calcium-activated potassium channels. *Anesth. Analg.* **90,** 727–732.
34. Rekling, J. C., Funk, G. D., Bayliss, D. A., Dong, X. W., and Feldman, J. L. (2000) Synaptic control of motoneuronal excitability. *Physiol. Rev.* **80,** 767–852.
35. Jonas, P., Bischofberger, J., and Sandkuhler, J. (1998) Corelease of two fast neurotransmitters at a central synapse. *Science* **281,** 419–424.
36. Hirota, K. and Roth S. H. (1997) Sevoflurane modulates both GABA$_A$ and GABA$_B$ receptors in area CA1 of rat hippocampus. *Brit. J. Anaesth.* **78,** 60–65.
37. Freund, F. G., Martin, W. E., and Hornbein, T. F. (1969) The H-reflex as a measure of anesthetic potency in man. *Anesthesiology* **30,** 642–647.
38. Mavroudakis, N., Vandesteene, A., Brunko, E., Defevrimont, M., and Zegers de Beyl, D. (1994) Spinal and brain-stem SEPs and H reflex during enflurane anesthesia. Electroencephalogr *Clin. Neurophysiol.* **92,** 82–85.
39. Kerz, T., Hennes, H. J., Feve, A., Decq P., Filipetti, P., and Duvaldestin, P. (2001) Effects of Propofol on H-reflex in Humans. *Anesthesiology* **94,** 32–37.
40. Kano, T. and Shimoji, K. (1974) The effects of ketamine and neuroleptanalgesia on the evoked electrospinogram and electromyogram in man. *Anesthesiology* **40,** 241–246.
41. Meinck, H. M., Mohlenhof, O., and Kettler, D. (1980) Neurophysiological effects of etomidate, a new short-acting hypnotic. *Electroencephalogr. Clin. Neurophysiol.* **50,** 515–522.
42. Zhou, H. H., Mehta, M., and Leis, A. A. (1997) Spinal cord motoneuron excitability during isoflurane and nitrous oxide anesthesia. *Anesthesiology* **86,** 302–307.
43. Rampil, I. J. and King, B. S. (1996) Volatile anesthetics depress spinal motor neurons. *Anesthesiology* **85,** 129–134.
44. King, B. S. and Rampil, I. J. (1994) Anesthetic depression of spinal motor neurons may contribute to lack of movement in response to noxious stimuli. *Anesthesiology* **81,** 1484–1492.
45. Friedman, Y., King, B. S., and Rampil, I. J. (1996) Nitrous oxide depresses spinal F waves in rats. *Anesthesiology* **85,** 135–141.
46. Antognini, J. F., Carstens, E., and Buzin, V. (1999) Isoflurane depresses motoneuron excitability by a direct spinal action: an F-wave study. *Anesth. Analg.* **88,** 681–685.
47. Zhou, H. H., Jin, T. T., Qin, B., and Turndorf, H. (1998) Suppression of spinal cord motoneuron excitability correlates with surgical immobility during isoflurane anesthesia. *Anesthesiology* **88,** 955–961.
48. Nicoll, R. A. and Madison, D. V. (1982) General anesthetics hyperpolarize neurons in the vertebrate central nervous system. *Science* **217,** 1055–1057.
49. Takenoshita, M. and Takahashi, T. (1987) Mechanisms of halothane action on synaptic transmission in motoneurons of the newborn rat spinal cord in vitro. *Brain Res.* **402,** 303–310.
50. Savola, M. K., Woodley, S. J., Maze, M., and Kendig, J. J. (1991) Isoflurane and an alpha 2-adrenoceptor agonist suppress nociceptive neurotransmission in neonatal rat spinal cord. *Anesthesiology* **75,** 489–498.
51. Wong, S. M. E., Cheng, G., Homanics, G., and Kendig, J. J. (2001) Enflurane actions on spinal cords from mice that lack the β3 subunit of the GABA$_A$ receptor. *Anesthesiology* **95,** 154–164.
52. Wong, S. M., Fong, E., Tauck, D. L., and Kendig, J. J. (1997) Ethanol as a general anesthetic: actions in spinal cord. *Eur. J. Pharmacol.* **329,** 121–127.
53. Tsutahara, S., Furumido, H., Ohta, Y., Harasawa, K., Yamamura, T., and Kemmotsu, O. (1996) [Effects of halothane, isoflurane, enflurane, and sevoflurane on the monosynaptic reflex response in the isolated spinal cord of newborn rats]. *Masui* **45,** 829–836.
54. Kendig, J. J., Kodde A., Gibbs L. M., Ionescu P., and Eger E. I. (1994) Correlates of anesthetic properties in isolated spinal cord: cyclobutanes. *Eur. J. Pharmacol.* **264,** 427–436.

55. Jewett, B. A., Gibbs, L. M., Tarasiuk, A., and Kendig, J. J. (1992) Propofol and barbiturate depression of spinal nociceptive neurotransmission. *Anesthesiology* **77,** 1148–1154.
56. Feng, J. and Kendig, J. J. (1995) Selective effects of alfentanil on nociceptive-related neurotransmission in neonatal rat spinal cord. *Brit. J. Anaesth.* **74,** 691–696.
57. Brockmeyer, D. M. and Kendig, J. J. (1995) Selective effects of ketamine on amino acid-mediated pathways in neonatal rat spinal cord. *Brit. J. Anaesth.* **74,** 79–84.
58. Hao, J. X., Sjolund, B. H., and Wiesenfeld-Hallin, Z. (1998) Electrophysiological evidence for an antinociceptive effect of ketamine in the rat spinal cord. *Acta Anaesthesiol. Scand.* **42,** 435–441.
59. Lodge, D. and Anis, N. A. (1984) Effects of ketamine and three other anaesthetics on spinal reflexes and inhibitions in the cat. *Brit. J. Anaesth.* **56,** 1143–1151.
60. Quinlan, J. J., Homanics, G. E., and Firestone, L. L. (1998) Anesthesia sensitivity in mice that lack the beta3 subunit of the gamma- aminobutyric acid type A receptor. *Anesthesiology* **88,** 775–780.
61. Lozier, A. P. and Kendig, J. J. (1995) Long-term potentiation in an isolated peripheral nerve-spinal cord preparation. *J. Neurophysiol.* **74,** 1001–1009.
62. Otsuka, M. and Yanagisawa, M. (1988) Effect of a tachykinin antagonist on a nociceptive reflex in the isolated spinal cord-tail preparation of the newborn rat. *J. Physiol.* **395,** 255–270.
63. Yanagisawa, M., Murakoshi, T., Tamai, S., and Otsuka, M. (1984) Tail-pinch method in vitro and the effects of some antinociceptive compounds. *Eur. J. Pharmacol.* **106,** 231–239.
64. Feng, J. and Kendig, J. J. (1996) Synergistic interactions between midazolam and alfentanil in isolated neonatal rat spinal cord. *Brit. J. Anaesth.* **77,** 375–380.
65. Wang, M. Y. and Kendig, J. J. (2000) Patch clamp studies of motor neurons in spinal cord slices: a tool for high-resolution analysis of drug actions. *Acta Pharmacologica Sinica* **21,** 481–576.
66. Cheng, G. and Kendig, J. J. (2000) Enflurane directly depresses glutamate AMPA and NMDA currents in mouse spinal cord motor neurons independent of actions on GABA$_A$ or glycine receptors. *Anesthesiology* **93,** 1075–1084.
67. Wang, M. Y., Rampil I. J., and Kendig, J. J. (1999) Ethanol directly depresses AMPA and NMDA glutamate currents in spinal cord motor neurons independent of actions on GABA$_A$ or glycine receptors. *J. Pharmacol. Exp. Ther.* **290,** 362–367.
68. Franks, N. P. and Lieb, W. R. (1993) Selective actions of volatile general anaesthetics at molecular and cellular levels. *Brit. J. Anaesth.* **71,** 65–76.
69. Franks, N. P. and Lieb, W. R. (1994) Molecular and cellular mechanisms of general anesthesia. *Nature* **367,** 607–614.
70. Tanelian, D. L., Kosek P., Mody, I., and MacIver, M. B. (1993) The role of the GABA$_A$ receptor/chloride channel complex in anesthesia. *Anesthesiology* **78,** 757–776.
71. de Sousa, S. L., Dickinson, R., Lieb, W. R., and Franks, N. P. (2000) Contrasting synaptic actions of the inhalational general anesthetics isoflurane and xenon. *Anesthesiology* **92,** 1055–1066.
72. Cheng, G. and Kendig, J. J. (2000) Pre- and postsynaptic volatile anesthetic actions on glycinergic transmission to special, unpublished data.
73. Zhang, Y., Wu, S., Eger, E. I., and Sonner, J. M. (2001) Neither GABA$_A$ nor strychnine-sensitive glycine receptors are the sole mediators of MAC for isoflurane. *Anesth. Analg.* **92,** 123–127.
74. Collins, J. G., Kendig, J. J., and Mason, P. (1995) Anesthetic actions within the spinal cord: contributions to the state of general anesthesia. *Trends Neurosci.* **18,** 549–553.

14
Simple Genetic Models for Anesthetic Action

Philip G. Morgan and Margaret Sedensky

INTRODUCTION

Since their introduction 150 yr ago, volatile anesthetics have revolutionized the practice of medicine. However, it is not clearly understood how the volatile anesthetics produce any of their most profound effects: loss of consciousness, amnesia, and lack of perception of pain. This uncertainty is greatly accentuated by the large number of potential targets that are affected by volatile anesthetics [1,2,3].

The "unitary hypothesis" of general anesthesia argues that all volatile anesthetics work via an identical site in all species [4,5]. During the past two decades, however, a great amount of evidence has been presented which is most consistent with multiple sites of volatile anesthetic action [6–13]. It is now clear that genetic mutations exist that distinguish between different volatile anesthetics, i.e., they alter sensitivity to some anesthetics differently than others. It follows that various molecular sites affect sensitivity to specific volatile anesthetics, and that the unitary hypothesis of general anesthesia is an oversimplification. Since it is probable that multiple targets contribute to the effects of anesthetics, a genetic approach is the most powerful way of sorting out which molecules contribute to specific anesthetic effects.

Ultimately, the phenomenon of anesthesia is a whole animal behavior, and as such, must eventually be studied at the level of the whole organism. Although many valuable approaches are being used to understand how volatile anesthetics work, the use of molecular genetics in a whole animal model possesses three powerful and unique advantages. First, our genes contain the blueprint for every molecular component of the anesthetic site of action. Therefore, the structure of an anesthetic site, regardless of its exact chemical nature (i.e., lipid, protein or both), is dictated by an invariant material (DNA) contained within virtually all cells. Second, a genetic approach is capable of correlating complicated behavior to a discreet set of molecular species, thus potentially greatly simplifying the study of behavior. Third, by screening for mutations that alter responses to anesthetics, nature directs the researcher to the important targets. As such, the data do not arise from preconceived ideas about what should be an anesthetic target. Other experimental designs make a "best guess" as to the nature of molecules that directly interact with volatile anesthetics, and then measure the effect of these agents on the suspect molecule. Even though these "guesses" are the end product of well-researched data, the results of such studies often leave doubts as to whether the effects represent phenomena incidental to the state of anesthesia or possibly are only partially responsible for the anesthetic state. That so many systems can be perturbed by these highly lipid-soluble compounds has contributed to some uncertainty as to which molecular species serves in vivo as an anesthetic target and how many might be important [14–17].

From: *Contemporary Clinical Neuroscience: Neural Mechanisms of Anesthesia*
Edited by: Joseph F. Antognini et al. © Humana Press Inc., Totowa, NJ

In contrast, molecular genetics can give information about molecules that are indisputably involved in the anesthetic response. The basic approach is to identify genes that code for molecules that directly control an animal's response to volatile anesthetics. This is generally done by exposing the animal to mutagens, and screening or selecting for offspring that are changed in their behavior in anesthetics. The mutagen has permanently affected the DNA of such an animal, and by virtue of this mutation can be identified and isolated, i.e., "cloned." This cloned gene, whose function can often be inferred from its structure, is necessarily responsible for the changed behavior for that anesthetic endpoint. Molecular data on the anesthetic site(s) of action, identified from whole animal responses, are absolutely necessary for advancement in our understanding of this fundamental question. The huge strides made in the field of molecular genetics now make such an approach possible. Since there will undoubtedly be some variation between organisms in the response to anesthetics, it is by comparing the results between these different systems that we are likely to understand the global mechanisms by which volatile anesthetics function.

Although still not a trivial undertaking, the task of dissecting the molecular mode of action of volatile anesthetics is substantially simplified by the use of genetic models. What should be the characteristics of such a tractable model? Researchers are generally faced with a tradeoff. A nervous system approximating that of humans is desirable, however a simple genetic system that can exploit the powerful tools of modern molecular genetic techniques is also needed. Mutagenesis, rapid gene mapping, the ability to direct mutagenesis, and the use of transgenic and mosaic animals are part of the current armamentarium of molecular genetics. In addition, a complete genetic sequence of the chromosomal DNA and a reasonable degree of homology of the genes from the organism to those of humans is also necessary. Finally, of course, the organism must have observable behaviors that are disrupted by anesthetics. Preferably these behaviors should be mediated by a nervous system. The relative advantages and disadvantages of different organisms are presented in Table 1.

BACKGROUND

Finding genes that control the whole animal response to volatile anesthetics is the crucial first step in a genetic approach to investigating the mechanism of action of anesthetics. Generally, in order to understand a gene's function, one has to first change a gene (i.e., make a mutation in that gene) to see the effect on the system. Thus, in the case of volatile anesthetics, one tries to change aspects of an animal's behavior by mutating the animal. Classical genetics then pinpoints that change to a single gene. Molecular genetics is, in turn, used to analyze the nature of the mutation, relating it to the normal function of the normal gene product.

An important point to remember is, whether the gene encodes a structural protein such as hemoglobin, a membrane-bound receptor such as an alpha-adrenergic receptor, or an enzyme such as pseudocholinesterase, it is the sequence of DNA that dictates the particular amino acids within the gene product. The structures of other molecules that are not proteins, such as lipids or sugars, are likewise determined by the ability of proteins (enzymes, the original gene products) to correctly synthesize them. All aspects of our physiology are ultimately dependent on the genetic material, and can be perturbed by changes in it. The processes of transcription and translation are essentially identical (i.e., conserved) across the animal and plant kingdoms, and were first described in simple genetic models. Somewhat surprisingly, the number of genes does not vary greatly between invertebrates, such as nematodes and fruit flies, and mammals, such as man. In fact, it would appear that the human genome is much smaller than previously assumed, and may be more similar to the genomes of nematodes and fruit flies than previously supposed. A relatively high percentage of genes is conserved even across this wide variation in complexity of animals. Thus, in many ways different-appearing organisms are very similar at the DNA level, and simple organisms often can be good initial models for molecular processes of more complex ones. This is particularly true if the physiologic process being studied appears to be conserved across species. In fact, most of our detailed

Table 1
Four Genetic Models for Anesthetic Action

	Advantages	*Disadvantages*
Yeast	Good classical genetics Sequenced genome	No nervous system Correct endpoint unclear
Worms	Good classical genetics Sequenced genome Simple nervous system	Correct endpoint unclear Simple nervous system
Flies	Good classical genetics Complicated nervous system	Correct endpoint unclear Complicated nervous system
Rodents	Targeted mutagenesis Complicated nervous system	Endpoints similar to humans Complicated nervous system

Table 1. The advantages and disadvantages are shown for four genetic models for studies of anesthetic action. The table centers on the value to studies involving nervous system function and does not reflect the usefulness of these organisms for studies of other developmental processes.

knowledge of the functioning of mammalian cellular machinery is derived directly from the brilliant studies of bacteria and viruses during the past 50 yr.

Genetics uses what may seem to most of us like a backward approach to answer a question. In classical genetics, one changes the experimental animal without knowing which variable (gene) caused the change, then looks for the altered variable (a mutated gene). Although one does not necessarily know what molecules caused that trait to change, it is clear a permanent change has occurred in the gene that controls that trait. As previously mentioned, the beauty of this approach is its lack of preconceptions as to the molecular nature of a given trait. However, if a complicated pathway or cascade of events leads to particular behavior, one may have mutated any one of a great number of genes that may contribute to that behavior. For example, mutations that change sensitivity to volatile anesthetics could arise from structural changes in molecules that are an anesthetic target, from elimination of enzymes that make these molecules, from changes in molecules that interact with an anesthetic target, from changes in molecules that make the anesthetic available to a target, or from changes which have no direct effect on anesthetic function but which raise or lower the general activity of an animal. Data are sorted out in part by collecting multiple mutations that affect anesthetic sensitivity and studying their interactions and relative importance in determining anesthetic sensitivity. Finally, one must identify, using molecular techniques, the protein products of these genes and deduce their functions from their structure and their interactions with other molecules.

Classical genetics can define the specific chromosomal region in which a gene is located. Advances in molecular biology now allow this information to be used to pinpoint a gene to a specific physical fragment of DNA. It is also possible to manipulate pieces of DNA such that they can be moved into novel environments to isolate their effects. For example, a normal gene can be introduced into a defective or mutant animal, giving rise to a normal animal. Such a technique is the first step in treating genetic diseases (i.e., the beginning of genetic therapeutics). A second use is to introduce a defective gene into a previously normal organism, to "genetically engineer" a mutation into an organism to study a gene's function. Introduction of specific mutations into an organism is referred to as targeted mutagenesis and illustrates an important point. Generally, organisms with rapid generation times and large numbers of offspring are used to perform random mutagenesis searching for mutations affecting a phenotype (such as altered anesthetic sensitivity). The most commonly used model organisms are yeast (*Saccharomyces cerevisiae*), the worm (*Caenorhabditis elegans*), and the fruit fly (*Drosophila melanogaster*). These are the studies that avoid preconceptions as to the correct answer. After these studies are done, it is often useful to create similar mutations in a more complicated organism, such as a mouse, to determine whether the mutation has similar effects in a mammal. Targeted mutagenesis cannot be used as an initial screen in mammals, but is a powerful technique for extending studies from a simple genetic model into more complicated animals.

CLASSICAL GENETICS

Gene Mapping

Traditionally, geneticists have tackled questions of inheritance by observing the passage of clearly identifiable traits from one generation to the next. An organism's observed features, its phenotype, must arise from the content of its genetic material, its genotype. Classical genetics relies on differences in phenotype (e.g., blue eyes vs brown eyes) as the probes for identifying different genes and locating their relative positions. These differences are ascribed to individual genes and positioned in the genome (all the DNA of an organism) only after genetic manipulations, usually matings, have been carried out.

In classical genetic animals such as fruit flies (*Drosophila*), one can usually mate an animal with a new mutation to an animal that carries strategically placed genetic markers. These markers are characteristics that are easy to see (such as eye color or wing configuration) that are known to be coded by DNA of specific regions of specific chromosomes. These markers are already "mapped," that is their positions on chromosomes are known. The number of offspring that show the new mutation in combination with these mapped genes eventually pinpoints the mutation to a specific region of a specific chromosome. If two mutations are in the same chromosome, the distance between them is specified in terms of map units. Two mutations that are one map unit apart are genetically very close to each other; they have about one chance in 100 of separating from each other by chromosomal recombination in each generation. The further apart two mutations are, the greater the number of map units between them.

Gene Interactions

A second, equally important aspect of classical genetics is to determine the interaction between genes. One may determine the effect of one mutation (A) on a second mutation, or (B) by constructing an animal containing both mutations. If such an animal has elements of both phenotypes, then A and B may function independently. If such an animal has the phenotype of only one mutation, that mutation is thought to be "downstream" of the other. Such information is useful in determining functional pathways involving many gene products. For example, if an animal carrying both mutations A and B looks identical to an animal carrying only mutation B, then B is said to be "downstream" of A in a common genetic pathway. In a genetic pathway, "downstream" means that one gene product, (in this case A) exerts its effects by functioning through a second one, (in this case B). When an animal has the B phenotype, it does not matter what the state of A is, because A's effects are dependent on a functioning B product. A mutation resulting in loss of the B product will always produce the B phenotype.

Gene Sequence

Once the coding sequence of a gene is known, one can begin to understand the function of the protein product. Genes coding for similar proteins in different organisms often have a similar order of bases (i.e., of A's, T's, G's, and C's). Proteins with similar functions usually have regions of identical or similar amino acids. By comparing these similarities, called homologies, one can often assign a function to a newly identified protein. A truly immense amount of sequence data has accumulated over the past 10 yr culminating with the recent sequencing of the yeast, nematode, fly, and human genomes *(18–21)*. By comparing newly identified sequences with other known genes, one can often identify homologies, which in turn often implies similar functions *(22,23)*. If no such homology exists, all is not lost. Certain aspects of a protein's structure and function (such as a membrane spanning region) give characteristic recognizable patterns of amino acids. Thus, much information can be gained from the sequence even in the absence of known homologies. It is certainly widely anticipated that in the future the ability to analyze existing data bases will expand greatly. The structure of a protein can then lead to conclusions about its function. The occasional truly novel gene product must wait until biochemical studies are done or other similar genes are characterized (possibly in another organism) to determine its function. In addition, the cloned gene often allows one to synthesize the protein product and study it directly in a variety of other surroundings. Thus, we have gone from a gross change in the whole animal to a specific gene and protein product, which can be isolated and studied independently of the organism.

SPECIFIC ORGANISMS

As described above in Gene Sequence, currently the genetic determinants of volatile anesthetics are being studied in four very different organisms: the yeast, *Saccharomyces cerevisiae*; the nematode, *Caenorhabditis elegans*; the fruit fly, *Drosophila melanogaster*; and the mouse, *Mus musculus*. Below, we detail these studies, from most simple to most complex animal model.

Saccharomyces cerevisiae (S. cerevisiae)

Keil and colleagues *(24)* have studied the effects of volatile anesthetics on yeast, *S. cerevisiae*. As the authors note, yeast has both advantages and disadvantages compared with more complex eukaryotes. Yeast offers superb, extremely powerful genetics that control a complicated life cycle. It possesses a very short generation time and a tremendous number of mapped genes. In addition, it was the first eukaryote to have its entire genome sequenced. Thus, for a molecular genetic approach to many questions of interest, it is unparalleled in its advantages.

Clearly to its disadvantage for our purposes, yeast do not have a nervous system. The precise mechanism of action of volatile anesthetics will therefore probably differ between yeast and higher eukaryotes. However, as Keil and colleagues state, any mutations isolated must "reflect molecular effects of the anesthetics *(25)*." Just as the basic interactions of volatile anesthetics with isolated proteins such as albumin can be instructive, the effects of volatile anesthetics on a living organism with an easily measurable response to the anesthetic can be very valuable. Determining the nature of the interactions between anesthetics and their targets will probably shed light on similar interactions in nervous systems, even if the targets, or their precise function, differ. The authors found that all volatile anesthetics inhibit growth in yeast, at concentrations approx 10× those required for surgical anesthesia in mammals. However, the inhibiting concentrations followed the Meyer-Overton relationship as noted for inhibition of the nervous system in more complex organisms. This inhibition was reversible after 24 h of exposure to the anesthetic *(24)*. In addition, the potencies of different volatile anesthetics were additive and nonimmobilizers had no effect on the growth of yeast *(25)*.

The authors screened for mutations conferring resistant to the inhibitory effect of volatile anesthetics. They isolated a single mutation, termed zzz4, which conferred resistance to 13% isoflurane (EC_{50} for isoflurane is 12% for wild type) and also had altered degradation of ubiquinated (see below) proteins *(24)*. Ubiquitin is a 76 amino acid polypeptide that is attached to other proteins to target them for degradation and is highly conserved in all animals studied including mammals. Keil and colleagues cloned and identified ZZZ4 as a membrane protein whose amino acid structure is similar (homologous) to a rodent phospholipase A1-activating protein (PLAP). PLAP itself is homologous to G-proteins, and so falls into one class of candidates proposed to be affected by volatile anesthetics *(26)*.

The authors have also identified two other genes which can be mutated to alter anesthetic sensitivity in yeast. One codes for a protein that binds ubiquitin ligase and the other one for the protein ubiquitin ligase itself *(26).* These findings and others reported by these authors clearly indicate a role for ubiquitin metabolism in controlling the sensitivity to volatile anesthetics in yeast. It remains to be seen whether homologs of this class of protein also affect anesthetic sensitivities in organisms with nervous systems. However, an interesting association of ubiquitin ligase with lipid rafts *(see* Section on Immobility) has been noted in MDCK (Madin-Darby canine kidney) cells *(27).* As will be discussed later, lipid rafts may relate data gathered for several proposed targets of volatile anesthetics.

Caenorhabditis elegans (C. elegans)

C. elegans is a nonparasitic nematode (roundworm) that is about 1 mm long. It is widely studied as an animal model for a variety of processes, from cell division and embryogenesis to aging and Alzheimer's disease. When first espoused as a scientific model system by Sydney Brenner, *C. elegans* was originally envisioned as the organism in which to pursue the molecular basis of behavior *(28).* The excellent genetics, superb catalog of known neuronal/muscular mutations, well-defined behaviors, invariant cell lineage and anatomy make this organism an exquisitely useful genetic model *(29–31).* This is coupled with a complete wiring diagram of every synapse of the hermaphrodite's 302 neurons makes the nematode unique for studies of nervous system function *(32). C. elegans* has other aspects that make it a good model for the study of behavioral processes in mammals. These include a surprising similarity of the underlying molecular basis of its nervous system when compared to that of mammals. The worm possesses many of the same neurotransmitters to mediate behavior as found in mammals (acetylcholine, serotonin, GABA, dopamine, glutamate, and peptides). The identified ion channels are also closely conserved between mammals and nematodes. In addition, about half of the genes sequenced have homologs in mammals, a staggering conservation of structure and function *(19,33).* While these similarities do not guarantee that molecular sites of anesthetic action will be identical in nematodes and mammals, they do point out that nature tends to continue to use similar motifs for similar functions throughout phylogeny. Thus, identification of the mechanisms of anesthetic action in nematodes are very likely to shed light on the mechanisms of anesthetic action in more complicated animals.

Anesthetic Endpoints

C. elegans responds to volatile anesthetics in a manner similar to mammals. Initial efforts to establish *C. elegans* as a useful model for anesthetic action involved exposing the worm to a variety of volatile anesthetics, and selecting a behavioral endpoint to represent the "anesthetic state" *(34–37).* Wild type worms, N2, move constantly in a sinuous motion on an agar plate. When exposed to volatile anesthetics, they first increase movement, become "excited", and lose their response to volatile attractants. This behavior proceeds to a progressive lack of coordination, followed by immobility and unresponsiveness to a tap to the snout. This progression of neurologic changes is reminiscent of the excitation, loss of the sense of smell, uncoordination, and loss of response to noxious stimuli seen in mammals *(36).* Two different endpoints have been used to measure anesthetic effects in *C. elegans.* One of these is radial dispersion, the ability of a nematode to move radially from a starting point in the center of a plate of agar towards a peripheral ring of food, *Escherichia coli* *(E. coli).* The percentage of nematodes reaching the peripheral ring of food in the presence of a volatile anesthetic serves as the endpoint *(37).* The second endpoint is complete immobility of the animal for 10 s *(36).* The loss of function associated with both endpoints is quickly reversed upon removal of the worms from the anesthetic agent; subsequent life-span, fertility, movement, chemotaxis, and mating are unaffected by exposure to these agents *(33,34,38).* The absolute dose of anesthetic required to cause immobility is higher than MAC in mammals, while that required for loss of radial dispersion is similar to MAC. The ratio of the LC_{50} to the EC_{50} for immobility is approx 2.5, similar to that for volatile anesthetics in mammals *(38)*, whereas that for radial dispersion is approx 20. Thus, strengths and weaknesses exist for both endpoints as a model specifically for MAC. However, both endpoints follow the Meyer-Overton rule very closely; a log-log plot of EC_{50}s vs O/Gs yields a very good straight line fit with a slope of -1 *(33,34)*. The nonanesthetic and "transition" lipid soluble gases studied by Koblin et al *(39)* failed to immobilize *C. elegans* (F4 and F6), or did so at a higher concentration than that predicted by their O/G (toluene) *(40)*. Stereoisomers of volatile anesthetics exhibit different potencies in *C. elegans* when immobility is used as an endpoint *(41)*. The effects of nonimmobilizers and stereoisomers on radial dispersion have not been reported.

A great deal of debate centers upon selection of anesthetic endpoints in mammalian studies, like loss of righting reflex vs tail clap in rodents. Even in a simple model, behavioral endpoints for the phenomena of "anesthesia" can be debated. In the wild, the nematode lives in a cool environment, (which may lead to different properties of the cell membrane in comparison to warm blooded animals) and is exposed to a variety of lipid soluble compounds. In addition, the wild type animal never stops moving, not surprising given that oxygenation of its tissues is presumably via simple diffusion. It seems unlikely that an animal with so many similarities to more complicated organisms, which behaves so similarly to mammals in volatile anesthetics, would have a radically different molecular interaction between a volatile anesthetic and its target. Studying different endpoints in *C. elegans* certainly has value in understanding how volatile anesthetics interact with a spectrum of targets. In mammals different endpoints like loss of recall are clearly affected at concentrations lower than MAC, and are the subject of meaningful study. The close adherence of both these *C. elegans* endpoints to the Meyer-Overton rule, the absolute reversibility of this exposure, and the lack of toxicity on any subsequent behaviors, make both very compelling choices as anesthetic endpoints. The advantages of *C. elegans* as a model must be weighed against the disadvantages that its differences from mammals represent. The findings resulting from the genetic studies are grouped below under the heading of the endpoint used to generate mutants.

Immobility

Morgan and Sedensky *(33,42)* originally mutagenized normal worms and then screened for mutations that altered anesthetic sensitivity using immobility as the endpoint. The first identified mutant with profound changes was *unc-79*. Mutations in *unc-79* cause a striking hypersensitivity to the four most lipid soluble volatile anesthetics, but either no change or resistance to other classes of volatile anesthetics, and an intermediate increase in sensitivity to diethylether. *unc-79* animals showed decreased binding of the anesthetic, halothane (Eckenhoff, R. G., personal communication). Because *unc-79* deviates from the Meyer-Overton rule, it follows that the unitary hypothesis is an oversimplification.

The X-linked mutation *unc-1(e580)* suppressed *unc-79*, i.e., when added to *unc-79* it restored to normal the hypersensitivity of *unc-79* to the most lipid soluble anesthetics *(43)*. *unc-1* also restored the resistance of *unc-79* to flurothyl and enflurane to normal, and left unchanged any responses that were identical between mutants and wild type. However, it did not return to baseline the changed response of *unc-79* to diethylether. *unc-1(e580)* is similar to N2 in anesthetic response, except for an approx 30% increase in sensitivity to diethylether and a 5–10% resistance to halothane. These data all support the interpretation of the original *unc-79* data, i.e. that multiple sites of action exist for volatile anesthetics.

unc-1 is a complicated gene, having four different classes of alleles *(44)*. The dominant alleles increases sensitivity to all volatile anesthetics. The recessive alleles primarily affect sensitivity to ether and halothane. Complex interactions between alleles in each class of *unc-1* indicate that the gene product, UNC-1, probably works as a multimeric protein that contains multiple copies of the UNC-1 protein *(44,45)*. The *unc-1* gene encodes a homolog of a human protein, *stomatin (46)*.

Stomatin is an integral membrane protein in humans that is expressed within many types of cells. *(47–49)* It controls sodium and potassium flux across membranes, though its exact mode of action is not known. We have also shown that the mutations in UNC-1 that affect sensitivity to anesthetics, reside in that part of the protein postulated to directly control ion flux. A protein with the intrinsic ability to fluoresce (green fluorescent protein, GFP) can be linked to the UNC-1 protein to "light up" cells that express the gene in a living animal *(45,50)* (Fig. 1). Expression of *unc-1*'s protein product is almost entirely within neurons in *C. elegans*, at all times of larval and adult development. Antibody staining with monoclonal antibodies to UNC-1 has confirmed this result *(51)*. It appears that the UNC-1 protein may be part of a protein complex involving a sodium channel within the plasma membrane that affects sensitivity to a wide range of volatile anesthetics. Genetic studies have shown that UNC-1 interacts with a class of epithelial sodium channels (termed ENaCs) and that mutations in these sodium channels (encoded by a gene called *unc-8*) also directly alter anesthetic sensitivity *(45,52)*. In addition, gap junction proteins (*unc-7* and *unc-9*) have been shown to interact in this pathway *(43,53)* (Fig. 2).

Recent work in mammals has indicated that stomatin is localized to lipid microdomains found in cell membranes termed "lipid rafts" *(54,55)*. Stomatin may be partly responsible for the formation and maintenance of these rafts *(56)*. Lipid rafts are microdomains in the cell membrane with increased amounts of sphingolipids and cholesterol. These domains are thought to localize multiple membrane proteins into complexes. It is known that glycosyl-phosphatidylinositol (GPI) anchored proteins and acylated proteins are localized in these domains in mammalian cells *(54,55)*. The list of proteins associated with lipid rafts includes ligand gated channels, G-protein coupled receptors, and members of the SNARE complex (the complex containing syntaxin, shown by Crowder to play a role in anesthetic sensitivity) *(27,37,57)*. Each of these has been postulated to be a target of volatile anesthetics. Thus, mutations in stomatin and stomatin-like proteins could exert their effects by disruption of membrane associated lipid domains and their associated protein complexes. Morgan and Sedensky isolated lipid rafts in *C. elegans* and found that stomatin also localizes to these domains. In addition, a mutation in a gene called *unc-24*, apparently blocks the movement of these rafts from the endoplasmic reticulum to the cellular membrane. Nematodes mutant in *unc-24* sequester UNC-1 in the endoplasmic reticulum and mimic the *unc-1* loss of function phenotype both in air and in anesthetics *(51)*.

A third mutation, *gas-1(fc21)*, causes *C. elegans* to be hypersensitive to all volatile anesthetics tested, despite normal motion in air *(58)*. The *gas-1* gene encodes the 49 kDa(IP) subunit of the mitochondrial NADH:ubiquinone-oxidoreductase (complex I of the respiratory chain) *(59)*. It is a member of a very large protein complex that is the first step of electron transport. Metabolic studies show that the function of complex I is reduced in gas-1 mutants and that anesthetics further decrease the function of this complex *(60)*. Interestingly, a mutation in complex II of the electron transport chain *(61)* (*mev-1*) does not affect the function of complex I and does not alter anesthetic sensitivity *(62)*. Complex II feeds electrons into the same acceptor as complex I, i.e., it is a separate way to donate electrons to Coenzyme Q. The finding that a mutation in complex I increases sensitivity of *C. elegans* to volatile anesthetics while a mutation in complex II does not, implicates this particular step in electron transport in the determination of anesthetic sensitivity. Additional mutations in these and other genes of electron transport will be needed to unravel this story.

The contribution of mitochondrial proteins to anesthetic response is particularly interesting since previous work in mammalian systems has also shown that complex I-dependent oxidative phosphorylation is sensitive to volatile anesthetics *(63,64)*. However, the pattern of oxidative phosphorylation inhibition in *gas-1* animals indicates that mitochondria probably affect secondary sites (perhaps UNC-1, UNC-8, and UNC-79) to cause changes in sensitivity *(60)*. Recently, a subset of patients with mitochondrial defects have been shown to be profoundly more sensitive to sevoflurane (Morgan and Sedensky, unpublished results), as judged by the concentration of the gas

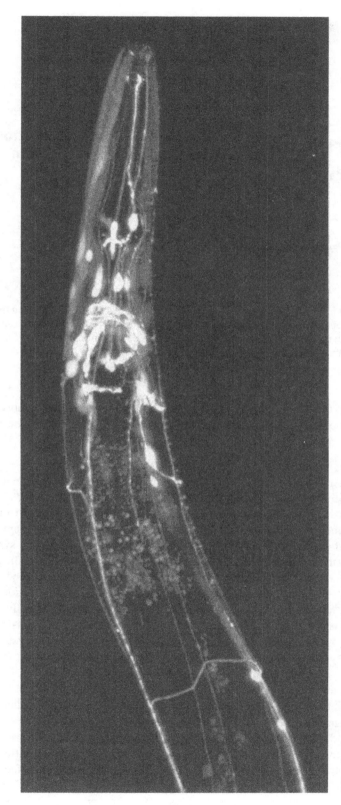

Fig. 1. The cellular expression of green fluorescent protein (GFP) is under the control of the *unc-1* promoter in *C. elegans*. The cells which normally express *unc-1* "light up" green in the living animal. This work demonstrates the usefulness of a simple, transparent animal in determining the specific cells in which a gene is expressed and the timing of that expression.

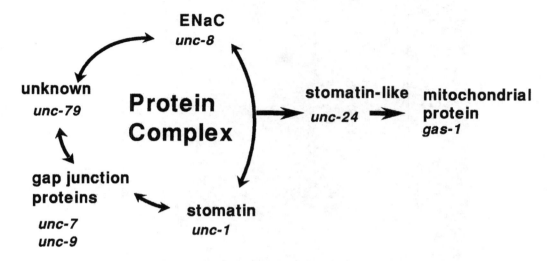

Fig. 2. The genes involved in controlling sensitivity to volatile anesthetics in *C. elegans* using immobility as the endpoint. Each of these genes is mentioned in the text and has unique effects on anesthetic sensitivity. The simplest explanation of the interaction of these genes is that they function in a protein complex. Similar interactions have been found for homologs of these genes in higher organisms. The role of *gas-1* in this pathway, if any, is unclear at present.

necessary to reach a BIS of 60. Thus, the findings in *C. elegans* are corroborated by observations in humans. This indicates the potential applicability of studies in a model organism to a human disease process.

Radial Dispersion

Crowder has screened nematodes carrying previously identified mutations in neuronal proteins of *C. elegans* for altered sensitivity to anesthetics using radial dispersion as the endpoint *(37)*. He found that a mutation in syntaxin dominantly conferred resistance to the volatile anesthetics isoflurane and halothane. Syntaxin is a member of the protein complex (Fig. 3), which controls presynaptic vesicular fushionfusion with the cell membrane resulting in neurotransmitter release into the synaptic cleft *(65)*. This complex is termed the SNARE complex, including the syntaxin-binding proteins, synaptobrevin, and SNAP-25 *(65,66)*. Mutations in these other proteins failed to produce volatile anesthetic hypersensitivity. The syntaxin allelic variation was striking, particularly for isoflurane, where a 33-fold range of sensitivities was seen. Both the resistant and hypersensitive mutations decrease synaptic transmission; thus, the indirect effect of reducing neurotransmission does not explain the anesthetic resistance. These results were consistent with a protein target for volatile anesthetics and implicate syntaxin as a possible anesthetic target. Crowder has also presented data showing that mammalian syntaxin is capable of binding halothane *(67)*.

It is interesting that the members of the SNARE complex have been found to be associated with lipid rafts and with ENaC channels *(27,68)*. Could the gene products identified using different endpoints interact in some fashion? *unc-1* animals are too uncoordinated to use in a radial dispersion assay. Syntaxin mutations do not alter anesthetic sensitivity when using immobility as an endpoint (Morgan, unpublished). However, the association of the SNARE complex, stomatin and ENaC channels with lipid rafts and with each other, suggests a common pathway or target affected by these mutations. These data are further emphasized by the fact that the system identified in yeast, the ubiquitin system, has also been shown to reside in lipid rafts *(69)*. Thus, proteins identified by diverse screens may implicate similar types of targets both in yeast and in *C. elegans*. However, the nature of any interaction is unclear at this time.

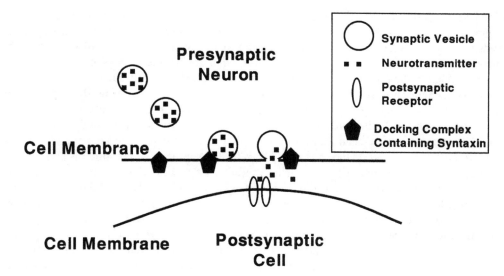

Fig. 3. A model for the function of the complex containing syntaxin in vesicular fusion and release of neurotransmitter at a nerve terminal. Syntaxin is part of the docking complex that both binds vesicles to the membrane and allows for their fusion with the membrane. As a result of the fusion, the neurotransmitter is released into the synaptic cleft. The docking complex contains several proteins in addition to syntaxin. However, at present, only syntaxin has been shown to affect anesthetic sensitivity and to bind volatile anesthetics.

Drosophila melanogaster

The advantages and disadvantages of using *Drosophila* as a genetic model are very similar to those for *Caenorhabditis*. As a genetic model, *Drosophila* is at least the equal of the nematode, with a high density of genetic markers, completely sequenced genome and easy to identify behaviors and physical markers. In addition, like in the nematode, there is a high degree of conservation between genes in the fly and in mammals. The nervous system is more complicated than that of the nematode, which serves as a mixed blessing. On the one hand, the behaviors of the fly are likely to result from an increased level of complexity in neuronal connections, more like that of a mammal. However, as might be expected, this increased complexity makes it more difficult to trace genetic changes to specific neurons or groups of neurons. As with any genetic model, the disadvantages must be weighed against the advantages and results interpreted carefully.

Drosophila has been used extensively by two laboratories studying the mechanism of action of volatile anesthetics. Gamo and colleagues pioneered the use of *Drosophila* by studying the sensitivity of the fly to diethyl ether using nonresponsiveness to touch as the endpoint *(70,71)*. The wild type Canton-S strain has an EC_{50} for ether of about 1.9 vol % in air. The authors then identified 14 mutations that altered the sensitivity of the flies to diethyl ether. The changes in EC_{50}s ranged from a decrease to 1.3% to an increase to 3.2% ether *(71)*. The identities of two of the genes have been confirmed. The first gene (para) encodes the alpha subunit of a sodium channel *(71)*. The second gene codes for calreticulin, a multifunctional calcium-binding protein in the endoplasmic reticulum of non-muscle cells. However, no further work on these genes has been reported. At present, it is unclear whether these genes interact in some way, or whether they represent two separate pathways that control response to ether.

Howard Nash at the NIMH has screened extensively for mutations that alter anesthetic sensitivity in *Drosophila*. However, he has used different endpoints than Gamo by scoring the posture or movement of the flies in anesthetics *(72,73)*. Using this mechanism, his laboratory identified a group of mutations, known as *har* mutants, which conferred resistance to halothane. At least four such mutations were identified on the X-chromosome. The *har* mutants have a common interesting feature with some of the mutants found in the nematode in that they alter sensitivity to some anesthetics differently than others. These findings are also most consistent with multiple sites of anesthetic action. Krishnan has identified two autosomal loci in *Drosophila* that alter anesthetic sensitivity *(74)*. These have been mapped to the third chromosome, but have not yet been identified.

Nash and colleagues also studied the use of other endpoints for measuring anesthetic sensitivity in flies *(75,76)*. They reported that the changes in sensitivity in *har* mutants are dependent on the assay used, i.e., the mutants exhibited differential changes in sensitivity when the endpoint was varied *(72,75)*. They used an intense beam of light *(76)* or direct electrical signals to the eye *(77)* to assess the effect of the har mutations on the capacity of fruit flies to sense a noxious stimulus and respond to it. These results were compared to the earlier studies using changes in posture and movement described above. Undoubtedly, such results represent layers of integrated neuronal interactions which produce a complex behavioral response. As previously discussed, complex behaviors can be changed by mutations that have indirect effects on the phenomenon of anesthesia. Nash and colleagues hope to isolate mutations that are as close as possible to the actual target of volatile anesthetics by studying a defined cellular physiology. Consequently, they have pursued the study of a variety of simple, well-defined reflexes of *Drosophila* in order to test the effects of volatile anesthetics on specific neuronal circuits. Nishikawa and Kidokoro studied the effects of two *har* mutations on synaptic transmission at the larval neuromuscular junction *(78)*. They found that halothane decreased the frequency of glutaminergic miniature excitatory junctional currents in the wild type synapse, but that halothane did not change the frequency in synapses from the mutants *har38* and *har85*. These results indicate that this glutamate-mediated pathway is important in determining halothane sensitivity in flies and that at least two of the *har* mutants alter sensitivity by affecting this pathway. The exact role of the genes in this pathway defined by *har38* and *har85* awaits molecular data characterizing their gene products.

Using the escape response as another well-defined neuronal circuit in which to test the effects of volatile anesthetics, Walcourt and Nash have shown that *mushroom body defect* (*mud*) mutants have an increased sensitivity to halothane *(77)*. These animals have a variety of changes in brain structure, although gross changes in brain anatomy did not correlate with anesthetic sensitivity. Similarly to the *har* mutants, changes in anesthetic sensitivity of *mud* mutants differ between the three tested anesthetics. Interestingly, several other mutations causing global changes in brain structure did not alter anesthetic sensitivity. Thus, the circuit affected by *mud* seems to be specifically sensitive to anesthetics and a good model for identifying genes affecting anesthetic response of a behavior with a much simpler level of complexity. Nash's group recently studied the affects of changes in the potassium channel encoded by the *Shaker* gene on the escape pathway *(79)*. They found that *Shaker* had profound effects on the response of this circuit to halothane. Using a well-defined neuronal circuit, such as the escape response, may in fact be very important in isolating an effect of volatile anesthetics that is close to the anesthetic target.

These studies emphasize both the power of genetic approaches and the importance of correlation of the findings to other methods of characterizing anesthetic action. In *Drosophila*, the classic genetic approach of Nash has been greatly aided by the neurophysiologic studies of the *har* mutants, the studies of flies with defined anatomical defects in the brain, and by studies of flies with changes in specific ion channels. As seen in nematodes, the initial findings implicate sites that are not obviously felt to be likely targets for volatile anesthetics. Only by using such unbiased approaches to determining genes affecting anesthetic response are we likely to truly understand the nature of anesthetic action.

MAMMALS

Mammals, like rats or mice, have behaviors that can unequivocally be related to human MAC. In addition, the organization of neuronal pathways in rodents more clearly approximate that of man. It is clearly desirable to use these convenient laboratory animals to investigate how volatile anesthetics

Targeted Mutagenesis

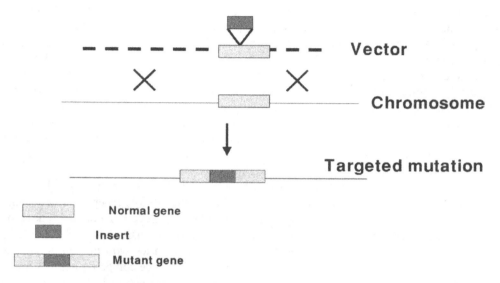

Fig. 4. A general plan for targeting genes for mutation in mice. There are multiple methods for generating such mutations, but this represents a very simple one. A homolog of the gene to be mutated is disrupted in a plasmid or other vector. This altered gene is then inserted in place of the normal gene on the chromosome by homologous recombination. This technique allows for specific genes to be mutated, but is not amenable to random mutagenesis.

work. In addition, the sequence of the mouse genome is currently nearing completion. However, compared to yeast, or worms, or flies, rodents are much more difficult to use as a model for classic sorts of genetic studies. Generation times are in terms of months rather than days, good genetic markers are comparatively few and far between, and the selection for observed behaviors is difficult. For example, no one would seriously consider exposing an inbred mouse strain to a mutagen and then screen for mutations that change the behavior of offspring in a volatile anesthetic. The numbers of animals necessary would be prohibitive in terms of both time and money. In the past, the changes in behavior that have been observed for rodents in volatile anesthetics have been the result of selective pressures kept on certain sorts of inbred lines that are the results of intense and time-consuming series of matings and selections that have taken many years to yield results.

On the other hand, a molecule that is already perceived to be important in the function of volatile anesthetics can be tested for its importance to the behavior of the whole animal in the mouse. This sort of approach, sometimes called "reverse genetics", targets the DNA that makes that molecule, and engineers an animal such that that particular molecule is absent in the genetically engineered mouse (Fig. 4). Also, various "wild type" strains, i.e., normal or nonmutated strains, have different anesthetic sensitivities that can be used to address the question of how volatile anesthetics work. In addition, recombinant inbred strains have already been made in the mouse and rat which change the sensitivity of the strains to alcohol or benzodiazepines. These have been studied for their effects on anesthetic sensitivity. Each of these approaches are discussed below. Clearly, with the recent sequencing of the human genome, (which turns out to be smaller than once thought) and the soon to be completed sequence of the mouse genome, an increasing ability to correlate genetic work in the mouse to human physiology is likely.

Mus musculus

Eger and colleagues measured the naturally occurring variability in anesthetic potency, defined by the minimum alveolar anesthetic concentrations (MACs) required to produce immobility in response to noxious stimuli. Fifteen commonly used laboratory mouse strains were studied *(80,81)*. They found that the range of MAC values was 39% for desflurane, 44% for isoflurane, and 55% for halothane. It is remarkable to realize that these strains, all of which are "normal," and all of which belong to the same species and therefore are nearly genetically identical, have such widely differing responses to different volatile anesthetics. One hundred forty-six statistically significant differences among the 15 strains were found for the three inhaled anesthetics (isoflurane, desflurane, and halothane). They concluded that multiple genes underlie the observed variability in anesthetic potency, once again consistent with the hypothesis that multiple targets exist for these anesthetics. These results also highlight one of the problems when using the mouse for genetics. One must be rigorous in identifying the wild-type strain from which mutations arose and use correct controls, because the wild-type strains themselves vary in their sensitivities.

Genetic studies of anesthetic action in mice originally centered on susceptibility of inbred strains to ethanol *(82,83)*. Multiple in vitro studies have implicated the $GABA_A$ receptor as contributing to the ethanol response *(84)*, though not unique in doing so *(83,85)*. Several laboratories have studied strains with increased sensitivity (LS for long sleep) and decreased sensitivity (SS for short sleep) to ethanol. The sensitivity of these strains to volatile anesthetics varies with the anesthetic studied. Erwin et al. found that sensitivity to ether did not increase in LS mice compared with SS mice *(86)*. Similarly, Baker found that sensitivity to halothane was not increased in LS mice *(7)*. However, Koblin and Deady showed that LS mice did have increased sensitivities to enflurane and isoflurane *(8)*. These studies are most consistent with multiple sites of anesthetic action for volatile anesthetics. However, at least nine genetic loci are estimated to vary between the LS and SS lines. While one of these involves the $GABA_A$ receptor, the identity of the remaining loci is unknown *(83,84)*. Similar results have recently been obtained using rat lines bred for sensitivity or resistance to ethanol. Firestone studied the response of these strains to halothane and to desflurane *(87)*. His group found that lines with differing sensitivities to ethanol had differing sensitivities to halothane for both loss of righting reflex (LORR) and for withdrawal to tail clamp. However, they only showed a difference to LORR for desflurane. They concluded that their data support the hypothesis that different anesthetic endpoints are produced by separate mechanisms. At least some of these mechanisms have multiple mechanisms for the different anesthetics.

Targeted mutations in the $GABA_A$ receptor have also been studied in the mouse. Firestone has created several knockouts affecting different subunits of the $GABA_A$ receptor. The authors tested whether genetically engineered mice that lack the β3 subunit of the $GABA_A$ receptor differed in their sensitivities to several general anesthetic agents. Mice completely lacking the beta-3 subunit of the $GABA_A$ receptor (b3 –/–) did not differ from wild-type mice (b3 +/+) in the obtunding response to enflurane and halothane, but were mildly resistant (10–20%) to enflurane and halothane as determined by tail clamp response *(88)*. However, these animals also demonstrated a generalized loss of nociception in the absence of anesthetic *(89)*. When the effects of loss of the alpha-6 subunit were tested, no differences between wild type and mutant were seen *(90)*. These results indicated that the $GABA_A$ receptor probably does contribute to the anesthetic response in the normal mouse. However, it is also clear that this receptor does not represent the only major anesthetic target.

SUMMARY

Genetic data are beginning to form the picture of the molecular sites that control anesthetic sensitivity. At present, the mutations identified are most consistent with protein targets, though a contribution by lipid species is still a possibility. Significant contributions to anesthetic response are probably made by the $GABA_A$ receptor and by the glutamate receptor. However, the genetic studies described above strongly suggest that anesthetic response is dependent on a much broader group of molecular targets or pathways. The finding of altered sensitivity in patients with mitochondrial disease underscores the applicability of these studies to the human population.

It is also interesting to note what genetic data fail to do. They do not identify a single protein or channel that is uniquely responsible for the effects of anesthetics. The many endpoints associated with the anesthetic state are probably the result of effects at different sites of anesthetic action. In addition, even when considering a defined simple endpoint, the different anesthetics behave differently from each other. This indicates that even with single endpoints, multiple targets or mechanisms are involved. We are beginning to identify physical properties which are common between possible anesthetic targets. However, additional genes that affect anesthetic sensitivity will certainly still be identified. Among those that have been characterized, there still exists a diversity that is difficult to mold into a common theme. The continuing advances in molecular characterization of the human genome will certainly accelerate the synthesis of knowledge gained from model systems to the human behavior.

Clearly genetic studies on whole animals are an absolute necessity to corroborate data that are obtained from a variety of in vitro paradigms. With the tremendous strides being made in the rapidly advancing field of molecular genetics, it is inevitable that our specialty will advance in understanding the very basic question of how volatile anesthetics work. The ideal volatile anesthetics can most easily emerge from a knowledge of the basic principles of the mechanism of action of volatile anesthetics. Not only might this type of research lead to rational drug design, we may be able to use these remarkable drugs to understand the nature of consciousness itself.

REFERENCES

1. Franks, N. P. and Lieb, W. R. (1994) Molecular and cellular mechanisms of general anaesthesia. *Nature* **367,** 607–614.
2. Kayser, E.-B., Morgan, P. G., and Sedensky, M. M. (1999) GAS-1: A mitochondrial protein controls sensitivity to volatile anesthetics in *C. elegans. Anesthesiology* **90,** 545–554.
3. van Swinderen, B., Saifee, O., Shebester, L., Roberson, R., Nonet, M. L., and Crowder, C. M. (1999) A neomorphic syntaxin mutation blocks volatile-anesthetic action in *Caenorhabditis elegans. Proc. Natl. Acad. Sci. USA* **96(5),** 2479–2484.
4. Tanifuji, Y., Eger, E. I., II, and Terrell, R. C. (1977) Some characteristics of an exceptionally potent inhaled anesthetic: Thiomethoxyflurane. *Anesth. Analg.* **56,** 387–391.
5. Koblin, D. D. (2000a) In Anesthesia, Mechanisms of Action, (Miller, R. D., ed.) Churchill Livingstone, New York, pp. 48–73.
6. Morgan, P. G., Sedensky, M. M., and Meneely, P. M. (1990) Multiple sites of action of volatile anesthetics in *Caenorhabditis elegans. PNAS* **87,** 2965–2968.
7. Baker, R., Melchior, C., and Deitrich, R. (1980) The effect of halothane on mice selectively bred for differential sensitivity to alcohol. *Pharmacol. Biochem. Behav.* **12,** 691–695.
8. Koblin, D. D. and Deady, J. E. (1981) Anaesthetic requirement in mice selectively bred for differences in ethanol Sensitivity. *Brit. J. Anaesth.* **53,** 5–10.
9. Simpson, V. J., Baker, R. C., and Timothy, B. S. (1993) Isoflurane but not halothane demonstrates diffential sleep time in long sleep and short sleep mice. *Anesthesiology* **79(3A),** A387.
10. Krishnan, K. S. and Nash, H. A. (1990) A genetic study of the anesthetic response: Mutants of *Drosophila melanogaster* altered in sensitivity to halothane. *Proc. Natl. Acad. Sci. USA* **87,** 8632–8636.
11. Gamo, S., Ogaki, M., and Nakashima-Tanaka, E. (1981) Strain differences in minimum anesthetic concentrations in *Drosophila melanogaster. Anesthesiology* **54,** 289–291.
12. MacIver, M. B. and Kendig, J. J. (1991) Anesthetic effects on resting membrane potential are voltage-dependent and agent-specific. *Anesthesiology* **74,** 83–88.
13. Sonner, J. M., Gong, D., and Eger, E. I., 2nd. (2000) Naturally occurring variability in anesthetic potency among inbred mouse strains. *Anesth. Analg.* **91,** 720–726.
14. Zhang, Y., Wu, S., Eger, E. I., 2nd, and Sonner, J. M. (2001) Neither GABA_A nor strychnine-sensitive glycine receptors are the sole mediators of MAC for isoflurane. *Anesth. Analg.* **92,** 123–127.
15. Yamakura, T. and Harris, R. A. (2000) Effects of gaseous anesthetics nitrous oxide and xenon on ligand-gated ion channels. Comparison with isoflurane and ethanol. *Anesthesiology 2000* **93,** 1095–1101.
16. Urban, B. W. and Friederich, P. (1998) Anesthetic mechanisms in-vitro and in general anesthesia. *Toxicol. Lett.* **100–101,** 9–16.
17. van Swinderen, B., Metz, L. B., Shebester, L. D., Mendel, J. E., Sternberg, P. W., and Crowder, C. M. (2001) Goalpha regulates volatile anesthetic action in *Caenorhabditis elegans. Genetics* **158,** 643–655.
18. Oliver, S. G. (1997) From gene to screen with yeast. *Curr. Opin. Genet. Dev.* **7,** 405–409.

19. Wilson, R. K. (1999) How the worm was won. The *C. elegans* genome sequencing project. *Trends Genet.* **15**, 51–58.
20. Celniker, S. E. (2000) The *Drosophila* genome. *Curr. Opin. Genet. Dev.* **10**, 612–616.
21. Lander, E. S., et al. (2001) Initial sequencing and analysis of the human genome. *Nature* **409**, 860–921.
22. Clark, M. S. (1999) Comparative genomics: the key to understanding the Human Genome Project. *Bioessays* **21**, 121–130.
23. No author listed. (2001) Harvesting the fruits of the human genome. *Nat. Genet.* **27**, 227, 228.
24. Keil, R. L., Wolfe, D., Reiner, T., Peterson, C. J., and Riley, J. L. (1996) Molecular genetic analysis of volatile anesthetic action. *Mol. Cell. Biol.* **16**, 3446–3453.
25. Wolfe, D., Hester, P., and Keil, R. L. (1998) Volatile anesthetic additivity and specificity in Saccharomyces cerevisiae. *Anesthesiology* **89**, 174–181.
26. Wolfe, D., Reiner, T., Keeley, J. L., Pizzini, M., and Keil, R. L. (1999) Ubiquitin metabolism affects cellular response to volatile anesthetics in yeast. *Mol. Cell. Biol.* **19**, 8254–8262.
27. Lafont, F., Verkade, P., Galli, T., et al. (1999) Raft association of SNAP receptors acting in apical trafficking in Madin-Darby canine kidney cells. *Proc. Natl. Acad. Sci. USA* **96**, 3734–3768.
28. Brenner, S. (1974) The genetics of *Caenorhabditis elegans. Genetics* **77**, 71–94.
29. Herman, R. K. (1988) Genetics of *C. elegans.* The Nematode *Caenorhabditis elegans.* (Wood, W. B., ed.) (Cold Spring Harbor, Cold Spring Harbor Laboratory Press) pp. 22–33.
30. Sulston, J. E. and Horvitz, H. R. (1977) Post-embryonic cell lineages of the nematode, *Caenorhabditis elegans. Dev. Biol.* **56**, 110–156.
31. Sulston, J. E., Schierenberg, E., White, J. G., and Thomson, J. N. (1983) The embryonic cell lineage of the nematode, *Caenorhabditis elegans. Dev. Biol.* **100**, 64–119.
32. White, J. G., Southgate, E., Thomson, J. N., and Brenner, S. (1986) The structure of the nervous system in *Caenorhabditis elegans. Philos. Trans. Roy. Soc. Lond.* **314B**, 1–340.
33. No authors listed. (1998) The genomic sequence of *C. elegans. Science* **282**, 2012–2018.
34. Morgan, P. G., Sedensky, M. M., Meneely, P. M., and Cascorbi, H. F. (1988) The effect of two genes on anesthetic response in the nematode *Caenorhabditis elegans. Anesthesiology* **69**, 246–251.
35. Crowder, C. M., Shebester, L. D., and Schedl, T. (1996) Behavioral effects of volatile anesthetics in *Caenorhabditis elegans. Anesthesiology* **85**, 901–912.
36. Morgan, P. G and Cascorbi, H. F. (1985) Effect of Anesthetics and a Convulsant on Normal and Mutant *Caenorhabditis elegans. Anesthesiology* **62**, 738–744.
37. van Swinderen, B., Saifee, O., Shebester, L., Roberson, R., Nonet, M. L., and Crowder, C. M. (1999) A neomorphic syntaxin mutation blocks volatile-anesthetic action in Caenorhabditis elegans. *Proc. Natl. Acad. Sci. USA* **96**, 2479–2484.
38. Kayser, B., Rajaram, S., Thomas, S., Morgan, P. G., and Sedensky, M. M. (1998) Control of anesthetic response in *C. elegans. Toxicol. Lett.* **100–101**, 339–346.
39. Koblin, D. D., Chortkoff, B. S., Laster, M. J., Eger, E. I., 2nd, Halsey, M. J., and Ionescu, P. (1994) Polyhalogenated and perfluorinated compounds that disobey the Meyer-Overton hypothesis. *Anesth. Analg.* **79**, 1043–1048.
40. Morgan, P. G., Radke, G. W., and Sedensky, M. M. (2000) Effects of Nonimmobilizers and Halothane on *Caenorhabditis elegans. Anesth. Analg.* **91**, 1007–1012.
41. Morgan, P. G, Usiak, M., and Sedensky, M. M. (1996) Genetic differences affecting the potency of stereoisomers of isoflurane. *Anesthesiology* **85**, 385–392.
42. Sedensky, M. M. and Meneely, P. M. (1987) Genetic analysis of halothane sensitivity in *C. elegans. Science* **236**, 952–954.
43. Morgan, P. G, Sedensky, M. M., and Meneely, P. M. (1990) Multiple sites of action of volatile anesthetics in *C. elegans. Proc. Natl. Acad. Sci. USA* **87**, 2965–2969.
44. Park, E. C. and Horvitz, H. R. (1986) Mutations with dominant effects on the behavior and morphology of the nematode Caenorhabditis elegans. *Genetics* **113**, 821–852.
45. Rajaram, S., Spangler, T. L., Sedensky, M. M., and Morgan, P. G. (1999) A Stomatin and a Degenerin Interact to Control Anesthetic Sensitivity in *C. elegans. Genetics* **153**, 1673–1682.
46. Rajaram, S., Sedensky, M. M., Morgan, P. G. (1998) A stomatin homologue controls sensitivity to volatile anesthetics in *C. elegans. Proc. Natl. Acad. Sci. USA* **95**, 8761–8766.
47. Stewart, G. W., Argent, A. C., and Dash, B. C. J. (1993) Stomatin: a putative cation transport regulator in red cell membrane. *Biochim. Biophys. Acta* **1225**, 15–25.
48. Stewart, G. W., et al. (1992) Isolation of cDNA coding for a ubiquitous membrane protein deficient in high NA^+, low K^+, stomatocytic erythrocytes. *Blood* **79**, 1593–1601.
49. Mannsfeldt, A. G., Carroll, P., Stucky, C., et al. (1999) Stomatin, a MEC-2-like protein, is expressed by mammalian sensory neurons. *Molec. Cell Neurosci.* **13**, 391–404.
50. Chalfie, M., Tu, Y., Euskirchen, G., Ward, W. W., and Prasher, D. C. (1994) Green fluorescent protein as a marker for gene expression. *Science* **263**, 802–805.
51. Sedensky, M. M, Siefker, J. M., Morgan, P. G. (2001) Stomatin homologues interact in Caenorhabditis elegans. *Am. J. Physiol. Cell Physiol.* **280**, C1340–C1348.
52. Tavernarakis, N., Shreffler, W., Wang, S., and Driscoll, M. (1997) *unc-8*, a DEG/ENaC family member, encodes a subunit of a candidate mechanically gated channel that modulates *C. elegans* locomotion. *Neuron* **18**, 107–119.
53. Phelan, P., Bacon, J. P., Davies, J. A., et al. (1998) Innexins: a family of invertebrate gap-junction proteins. *Trends Genet.* **14(9)**, 348, 349.
54. Lipardi, C., Nitsch, L., and Zurzolo, C. (2000) Detergent-insoluble GPI-anchored proteins are apically sorted in Fischer rat thyroid cells, but interference with cholesterol or sphingolipids differentially affects detergent insolubility and apical sorting. *Mol. Biol. Cell* **11**, 531–542.

55. Hooper, N. M. (1999) Detergent-insoluble glycosphigolipid/cholesterol-rich membrane domains, lipid rafts and caveolae. *Molec. Emb. Biol.* **16,** 145–156.

56. Snyers, L., Umlauf, E., and Prohaska, R. (1999) Association of stomatin with lipid-protein complexes in the plasma membrane and the endocytic compartment. *Eur. J. Cell Biol.* **78,** 802–812.

57. Moffett, S,. Brown, D. A., and Linder, M. E. (2000) Lipid-dependent targeting of G proteins into rafts. *J. Biol. Chem.* **275,** 2191–2198.

58. Morgan, P. G. and Sedensky, M. M. (1994) Mutations conferring new patterns of sensitivity to volatile anesthetics in *C. elegans. Anesthesiology* **81,** 888–898.

59. Kayser, E.-B., Morgan, P. G., and Sedenskym, M. M. (1999) GAS-1: A mitochondrial protein controls sensitivity to volatile anesthetics in *C. elegans. Anesthesiology* **90,** 545–554.

60. Kayser, E. B., Morgan, P. G., Hoppel, C. L., and Sedensky, M. M. (2001) Mitochondrial Expression and Function of GAS-1 in Caenorhabditis elegans. *J. Biol. Chem.* **122,** 1187–1201.

61. Ishii, N., Fujii, M., Hartman, P. S., et al. (1998) A mutation in succinate dehydrogenase cytochrome b causes oxidative stress and ageing in nematodes. *Nature* **394,** 694–697.

62. Hartman, P. S., Ishii, N., Kayser, E. B., Morgan, P. G., and Sedensky, M. M. (2001) Varied phenotypes caused by mutations altering mitochondrial complex I or complex II subunits in *Caenorhabditis elegans. Mech. Aging Dev.* In Press.

63. Cohen, P. J. (1973) Effects of anesthetics on mitochondrial function. *Anesthesiology* **39,** 153–164.

64. Harris, R. A., Munroe, J., Farmer, B., Kim, K. C., and Jenkins, P. (1971) Action of halothane upon mitochondrial respiration. *Arch. Biochem. Biophys.* **142,** 435–444.

64a. Morgan, P. G., Hoppel, C. L., and Sedensky, M. M. (2002) Mitochondrial defects and anesthetic sensitivity. *Anesthesiology* **96,** 1268–1269.

65. Koushika, S. P. and Nonet, M. L. (2000) Sorting and transport in *C. elegans*: A model system with a sequenced genome. *Curr. Opin. Cell Biol.* **12,** 517–523.

66. Rand, J. B. and Nonet, M. L. (1997) Synaptic Transmission. in *C. elegans II.* (Riddle, D. L., Blumenthal, T., Meyer, B. J., and Priess, J. R., eds.) Cold Spring Harbor, Cold Spring Harbor Laboratory Press, pp. 611–643.

67. Crowder, C. M. and Berilgen, J. (2000) Isoflurane Binds the Rat Synaptic Protein SNAP-25 at Clinical Concentrations. *Anesthesiology* A806.

68. Qi, J., Peters, K. W., Liu, C., Wang, J. M., Edinger, R. S., Johnson, J. P., Watkins, S. C., and Frizzell, R. A. (1999) Regulation of the amiloride-sensitive epithelial sodium channel by syntaxin 1A. *J. Biol. Chem.* 274, 30,345–30,348.

69. Plant, P. J., Lafont, F., Lecat, S., Verkade, P., Simons, K., and Rotin, D. (2000) Apical membrane targeting of Nedd4 is mediated by an association of its C2 domain with annexin XIIIb. *J. Cell Biol.* **149,** 1473–1484.

70. Gamo, S., Ogaki, M., and Nakashima-Tanaka, E. (1981) Strain differences in minimum anesthetic concentrations in Drosophila melanogaster. *Anesthesiology* **54,** 289–293.

71. Gamo, S., Dodo, K., Matakatsu, H., and Tanaka, Y. (1998) Molecular genetical analysis of Drosophila ether sensitive mutants. *Toxicol. Lett.* **100–101,** 329–337.

72. Krishnan, K. S. and Nash, H. A. (1990) A genetic study of the anesthetic response: mutants of Drosophila melanogaster altered in sensitivity to halothane. *Proc. Natl. Acad. Sci. USA* **87,** 8632–8636.

73. Campbell, D. B. and Nash, H. A. (1994) Use of *Drosophila* mutants to distinguish among volatile general anesthetics. *Proc. Natl. Acad. Sci. USA* **91,** 2135–2139.

74. Madhavan, M. C., Kumar, R. A., and Krishnan, K. S. (2000) Genetics of anesthetic response: autosomal mutations that render *Drosophila* resistant to halothane. *Pharmacol. Biochem. Behav.* **67,** 749–757.

75. Guan, Z., Scott, R. L., and Nash, H. A. (2000) A new assay for the genetic study of general anesthesia in *Drosophila melanogaster*: use in analysis of mutations in the X-chromsomal 12E region. *J. Neurogen.* **14,** 25–42.

76. Campbell, J. L. and Nash, H. A. (1998) The visually induced jump response of *Drosophila melangaster* is sensitive to volatile anesthetics. *J. Neurogen.* **12,** 241–251.

77. Walcourt, A. and Nash, H. A. (2000) Genetic effects on an anesthetic sensitive pathway in the brain of *Drosophila. J. Neurobiol.* **42,** 69–78.

78. Nishikawa, K. and Kidokoro, Y. (1999) Halothane presynaptically depresses synaptic transmission in wild-type *Drosophila* larvae but not in *halothane-resistant* (*har*) mutants. *Anesthesiology* **90,** 1691–1697.

79. Walcourt, A., Scott, R. L., and Nash, H. A. (2001) Blockage of one class of potassium channel alters the effectiveness of halothane in a brain circuit of *Drosophila. Anesth. Analg.* **92,** 535–541.

80. Sonner, J. M., Gong, D., Li, J., Eger, E. I., 2nd, and Laster, M. J. (1999) Mouse strain modestly influences minimum alveolar anesthetic concentration and convulsivity of inhaled compounds. *Anesth. Analg.* **89,** 1030–1034.

81. Sonner, J. M., Gong, D., Eger, and E. I., 2nd. (2000) Naturally occurring variability in anesthetic potency among inbred mouse strains. Anesth. Analg. **91,** 720–726.

82. Demarest, K., McCaughran, J., Jr., Mahjubi, E., Cipp, L., and Hitzemann, R. (1999) Identification of an acute ethanol response quantitative trait locus on mouse chromosome 2. *J. Neurosci.* **19,** 549–561.

83. Browman, K. E. and Crabbe, J. C. (2000) Quantitative trait loci affecting ethanol sensitivity in BXD recombinant inbred mice. *Alcoh. Clin. Exp. Res.* **24,** 17–23.

84. Hood, H. M. and Buck, K. J. (2000) Allelic variation in the GABA A receptor gamma2 subunit is associated with genetic susceptibility to ethanol-induced motor incoordination and hypothermia, conditioned taste aversion, and withdrawal in BXD/Ty recombinant inbred mice. *Alcoh. Clin. Exp. Res.* **24,** 1327–1334.

85. Hanania, T., Negri, C. A, Dunwiddie, T. V., and Zahniser, N. R. (2000) *N*-methyl-D-aspartate receptor responses are differentially modulated by noncompetitive receptor antagonists and ethanol in inbred long-sleep and short-sleep mice: behavior and electrophysiology. *Alcoh. Clin. Exp. Res.* **24,** 1750–1758.

86. Erwin, V. G., Heston, W. D., McClearn, G. E., and Deitrich, R. A. (1976) Effect of hypnotics on mice genetically selected for sensitivity to ethanol. *Pharmacol. Biochem. Behav.* **4,** 679–683.

87. Firestone, L. L., Korpim, E. R., Niemi, L., Rosenberg, P. H., Homanics, G. E., and Quinlan, J. J. (2000) Halothane and desflurane requirements in alcohol-tolerant and -nontolerant rats. *Brit. J. Anaesth.* **85,** 757–762.

88. Quinlan, J. J., Homanics, G. E., and Firestone, L. L. (1998) Anesthesia sensitivity in mice that lack the beta3 subunit of the gamma-aminobutyric acid type A receptor. *Anesthesiology* **88,** 775–780.

89. Ugarte, S. D., Homanics, G. E., Firestone, L. L., and Hammond, D. L. (2000) Sensory thresholds and the antinociceptive effects of GABA receptor agonists in mice lacking the beta3 subunit of the $GABA_A$ receptor. *Neuroscience* **95,** 795–806.

90. Homanics, G. E., Ferguson, C., Quinlan, J. J., et al. (1997) Gene knockout of the alpha6 subunit of the gamma-aminobutyric acid type A receptor: lack of effect on responses to ethanol, pentobarbital, and general anesthetics. *Mol. Pharmacol.* **51,** 588–596.

15

Genetic Dissection of Anesthetic Action

Gregg E. Homanics and Leonard L. Firestone

INTRODUCTION

In vitro model systems are inarguably of great utility, but all in vitro systems suffer from an obvious inability to accurately model the behavioral state of general anesthesia. Because general anesthesia is characterized by amnesia and immobility, the only truly accurate system to model such a state is the whole, intact living organism. To date, several different model organisms and numerous genetic approaches have been utilized to gain an understanding of mechanisms of general anesthesia. The model organisms include the roundworm *Caenorhabditis elegans*, the fruit fly *Drosophilia melanogaster*, the laboratory mouse, and the laboratory rat. The genetic approaches are quite varied and range from analyzing existing animal lines to creating genetically engineered organisms that harbor precise, predetermined mutations (*see* Table 1).

This chapter is by no means meant to be an exhaustive review of all work related to anesthetic mechanisms that have utilized genetic approaches. Instead, our intent is to introduce different genetic methods that have been or might be employed. In some instances we have elected to highlight particularly illustrative examples. Space also does not permit us to go into technical details. However, we have tried to direct the reader to relevant publications for such information.

COMPARISON OF MODEL ORGANISMS

The nematode *C. elegans* is a great model organism for genetic studies. This relatively simple invertebrate has been characterized in great detail. The ~97 megabasepair genome has been sequenced and encodes ~19,000+ genes (1). The nervous system of the adult worm contains only 302 individually identifiable neurons. In addition, *C. elegans* are inexpensive, highly fecund, easy to maintain, have a short generation time, and are easy to modify genetically. Some worm behaviors have been demonstrated to be sensitive to clinical concentrations of anesthetics (e.g., coordinated movement, mating behavior, chemotaxis), whereas other behaviors occur at supraclinical concentrations (e.g., immobility) (2).

The fruit fly is also a terrific model organism for genetic studies. This organism is slightly more complex than the worm. The *Drosophila* nervous system is composed of ~10,000 neurons. The DNA sequence of the genome is ~120 megabases but surprisingly only contains ~13,000 potential genes (3). This organism is also easy to maintain, highly fecund, has a short generation time, and is easy to modify genetically. Anesthetic sensitive behaviors in *Drosophila* that have been studied include negative geotaxis, immobility, and movement in response to a noxious stimulus (e.g., light beam).

Though lower invertebrate systems are very useful for genetic studies of anesthetic mechanisms, they are somewhat limited in that the anesthetic induced endpoints are different from those directly

From: *Contemporary Clinical Neuroscience: Neural Mechanisms of Anesthesia*
Edited by: Joseph F. Antognini et al. © Humana Press Inc., Totowa, NJ

Table 1
Genetic Approaches to Investigating Anesthetic Mechanisms

Forward genetics	*Reverse genetics*	*Emerging genetic approaches*
Genetic selection	Transgenics	Database mining
Inbred strains	Known mutant screens	Microarray analysis
Recombinant inbred strains	Global gene knockouts	Conditional gene knockouts
QTL analysis	Knock-ins	
Random mutagenesis		
Screen spontaneous mutants		

relevant to humans. Also, because of the evolutionary distance between humans and invertebrates, it is not yet clear if mechanisms of anesthesia have been conserved. Thus, anesthetic targets in invertebrates may not be directly applicable to humans. Nonetheless, invertebrate studies still can provide key insight into how anesthetics exert their effects in vertebrates.

In terms of evolution, mice and rats are the closest species to humans that are easily used for genetic studies of anesthetic mechanisms. Molecular targets that mediate anesthesia in these models will almost certainly be directly pertinent to human anesthesia. Similar to the human, the genome of the mouse and rat is considerably larger than the invertebrates; the mouse genome is estimated to be ~3,000 megabasepairs and harbors ~100,000 genes *(4)*. Genomic sequencing projects for both the mouse and the rat are currently underway; a draft version of the mouse genome should be completed in 2002, and the rat should be completed shortly thereafter. The central nervous system is also much more complex than the invertebrates; it is estimated to be composed of ~10^{11} neurons. Importantly, rodents are sensitive to clinically relevant concentrations of anesthetic agents and the behavioral endpoints that can be monitored are similar to those that are clinically relevant to humans.

Which model organism is the best for the genetic dissection of anesthetic mechanisms? The answer is that no single organism by itself is the best. Each organism has advantages and disadvantages. Invertebrates are excellent for screening and identifying candidate targets/pathways. Vertebrates are also great for target identification but results from these models have the distinct advantage of being directly relevant to humans.

GENETICALLY SELECTED LINES OF ORGANISMS

Lines of organisms with divergent responses to various anesthetic compounds have been produced by selective breeding of those animals that display extreme responses. Such experiments conclusively establish that anesthetic responses are under genetic control. This line of research has been extensively applied to the investigation of drug and alcohol responses in rodents (for reviews, *see* refs. *5,6*). Numerous lines of animals have been produced that have alterations in sensitivity, tolerance, dependence, and other drug induced behavioral endpoints. Some, but clearly not all lines that have been selected for a given response to one drug also show cross sensitivity to other drugs. This suggests that there is some overlap in the mechanisms of action for these various drugs, but clearly all of the drugs are not operating through exactly the same targets. Despite decades of characterization, key molecular targets that explain how these drugs exert their effects have not been uncovered from studying selected lines. This difficulty in moving from a phenotype (altered sensitivity to various drugs) to the underlying genotype (the genetic change responsible for the altered drug response) is a significant limitation of this approach.

INBRED MOUSE STRAINS

There are currently several hundred inbred mouse strains in existence. These strains are lines of animals that have been produced by brother-sister mating for over 20 generations. Because each line is inbred, all animals within a line are for all practical purposes genetically identical. This means that for any given gene, no functional variation between animals within the line is present. However, because each line of inbred animals has been created and maintained in genetic isolation, numerous genotypic and phenotypic differences between inbred lines exist.

Investigators have compared anesthetic responses among various inbred mouse lines *(7,8)*. These studies have revealed several important findings regarding the mechanism of action of general anesthetics. First, there is considerable variablility among inbred mouse lines in terms of anesthetic sensitivity. This clearly establishes that there is a genetic basis for anesthetic responsiveness. This also widens the possibility that various inbred stains can be used for other genetic approaches, such as those detailed below. Secondly, these studies have revealed that multiple genes influence the variability in response to anesthetics.

RECOMBINANT INBRED LINES

Recombinant inbred lines are a special type of inbred organism. Production of a recombinant inbred line starts with two distinct inbred lines. Crossing of these two lines results in genetically homogenous F_1 offspring; all animals are heterozygous at each polymorphic locus. Subsequent crossing of F_1 animals results in an F_2 generation, in which each animal is genetically distinct. Inbreeding of animals from the F_2 generation, for approximately 20 generations, results in recombinant inbred lines of animals. Numerous panels of recombinant inbred mouse strains derived from a variety of parental inbred stains have been produced and are available, some from commercial sources such as The Jackson Laboratory (Bar Harbor, ME). Details of recombinant inbred mouse production and breeding strategies can be found in an excellent book by Silver *(4)*. Recombinant inbred strains are important for mapping studies (*see* below).

QUANTITATIVE TRAIT LOCI MAPPING

As genetic approaches have definitively established that anesthetic sensitivity is under direct genetic control, it has been impossible to move from the phenotype to the genotype despite decades of intense effort. Recently, genetics, molecular biology, and statistical approaches have been synergistically combined to create a novel approach that attempts to elucidate the genotypic changes that account for various phenotypes. This is the quantitative trait locus (QTL) mapping approach. In the anesthesiology field, QTL analysis is being used to zero in on those chromosomal regions that lead to quantitative variation in anesthetic sensitivity in various genetic lines of organisms. Since a lucid overview of QTL mapping has recently been published *(9)*, methodological details will not be covered in this section. A recent review of the QTL's that have been identified to date for a variety of alcohol and drug responses has also recently appeared *(10)*.

QTL studies in *C. elegans* have been used to map chromosomal regions that regulate halothane sensitivity of coordinated movement and male mating behaviors *(11)*. These worm behaviors were chosen because they are affected by concentrations of anesthetics that approximate clinically relevant concentrations in vertebrates. Starting with recombinant-inbred strains, QTL mapping was able to identify one major and five weaker loci that accounted for most of the variability in halothane sensitivity between strains. The major locus mapped to the middle of chromosome V and accounted for ~40% of the phenotypic variance. With the recent completion of the *C. elegans* genome *(1)*, it should be possible to rapidly screen the genes present within this QTL to identify the gene(s) responsible for the phenotype.

The mouse has also recently been enlisted for mapping QTLs for anesthetic sensitivity. Perhaps the most advanced study published to date is that of Simpson et al. *(12)*. These investigators utilized the much studied Long-Sleep (LS) and Short-Sleep (SS) mouse lines and their recombinant inbred derivatives. These mouse lines were originally selected for differences in sensitivity to ethanol. Subsequently, these mouse lines were also shown to differ in sensitivity to propofol. In this study, QTL analysis was able to identify a ~2.5 centimorgan (~5000 kb) region on mouse chromosome 7 that accounts for nearly all of the variability in propofol sensitivity between the LS and SS mouse lines. While this chromosomal region is very small by mapping standards, it is still estimated to contain about 150 genes. Thus, despite having eliminated nearly 99.8% of the genome from explaining the differences in propofol sensitivity between these mouse lines, a major undertaking will still be required to pinpoint the genetic alteration responsible for this interesting phenotypic difference.

LARGE-SCALE RANDOM MUTAGENESIS SCREENS

A classic forward genetics approach to isolate mutants with altered phenotypes involves large-scale random mutagenesis of the germline genome and subsequent screening of mutant offspring for interesting phenotypic alterations. Mutagensis screens in *Drosophila* have been utilized for many years to isolate genes affecting behavior. In the past decade, these screening techniques have been applied to isolate mutant fruit flies that have alterations in responses to anesthetics *(13)*. In that study, male flies were chemically mutagenized and subsequently mated. Offspring were screened for altered sensitivity to the induction of halothane anesthesia in an inebriometer. Four different halothane resistant mutants were isolated from ~20,000 mutagenized flies. More recently, these resistant mutant flies were tested for response to different anesthetics *(14)*. This study revealed that each of the mutations affects potency of the various anesthetics differently. This presents a strong argument against a unitary theory of anesthesia.

Though mutagenesis screens are most efficiently conducted in small organisms with very short generation times, large-scale mutagensis has also been successfully applied to the mouse (for review, *see* ref. *15*) for such phenotypic endpoints as circadian rhythm. While it is obviously difficult and expensive to produce and screen thousands of mutagenized mice, it is not impossible *(16)*. There are currently several large-scale mutagenesis/behavioral phenotype screens being conducted in the mouse around the world that are producing huge numbers of mutant animals. However, to our knowledge, no one is capitalizing on these valuable reagents to screen for anesthetic induced phenotypes.

REVERSE GENETICS

As illustrated by the many examples mentioned above, considerable effort has been expended toward attempting to identify anesthetic sites of action using a forward genetics approach in various complementary model organisms. With this approach, an attempt is made to deduce the molecular basis for an observed phenotype. All of these studies start with organisms that have an altered response to a drug of interest. As considerable progress has been made using this approach, uncovering the genetic basis for the observed phenotype has rarely been possible, to date. An alternative and complementary approach termed reverse genetics attacks the problem from the opposite direction. Organisms with known genetic alterations are first identified or created, then studied for the impact of the genetic alteration on the phenotype of interest. This approach has also revealed much about the mechanisms of action for various drugs.

SCREENS OF CHARACTERIZED MUTANTS

One particularly useful approach that has been employed to study anesthetic action was to screen organisms that have previously characterized mutations in known genes for altered anesthetic sensitivity. Typically, one begins by selecting a panel of mutant organisms that have genetic alterations in candidate genes. For example, using mutant stocks of the nematode, van Swinderen and collegues *(17)* screened several mutant lines that have defects in the synaptic machinery. In the *md130* mutant line, which has a mutation in the neuronal syntaxin gene, the ED_{50} for isoflurane induced loss of coordinated movement was increased nearly 6-fold compared to controls. Resistance to halothane was also observed, but the increased ED_{50} was not as dramatic. To date, these mutant worms are the most resistant organism identified in terms of response to volatile agents. The mechanism by which the *md130* syntaxin mutation confers resistance to volatile anesthetics is still not entirely clear.

Although the *md130* mutation reduces neurotransmission, other mutations which also reduce synaptic transmission, including several different reduction-of-function syntaxin mutants, surprisingly have hypersensitivity to isoflurane and halothane. Nonetheless, it is apparent from these studies that the synaptic machinery is involved, either directly or indirectly, in mediating and/or modulating volatile anesthetic action. Further analysis of these and other mutants should shed additional light on this.

Rodents with mutations in known genes have also been used to investigate anesthetic action. The alcohol nontolerant (ANT) rat line was originally identified on the basis of alcohol induced ataxia *(18)*, but was later demonstrated to also be more sensitive to benzodiazepines and barbiturates *(19)*. This spontaneous rat mutant was subsequently shown to have a point mutation in the α6 subunit of the GABA$_A$-R *(20)*. Recently, this rat line was screened for alterations in response to volatile anesthetics *(21)*. This study revealed that ANT rats were more sensitive to both halothane and desflurane on the loss of righting reflex assay. In contrast, using the tail clamp/withdrawal endpoint, ANT rats were more sensitive than controls to halothane, but not desflurane. These data suggest that different anesthetic induced behavioral endpoints are mediated by separate sites or mechanisms.

Despite the progress that has been made with screening mutant organisms, a few caveats exist that limit the conclusions of such studies in some instances. For example, even though the ANT rat line has been conclusively demonstrated to harbor a specific point mutation in the α6 subunit of the GABA$_A$-R *(20)*, it is also possible that other mutations coexist in this rat line. Without having any way of knowing what the possible additional mutations are and if any of them are linked to the GABA$_A$-R α6 mutation, one cannot be sure which genetic alteration is really at the root of the observed change in drug response. A potential approach to definitively establish if indeed the α6 mutation is responsible for the phenotype would be to create transgenic or gene knock-in animals (*see* below) that differ from controls only by the presence of that mutation. While such an approach has yet to be enlisted for the ANT phenotype in rats, transgenic rescue of the *md130* syntaxin mutation in worms conclusively demonstrated that the alteration in syntaxin was the mutated target responsible for the phenotype *(17)*.

TRANSGENIC ORGANISMS

Transgenic organisms are those organisms that have had additional DNA stably added to their genome with the most frequent intent being to overexpress/missexpress a gene of interest. Although the techniques used to generate various transgenic organisms differ from model to model, it should be appreciated that those organisms that are of interest to anesthesia research can be efficiently modified by transgenesis.

In *C. elegans*, transgenics have been used with great success. As mentioned above, transgenic rescue of a syntaxin mutant was used to convincingly demonstrate the involvement of this mutation in altered volatile anesthetic responses *(17)*.

Other investigators have created transgenic worms to identify a mutation in a gene that also alters sensitivity to volatile anesthetics *(22)*. To identify the gene responsible for the altered phenotype of *unc-1* mutant worms, a transgenic rescue experiment was undertaken. With this approach, a cosmid clone was identified that restored the mutant phenotype to wild type. The smallest fragment from this cosmid that was capable of rescue was determined to contain portions of two different genes. To identify which of these candidate genes was responsible for the phenotype, the investigators next sequenced these two genes from normal and mutant flies. From the sequencing analysis, it was concluded that a homolog of the human stomatin gene was the *unc-1* gene responsible for the change in anesthetic sensitivity. The human stomatin gene encodes a membrane protein that is probably associated with a sodium channel. Whether or not *unc-1* (or stomatin) is a direct or indirect target of anesthetics in worms (and humans) awaits further investigation. This same group of investigators also used transgenic overexpression of various *unc-1* reporter and translational fusion constructs to demonstrate that the *unc-1* gene could rescue the mutant phenotype, and reveal the anatomic pattern of *unc-1* expression *(23)*.

Transgenics have also been used to screen for genetic pathways that if modified, lead to an altered drug response in vertebrates. For example, the neurotransmitter serotonin has been strongly implicated in modulating behavioral sensitivity to ethanol. To address the functional role of the 5-HT$_3$ subtype of serotonin receptor, Engel and Allan *(24)* created transgenic mice that overexpressed the 5-HT$_3$ gene in the forebrain. These investigators found that the transgenic mice were more sensitive to low dose ethanol-induced activity, but were normally sensitive to high dose ethanol-induced sedation. Not only does this study enlighten our understanding of serotonin receptors and ethanol-induced behavioral responses, but this study also reveals that different behavioral responses to the same drug are under control of different genetic mechanisms.

GLOBAL GENE KNOCKOUT MICE

In contrast to transgenic organisms in which a gene of interest is added so that it can be overexpressed, a gene knockout organism has been engineered so that it lacks a specific gene product. The creation and analysis of designer organisms that differ from controls by a single mutation in a known gene provides for an extremely powerful approach to determine the function of that gene's product in an intact organism. Gene knockout technology is available for the mouse, fly, and worm. To date, only gene knockout mice have been developed for the express purpose of understanding anesthetic action.

To create gene knockouts in mice, one has to first modify the gene of interest by homologous recombination (or more informally known as gene targeting) in embryonic stem cells in culture. Once correctly targeted embryonic stem cells are identified and molecularly characterized, they are used to create chimeric mice that have germ cells derived from the targeted stem cells. Mating of these germline competent chimeras allows one to produce lines of mice harboring the gene targeted locus. Methodological details of gene knockout technology are available *(25,26)*.

A rapidly expanding zoo of genetically engineered mice has been utilized to investigate the mechanistic basis for the diverse behavioral effects of anesthetics and alcohol (for reviews, *see* refs. *27,28*). In the paragraphs that follow, we present some of our results with GABA$_A$-R gene knockout animals. These studies were selected because they highlight the potential and the perils of gene knockout studies.

Recently, we produced mice that completely and specifically lack the δ subunit of the GABA$_A$-R *(29)*. These mice were found to have normal responses to a wide variety of anesthetics, including volatile agents such as halothane and enflurane, and injectable agents such as pentobarbital, propofol, midazolam, etomidate, and ketamine (*see* Fig. 1). However, quite surprisingly, δ subunit deficient mice were found to be highly insensitive to several different effects of several different neuroactive steroid compounds. Thus, this single precise genetic change appears to impart a remarkably specific and selective change in the cellular and whole animal responses to a specific class of anesthetic compounds, the neurosteroids. A caveat to this study is that despite only making a specific genetic lesion in the δ subunit of the GABA$_A$-R, we have uncovered that the abundance of several other subunits of the GABA$_A$-R is altered in the brains of these mice *(30)*. Compensatory changes such as this do not discredit gene knockout studies, but they force the cautious interpretation of results.

Some time ago, we produced mice that specifically lacked the β3 subunit of the GABA$_A$-R *(31)*. Progress at understanding the importance of GABA$_A$-R isoforms that contain the β3 subunit have been hampered because most β3 deficient mice died as neonates. Nonetheless, we have successfully produced enough β3 knockout animals that survive to adulthood to allow us to investigate the contribution of this subunit to anesthetic responses. Knockout animals were found to be more resistant than wild type controls to the effects of volatile agents on the tail clamp/withdrawal behavioral endpoint, but knockouts and controls did not differ on the loss of righting reflex response to these same anesthetics *(32)*. Knockouts were also more resistant to other sedatives such as etomidate and midazolam in sleep time assays. However, knockouts and controls were equally sensitive to ethanol

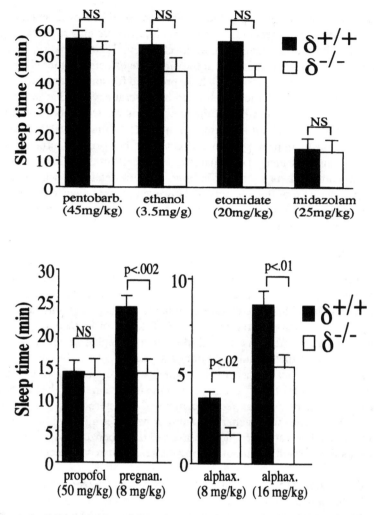

Fig. 1. Sleep time of wild type (+/+) and GABA$_A$ receptor delta subunit deficient (–/–) mice in response to injection of various sedative/hypnotic agents.

and pentobarbital. These studies indicate that different anesthetics produce their effects by different molecular mechanisms, and furthermore, that the different behavioral effects of these drugs are also mediated by different mechanisms.

Since we demonstrated that MAC is increased in the β3 knockout animals *(32)* and MAC is determined primarily in the spinal cord *(see* ref. *33)*, we analyzed the sensitivity of spinal cord responses to enflurane using electrophysiologic techniques *(34)*. This study revealed that knockout of the β3 subunit did not alter enflurane sensitivity of the cord. Interestingly, in these mutant animals, the contribution of GABA$_A$-Rs in mediating enflurane's actions seem to have been reduced. An increase in glycinergic inhibition in the cord was also noted, but this neurotransmitter pathway did not appear to be a substitute target of the anesthetic. These findings suggest that individual components of the anesthetic mechanism(s) are plastic and can compensate and adapt to various perturbations.

Mice lacking the β3 subunit have also been used to investigate the role of GABA and GABA$_A$-Rs in nociception *(35)*. The knockout mice were found to display thermal hyperalgesia and tactile allodynia. Administration of a GABA$_A$-R agonist produced antinociception in control animals, but failed to do so in β3 knockouts. Surprisingly, the antinociceptive effects of subcutaneous or intrathecal administration of a GABA type B receptor agonist (baclofen) were also reduced in the β3 deficient mice. This unexpected observation suggests that developmental compensation may have occurred, altering the neuronal circuits that mediate the antinociceptive effects of other classes of analgesics.

Though global gene knockout mice certainly have provided for some dramatic and exciting insight into anesthetic mechanisms, such studies are limited by several caveats that make interpretation of the results difficult. The main concern is that the gene that is rendered nonfunctional is eliminated from all cells of the animal throughout the animal's lifetime. As mentioned, it is clear that elimination of a single gene product can have profound effects on other genes, neurons, and even neuronal circuits. In addition, because the gene is eliminated from all cells of the animal, even if an interesting anesthesia-induced phenotype is observed, it is impossible to determine which cell type or which brain region is the key mediator of that phenotype. However, recent advances in genetic engineering, as discussed in the Section on Conditional Knockout Mice, that permit more subtle mutations offer hope that such limitations can be minimized or perhaps even eliminated.

GENE KNOCK-IN MICE

Genetically engineered mice, called "gene knock-in animals", are those animals that have an intentional mutation introduced into an endogenous gene that does not ablate the function of the gene, but merely alters its function. This type of subtle mutation has been demonstrated to be immensely powerful for the genetic dissection of the mechanism of action of benzodiazepines *(36–38)*. These drugs were known to exert their effects through the benzodiazepine sensitive $GABA_A$-Rs, namely those iosforms that contain as their α subunit either al1, α2, α3, or α5, but not α4 or α6. However, before these gene knock-in studies, it was not clear which specific subunits were responsible for each of the various behavioral effects of these drugs. To test the involvement of these subunits in benzodiazepine induced behavioral responses, separate mouse lines harboring single amino acid point mutations in most of these genes were generated using gene targeting technology in embryonic stem cells. The point mutations that were introduced converted these benzodiazepine sensitive subunits to benzodiazepine insensitive subunits, without altering the sensitivity of the receptors to the endogenous ligand, GABA.

In the genetically engineered mice that harbored the benzodiazepine insensitive α1 subunit, diazepam was no longer capable of inducing sedation or amnesia *(36,37)*. In contrast, the anxiolytic, myorelaxant, motor impairing, and ethanol potentiating effects of diazepam were still intact. In the knock-in mice that harbored a benzodiazepine insensitive α2 subunit, diazepam induced anxiolysis was ablated, but diazepam's sedative, motor impairing, and anticonvulsive effects were still intact *(38)*. In mice that harbored the α3 knock-in mutation, no changes in benzodiazepine induced behavioral responses have been identified *(38)*. Mice with a benzodiazepine insensitive α5 subunit have not yet been reported in the literature.

These gene knock-in studies serve as an excellent example of the power of this genetic approach. It is very important to realize that it is possible to create animals that harbor mutant receptors that respond normally to their endogenous gene product. It is only in the presence of exogenous modulators of channel function that the mutation exerts alterations in normal channel function. This is important in that in the absence of exogenous modulator, the channels (and the entire organism) will function normally. Thus, developmental compensation is not an issue with these sorts of studies.

Furthermore, these knock-in studies are important in that they reveal that the various behavioral responses to benzodiazepines are mediated by separate and distinct mechanisms. The same sort of genetically dissectable mechanisms are likely to also exist for various anesthetics. For example, it is probable that the amnestic effects of a given drug are mediated by a separate mechanism than the immobilizing effects. Now that various point mutations that eliminate sensitivity of $GABA_A$-Rs to volatile *(39)* and injectible *(40,41)* anesthetic have been identified in vitro, a similar gene knock-in

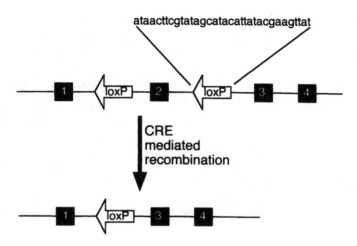

ataacttcgtatagcatacattatacgaagttat

CRE
mediated
recombination

Fig. 2. Cre/loxP conditional gene targeting. Targeted locus illustrating insertion of loxP sites into intron DNA (exons are represented by numbered black boxes). Following cre mediated recombination, one loxP site and the intervening DNA will be deleted and degraded rendering the gene nonfunctional.

approach should allow for the genetic dissection of the contribution of various $GABA_A$-R subunits to various anesthetic induced behavioral responses.

CONDITIONAL KNOCKOUT MICE

Another recently developed and rapidly evolving genetic technology that is likely to dramatically enhance our understanding of anesthetic mechanisms is that of conditional gene knockouts. With this technology, it is now possible to create gene knockout animals in which the gene of interest is rendered nonfunctional only in specific subsets of cells in the animal and/or only after a specific time in the animal's life. By creating tissue specific and developmentally regulated gene knockouts, many of the limitations of conventional global knockout technology are circumvented. For example, by allowing the animals to proceed through development and into adulthood with a functionally normal genome, inactivating the gene of interest only after critical periods of neuronal development have passed, issues of developmental compensation can be avoided. Also, by inactivating genes only in specific populations of cells in the brain, critical insight into those cells, tissues, and circuits that are critical for behavioral phenotypes should be readily dissected.

Like global gene knockouts, conditional knockout mice are also created using gene targeting in murine embryonic stem cells. Details of this technology are available elsewhere *(42,43)*. Briefly, using gene targeting, the gene of interest is modified so that an important part of that gene's coding DNA (exonic DNA) is flanked by loxP sites *(see* Fig. 2). LoxP sites are specific 34 basepair DNA sequences that by themselves are innocuous, i.e., a gene that is merely flanked by loxP sites will continue to function like a wild type gene. However, these sites are recognized by a DNA recombinase called cre. In cells that have a loxP flanked gene and also the cre recombinase protein, cre will enzymatically catalyze a recombination reaction between the loxP sites. The net result is that the intervening DNA will be excised and degraded. If that intervening DNA is critical for gene function, the recombined gene will be rendered nonfunctional. Thus, one can go from a wild type gene to a null gene simply by introducing cre recombinase. The key for creating tissue-specific and/or developmentally-regulated knockout animals with this approach is to restrict production of cre recombinase only to those tissues and/or times where recombination is desired. Most frequently, this is achieved in mice by utilizing transgenic mice that harbor a cre transgene that is under transcriptional control of a tissue-specific and/or developmentally regulated promoter.

To date, no publications describing the application of conditional knockouts to anesthetic mechanisms research have appeared. However, the usefulness of this type of genetically engineered animal to investigate complex phenomena in the neuroscience field are starting to appear in the literature *(44,45)*. Such an approach should be tremendously fruitful for anesthetic mechanism research. For example, knocking out genes that are candidate targets for anesthetics (e.g., ligand gated ion channels) in tissues that are thought to be important for various anesthetic responses (e.g., hippocampus for amnestic effects or spinal cord for immobilizing effects), will undoubtedly provide novel insight.

Very recently, the most advanced conditional knockout technique has appeared *(46)*. This third generation knockout is inducible, reversible, and tissue-specific. To accomplish this, a tissue-specific knockout was combined with an exogenously regulated transgene. This approach allows the investigator to control the activity (or inactivity) of the gene of interest in the tissue of interest simply by the removal (or addition) of a nontoxic drug to the animal's drinking water. The potential of this technology is enormous.

FUTURE DIRECTIONS

Previous studies using genetic approaches to anesthetic mechanisms have demonstrated the utility and power of these approaches and it is highly likely that many of the model organisms described above will continue to be utilized. However, to date genetic studies have focused in on the effects of individual genes (or at most only a few genes). This will change in the near future. We are rapidly racing into the age of genomics in which entire genomes are sequenced and cataloged in huge databases. Working drafts of the human, worm *(1)*, fruit fly *(3)*, and numerous other lower species have already been completed and great effort is being expended to sequence the genomes of other model organisms such as the mouse, rat, and monkey. With genomic information and associated technologies, it is now possible to being to analyze the effects of not just one or two genes in isolation, but instead one can analyze the dynamic interaction of hundreds and thousands of genes.

These rapidly expanding genetic databases are more and more frequently being searched to identify novel genes of interest. For example, Davies et al. *(47)* searched an expressed sequence tagged database with a $GABA_A$-R peptide consensus sequence to identify a previously unknown $GABA_A$-R subunit. This novel subunit named epsilon, was subsequently demonstrated to confer insensitivity to intravenous anesthetics in recombinant expression systems. Thus, by simply searching computer databases of sequence information from various genomic sequencing projects, it is possible to rapidly uncover insight into anesthetic mechanisms. A limitation of this approach is that database searches are biased toward sequences that are homologous to known candidate targets of anesthetics.

One emerging genetic technology that should be utilized in the anesthetic mechanisms field is microarray technology. With this approach, either cDNAs or oligonucleotides that correspond to various genes are spotted onto small glass slides. At present, several thousands different genes are typically represented on each slide. These arrays are then probed with mRNA samples isolated from various test specimens. By comparing the intensity of hybridization to each gene between test specimens, it is possible to estimate the extent of expression of each gene in the specimens. Thus, using sophisticated computer analysis one can rapidly determine if expression of particular genes or gene pathways are altered between specimens. A very important point to realize is that with this methodology thousands of genes are simultaneously screened without a *priori* biases about which genes may be important. This sort of data mining approach is already beginning to yield dividends in the search for the genetic underpinnings for alcoholism *(48)*, schizophrenia *(49)*, and various other complex, mutifactorial neuroscience-related phenomena.

How might array technology and genomics be applied to anesthetic mechanisms research? As should be obvious from the preceeding sections of this chapter, a wealth of diverse genetic resources exits that display altered responses to various anesthetics. However, a major impediment to progress has been the search for the needle in the haystack, that is to find the genetic change(s) that leads to the observed phenotype. Perhaps microarrays could be utilized to get a handle on some genes that control anesthetic sensitivity. For example, one could compare pertinent brain regions from recombinant inbred panels that differ in anesthetic responses. With this approach, one should be able to identify genes that are differentially expressed between sensitive and resistant lines. Certainly not all of the genes identified will be involved in the anesthetic phenotype; other genes may also differ between lines. Nonetheless, this approach offers an unbiased attempt to gain insight into the molecular pathways that control anesthetic sensitivity, some of which may not be intuitively obvious.

CONCLUSIONS AND COMMENTS

The use of genetic approaches to dissect the mechanisms of action of anesthetic compounds has a rich and productive history. Studying animal behavioral responses are critical to understanding how a complex behavioral response such as anesthesia is produced. By using genetically tractable model systems, insight into the molecular mechanisms that allow chemically diverse drugs to exert their common effects on the central nervous system is being made.

It is now clear that genetic studies have raised serious concerns about the plausibility of a unitary mechanism of action for anesthetic agents. Convergent evidence using various genetic approaches in worms, flies, and rodents has indicated that a unitary mechanism of action is unlikely. From these studies, it appears that there are likely to be multiple mechanisms to achieve anesthesia and also that some drugs may use different mechanisms.

It is also worth considering the following: In the invertebrate model systems with their relatively simple genomes and nervous systems, mutant organisms with huge differences in anesthetic sensitivity have been uncovered. For example, the most resistant worm identified is ~6-fold more resistant to halothane compared to controls. In contrast, in organisms that have much more complex nervous systems such as rodents (and humans), changes in anesthetic sensitivity have been much more modest. We posit that in the simple model systems, single genetic alterations often lead to huge effects because these model organisms are unable to invoke compensatory changes. In contrast, in complex higher eukaryotes, substantial redundancy exists that masks the effects of the genetic alteration. It is also plausible that in these highly complex nervous systems, an ensemble of mechanisms that individually contribute only a small part to the whole animal behavioral endpoint achieves anesthesia. Furthermore, it is also probable that the mechanisms for achieving the state of general anesthesia are malleable. For example, the mutant mouse approach has failed to achieve an exceptionally large change in response to volatile agents. This may be telling us that in the absence of a given gene product, the mammalian brain is so adaptable that compensatory changes take place that limit the impact of the genetic modification. In other words, the mechanism of anesthetic action is shifted to other targets. In fact, evidence from the $GABA_A$-R $\beta 3$ subunit knockout mouse seems to support this. As these mice do indeed have significant changes in some responses to volatile agents *(32)*, it is also clear that the apparent contribution of the GABA pathway to anesthesia has been decreased *(34)*. Thus, in the higher vertebrate models we may be searching for a moving target that may only be clearly elucidated by stacking multiple genetic alterations in the same organism.

In closing, genetic approaches have proved to be of great value in dissecting mechanisms of anesthesia, and it is certain that they will continue to be critical to advancement of our field. The emerging technologies for genetically modifying organisms, as well as genomic technologies are likely to provide the next great advances. Certainly, the future for the genetic dissection of anesthetic mechanisms is bright.

REFERENCES

1. The C. Elegans Sequencing Consortium. (1998) Genome sequence of the nematode C. elegans: a platform for investigating biology. *Science* **282**, 2012–2018.

2. Crowder, C. M., Shebester, L. D., and Schedl, T. (1996) Behavioral effects of volatile anesthetics in Caenorhabditis elegans. *Anesthesiology* **85,** 901–912.
3. Adams, M. D., Celniker, S. E., Holt, R. H., et al. (2000) The genome sequence of Drosophila melanogaster. *Science* **287,** 2185–2195.
4. Silver, L. (1995) Mouse Genetics: Concepts and Applications, Oxford University Press, Inc., New York, pp. 207–226.
5. Crabbe, J. C., Belknap, J. K., and Buck, K. J. (1994) Genetic animal models of alcohol and drug abuse. *Science* **264,** 1715–1723.
6. Crabbe, J. C. and Belknap, J. K. (1992) Genetic approaches to drug dependence. *Trends Pharmacol. Sci.* **13,** 212–219.
7. Sonner, J. M., Gong, D., and Eger, E. I., 2nd (2000) Naturally occurring variability in anesthetic potency among inbred mouse strains. *Anesth. Analg.* **91,** 720–726.
8. Crabbe, J. C. and Harris, R. A. (1991) (Plenum Press) The genetic basis of alcohol and drug actions, New York.
9. Crowder, C. M. (1998) Mapping anesthesia genes: why and how? *Anesthesiology* **88,** 293–296.
10. Crabbe, J. C., Phillips, T. J., Buck, K. J., Cunningham, C. L., and Belknap, J. K. (1999) Identifying genes for alcohol and drug sensitivity: recent progress and future directions. *Trends Neurosci.* **22,** 173–179.
11. van Swinderen, B., Shook, D. R., Ebert, R. H., et al. (1997) Quantitative trait loci controlling halothane sensitivity in Caenorhabditis elegans. *Proc. Natl. Acad. Sci. USA* **94,** 8232–8237.
12. Simpson, V. J., Rikke, B. A., Costello, J. M., Corley, R., and Johnson, T. E. (1998) Identification of a genetic region in mice that specifies sensitivity to propofol. *Anesthesiology* **88,** 379–389.
13. Krishnan, K. S. and Nash, H. A. (1990) A genetic study of the anesthetic response: mutants of Drosophila melanogaster altered in sensitivity to halothane. *Proc. Natl. Acad. Sci. USA* **87,** 8632–8636.
14. Campbell, D. B. and Nash, H. A. (1994) Use of Drosophila mutants to distinguish among volatile general anesthetics. *Proc. Natl. Acad. Sci. USA* **91,** 2135–2139.
15. Takahashi, J. S., Pinto, L. H., and Vitaterna, M. H. (1994) Forward and reverse genetic approaches to behavior in the mouse. *Science* **264,** 1724–1733.
16. Nolan, P. M., Kapfhamer, D., and Bucan, M. (1997) Random mutagenesis screen for dominant behavioral mutations in mice. *Methods* **13,** 379–395.
17. van Swinderen, B., Saifee, O., Shebester, L., Roberson, R., Nonet, M. L., and Crowder, C. M. (1999) A neomorphic syntaxin mutation blocks volatile-anesthetic action in Caenorhabditis elegans. *Proc. Natl. Acad. Sci. USA* **96,** 2479–2484.
18. Eriksson, K. and Rusi, M. (1981) in Development of animal models as pharmacogenetic tools, (McCLearn, G. E., Deitrich, G. E., and Erwin, G., eds.) (US Government Printing Office, Washington DC), pp. 87–117.
19. Hellevuo, K., Kiianmaa, K., Juhakoski, A., and Kim, C. (1987) Intoxicating effects of lorazepam and barbital in rat lines selected for differential sensitivity to ethanol. *Psychopharmacology* **91,** 263–267.
20. Korpi, E. R., Kleingoor, C., Kettenmann, H., and Seeburg, P. H. (1993) Benzodiazepine-induced motor impairment linked to point mutation in cerebellar GABA-A receptor. *Nature* **361,** 356–359.
21. Firestone, L. L., Korpi, E. R., Niemi, L., Rosenberg, P. H., Homanics, G. E., and Quinlan, J. J. (2000) Halothane and desflurane requirements in alcohol-tolerant and -nontolerant rats. *Br. J. Anaesth.* **85,** 757–762.
22. Rajaram, S., Sedensky, M. M., and Morgan, P. G. (1998) Unc-1: a stomatin homologue controls sensitivity to volatile anesthetics in Caenorhabditis elegans. *Proc. Natl. Acad. Sci. USA* **95,** 8761–8766.
23. Rajaram, S., Spangler, T. L., Sedensky, M. M., and Morgan, P. G. (1999) A stomatin and a degenerin interact to control anesthetic sensitivity in Caenorhabditis elegans. *Genetics* **153,** 1673–1682.
24. Engel, S. R. and Allan, A. M. (1999) 5-HT3 receptor over-expression enhances ethanol sensitivity in mice. *Psychopharmacology (Berl)* **144,** 411–415.
25. Galli-Taliadoros, L. A., Sedgwick, J. D., Wood, S. A., and Korner, H. (1995) Gene knock-out technology: a methodological overview for the interested novice. *J. Immunol. Methods* 181, 1–15.
26. Wasserman, P. M. and DePamphilis, M. L. (1993) in Methods in Enzymology, (Abelson, J. N. and Simon, M. I., eds.) (Academic Press, Inc., New York), Vol. 225.
27. Homanics, G. E., Quinlan, J. J., Mihalek, R. M., and Firestone, L. L. (1998) Alcohol and anesthetic mechanisms in genetically engineered mice. *Front. Biosci.* **3,** d548–d558.
28. Homanics, G. E. (2000) In Genetic manipulation of receptor expression and function, (Accili, D., ed.) (John Wiley & Sons, Inc., New York), pp. 93–110.
29. Mihalek, R. M., Banjeree, P. K., Korpi, E., et al. (1999) Attenuated sensitivity to neuroactive steroids in GABA type A receptor delta subunit knockout mice. *Proc. Natl. Acad. Sci. USA* **96,** 12,905–12,910.
30. Tretter, V., Hauer, B., Nusser, Z., et al. (2001) Targeted disruption of the GABAa receptor delta subunit gene leads to upregulation of gamma2 subunit-containing receptors in cerebellar granule cells. *JBC* **276,** 10,532–10,538.
31. Homanics, G. E., Delorey, T. M., Firestone, L. L., et al. (1997) Mice devoid of γ-aminobutyrate type A receptor β3 subunit have epilepsy, cleft palate, and hypersensitive behavior. *Proc. Natl. Acad. Sci. USA* **94,** 4143–4148.
32. Quinlan, J. J., Homanics, G. E., and Firestone, L. L. (1998) Anesthesia sensitivity in mice lacking the β3 subunit of the GABA$_A$ receptor. *Anesthesiology* **88,** 775–780.
33. Antognini, J. F., and Carstens, E. (1998) Macroscopic sites of anesthetic action: brain versus spinal cord. *Toxicol. Lett.* **100–101,** 51–58.
34. Wong, S. M. E., Cheng, G., Homanics, G., E., and Kendig, J. J. (2001) Enflurane actions on spinal cords from mice that lack the B3 subunit of the GABA$_A$ receptor. *Anesthesiology* **95,** 154–164.

35. Ugarte, S. D., Homanics, G. E., Firestone, L. L., and Hammond, D. L. (2000) Sensory thresholds and the antinociceptive effects of GABA receptor agonists in mice lacking the β3 subunit of the GABA$_A$ receptor. *Neuroscience* **95,** 795–806.
36. McKernan, R. M., Rosahl, T. W., Reynolds, D. S., et al. (2000) Sedative but not anxiolytic properties of benzodiazepines are mediated by the GABA$_A$ receptor alpha1 subtype. *Nat. Neurosci.* **3,** 587–592.
37. Rudolph, U., Crestani, F., Benke, D., et al. (1999) Benzodiazepine actions mediated by specific gamma-aminobutyric acid(A) receptor subtypes. *Nature* **401,** 796–800.
38. Low, K., Crestani, F., Keist, R., et al. (2000) Molecular and neuronal substrate for the selective attenuation of anxiety. *Science* **290,** 131–134.
39. Mihic, S., Ye, Q., Wick, M., et al. (1997) Molecular sites of volatile anesthetic action on GABA$_A$ and glycine receptors. *Nature* **389,** 385–389.
40. Moody, E. J., Knauer, C., Granja, R., Strakhova, M., and Skolnick, P. (1997) Distinct loci mediate the direct and indirect actions of the anesthetic etomidate at GABA$_A$ receptors. *J. Neurochem.* **69,** 1310–1313.
41. Belelli, D., Lambert, J. J., Peters, J. A., Wafford, K., and Whiting, P. J. (1997) The interaction of the general anesthetic etomidate with the gamma-aminobutyric acid type A receptor is influenced by a single amino acid. *Proc. Natl. Acad. Sci. USA* **94,** 11,031–11,036.
42. Torres, R. M. and Kuhn, R. (1997) Laboratory protocols for conditional gene targeting (Oxford University Press, Oxford).
43. Tsien, J. Z., Chen, D. F., Gerber, D., et al. (1996) Subregion- and cell type-restricted gene knockout in mouse brain. *Cell* **87,** 1317–1326.
44. Tsien, J. Z., Huerta, P. T., and Tonegawa, S. (1996) The essential role of hippocampal CA1 NMDA receptor-dependent synaptic plasticity in spatial memory. *Cell* **87,** 1327–1338.
45. Bruning, J. C., Gautam, D., Burks, D. J., et al. (2000) Role of brain insulin receptor in control of body weight and reproduction *Science* **289,** 2122–2125.
46. Shimizu, E., Tang, Y. P., Rampon, C., and Tsien, J. Z. (2000) NMDA receptor-dependent synaptic reinforcement as a crucial process for memory consolidation. *Science* **290,** 1170–1174.
47. Davies, P. A., Hanna, M. C., Hales, T. G., and Kirkness, E. F. (1997) Insensitivity to Anaesthetic Agents Conferred By a Class Of GABA$_A$ Receptor Subunit. *Nature* **385,** 820–823.
48. Lewohl, J. M., Wang, L., Miles, M. F., Zhang, L., Dodd, P. R., and Harris, R. A. (2000) Gene expression in human alcoholism: microarray analysis of frontal cortex. *Alcohol. Clin. Exp. Res.* **24,** 1873–1882.
49. Mirnics, K., Middleton, F. A., Marquez, A., Lewis, D. A., and Levitt, P. (2000) Molecular characterization of schizophrenia viewed by microarray analysis of gene expression in prefrontal cortex. *Neuron* **28,** 53–67.

V Cellular and Molecular Mechanisms

16

General Anesthetic Effects on GABA$_A$ Receptors

Robert A. Pearce

INTRODUCTION

Cells of the brain communicate with each other using a wide variety of chemical neurotransmitters. These molecules are stored in vesicles, and in response to electrical signals, they are released at synapses, specialized junctions between neurons. Synapses are classified as excitatory or inhibitory depending upon the effect of the released transmitter on the postsynaptic cell to which it binds. Excitatory transmitters, for example glutamate and acetylcholine, cause depolarization, typically by opening cation channels that pass a net positive charge into postsynaptic neurons. Conversely, inhibitory transmitters, such as γ-aminobutyric acid (GABA) and glycine, reduce postsynaptic activity, primarily via activation of chloride-selective ion channels that serve to hold the neuron at hyperpolarized potentials, below the threshold for action potential initiation. Receptors that contain an integral ion channel are termed ionotropic receptors, and general anesthetics have been found to act via both depression of excitatory and enhancement of inhibitory ionotropic receptors.

The most prevalent type of inhibitory ionotropic receptor in the brain is the GABA$_A$ receptor. It is activated by the natural amino acid transmitter GABA and its conformationally restricted analogs muscimol and 4,5,6,7-tetrahydroisoxazolo(5,4-c)pyridin-3-ol (THIP), and inhibited by the competitive antagonist bicuculline and the noncompetitive antagonist picrotoxin. A related but pharmacologically distinct type of GABA receptor was originally termed the GABA$_C$ receptor. The ρ subunits that make up this receptor are found primarily in the retina (hence ρ). Molecular cloning studies have now made it clear that this receptor is closely related to ionotropic GABA$_A$ receptors. Therefore, it has been proposed that it be classified as a part of this family, and that the older terminology be abandoned (1). Because this subunit forms functionally active homomultimers it has become an important experimental tool in the study of GABA$_A$ receptor pharmacology.

STRUCTURE OF THE GABA$_A$ RECEPTOR

The GABA$_A$ receptor is heteromeric, multimeric membrane protein that contains binding sites for the transmitter GABA, as well as for a large number of modulatory substances such as benzodiazepines, barbiturates, neurosteroids, and a wide variety of other drugs with anesthetic properties (for a recent comprehensive review of GABA$_A$ receptor structure and stoichiometry see refs. 1–3). It is a member of a large family of related receptors that includes the nicotinic acetylcholine receptor (nAChR), the 5-HT3$_A$ (serotonin) receptor, and the glycine receptor. Of these related proteins, the structure of the nAChR has been worked out in the greatest detail (owing in large part to its abundance in the Torpedo electric organ), but many of the findings regarding the general structure of this receptor have been confirmed directly for the GABA$_A$ receptor.

From: *Contemporary Clinical Neuroscience: Neural Mechanisms of Anesthesia*
Edited by: Joseph F. Antognini et al. © Humana Press Inc., Totowa, NJ

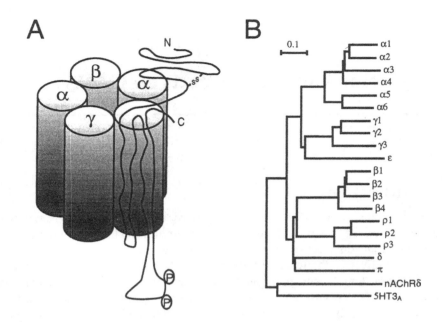

Fig. 1. Structure of the GABA$_A$ receptor. **(A)** Topology of the receptor/ionophore complex. Five subunits are arranged around a central pore. Each subunit has four membrane-spanning segments, with five alpha-helical M2 segments (one from each subunit) lining the pore. The GABA binding site is formed by residues from the N-terminal region of adjacent alpha and beta subunits. **(B)** Dendrogram showing the relationships between different families of GABA$_A$ receptor subunits, based upon amino acid similarities. The beta4 subunit is from the chicken, epsilon from human, the rest from rat sequences. (Adapted from ref. *1*).

The receptor is composed of five separate subunits arranged around a central pore (Fig. 1A). First demonstrated for the nAChR *(4)*, this topology has been confirmed recently for the GABA$_A$ receptor via electron microscopic image analysis of purified brain receptors, which showed a dominant fivefold symmetry *(5)*. Studies of molecular weight and stoichiometry are consistent with this structure as well *(6,7)*.

Molecular cloning has so far revealed 19 separate types of subunits from which GABA$_A$ receptors may be constructed. On the basis of sequence homology these subunits have been grouped into families, designated α1–α6, β1–β4, γ1–γ3, δ, ε, π, and ρ1–ρ3 (Fig. 1B). In addition, splice variants of the γ2 and α6 subunits have been identified *(8,9)*. Each subunit contains 400–450 base pairs, for a molecular weight of approx 50 kDa. All have the same topology, consisting of a large extracellular N-terminal domain, four transmembrane segments (designated TM1–TM4), and an extracellular C-terminus. A large intracellular loop between TM3–TM4 contains sites for phosphorylation and also appears to be involved in receptor targeting via binding domains that interact with intracellular proteins.

The precise subunit composition and stoichiometry of native GABA$_A$ receptors has been the subject of numerous investigations. The best evidence to date indicates that two α, two β, and one γ subunit combine to form the majority of receptors in the brain, but other stoichiometries have also been suggested (reviewed in ref. *2*). Given the large number of subunits that may be combined to form receptors, it is evident that the potential exists for a very large number of receptor subtypes, particularly considering that individual receptors may contain more than one type of α, β, or γ subunit *(10)*. However, immunoprecipitation, co-localization, and expression studies indicate that the number of distinct receptor types is on the order of tens of different types of receptors *(2,11)*.

SUBUNIT DISTRIBUTION

There is substantial regional heterogeneity in the expression pattern of GABA$_A$ receptors, as demonstrated using *in situ* hybridization *(12,13)* and immunohistochemistry *(14)*. Some subunits, such as the γ2, are widely distributed throughout the brain, whereas others have a tightly restricted expression pattern, such as the α6 receptor, found exclusively in the granule cells of the cerebellum *(15)*. Of the α subunits, the α1 subtype is the most widely distributed, and accounts for 75–90% of all α subunits in the brain. The β1 and β3 subunits are expressed most heavily in the hippocampus and cerebellum, whereas β2 is more heavily expressed in cerebellum. Cerebral cortex has intermediate levels of β1–β3.

Although the great majority of receptors throughout the brain are believed to consist of a combination of α, β, and γ subunits, other subunits are also present in distinct brain regions, and may substitute for the γ subunit *(16)*. The δ subunit is found predominantly in cerebellum, but also at lower levels in thalamus. The ε subunit, reported to confer insensitivity to a number of different anesthetics, is present in the thalamus and subthalamic nuclei, as well as the amygdala. The ρ subunit, the only subunit that forms functional homomeric receptors, was originally thought to be expressed exclusively in retina. However, it is now known to be present as well at low levels in various regions of the brain including the hippocampus and the cerebellum *(17)*. The π subunit is expressed primarily outside of the brain.

In addition to regional heterogeneity of expression, there is also evidence for differential subcellular distribution of different GABA$_A$ receptor isoforms. The determinants of targeting are not entirely clear, but may include isoforms of α *(18)*, β *(19)*, or γ *(20,21)* subunits, as well as variety of intracellular proteins that promote clustering via interactions with γ subunits *(20,21)*. These targeting mechanisms lead to subcellular specialization of physiological responses to GABA. For example, extrasynaptic receptors in cerebellar granule cells have a unique composition that produces high affinity for GABA and little desensitization, thus enabling them to respond to the ambient concentration of GABA within the glomerulus to produce a tonic GABA$_A$ current *(15,22)*.

SUBUNIT SPECIFICITY OF ANESTHETIC ACTIONS

Subunit-specific differences between the actions of a wide variety of anesthetics have been found, but often these differences are manifest as quantitative differences in sensitivity rather than qualitative differences in effects. It has been noted that interpretation of experiments designed to detect quantitative differences in anesthetic action is complicated by the strong dependence of effects on GABA concentration, together with the different sensitivities of receptors composed of different subunits *(23)*. Nevertheless, in some cases there are clear requirements for the presence of specific subunits. The best example is the absolute requirement for both the γ and α subunits to see benzodiazepine potentiation of GABA-gated currents *(1)*. As discussed below, this is likely to be due to the existence of a binding site at the interface between these subunits.

Other notable subunit-specific drug interactions occur for a variety of drugs with the β subunit. The anticonvulsant loreclezole and the anesthetic etomidate have both been shown to exhibit strong preference for β2 and β3 over β1-containing receptors when co-expressed with α and γ subunits *(24–26)*, and this preference has been traced to a single amino acid within the TM3 domain. Interestingly, the difference between β3 homomeric receptors, which cannot be activated by GABA but are directly activated by pentobarbital, and β1 homomeric receptors, which are not activated by either agent, has been traced to this same residue *(27)*. Although this residue was found to influence sensitivity of heteromeric receptors to etomidate and loreclezole, there was no influence for pentobarbital.

In contrast to the relatively indiscriminate action of general anesthetics on heteromeric GABA$_A$ receptors composed of a wide variety of subunit combinations (primarily αβ or αβγ), it was reported that co-expression of the ε subunit together with α and β subunits produces receptors that are insensitive to a number of intravenous agents, including pentobarbital, propofol, and neurosteroids *(28)*. Whether this insensitivity extends to volatile agents has not yet been tested.

BINDING SITES

A notable feature of $GABA_A$ receptors is the large number of ligands that bind to this receptor and alter its activity. Determining the sites at which different agents bind to the receptor is of considerable interest, but progress has been hindered by a number of limitations. Unlike the nAChR, there is no readily available source of biochemically homogeneous receptors. Also, the strong coupling between agonist or drug binding and receptor gating makes interpretations of mutagenesis studies difficult, because mutations that alter gating also will affect binding and vice-versa. Finally, the low affinity of many agents, including the majority of anesthetics that are of interest, makes the use of photoaffinity studies to define binding sites much more difficult. Nevertheless, amino acid residues involved in binding of GABA and benzodiazepines, both of which have high affinity for the receptor, have been identified. In addition, progress is being made in identifying residues important for the action of a number of anesthetic agents, primarily through the use of chimeric subunit and site-directed mutagenesis studies.

GABA

The binding site for GABA has been localized to the N-terminal domains of α and β subunits *(29–31)*. Within each of these N-terminal regions, multiple domains may contribute to the binding site, with two domains of the β subunit, and one domain of the α subunit forming a binding pocket. This configuration is based in part on homology with the nAChR, where it is thought that the agonist binding pocket is located at the interface between adjacent subunits *(32)*, and is supported by photoaffinity labeling with the GABA analog muscimol *(31)*. An alternating pattern of residues accessible to modification by cysteine-reactive agents suggests a β sheet secondary structure for the α subunit domain *(33)*. If two α and two β subunits are incorporated into receptors, two agonist binding sites are expected to be present, consistent with the typical finding that hill coefficients for activation of receptors are between one and two.

Benzodiazepines

The binding site for benzodiazepines has also been proposed to lie at the interface between two subunits. In this case, it is the α and γ subunits that contribute residues within the N-terminal regions for binding *(34–37)*. This is the binding site for not only classic benzodiazepines such as diazepam, but also for a variety of other neuroactive compounds including the sedative imidazopyridine zolpidem *(1,38)*. By binding to this site, agonists such as diazepam and zolpidem reduce GABA EC_{50}, inverse agonists increase GABA EC_{50}, and antagonists such as flumazenil do not alter GABA EC_{50}, but prevent actions of agonists and inverse agonists. A receptor with two α, two β, and one γ subunit would thus be expected to have a single benzodiazepine binding site, consistent with the finding that hill coefficients for receptor modulation by these drugs are approximately 1.

Volatile Anesthetics

In contrast to the binding sites that have been proposed for GABA and benzodiazepines, which are formed by residues of the N-terminal domain, it has been proposed that volatile agents (and a large number of structurally unrelated intravenous agents) bind to residues within the transmembrane regions of receptors. The initial identification of a putative volatile anesthetic binding site was accomplished through the use of chimeric receptors formed from $GABA_A$ ρ subunits and glycine $\alpha 1$ subunits, both of which form functional homomeric receptors in mammalian heterologous expression systems. Specific residues within the TM2 and TM3 domains were identified that are required for enflurane and ethanol enhancement of GABA-activated currents *(39)*. Mutation of analogous residues in the GABA_A receptor α2 subunit (S270 in TM2 and A291 in TM3) yielded receptors insensitive to isoflurane, but sensitive to propofol and halothane. These residues were thought to be located near the extracellular end of the channel, on the side of the alpha helix facing away from the pore.

The finding that a separate residue in TM1 (L232) conferred insensitivity to halothane, but not isoflurane, suggested initially that separate binding sites exists for ether and alkane anesthetics *(40)*. However, subsequent studies in which amino acid side chains at multiple locations were systematically mutated to residues of different molecular volumes showed that mutations of any of the sites can affect anesthetic sensitivity to other agents as well *(41)*. The finding that the cutoff volumes of volatile agents of different molecular size (isoflurane>halothane>chloroform) are predicted by the net change in molecular volume of the mutated residues led to the conclusion that there exists a common volatile anesthetic binding cavity with a molecular volume of 250–370 Å^3 that it is lined by residues in TM1, TM2, and TM3, and that for some anesthetics (e.g., chloroform) the cavity may be occupied by two molecules simultaneously *(41)*.

It can be problematic to infer binding sites solely from mutational studies, because changes in gating properties or other structurally unrelated domains may influence the ability of receptors to bind to or respond to drugs either via allosteric alterations in protein conformation or other structural rearrangements. Although their low potency, and hence rapid unbinding rate, has so far prevented the use of photoaffinity labeling techniques, as confirmation of binding at this site, Mascia et al. *(42)* used a combination of cysteine substitution at the S270 site in TM2 together with an alkanethiol anesthetic that can react with cysteines to provide evidence that this residue is part of an anesthetic binding site. They found that the alkanethiol anesthetic produced a similar enhancement of function for wildtype GABA_A receptors as conventional anesthetics, and that exposure of the S270C mutant to either the alkanethiol anesthetic or to the derivitizing agent propyl methanesulfonate produced an irreversible enhancement of receptor function, and prevented further enhancement by isoflurane. This result, together with the mutational analysis demonstrating that molecular volumes correlate well with cutoff effects *(41)*, provides further evidence that anesthetics bind directly to a pocket within the receptor protein to exert their effects. It has been noted also that this molecular volume agrees closely with values obtained using cycloalkanols to estimate molecular dimensions of anesthetic target sites in tadpoles in vivo *(41,43)*.

Barbiturates, Etomidate, and Propofol

Using approaches, similar to those described in Volatile Anesthetics for volatile agents, mutagenesis studies have led to the identification of amino acid residues within the transmembrane domains that influence sensitivity to a number of intravenous anesthetics. Prior to identification of these critical transmembrane sites, a variety of pharmacological studies had provided evidence that barbiturate and other anesthetic binding sites are distinct from the GABA binding site *(44)*. The subsequent demonstration that mutation of residues at the GABA binding site in the N-terminal domain abolished responses to GABA, but did not prevent direct channel activation by pentobarbital, is consistent with the notion that separate binding sites exist for GABA and barbiturates *(30, see* also ref. *45)*.

In general, the residues that influence sensitivity to these multiple intravenous agents have been found to be distinct from those that influence sensitivity to volatile agents. However, it is intriguing that they are present at equivalent positions, near the extracellular ends of TM1, TM2, and TM3, as those that have been proposed as the volatile anesthetic binding site discussed above. Thus, single amino acid residues within TM3 of the β subunit determine sensitivity to etomidate *(25)* and the anticonvulsant loreclezole *(24)*. Mutations at a site one turn of the alpha helix closer to the extracellular mouth of the pore alter sensitivity to barbiturates *(46–48)* and propofol *(47)*. Similarly, a conserved glycine residue on the first turn of the TM1 region of the β2 subunit influences efficacy of a number of intravenous anesthetics, including pentobarbital, alphaxalone, etomidate, and propofol *(49)*.

The underlying mechanism by which sensitivity to multiple agents is influenced by these closely related residues is not known. As discussed above for volatile anesthetics, these sites may represent drug binding sites, perhaps within clefts that extend deep into the protein, outside of the ion permeation pathway *(50)*. Alternatively, this region may be part of or functionally coupled to the gating machinery of the channel, so that mutations could alter modulatory influences via allosteric mechanisms. This possibility is consistent with the finding that mutations near this site abolish benzodiazepine modulation of GABA-activated channels, but do not prevent benzodiazepine binding itself *(51)*. It is also possible that multiple binding sites are present even for single agents, each site responsible for a different aspect of drug action (modulation, direct activation, or block) *(52–54)*.

Neurosteroids

Despite the presence of an apparently large number of modulatory drug binding sites on the GABA$_A$ receptor, it is remarkable that for most sites no endogenous ligands have been identified. The exception is neurosteroids, of which a large number of related compounds, including several metabolites of progesterone and corticosterone, have been found to have potent actions in modulating or directly activating GABA$_A$ receptors (reviewed in ref. *55*). Examples of neurosteroids include the anesthetic alphaxalone, which has been used clinically for induction and maintenance of anesthesia *(56)*, as well as the naturally occurring progesterone metabolites pregnanolone (3α-hydroxy-5β-pregnan-20-one) and allopregnanolone (3α-hydroxy-5α-pregnan-20-one), and the corticosterone metabolite THDOC (3α,21-dihydroxy-5α-pregnan-20-one). The binding site (or sites) for these agents has not been identified, but is thought to be distinct from that for barbiturates and benzodiazepines *(57)*. Based upon displacement of TBPS from the picrotoxin site it has been proposed that multiple sites exist, and studies of enantioselectivity are consistent with this suggestion, although it is possible that a single class of sites exists that can accommodate multiple enantiomers *(58)*. In addition to these positive modulators, steroids with potent antagonistic properties exist, most notably pregnenolone sulfate (PS) *(59)*. It was proposed that this compound acts as an endogenous antagonist of the GABA$_A$ receptor, but again its binding site has not been identified.

SPECIFIC BEHAVIORAL ACTIONS MAY BE LINKED TO SPECIFIC SUBUNITS

Drugs that modulate GABA$_A$ receptors have many different clinical uses, suggesting that they target multiple functionally distinct circuits in the brain. This is perhaps not surprising given the broad anatomical distribution of GABA$_A$ receptors. However, given the evidence that pharmacologically distinct receptor subtypes can be formed by combining different subunits, it is somewhat surprising that there is such a great degree of overlap in the spectrum of actions seen for most agents. Often, this leads to undesirable side effects. For example, the use of anticonvulsant barbiturates and benzodiazepines is limited by the sedation that often accompanies administration of higher doses. Motor coordination can be impaired by hypnotics and anticonvulsants, and sedation limits the use of diazepam as an anxiolytic and muscle relaxant.

It has proved relatively difficult to create drugs with more specific behavioral actions. This might be owing to the presence of a strong functional heterogeneity in receptor types involved in complex behaviors, or it could simply reflect the lack of development of drugs with adequate subunit specificity. Recent experimental evidence suggests that the latter may be the explanation, as specific behavioral consequences have been tied to benzodiazepine effects on receptors containing specific α subunits. Taking advantage of the requirement for a specific amino acid residue in order to maintain benzodiazepine sensitivity (His 101 of the α subunit), Rudolph et al. *(60)* created transgenic mice in which one type of α subunit that had been previously sensitive was rendered benzodiazepine-insensitive via mutation at this site. Remarkably, they found that mice with benzodiazepine-insensitive α1 receptors did not show the sedative, amnestic, and in part, the anticonvulsant responses to diazepam that are seen in wild type mice. However, the anxiolytic, myorelaxant, motor-impairing, and ethanol-potentiating responses were all maintained, suggesting that these behaviors are mediated by different receptor subtypes in distinct neuronal circuits. Complementary studies in which α2 receptors were rendered benzodiazepine-insensitive demonstrated that the anxiolytic properties of diazepam, but not the other behavioral actions, were mediated by receptors containing α2 subunits *(61)*. Taken together, these results indicate that specific behavioral responses may be closely enough associated with distinct GABA_A receptor subtypes that the design of more subtype-specific drugs may well lead to substantial improvements in effect/side-effect profiles.

PHYSIOLOGICAL PROPERTIES AND ANESTHETIC ACTIONS

Interest in the GABA_A receptor, at least in terms of understanding anesthetic mechanisms, derives in large part from its major role as a mediator of synaptic inhibition in the brain. It is present in the membranes of all (or nearly all) neurons in the brain, and its activity is enhanced by a wide variety of anesthetics, both intravenous and volatile *(62,63)*. At receptors in the brain, anesthetic enhancement results in prolongation of the decay of the inhibitory postsynaptic potential (IPSP), or in voltage clamp experiments, the inhibitory postsynaptic current (IPSC). Depending upon the experimental paradigm, this enhancement may be manifest as an increase in the current that is elicited, as occurs when low nonsaturating concentrations of GABA are applied to receptors, or as an increase in the decay time constant of the receptors, as is seen when brief saturating concentrations of GABA are applied *(64)*.

Even in the absence of anesthetics or other drugs, the response of GABA_A receptors to agonist application is complex. When GABA is applied for prolonged periods (hundreds of milliseconds to seconds) at a low concentration, channels activate slowly until there is a steady-state current (Fig. 2A). If higher concentrations are applied, channels open more rapidly and to a greater extent. However, in the continued presence of GABA, current declines. This decline is termed desensitization, and depending on the subunit composition of the receptors, it occurs on the order of milliseconds to seconds *(16,65,66)*. Even at synapses where transmitter is present only for a brief duration (<1 ms), desensitization may occur, resulting in complex deactivation kinetics *(67)* and use-dependent depression *(68)*. Responses to brief pulse applications of GABA generally have been found to resemble the responses of receptors at synapses *(67,69)*, but quantitative differences have been noted (Fig. 2B), reflecting perhaps differences in receptor subunit composition between subsynaptic and extrasynaptic receptors *(70)*.

ENHANCEMENT OF GABA RESPONSES BY ANESTHETICS

Concentration-response curves are often used to characterize the electrophysiological responses or binding characteristics of receptors to agonist application. The concentration at which GABA_A receptor responses are half-maximal (EC_{50}) is typically 5–50 μ*M* for physiological responses, and 5–50 n*M* in binding studies. The difference in these values is thought to reflect the higher affinity of desensitized receptors for GABA, as occurs during equilibrium binding studies. Nevertheless, it is found that positive modulators, including benzodiazepines, barbiturates, volatile anesthetics, propofol, neurosteroids, etomidate, and other intravenous agents, all shift the concentration-response curve to the left, in qualitatively and even quantitatively similar fashions. Maximal responses to high concentrations are not typically enhanced. In most cases, the application of anesthetic agents in the presence of a saturating concentration of GABA leads to a depression of peak responses despite an increase in apparent affinity. The exception to this rule is for benzodiazepines, in which case peak responses may be increased, even with saturating GABA concentrations. The shift in apparent agonist affinity means that responses to lower concentrations are increased to a greater extent than are higher concentration responses. When responses to drugs of receptors of different GABA sensitivity are compared, this becomes an important consideration, and it is important to compare effects on equieffective concentrations. Typically, enhancement of EC_5 to EC_{20} concentrations are tested.

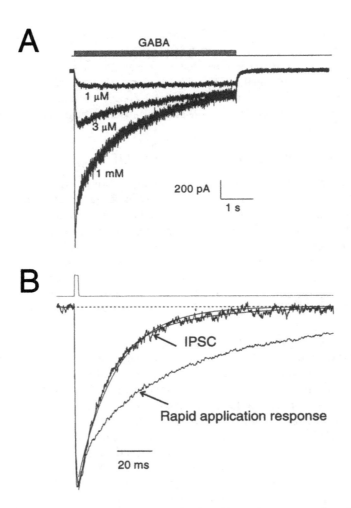

Fig. 2. Response of GABA$_A$ receptors to agonist application. (**A**) As the concentration of GABA is increased, receptors activate more rapidly, and desensitization (a reduction in open probability in the continued presence of agonist) occurs more rapidly and to a greater extent. These recordings are from receptors composed of α1 and β2 subunits expressed in HEK293 cells (Unpublished data; Li, T. B. and Pearce, R. A.). (**B**) Response of native receptors from hippocampal CA1 neurons. In response to a brief pulse of GABA, excised receptors activate rapidly and then deactivate with biexponential kinetics. This deactivation is slower than the time course of IPSCs recorded from these cells due to the presence of extrasynaptic receptors with different kinetics than the subsynaptic receptors that underlie the IPSC. (Adapted from ref. *70*).

Accompanying the increase in apparent GABA affinity is a slowing of the deactivation time course in response to brief pulse applications of GABA (Fig. 3A–C) *(64,71,72)*. Presumably, these two manifestations of enhancement arise from a single molecular drug action *(64)*. This hypothesis is supported primarily by the nearly universal correspondence between the two effects. The similarity between prolongation of IPSCs and deactivation following brief GABA pulses (Fig. 3A,C) suggests that anesthetics alter the time course of synaptic inhibition, primarily via alterations in intrinsic receptor kinetics.

The ability of general anesthetics to prolong synaptic inhibition led to suggestions that enhanced inhibition may contribute to the effects of pentobarbital and halothane *(73–75)*. It has not been until the past decade that it has become clear that this is a general principle, which applies to a wide variety of intravenous and general anesthetics *(63,76)*. A prolonged duration of inhibition has now been seen

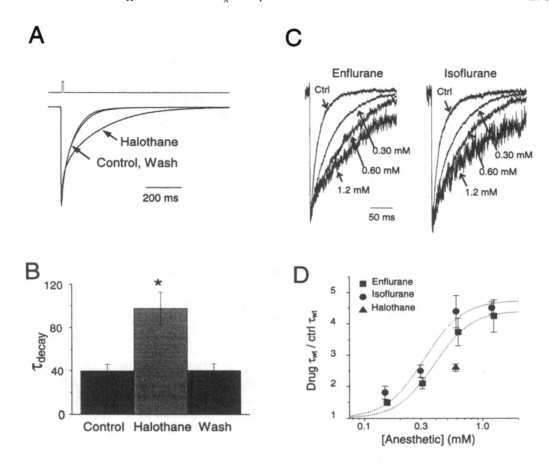

Fig. 3. Prolonged deactivation of GABA$_A$ receptors by volatile anesthetics. **(A,B)** Deactivation of expressed α1β2γ2s receptors is prolonged by halothane (0.8%, ≈ 0.43 mM). Responses were normalized to the peak of the response. **A, B** Adapted from Li and Pearce, 2000 *(64)*. **C, D.** Hippocampal CA1 pyramidal neuron IPSCs are prolonged by enflurane, isoflurane, and halothane. Responses in **C** were normalized to the peak current. (Adapted from ref. *[86]*).

in vivo for volatile anesthetics *(77,78)*, benzodiazepines *(79,80)*, barbiturates *(75,77,79–81)*, propofol *(82)*, and etomidate *(81)*, and in vitro in cultured neuron and slice preparations for volatile agents *(83–86)*, benzodiazepines *(87)*, barbiturates *(83)*, neurosteroids *(88)*, propofol *(89)*, and etomidate *(90)*. This commonality in anesthetic effects on synaptic inhibition, together with the excellent correlation between EC$_{50}$ values for actions in vivo and in vitro *(62)*, are important findings that have contributed to the acceptance of the GABA$_A$ receptor as a relevant anesthetic target *(63,91)*.

DIRECT RECEPTOR ACTIVATION BY ANESTHETICS

Many anesthetics have been found to not only enhance responses of GABA-activated channels, but also at slightly higher concentrations, to cause channels to open in the absence of GABA. This "direct channel gating" is seen with many anesthetics, including volatile *(86,92,93)* and intravenous agents *(94–98)*. One notable exception is benzodiazepines, which do not directly activate channels until concentrations are several orders of magnitude greater than required to enhance GABA-activated current *(99)*. It is interesting that benzodiazepines are somewhat unique in this regard, just as they have a unique binding site away from the TM2/TM3 region that influences the anesthetic sensitivity of other agents.

The best-characterized drug with regard to direct activation is pentobarbital. Although some characteristics are different than those of GABA-activated channels, there are also several striking similarities. Single channel openings produced by pentobarbital and GABA are similar in conductance *(100,101)*, and open times can be similar to those produced by low concentrations of GABA *(95,100,101)*, suggesting that the structure of the open states induced by these agents are similar. It is also interesting that the GABA binding site competitive antagonists bicuculline and gabazine also inhibit pentobarbital-activated channels, suggesting that allosteric coupling between the open channel configuration and GABA binding site is preserved in pentobarbital-activated channels *(102)*.

For most receptor combinations that have been studied, the opening efficacy of pentobarbital and other drugs is lower than that of GABA. However, for some combinations, such as homomeric β2 or β3 receptors, which do not open in response to GABA but are directly activated by pentobarbital *(103)*, evidently efficacy can be higher. The different apparent affinities of pentobarbital for direct activation and modulation of GABA-activated currents may indicate that binding sites for these two actions are distinct *(101)*. Alternatively, this may arise from a change in affinity at a single site caused by occupancy of the GABA binding site. The observation that the ability of pentobarbital to directly activate channels is maintained, despite the presence of a mutation in the TM2 domain that prevents enhancement of GABA-gated currents *(53)* would appear to support the former. The presence of distinct sites for modulation and direct activation has also been suggested for etomidate and propofol, based on different apparent affinities and on the selective effects of mutations *(52,54)*.

The ability of various anesthetics to activate channels directly is of considerable interest with regard to understanding molecular mechanisms of anesthetic action, but does it have any functional relevance? Experimental evidence addressing this question is lacking. This is certainly a plausible suggestion, and is supported by the ability of GABA analogs that cross the blood-brain barrier and directly activate receptors to produce anesthesia *(104)*. There is accumulating evidence for extrasynaptic GABA receptors, which may be present in greater numbers than subsynaptic receptors *(70,105,106)*, so direct activation of these receptors may have a substantial effect. However, there is evidence for micromolar levels of GABA in the extracellular space *(107)*, which is a high enough concentration that it may be difficult to separate enhancement of GABA-activated currents and direct activation in the physiological setting.

CHANNEL BLOCK BY ANESTHETICS

In addition to positive modulation of GABA-activated currents and direct channel activation, many anesthetics also have a blocking action, not only on GABA$_A$ receptors, but also on a variety of ligand- and voltage-activated channels *(108–111)*. This relative lack of target specificity and relatively high concentration requirement have led to the suggestion that blocking may result not from binding to specialized high affinity sites, but rather to some common or universal motif that has been conserved in many ion channels *(101)*.

Depending on the experimental paradigm, block may be manifest as 1) a decrease in IPSC amplitude *(86)* or a reduction in peak current when high GABA concentrations are applied *(64)*, 2) as a rebound or "surge" current following the rapid termination of anesthetic exposure, particularly when channels have been activated directly by anesthetic *(93,95)*, 3) as a rapid and reversible reduction in current when anesthetic is applied during deactivation *(64)*, or 4) as a reduction in the open duration in single channel recordings *(101)*. Unlike modulation and direct activation, amino acid residues critical for channel block have not been identified thus far.

Compared to the number of studies of other anesthetic effects, there have been relatively few detailed studies of the phenomenon of channel block by general anesthetics. The existing data do not appear to be consistent with a simple open channel blocking scheme, as was proposed for local anesthetic block of muscle acetylcholine receptors *(112)*. Rather, for the nAChR, a model has been proposed whereby anesthetics bind and interrupt current flow (though not necessarily via a pore "plugging" mechanism), and that binding and unbinding rates are not influenced by the state of the channel, but that their frequency dictates the nature of the block by different drugs *(113)*. Similarly, in detailed studies of GABA$_A$ receptor block by pentobarbital, it was observed that block does not influence entry into the desensitized state, and that blocked duration increases with increasing concentration of pentobarbital *(101)*. These findings led to the suggestion that multiple blocking sites are present, but that occupancy of a single site is sufficient to prevent current flow.

What might be the functional relevance of this blocking action? Other drugs that block the GABA$_A$ receptor typically produce convulsions, and this may be the case for some anesthetics. It has been found that enflurane, which is epileptogenic at high concentrations, strongly reduces somatic inhibition in hippocampal CA1 neurons, whereas halothane and isoflurane, which do not cause seizures, cause smaller reductions *(85,86)*. Even if block does not lead to seizures, it is possible that this action increases anesthetic requirement for some drugs. This suggestion is supported by the better correlation with MAC for net current through GABA$_A$ receptors than for peak current amplitudes or decay rates *(86)*.

KINETIC PROPERTIES AND ANESTHETIC MODULATION

Because of the brief time course and high concentration of transmitter to which synaptic GABA$_A$ receptors are exposed, intrinsic kinetic properties determine the time course of inhibition *(67,114)*. Similarly, prolongation of inhibition by anesthetics arises from alterations in the rates of transitions made by anesthetic-bound receptors. Evidently, linking drug binding to changes in kinetic properties will be an important step in elucidating the mechanism of action of general anesthetics.

Studies aimed at understanding the kinetic basis of channel function and anesthetic action have been carried out at microscopic (single channel) and macroscopic (ensembles of many channels) levels. On the basis of these studies, kinetic models have been developed to explain various aspects of the baseline and drug-altered behavior of channels. In single channel recordings from mouse spinal cord neurons and chick cerebral neurons in culture, up to three open and five closed states were seen when receptors were exposed to low concentrations of GABA *(115,116)*. Detailed analysis of the patterns of openings, including the effect of agonist concentration on open and closed times and burst durations, suggested a model incorporating sequential binding of two molecules of GABA, transitions between two adjacent closed fully liganded receptors, long-lived open states associated only with doubly liganded receptors, and brief closures during openings. Within this framework, it was concluded that barbiturates and benzodiazepines, both of which enhanced channel opening, operated through quite distinct mechanisms *(117)*. Barbiturates shifted the balance between the two doubly liganded states to favor transitions to the longer-lived state without altering the kinetic properties of the open states directly. Benzodiazepines did not alter gating transitions *per se*, but rather increased the microscopic binding rate for GABA, resulting in a larger proportion of channels that are fully liganded and thus have a higher open probability (Fig. 4).

With the advent of rapid application techniques, agonists and drugs could be applied with millisecond precision. It was quickly recognized that macroscopic properties can be quite complex, with multiple desensitized states *(65)* that may influence the time course of synaptic currents *(67)* (Fig. 4B). In addition, it has become clear that different subunits produce different kinetic properties, including deactivation and desensitization rates *(118)*. Studies in which both microscopic and macroscopic channel properties have been measured in a single preparation are providing new details regarding unique kinetic features of channels that are conferred by specific receptor subunits, and even specific amino acid residues *(16,119)*. It appears that all types of subunits influence the kinetic properties of heteromeric receptors, with striking differences between macroscopic desensitization and deactivation, as well as single channel properties *(16,120,121)*.

There have been a number of studies of how anesthetics affect the macroscopic kinetic properties of various receptors, both recombinant and native. Based on single channel kinetics the suggestion

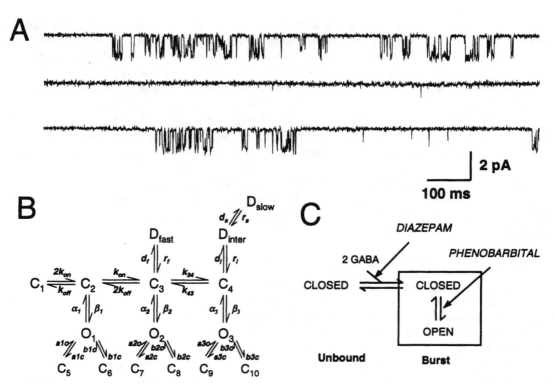

Fig. 4. Microscopic kinetic characteristics of GABA$_A$ receptors. **(A)** Single channel currents during the application of 1 mM GABA to an outside-out membrane patch containing α1β3γ2L subunits expressed in mouse L929 fibroblasts. Note that openings occur in bursts, with long closed intervals between bursts that represent entry into desensitized states. **(B)**. A kinetic model for the α1β3γ2L isoform that was derived from steady-state single channel and rapid kinetic analysis from outside-out membrane patches. **A, B**. Adapted from ref. *(16)*. **(C)**. Proposed mechanisms for diazepam and phenobarbital action in a simplified burst model, based on drug effects on receptors from dissociated mouse spinal neurons. (Adapted from ref. *[117]*).

that benzodiazepines increase the agonist binding rate was supported by a study demonstrating that activation rate is increased, but deactivation is not slowed in the presence of diazepam *(122)*. This finding is difficult to reconcile with the concept that transmitter transients are brief and saturating, since IPSC decay is slowed by benzodiazepines *(87)*. It may be that for some synapses, continued rebinding of low concentrations of transmitter continues to occur during the deactivation phase, or that postsynaptic receptors are not fully occupied by transmitter under control conditions *(123)*.

Other studies have implicated different kinetic steps for the actions of various drugs. Neurosteroids were found to slow the rate of slow desensitization, and to slow rates of entry and recovery from the fast desenstitized state, as assessed by pairs of high concentration pulses *(71)*. Based on these results it was suggested that IPSCs may be prolonged solely via ability to alter desensitization. However, subsequent modeling studies revealed that the rate of recovery using paired pulses is sensitive to alterations in unbinding rate *(64,72)*, so at least this additional mechanism should also be considered. Like neurosteroids, propofol and halothane were both found to slow recovery from paired pulse depression, as well as slow deactivation *(64,72)*. Whereas propofol altered fast and slow desensitization, halothane had no effect. It was concluded from these studies that halothane slows desensitization by slowing the agonist unbinding rate *(64)*, that this action is shared by propofol *(72)*, and that in addition, propofol slows transitions into desensitized states. Overall, it is striking that these different drugs display such similarities in a number of macroscopic actions, although there may be differences as well. Again, as observed for the effects on direct activation, benzodiazepines appear to be somewhat unique compared to the other anesthetics studied here, a difference that correlates with its unique binding site.

FUNCTIONAL ROLES OF GABAERGIC INHIBITION

From the above discussion, it is apparent that anesthetics affect GABA$_A$ receptors in a number of ways. Which of these contribute to the state of "anesthesia"? The answer to this question is unknown. It seems likely that the ability of anesthetics to prolong the time course of inhibitory synaptic currents is functionally significant. It is also possible that enhancement of tonic or "background" current produced by ambient levels of GABA, direct activation of channels, alterations in desensitization, or even channel block all play important roles. If "anesthesia" consists of a collection of different effects, such as amnesia, analgesia, hypnosis, immobility, etc., each of which is produced via different mechanisms at different sites in the nervous system *(124)*, then the different anesthetic actions on GABA$_A$ receptors might be functionally significant for some effects and not others.

Based upon current concepts regarding the functional roles of GABA$_A$ receptors and inhibition, a number of possible links between inhibition and "anesthesia" may be considered. It may be that simply by enhancing ongoing inhibition, without particular regard to the timing or location of inhibitory inputs, the ability of principal or projection neurons to generate action potentials and communicate effectively with other neurons will be degraded. This concept fits well with "rate coding" theories of information processing, wherein summation of excitatory and inhibitory activity over a relatively broad time window determines the net firing rate *(125)*. This type of temporally nonspecific depression may be particularly effective if the activity of GABA$_A$ receptors near the spike initiation zone is enhanced. There is indeed evidence that tonic inhibition arises from synapses close to the soma *(126,127)*, and that certain classes of interneurons, such as basket cells and chandelier cells, make large numbers of synapses on the soma and axon initial segment of pyramidal cells *(128)*. In addition, there is evidence for large numbers of extrasynaptic somatic receptors *(70)*. Therefore, direct receptor activation or enhancement of tonically active somatic receptors may be powerful enough to prevent action potential firing and thereby disrupt effective neural communication. However, there is increasing evidence that not just firing rate, but the specific temporal relationships between synaptic inputs determines the firing rate and patterns of certain neurons *(129)*, and millisecond differences in timing have been found to be critical in some aspects of integrative cellular function, such as plasticity *(130)*. It may be that in some circuits, such as autonomic control centers, pain pathways, or spinal cord, rate coding is utilized extensively, and non-specific enhancement of depression by anesthetics plays a major role, but that in other circuits, such as in cerebral cortex, this mechanism is less important.

Although somatic inhibition may be well suited to control action potential firing, dendritic inhibition may be involved in other aspects of integrative neuronal function, such as coincidence detection and control of synaptic plasticity. Several classes of GABAergic interneurons innervate proximal or distal dendritic regions of pyramidal neurons *(128)*, and somatic and dendritic receptors may be physiologically, pharmacologically, and functionally distinct *(131,132)*. By virtue of its location and duration, it has been proposed that a long-lasting dendritic inhibitory current seen in hippocampal CA1 and piriform cortex pyramidal neurons controls synaptic plasticity by preventing the local dendritic depolarization that is required for NMDA receptor activation during high frequency excitatory synaptic input *(131,133,134)*. Alternatively, the ability of backpropagating action potentials to enhance calcium entry through NMDA receptors during paired presynaptic and postsynaptic stimulation may be selectively modulated by interneurons such as bistratified cells that target proximal dendrites *(135)*. Thus, by selectively targeting different regions of cells, segregated somatic and dendritic inhibitory circuits may act to create distinct functional zones. Their selective modulation by anesthetic agents might then selectively regulate different aspects of neuronal function (downstream communication via forward propagating action potentials vs coincidence detection via backwards propagating action potentials vs synaptic plasticity in response to high frequency input).

Another possible functional link between enhanced $GABA_A$ receptor activity and "anesthesia" has been suggested by the discovery that oscillations in the brain are generated by circuits composed of GABAergic interneurons, and that oscillation frequency is determined in large part by the rate of decay of the inhibitory synaptic connections *(136)*. Although the precise functional roles of brain oscillations remains somewhat speculative, their significance in brain function is becoming more widely accepted. It has been proposed that through the synchronous activity of widespread interneurons networks, coordinated oscillatory activity provides a "context" for the "content" carried by principal neurons *(137)*. High frequency (~40 Hz) "gamma" oscillations found throughout the cerebral cortex have been hypothesized to play a role in perceptual binding *(138,139)*, and several anesthetic agents were found to slow the frequency and/or disrupt synchrony of such oscillations in vitro *(140)*, just as high frequency components of EEG activity are slowed in human subjects *(141)*. Lower frequency (~8 Hz) "theta" oscillations are most prominent in the hippocampus, a structure that is important for memory formation, and stimulus paradigms based on the theta frequency are particularly effective at altering synaptic strength *(142,143)*. Taken together, these findings thus suggest that anesthetic modulation of $GABA_A$-mediated synaptic inhibition may alter coordinated oscillatory firing of interneurons, and thereby disrupt the timing that is critical for information processing in neuronal circuits *(130,144)*.

REFERENCES

1. Barnard, E. A., Skolnick, P., Olsen, R. W., et al. (1998) International union of pharmacology - xv - subtypes of gamma-aminobutyric acid(A) Receptors - classification on the basis of subunit structure and receptor function. *Pharmacolo. Rev.* **50,** 291–313.
2. Sieghart, W., Fuchs, K., Tretter, V., et al. (1999) Structure and subunit composition of $GABA_A$ receptors. *Neurochem. Internat.* **34,** 379–385.
3. Mehta, A. K. and Ticku, M. K. (1999) An update on $GABA_A$ receptors. *Brain Res. - Brain Res. Rev.* **29,** 196–217.
4. Unwin, N. (1993) Neurotransmitter action: opening of ligand-gated ion channels. *Cell* **72 Suppl.,** 31–41.
5. Nayeem, N., Green, T. P., Martin, I. L., and Barnard, E. A. (1994) Quaternary structure of the native $GABA_A$ receptor determined by electron microscopic image analysis. *J. Neurochem.* **62,** 815–818.
6. Chang, Y. C., Wang, R. P., Barot, S., and Weiss, D. S. (1996) Stoichiometry of a recombinant $GABA_A$ receptor. *J. Neurosci.* **16,** 5415–5424.
7. Tretter, V., Ehya, N., Fuchs, K., and Sieghart, W. (1997) Stoichiometry and assembly of a recombinant $GABA_A$ receptor subtype. *J. Neurosci.* **17,** 2728–2737.
8. Kofuji, P., Wang, J. B., Moss, S. J., Huganir, R. L., and Burt, D. R. (1991) Generation of two forms of the gamma-aminobutyric acidA receptor gamma 2-subunit in mice by alternative splicing. *J. Neurochem.* **56,** 713–715.
9. Korpi, E. R., Kuner, T., Kristo, P., et al. (1994) Small N-terminal deletion by splicing in cerebellar alpha 6 subunit abolishes $GABA_A$ receptor function. *J. Neurochem.* **63,** 1167–1170.
10. Verdoorn, T. A. (1994) Formation of heteromeric γ-aminobutyric acid type A receptors containing two different alpha subunits. *Mol. Pharmacol.* **45,** 475–480.
11. McKernan, R. M. and Whiting, P. J. (1996) Which $GABA_A$-receptor subtypes really occur in the brain? *Trends Neurosci.* **19,** 139–143.
12. Laurie, D. J., Seeburg, P. H., and Wisden, W. (1992) The distribution of 13 $GABA_A$ receptor subunit mRNAs in the rat brain. II. Olfactory bulb and cerebellum. *J. Neurosci.* **12,** 1063–1076.
13. Wisden, W., Laurie, D. J., Monyer, H., and Seeburg, P. H. (1992) The distribution of 13 $GABA_A$ receptor subunit mRNAs in the rat brain. I. Telencephalon, diencephalon, mesencephalon. *J. Neurosci.* **12,** 1040–1062.
14. Sperk, G., Schwarzer, C., Tsunashima, K., Fuchs, K., and Sieghart, W. (1997) $GABA_A$ receptor subunits in the rat hippocampus I: immunocytochemical distribution of 13 subunits. *Neuroscience* **80,** 987–1000.
15. Nusser, Z., Sieghart, W., and Somogyi, P (1998) Segregation of different $GABA_A$ receptors to synaptic and extrasynaptic membranes of cerebellar granule cells. *J. Neurosci.* **18,** 1693–1703.
16. Haas, K. F. and Macdonald, R. L. (1999) $GABA_A$ receptor subunit γ2 and δ subtypes confer unique kinetic properties on recombinant $GABA_A$ receptor currents in mouse fibroblasts. *J. Physiol.* **514,** 27–45.
17. Boue-Grabot, E., Roudbaraki, M., Bascles, L., Tramu, G., Bloch, B., and Garret, M. (1998) Expression of GABA receptor rho subunits in rat brain. *J. Neurochem.* **70,** 899–907.
18. Fritschy, J. M., Johnson, D. K., Mohler, H., and Rudolph, U. (1998) Independent assembly and subcellular targeting of $GABA_A$-receptor subtypes demonstrated in mouse hippocampal and olfactory neurons in vivo. *Neurosci. Lett.* **249,** 99–102.
19. Connolly, C. N., Wooltorton, J. R. A., Smart, T. G., and Moss, S. J. (1996) Subcellular Localization of γ-Aminobutyric Acid Type A Receptors Is Determined by Receptor β Subunits. *Proc. Natl. Acad. Sci. USA* **93,** 9899–9904.

20. Essrich, C., Lorez, M., Benson, J. A., Fritschy, J. M., and Luscher, B. (1998) Postsynaptic clustering of major GABA$_A$ receptor subtypes requires the gamma 2 subunit and gephyrin. *Nat. Neurosci.* **1,** 563–571.
21. Baer, K., Essrich, C., Benson, J. A., Benke, D., Bluethmann, H., Fritschy, J. M., and Luscher, B. (1999) Postsynaptic clustering of gamma-aminobutyric acid type A receptors by the gamma3 subunit in vivo. *Proc. Natl. Acad. Sci. USA* **96,** 12,860–12,865.
22. Brickley, S. G., Cull-Candy, S. G., and Farrant, M. (1999) Single-channel properties of synaptic and extrasynaptic GABA$_A$ receptors suggest differential targeting of receptor subtypes. *J. Neurosci.* **19,** 2960–2973.
23. Harris, R. A., Mihic, S. J., Dildy-Mayfield, J. E., and Machu, T. K. (1995) Actions of anesthetics on ligand-gated ion channels: role of receptor subunit composition. *FASEB J.* **9,** 1454–1462.
24. Wingrove, P. B., Wafford, K. A., Bain, C., and Whiting, P. J. (1994) The modulatory action of loreclezole at the gamma-aminobutyric acid type A receptor is determined by a single amino acid in the beta 2 and beta 3 subunit. *Proc. Natl. Acad. Sci. USA* **91,** 4569–4573.
25. Belelli, D., Lambert, J. J., Peters, J. A., Wafford, K., and Whiting, P. J. (1997) The interaction of the general anesthetic etomidate with the γ-aminobutyric acid type A receptor is influenced by a single amino acid. *Proc. Natl. Acad. Sci. USA* **94,** 11,031–11,036.
26. Katz, B. (1962) The transmission of impulses from nerve to muscle, and the subcellular unit of synaptic action. *Proc. Royal Soc. London - B: Biol. Sci.* **155,** 455–479.
27. Cestari, I. N., Min, K. T., Kulli, J. C., and Yang, J. (2000) Identification of an amino acid defining the distinct properties of murine beta1 and beta3 subunit-containing GABA$_A$ receptors. *J. Neurochem.* **74,** 827–838.
28. Davies, P. A., Hanna, M. C., Hales, T. G., and Kirkness, E. F. (1997) Insensitivity to anaesthetic agents conferred by a class of GABA$_A$ receptor subunit. *Nature* **385,** 820–823.
29. Sigel, E., Baur, R., Kellenberger, S., and Malherbe, P. (1992) Point mutations affecting antagonist affinity and agonist dependent gating of GABA$_A$ receptor channels. *EMBO J.* **11,** 2017–2023.
30. Amin, J. and Weiss, D. S. (1993) GABA$_A$ receptor needs two homologous domains of the beta-subunit for activation by gaba but not by pentobarbital. *Nature* **366,** 565–569.
31. Smith, G. B., and Olsen, R. W. (1994) Identification of a [^{3}H]muscimol photoaffinity substrate in the bovine gamma-aminobutyric acidA receptor alpha subunit. *J. Biol. Chem.* **269,** 20,380–20,387.
32. Karlin, A. and Akabas, M. H. (1995) Toward a structural basis for the function of nicotinic acetylcholine receptors and their cousins. *Neuron* **15,** 1231–1244.
33. Boileau, A. J., Evers, A. R., Davis, A. F., and Czajkowski, C. (1999) Mapping the agonist binding site of the GABA$_A$ receptor: evidence for a beta-strand. *J. Neurosci.* **19,** 4847–4854.
34. Smith, G. B. and Olsen, R. W. (1995) Functional domains of GABA$_A$ receptors. *Trends Pharmacol. Sci.* **16,** 162–168.
35. Duncalfe, L. L. and Dunn, S. M. (1996) Mapping of GABA$_A$ receptor sites that are photoaffinity-labelled by [^{3}H]flunitrazepam and [^{3}H]Ro 15-4513. *Eur. J. Pharmacol.* **298,** 313–319.
36. Sigel, E. and Buhr, A. (1997) The benzodiazepine binding site of GABA$_A$ receptors. *Trends Pharmacol. Sci.* **18,** 425–429.
37. Kucken, A. M., Wagner, D. A., Ward, P. R., Boileau, J. A., and Czajkowski, C. (2000) Identification of benzodiazepine binding site residues in the gamma2 subunit of the gamma-aminobutyric acid(A) receptor. *Mol. Pharmacol.* **57,** 932–939.
38. Maric, D., Maric, I., Wen, X., et al. (1999) GABA$_A$ receptor subunit composition and functional properties of Cl$^-$ channels with differential sensitivity to zolpidem in embryonic rat hippocampal cells. *J. Neurosci.* **19,** 4921–4937.
39. Mihic, S. J., Ye, Q., Wick, M. J., et al. (1997) Sites of alcohol and volatile anaesthetic action on GABA$_A$ and glycine receptors. *Nature* **389,** 385–389.
40. Greenblatt, E. P. and Meng, X. (1997) Differential modulation of chimeric inhibitory receptors by halothane versus isoflurane. *Anesthesiology* **87,** A704.
41. Jenkins, A., Greenblatt, E. P., Faulkner, H. J., et al. (2001) Evidence for a common binding cavity for three general anesthetics within the GABA$_A$ receptor. *J. Neurosci.* **21Rc136,** 1–4.
42. Mascia, M. P., Trudell, J. R., and Harris, A. (2000) Specfic binding sites for alcohols and anesthetics on ligand-gated ion channels. *Proc. Natl. Acad. Sci. USA* **97,** 9305–9310.
43. Curry, S., Moss, G. W., Dickinson, R., Lieb, W. R., and Franks, N. P. (1991) Probing the molecular dimensions of general anaesthetic target sites in tadpoles (Xenopus laevis) and model systems using cycloalcohols. *Brit. J. Pharmacol.* **102,** 167–173.
44. Macdonald, R. L. and Olsen, R. W. (1994) GABA$_A$ receptor channels. *Annu. Rev. Neurosci.* **17,** 569–602.
45. Uchida, I., Cestari, I. N., and Yang, J. (1996) The differential antagonism by bicuculline and SR95531 of pentobarbitone-induced currents in cultured hippocampal neurons. *Eur. J. Pharmacol.* **307,** 89–96.
46. Birnir, B., Tierney, M. L., Dalziel, J. E., Cox, G. B., and Gage, P. W. (1997) A structural determinant of desensitization and allosteric regulation by pentobarbitone of the gabaa receptor. *J. Membr. Biol.* **155,** 157–166.
47. Krasowski, M. D., Koltchine, V. V., Rick, C. E., Ye, Q., Finn, S. E., and Harrison, N. L. (1998) Propofol and other intravenous anesthetics have sites of action on the gamma-aminobutyric acid type A receptor distinct from that for isoflurane. *Mol. Pharmacol.* **53,** 530–538.
48. Amin, J. (1999) A single hydrophobic residue confers barbiturate sensitivity to gamma-aminobutyric acid type C receptor. *Mol. Pharmacol.* **55,** 411–423.
49. Carlson, B. X., Engblom, A. C., Kristiansen, U., Schousboe, A., and Olsen, R. W. (2000) A single glycine residue at the entrance to the first membrane-spanning domain of the gamma-aminobutyric acid type A receptor beta(2) subunit affects allosteric sensitivity to GABA and anesthetics. *Mol. Pharmacol.* **57,** 474–484.
50. Wiliams, D. B. and Akabas, M. H. (1999) gamma-aminobutyric acid increases the water accessibility of M3 membrane-spanning segment residues in gamma-aminobutyric acid type A receptors. *Biophys. J.* **77,** 2563–2574.

51. Boileau, A. J., Kucken, A. M., Evers, A. R., and Czajkowski, C. (1998) Molecular dissection of benzodiazepine binding and allosteric coupling using chimeric γ-aminobutyric acid$_A$ receptor subunits. *Mol. Pharmacol.* **53,** 295–303.

52. Moody, E. J., Knauer, C., Granja, R., Strakhova, M., and Skolnick, P. (1997) Distinct loci mediate the direct and indirect actions of the anesthetic etomidate at GABA$_A$ receptors. *J. Neurochem.* **69,** 1310–1313.

53. Dalziel, J. E., Cox, G. B., Gage, P. W., and Birnir, B. (1999) Mutant human alpha(1)beta(1)(T262Q) GABA$_A$ receptors are directly activated but not modulated by pentobarbital. *Eur. J. Pharmacol.* **385,** 283–286.

54. Fukami, S., Uchida, I., Takenoshita, M., Mashimo, T., and Yoshiya, I. (1999) The effects of a point mutation of the beta2 subunit of GABA$_A$ receptor on direct and modulatory actions of general anesthetics. *Eur. J. Pharmacol.* **368,** 269–276.

55. Lambert, J. J., Belelli, D., Hill-Venning, C., Callachan, H., and Peters, J. A. (1996) Neurosteroid modulation of native and recombinant gabaa receptors. *Cell. Molec. Neurobiol.* **16,** 155–174.

56. Clarke, R. S. (1992) Steroid anaesthesia. *Anesthesia* **47,** 285–286.

57. Turner, D. M., Ransom, R. W., Yang, J. S., and Olsen, R. W. (1989) Steroid anesthetics and naturally occurring analogs modulate the gamma-aminobutyric acid receptor complex at a site distinct from barbiturates. *J. Pharmacol. Exp. Ther.* **248,** 960–966.

58. Covey, D. F., Nathan, D., Kalkbrenner, M., et al. (2000) Enantioselectivity of pregnanolone-induced gamma-aminobutyric acid(A) receptor modulation and anesthesia. *J. Pharmacol. Exp. Ther.* **293,** 1009–1016.

59. Majewska, M. D. and Schwartz, R. D. (1987) Pregnenolone-sulfate: an endogenous antagonist of the gamma-aminobutyric acid receptor complex in brain? *Brain Res.* **404,** 355–360.

60. Rudolph, U., Crestani, F., Benke, D., et al. (1999) Benzodiazepine actions mediated by specific gamma-aminobutyric acid(A) receptor subtypes. *Nature* **401,** 796–800.

61. Low, K. (2000) Molecular and neuronal substrate for the selective attenuation of anxiety. *Science* **290,** 936.

62. Zimmerman, S. A., Jones, M. V., and Harrison, N. L. (1994) Potentiation of GABA$_A$ receptor Cl⁻ current correlates with in vivo anesthetic potency. *J. Pharmacol. Exp. Ther.* **270,** 987–991.

63. Franks, N. P. and Lieb, W. R. (1994) Molecular and cellular mechanisms of general anaesthesia. *Nature* **367,** 607–614.

64. Li, X. and Pearce, R. A. (2000) Effects of halothane on GABA$_A$ receptor kinetics: evidence for slowed agonist unbinding. *J. Neurosci.* **20,** 899–907.

65. Celentano, J. J. and Wong, R. K. (1994) Multiphasic desensitization of the GABA$_A$ receptor in outside-out patches. *Biophysical. J.* **66,** 1039–1050.

66. Dominguez-Perrot, C., Feltz, P., and Poulter, M. O. (1996) Recombinant GABA$_A$ receptor desensitization: the role of the gamma 2 subunit and its physiological significance. *J. Physiol.* **497,** 145–159.

67. Jones, M. V. and Westbrook, G. L. (1995) Desensitized states prolong GABA$_A$ channel responses to brief agonist pulses. *Neuron* **15,** 181–191.

68. Pearce, R. A., Grunder, S. D., and Faucher, L. D. (1995) Different mechanisms for use-dependent depression of two gaba(a)-mediated ipscs in rat hippocampus. *J. Physiol. (Lond.)* **484,** 425–435.

69. Puia, G., Costa, E., and Vicini, S. (1994) Functional diversity of GABA-activated Cl⁻ currents in Purkinje versus granule neurons in rat cerebellar slices. *Neuron* **12,** 117–126.

70. Banks, M. I. and Pearce, R. A. (2000) Kinetic differences between synaptic and extrasynaptic GABA$_A$ receptors in CA1 pyramidal cells. *J. Neurosci.* **20,** 937–948.

71. Zhu, W. J. and Vicini, S. (1997) Neurosteroid prolongs GABA$_A$ channel deactivation by altering kinetics of desensitized states. *J. Neurosci.* **17,** 4022–4031.

72. Bai, D., Pennefather, P. S., MacDonald, J. F., and Orser, B. A. (1999) The general anesthetic propofol slows deactivation and desensitization of GABA$_A$ receptors. *J. Neurosci.* **19,** 10,635–10,646.

73. Miyahara, J. T., Esplin, D. W., and Zablocka, B. (1966) Differential effects of depressant drugs on presynaptic inhibition. *J. Pharmacol. Exp. Ther.* **154,** 119–127.

74. Ribak, C. E., Vaughn, J. E., and Saito, K. (1978) Immunocytochemical localization of glutamic acid decarboxylase in neuronal somata following colchicine inhibition of axonal transport. *Brain Res.* **140,** 315–332.

75. Nicoll, R. A., Eccles, J. C., Oshima, T., and Rubia, F. (1975) Prolongation of hippocampal inhibitory postsynaptic potentials by barbiturates. *Nature* **258,** 625–627.

76. Tanelian, D. L., Kosek, P., Mody, I., and MacIver, M. B. (1993) The role of the GABA$_A$ receptor/chloride channel complex in anesthesia. *Anesthesiology* **78,** 757–776.

77. Nicoll, R. A. (1972) The effects of anaesthetics on synaptic excitation and inhibition in the olfactory bulb. *J. Physiol. (Lond.)* **223,** 803–814.

78. Pearce, R. A., Stringer, J. L., and Lothman, E. W. (1989) Effect of volatile anesthetics on synaptic transmission in the rat hippocampus. *Anesthesiology* **71,** 591–598.

79. Wolf, P. and Haas, H. L. (1977) Effects of diazepines and barbiturates on hippocampal recurrent inhibition. *Naunyn-Schmiedebergs Arch. Pharmacol.* **299,** 211–218.

80. Rock, D. M. and Taylor, C. P. (1986) Effects of diazepam, pentobarbital, phenytoin and pentylenetetrazol on hippocampal paired-pulse inhibition in vivo. *Neurosci. Lett.* **65,** 265–270.

81. Proctor, W. R., Mynlieff, M., and Dunwiddie, T. V. (1986) Facilitatory action of etomidate and pentobarbital on recurrent inhibition in rat hippocampal pyramidal neurons. *J. Neurosci.* **6,** 3161–3168.

82. Albertson, T. E., Tseng, C. C., and Joy, R. M. (1991) Propofol modification of evoked hippocampal dentate inhibition in urethane-anesthetized rats. *Anesthesiology* **75,** 82–90.

83. Gage, P. W. and Robertson, B. (1985) Prolongation of inhibitory postsynaptic currents by pentobarbitone, halothane and ketamine in CA1 pyramidal cells in rat hippocampus. *Brit. J. Pharmacol.* **85,** 675–681.

84. Mody, I., Tanelian, D. L., and MacIver, M. B. (1991) Halothane enhances tonic neuronal inhibition by elevating intracellular calcium. *Brain Res.* **538,** 319–323.
85. Pearce, R. A. (1996) Volatile anesthetic enhancement of paired-pulse depression investigated in the rat hippocampus in vitro. *J. Physiol. (Lond.)* **492.3,** 823–840.
86. Banks, M. I. and Pearce, R. A. (1999) Dual actions of volatile anesthetics on GABA$_A$ IPSCs: dissociation of blocking and prolonging effects. *Anesthesiology* **90,** 120–134.
87. Mellor, J. R. and Randall, A. D. (1997) Frequency-dependent actions of benzodiazepines on GABA$_A$ receptors in cultured murine cerebellar granule cells. *J. Physiol.* **503,** 353–369.
88. Wang, M. D., Backstrom, T., and Landgren, S. (2000) The inhibitory effects of allopregnanolone and pregnanolone on the population spike, evoked in the rat hippocampal CA1 stratum pyramidale in vitro, can be blocked selectively by epiallopregnanolone. *Acta Physiol. Scandin.* **169,** 333–341.
89. Albertson, T. E., Walby, W. F., Stark, L. G., and Joy, R. M. (1996) The effect of propofol on ca1 pyramidal cell excitability and GABA$_A$-mediated inhibition in the rat hippocampal slice. *Life Sci.* **58,** 2397–2407.
90. Ashton, D. and Wauquier, A. (1985) Modulation of a GABA-ergic inhibitory circuit in the in vitro hippocampus by etomidate isomers. *Anesth. Analg.* **64,** 975–980.
91. Krasowski, M. D. and Harrison, N. L. (1999) General anaesthetic actions on ligand-gated ion channels. *Cell. Mol. Life Sci.* **55,** 1278–1303.
92. Yang, J., Isenberg, K. E., and Zorumski, C. F. (1992) Volatile anesthetics gate a chloride current in postnatal rat hippocampal neurons. *FASEB J.* **6,** 914–918.
93. Wu, J., Harata, N., and Akaike, N. (1996) Potentiation by sevoflurane of the γ-aminobutyric acid induced chloride current in acutely dissociated CA1 pyramidal neurons from rat hippocampus. *Brit. J. Pharmacol.* **119,** 1013–1021.
94. Mathers, D. A. and Barker, J. L. (1980) (–)Pentobarbital opens ion channels of long duration in cultured mouse spinal neurons. *Science* **209,** 507–509.
95. Rho, J. M., Donevan, S. D., and Rogawski, M. A. (1996) Direct activation of GABA$_A$ receptors by barbiturates in cultured rat hippocampal neurons. *J. Physiol.* **497,** 509–522.
96. Hara, M., Kai, Y., and Ikemoto, Y. (1993) Propofol activates GABA$_A$ receptor-chloride ionophore complex in dissociated hippocampal pyramidal neurons of the rat. *Anesthesiology* **79,** 781–788.
97. Orser, B. A., Wang, L. Y., Pennefather, P. S., and MacDonald, J. F. (1994) Propofol modulates activation and desensitization of GABA$_A$ receptors in cultured murine hippocampal neurons. *J. Neurosci.* **14,** 7747–7760.
98. Adodra, S. and Hales, T. G. (1995) Potentiation, activation and blockade of gabaa receptors of clonal murine hypothalamic gt1-7 neurones by propofol. *Brit. J. Pharmacol.* **115,** 953–960.
99. Walters, R. J., Hadley, S. H., Morris, K. D., and Amin, J. (2000) Benzodiazepines act on GABA$_A$ receptors via two distinct and separable mechanisms. *Nat Neurosci.* **3,** 1274–1281.
100. Jackson, M. B., Lecar, H., Mathers, D. A., and Barker, J. L. (1982) Single channel currents activated by gamma-aminobutyric acid, muscimol, and (–)-pentobarbital in cultured mouse spinal neurons. *J. Neurosci.* **2,** 889–894.
101. Akk, G. and Steinbach, J. H. (2000) Activation and block of recombinant GABA$_A$ receptors by pentobarbitone: a single-channel study. *Brit. J. Pharmacol.* **130,** 249–258.
102. Ueno, S., Bracamontes, J., Zorumski, C., Weiss, D. S., and Steinbach, J. H. (1997) Bicuculline and gabazine are allosteric inhibitors of channel opening of the GABA$_A$ receptor. *J. Neurosci.* **17,** 625–634.
103. Cestari, I. N., Uchida, I., Li, L., Burt, D., and Yang, J. (1996) The agonistic action of pentobarbital on GABA$_A$ β-subunit homomeric receptors. *Neuroreport* **7,** 943–947.
104. Cheng, S. C. and Brunner, E. A. (1985) Inducing anesthesia with a gaba analog, thip. *Anesthesiology* **63,** 147–151.
105. Nusser, Z., Roberts, J. D., Baude, A., Richards, J. G., and Somogyi, P. (1995) Relative densities of synaptic and extrasynaptic GABA$_A$ receptors on cerebellar granule cells as determined by a quantitative immunogold method. *J. Neurosci.* **15,** 2948–2960.
106. Scotti, A. L. and Reuter, H. (2001) Synaptic and extrasynaptic gamma-aminobutyric acid A receptor clusters in rat hippocampal cultures during development. *Proc. Natl. Acad. Sci. USA* **98,** 3489–3494.
107. Lerma, J., Herranz, A. S., Herreras, O., Abraira, V., Martin, D., and Rio, R. (1986) In vivo determination of extracellular concentration of amino acids in the rat hippocampus. A method based on brain dialysis and computerized analysis. *Brain Res.* **384,** 145–155.
108. Dilger, J. P., Boguslavsky, R., Barann, M., Katz, T., and Vidal, A. M. (1997) Mechanisms of barbiturate inhibition of acetylcholine receptor channels. *J. Gen. Physiol.* **109,** 401–414.
109. Taverna, F. A., Cameron, B. R., Hampson, D. L., Wang, L. Y., Macdonald, and J. F. (1994) Sensitivity of AMPA receptors to pentobarbital. *Eur. J. Pharmacol.* **267,** R3–R5.
110. Ffrench-Mullen, J. M., Barker, J. L., and Rogawski, M. A. (1993) Calcium current block by (–)-pentobarbital, phenobarbital, and CHEB but not (+)-pentobarbital in acutely isolated hippocampal CA1 neurons: comparison with effects on GABA-activated Cl⁻ current. *J. Neurosci.* **13,** 3211–3221.
111. Todorovic, S. M., Perez-Reyes, E., and Lingle, C. J. (2000) Anticonvulsants but not general anesthetics have differential blocking effects on different T-type current variants. *Mol. Pharmacol.* **58,** 98–108.
112. Neher, E. and Steinbach, J. H. (1978) Local anaesthetics transiently block currents through single acetylcholine-receptor channels. *J. Physiol. (Lond.)* **277,** 153–176.
113. Dilger, J. P., Vidal, A. M., Mody, H. I., and Liu, Y. (1994) Evidence for direct actions of general anesthetics on an ion channel protein: A new look at a unified mechanism of action. *Anesthesiology* **81,** 431–442.
114. Clements, J. D. (1996) Transmitter timecourse in the synaptic cleft: its role in central synaptic function. *Trends Neurosci.* **19,** 163–171.

115. Macdonald, R. L., Rogers, C. J., and Twyman, R. E. (1989) Kinetic properties of the GABA$_A$ receptor main conductance state of mouse spinal cord neurones in culture. *J. Physiol. (Lond.)* **410,** 479–499.

116. Weiss, D. S. and Magleby, K. L. (1989) Gating scheme for single GABA-activated Cl⁻ channels determined from stability plots, dwell-time distributions, and adjacent- interval durations. *J. Neurosci.* **9,** 1314–1324.

117. Twyman, R. E., Rogers, C. J., and Macdonald, R. L. (1989) Differential regulation of g-aminobutyric acid receptor channels by diazepam and phenobarbital. *Ann. Neurol.* **25,** 213–220.

118. Zhuo, M., Small, S. A., Kandel, E. R., and Hawkins, R. D. (1993) Nitric oxide and carbon monoxide produce activity-dependent long-term synaptic enhancement in hippocampus. *Science* **260,** 1946–1950.

119. Fisher, J. L. and Macdonald, R. L. (1998) The role of an alpha subtype M2-M3 His in regulating inhibition of GABA$_A$ receptor current by zinc and other divalent cations. *J. Neurosci.* **18,** 2944–2953.

120. Gingrich, K. J., Roberts, W. A., and Kass, R. S. (1995) Dependence of the GABA$_A$ receptor gating kinetics on the alpha- subunit isoform–implications for structure-function relations and synaptic transmission. *J. Physiol. (Lond.)* **489,** 529–543.

121. Fisher, J. L. and Macdonald, R. L. (1997) Functional properties of recombinant GABA$_A$ receptors composed of single or multiple beta subunit subtypes. *Neuropharmacology* **36,** 1601–1610.

122. Lavoie, A. M. and Twyman, R. E. (1996) Direct evidence for diazepam modulation of GABA$_A$ receptor microscopic affinity. *Neuropharmacology* **35,** 1383–1392.

123. Perrais, D. and Ropert, N. (1999) Effect of zolpidem on miniature IPSCs and occupancy of postsynaptic GABA$_A$ receptors in central synapses. *J. Neurosci.* **19,** 578–588.

124. Eger, E. I., Koblin, D. D., Harris, R. A., et al. (1997) Hypothesis: inhaled anesthetics produce immobility and amnesia by different mechanisms at different sites. *Anesth. Analg.* **84,** 915–918.

125. Konig, P., Engel, A. K., and Singer, W. (1996) Integrator or coincidence detector? The role of the cortical neuron revisited. *Trends Neurosci.* **19,** 130–137.

126. Soltesz, I., Smetters, D. K., and Mody, I. (1995) Tonic inhibition originates from synapses close to the soma. *Neuron* **14,** 1273–1283.

127. Banks, M. I., Li, T. B., and Pearce, R. A. (1998) The synaptic basis of GABA$_A$, slow. *J. Neurosci.* **18,** 1305–1317.

128. Freund, T. F. and Buzsaki, G. (1996) Interneurons of the Hippocampus. *Hippocampus* **6,** 347–470.

129. Gauck, V. and Jaeger, D. (2000) The control of rate and timing of spikes in the deep cerebellar nuclei by inhibition. *J. Neurosci.* **20,** 3006–3016.

130. Markram, H., Lubke, J., Frotscher, M., and Sakmann, B. (1997) Regulation of synaptic efficacy by coincidence of postsynaptic APs and EPSPs. *Science* **275,** 213–215.

131. Pearce, R. A. (1993) Physiological evidence for two distinct GABA$_A$ responses in rat hippocampus. *Neuron* **10,** 189–200.

132. Kapur, A., Pearce, R. A., Lytton, W. W., and Haberly, L. B. (1997) GABA$_A$-Mediated IPSCs in piriform cortex have fast and slow components with different properties and locations on pyramidal cells. *J. Neurophysiol.* **78,** 2531–2545.

133. Kapur, A., Pearce, R. A., and Haberly, L. B. (1993) Regulation of an NMDA-mediated EPSP by a slow dendritic GABA$_A$-mediated IPSC in piriform cortex. *Soc. Neurosci.* **19,** 1521.

134. Miller, M. S., and Gandolfi, A. J. (1979) A rapid, sensitive method for quantifying enflurane in whole blood. *Anesthesiology* **51,** 542–544.

135. Halasy, K., Buhl, E. H., Lorinczi, Z., Tamas, G., and Somogyi, P. (1996) Synaptic target selectivity and input of gabaergic basket and bistratified interneurons in the ca1 area of the rat hippocampus. *Hippocampus* **6,** 306–329.

136. Traub, R. D., Whittington, M. A., Colling, S. B., Buzsaki, G., and Jefferys, J. G. R. (1996) Analysis of gamma rhythms in the rat hippocampus in vitro and in vivo. *J. Physiol. (Lond.)* **493,** 471–484.

137. Buzsaki, G. and Chrobak, J. J. (1995) Temporal structure in spatially organized neuronal ensembles: a role for interneuronal networks. *Curr. Opin. Neurobiol.* **5,** 504–510.

138. Joliot, M., Ribary, U., and Llinas, R. (1994) Human oscillatory brain activity near 40 Hz coexists with cognitive temporal binding. *Proc. Natl. Acad. Sci. USA* **91,** 11,748–11,751.

139. Gray, C. M. (1994) Synchronous oscillations in neuronal systems: mechanisms and functions. *J. Computat. Neurosci.* **1,** 11–38.

140. Faulkner, H. J., Traub, R. D., and Whittington, M. A. (1998) Disruption of synchronous gamma oscillations in the rat hippocampal slice: a common mechanism of anaesthetic drug action. *Brit. J. Pharmacol.* **125,** 483–492.

141. Andrade, J., Sapsford, D. J., Jeevaratnum, D., Pickworth, A. J., and Jones, J. G. (1996) The coherent frequency in the electroencephalogram as an objective measure of cognitive function during propofol sedation. *Anesth. Analg.* **83,** 1279–1284.

142. Larson, J., Wong, D., and Lynch, G. (1986) Patterned stimulation at the theta frequency is optimal for the induction of hippocampal long-term potentiation. *Brain Res.* **368,** 347–350.

143. Huerta, P. T. and Lisman, J. E. (1995) Bidirectional synaptic plasticity induced by a single burst during cholinergic theta oscillation in CA1 in vitro. *Neuron* **15,** 1053–1063.

144. Koester, H. J. and Sakmann, B. (1998) Calcium dynamics in single spines during coincident pre- and postsynaptic activity depend on relative timing of back-propagating action potentials and subthreshold excitatory postsynaptic potentials. *Proc. Natl. Acad. Sci. USA* **95,** 9596–9601.

17

Nicotinic Acetylcholine Receptors and Anesthetics

Stuart A. Forman, Pamela Flood, and Douglas Raines

INTRODUCTION

Nicotinic acetylcholine receptors (nAChRs) are a diverse group of membrane proteins found in many types of excitable tissue, including brain, autonomic ganglia, and muscle. Acetylcholine (ACh), the endogenous ligand for these receptors, binds to agonist sites on nAChRs, causing opening of an intrinsic transmembrane cation channel and depolarization of neurons or muscle cells. Muscle nAChRs mediate fast neuromuscular transmission. Cholinergic transmission in the autonomic nervous system (ANS) regulates cardiac output, vascular tone, body temperature, blood glucose, osmolality, respiration, and gastrointestinal tract activity. The roles of nAChRs in neurons and glial cells of the CNS are not fully defined, but they appear to play roles in many functions altered by anesthetics, including memory, arousal, and pain.

Many general anesthetics alter neuronal nAChR functions at lower concentrations than required to ablate movement responses to surgical stimulation (e.g., MAC). Thus, neuronal nAChRs may play key roles in general anesthesia and specifically in behaviors that are observed at low anesthetic concentrations. The structural and functional characteristics of muscle nAChRs and their close homologs from electroplaques of rays and eels are known in more detail than other ligand-gated ion channels. These nAChRs have proven to be valuable models for studying the molecular mechanisms by which anesthetics alter ion channel functions.

This chapter presents a brief review of the general structure and function of nAChRs, as well as a summary of the functional effects of general anesthetics on these proteins. We also review data addressing the mechanisms of anesthetic actions on nAChRs.

MOLECULAR STRUCTURE OF NACHRS

Prototypical Ligand-Gated Ion Channels

Nicotinic AChRs are a branch of a superfamily of anesthetic-sensitive ligand-gated ion channels (LGICs) that also include serotonin receptors (5-HT$_3$Rs), GABA type A receptors (GABA$_A$Rs), and glycine receptors (GlyRs) (1,2). All these LGICs contain both neurotransmitter binding sites and transmembrane ion channels formed from five homologous subunits. Structural and functional paradigms for all LGICs are based largely on studies of nAChRs from electroplaques of *Torpedo* rays and skeletal muscle, which were discovered much earlier than the other receptors.

From: *Contemporary Clinical Neuroscience: Neural Mechanisms of Anesthesia*
Edited by: Joseph F. Antognini et al. © Humana Press Inc., Totowa, NJ

Size and Shape

Both electric eels *Electrophorus* and rays *Torpedo* possess specialized organs, electroplaques, containing nAChRs at concentrations that are 10,000-fold higher than muscle or brain, enabling isolation of purified protein for biochemical and biophysical studies. The *Torpedo* electroplaque nAChR is a 290 kDa glycoprotein comprised of α, β, γ, and δ subunits (437–501 amino acids/subunit), with a stoichiometry of $2\alpha:\beta:\gamma:\delta$. The α subunits bind to agonists and alpha-bungarotoxin (BTX), a high-affinity inhibitor isolated from snake venom *(3)*.

Electron photomicrographs of frozen *Torpedo* electroplaque membranes show the general size and shape of nAChR *(4)*. At a resolution of 9 Å, the receptor is observed to be 125 Å in length and 80 Å at its widest. The receptor extends approx 60 Å above the phospholipid headgroups on the synaptic side of the membrane and 20 Å below on the cytoplasmic side. There is a pseudo-5-fold symmetry throughout the length of the nAChR, reflecting the symmetric arrangement of five subunits around an extracellular vestibule that funnels into the central ion channel.

Subunit Structure

Hydropathy analysis of nAChR subunit amino acid sequences displays four hydrophobic domains of sufficient size to cross cell membranes *(3,5,6)*. The transmembrane domains (TM1–TM4) are flanked at the amino terminus by a large (approx 200 amino acids) extra-cytoplasmic domain (ECD) containing an inter-cysteine disulfide bond separated by 13 amino acids, and by a small cytoplasmic carboxy-terminus. A large intracellular domain is located between TM3 and TM4. The shared topology of nAChR subunits (and that of related LGICs) is that depicted in Fig. 1.

The Agonist Sites

Torpedo nAChR α subunits (and other nAChR α subunits) contain disulfide bonds at positions 192–193 that are required for agonist function. Covalent labeling of *Torpedo* nAChR protein with agonists and competitive antagonists occurs at these cysteines and nearby tyrosines in the ECD of α subunits *(7–9)*. Homologous structures in γ and δ subunits are also identified by covalent incorporation of competitive antagonists *(10)*. The roles of these amino acids in agonist binding has been confirmed by mutational/functional studies of recombinant nAChRs expressed in *Xenopus* oocytes and mammalian cells. Thus, the ACh binding sites are thought to be formed by several loops of amino acids within the ECDs, at the α/γ and α/δ subunit interfaces.

Recent photomicrographic analyses visualize cavities in the ECD of each α-subunit, sufficiently large to accommodate an agonist molecule. These cavities are located approx 30 Å above the membrane surface and a 10–15 Å tunnel leads to each cavity from the extracellular pore vestibule, presumably representing the pathways that agonists follow to their binding sites *(11)*.

The Transmembrane Pore

The intrinsic cation pore of nAChRs is visualized as a narrow hypodense tunnel passing across the membrane along the receptor's central axis. In closed nAChRs, dense "bent-rod" structures are visualized near the middle of the pore, narrowing the ion channel. Images of nAChRs frozen in the open state show these rods rotated away from the pore axis *(12)*.

Photo-affinity labeling with nAChR channel blockers suggested that the TM2 domains of all five nAChR subunits form the lining of the transmembrane channel *(13,14)*. The amino acid sequences of TM2 domains are remarkably conserved and in particular, all TM2 domains from LGICs contain a leucine in the ninth position from the intracellular end *(15)*. TM2 mutations affect the nAChR's sensitivity to channel blockers, single channel ion conductance, and the amount of time the channel stays open after gating. Scanning cysteine mutagenesis and chemical accessibility (SCAM) studies suggest that the secondary structure of nAChR TM2 domains is mostly α-helical *(16)*. It has been

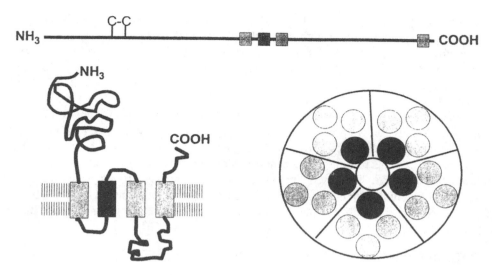

Fig. 1. Structural motifs of nicotinic acetylcholine receptors and related ligand-gated ion channels. *Top:* The amino acid domains of an isolated nAChR subunit are depicted as a linear chain. The N-terminal domain contains a disulfide loop, and the four predicted transmembrane domains (TM1–TM4) are shown as boxes. TM2 domains are shaded dark. *Lower left:* The transmembrane topography of nAChR subunits is shown, including extracellular N-terminus and C-terminus, four transmembrane domains, and a large intracellular loop between TM3 and TM4. *Lower right:* An end-on view of the nAChR pentamer is depicted. Note that the five TM2 domains (dark circles) surround the central ion channel.

suggested that the bent-rod structures in *Torpedo* nAChRs represent TM2 domains, and that the kinks in these rods correspond to the highly conserved ring of leucines.

The Lipid-Protein Interface

Photo-affinity labeling studies using hydrophobic probes such as 3-(trifluoromethyl-)-3-(m-[^{125}I]iodophenyl) diazirine ([^{125}I]TID) and 1-azidopyrene (1-AP) suggest that the TM4 transmembrane domain is in direct contact with the lipid bilayer portion of the membrane *(17,18)*. From the pattern of label incorporation, it appears likely that the TM4 secondary structure is mostly α-helical. The structures and arrangements of the TM1 and TM3 domains are less clear, but structural models frequently assume that they contain considerable β structure, and are located between the TM2 and TM4 domains.

Subunit Composition of Different nAChRs

Analysis of the genes encoding nAChR subunits from a variety of organisms suggests that they all derived from a common progenitor gene about 2 billion years ago *(2)*. Genetically, nAChR subunits form 5 genetically related groups, four of which, α, β, γ, and δ correspond with the biochemically identified *Torpedo* subunits. The fifth type, ε, is similar to the γ subunit. The α subunits ($α_{1-9}$) are thought to be most similar to the common progenitor subunit, because they are necessary for neurotransmitter binding, and some α subunits can form functional channels in the absence of other subunit types. Other nAChR subunits ($β_{1-4}$, $γ_1$, $δ_1$, $ε_1$) do not form functional channels in the absence of α subunits.

Like *Torpedo* nAChRs, vertebrate fetal muscle nAChRs contain $α_1$, $β_1$, $γ_1$, and $δ_1$ subunits, in a ratio of 2α:β:γ:δ. In mature muscle, the $γ_1$ subunit is replaced with $ε_1$. Muscle nAChRs also bind BTX with high affinity.

The subunit composition of neuronal nAChR pentamers is variable. Studies in *Xenopus* oocytes reveal that α_{2-6} subunits combine with β_{2-4} subunits to form heteromeric receptors, while α_{7-9} subunits can form homomeric nAChRs *(19)*. Homomeric channels containing α_7, α_8, or α_9 subunits are inhibited by α-BTX and have similar electrophysiological and pharmacological properties to BTX-sensitive nAChRs from brain. *In situ* hybridization suggests that homomeric α_7 nAChRs are the dominant BTX-sensitive form in the brain *(19)*.

CNS nAChRs that are insensitive to BTX most likely contain mixtures of α and β subunits with a stoichiometry of $2\alpha{:}3\beta$. Recombinant expression studies demonstrate a multitude of functional combinations of heteromeric subunit isoforms, including combinations with two different α subunits or multiple β isoforms, but determining the actual subunit composition of neuronal nAChRs has proven difficult. Most neuronal nAChRs, including those from hippocampal neurons, have functional properties like those of recombinant $\alpha_4\beta_2$ nAChRs, while nAChRs from the medial habenula behave like recombinant $\alpha_3\beta_4$ or $\alpha_3\beta_2$ nAChRs. Ganglionic (ANS) nAChRs generally contain α_3 and β_4 subunits and may also be composed of α_5, α_7 and/or β_2 nicotinic subunits *(20)*.

FUNCTIONS OF NICOTINIC RECEPTORS

Agonist-Induced Gating and Desensitization

Biochemical tracer ion flux studies in *Torpedo* electroplaque membrane vesicles and electrophysiological studies of muscle endplates indicate that the binding of two agonist molecules to (closed) resting state nAChRs induces receptors to undergo a very rapid conformational transition to an open channel state that allows transmembrane ion permeation *(21)*. Early recordings of spontaneous excitatory postsynaptic currents (EPSCs) from voltage-clamped muscles demonstrated very rapid depolarization and subsequent current decay. The rapidity of current decay is due in part to the extraordinarily brief lifespan of ACh in the synapse. Acetylcholinesterase degrades the neurotransmitter within a millisecond, leading to ligand dissociation and deactivation of nAChRs. However, when exogenous ACh is applied for longer periods to motor endplates, rapid activation is followed by a slower current decay, termed "desensitization". Desensitization of agonist-bound nAChRs leads to inactive receptor conformations in two-steps. A fast step occurs over hundreds of milliseconds (fast desensitization) and a slow process occurs over seconds to minutes (slow desensitization). After removal of ACh, desensitized nAChRs return to an activatable resting conformation without re-opening, indicating that resting and desensitized states can directly interchange *(22)*.

Patch-clamp techniques enable recording of the currents associated with individual nAChR channels. These single channel current recordings demonstrate a large conductance of about 50 pS, and variable channel open times. The distribution of open times from equilibrium channel recordings shows at least two exponential components, indicating multiple open states that close at different rates. "Bursts" of channel openings at low ACh demonstrate multiple closures and re-openings, representing closure of ligand-bound receptors and subsequent re-openings before burst termination by dissociation of agonist. "Clusters" of channel openings have also been described at very high ACh, which are apparently initiated when a single nAChR opens from a desensitized state. Multiple closures and re-openings are observed, as with bursts, but since rebinding instantly follows agonist dissociation, clusters are presumably terminated by the active channel returning to a desensitized state *(23)*.

Agonist Affinity Changes Associated with State-changes

Agonist pre-exposure greatly increases the binding of [³H]-ACh to *Torpedo* electroplaque membranes, indicating that desensitized receptors bind ACh more tightly than do resting receptors. Furthermore, even in the absence of agonist, ~20% of *Torpedo* receptors exist in the high-affinity desensitized state.

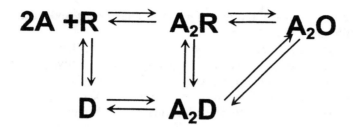

Fig. 2. A simplified kinetic scheme for nAChR gating and desensitization. Five nAChR states are shown, linked by known transitions represented as arrows. The R state is the resting (activable) state. Upon binding of two agonist (A) molecules, the receptor forms a pre-open (A_2R) state, that rapidly gates to the active open-channel (A_2O) state. Desensitized (D) receptors are in equilibrium with resting receptors. Desensitization also occurs from pre-open and open states, leading to the stable agonist-bound desensitized state (A_2D).

Stopped-flow techniques using the fluorescent agonist Dns-C_6-cho and *Torpedo* membranes permit kinetic analysis of agonist binding and receptor desensitization. Under conditions of fluorescence energy transfer from receptors to Dns-C_6-cho, increased fluorescence is observed when nAChRs bind Dns-C_6-cho with high affinity. When *Torpedo* nAChR-rich membranes are rapidly mixed with Dns-C_6-cho, an initial rapid fluorescence enhancement reflecting Dns-C_6-cho binding to desensitized nAChRs is followed by slower additional Dns-C_6-cho binding as resting nAChRs first open and then desensitize.

Kinetic Gating Model

The essential features of nAChR gating and desensitization behavior are illustrated in Fig. 2. In this scheme, R is the resting (unbound) receptor, and A is agonist. Binding of two agonists proceeds sequentially to form A_2R (the pre-open state), followed by opening (A_2O). Inactive desensitized (D) receptors are in equilibrium with resting receptors, and bind agonist with high affinity, but do not open. Agonist-induced desensitization proceeds from the open state, leading to A_2D.

Comparing Neuronal and Muscle nAChR Currents

ACh-activated currents have been recorded from autonomic ganglia and related tissue (e.g., adrenal chromaffin cells), as well as neurons and glia, but direct recordings of EPSPs in brain have been difficult to obtain. This is likely because brain nAChRs are primarily pre-synaptic, rather than post-synaptic. Recordings of nicotinic currents from pre-synaptic nerve terminals *(24)* have been reported.

Neuronal nAChRs display single channel conductances of 30–40 pS, but unlike muscle nAChRs, neuronal channels are strongly inwardly rectifying, owing to voltage-dependent closure rates. General behaviors of macroscopic currents (i.e., low cation selectivity, rapid activation, desensitization, and deactivation) are similar to those of muscle nAChRs, indicating that the underlying modes of receptor function are conserved. However, variable properties of macroscopic and single-channel neuronal nAChR currents are associated with different subunit compositions, seen in electrophysiologic experiments on recombinant nAChRs. In particular, the homomeric channels formed by α_7 subunits have high calcium conductance and desensitize extremely rapidly, features similar to glutamate receptors.

NICOTINIC RECEPTOR ROLES IN ANESTHESIA

The roles of nAChRs as targets of anesthetic drugs reflect their wide variety and distribution in excitable tissues. Muscle nAChRs are the targets for both depolarizing and nondepolarizing neuromuscular blocking compounds, while noncompetitive inhibition of muscle nAChRs contributes to the clinically observed relaxant activity of volatile anesthetics and other compounds (e.g., aminoglycoside antibiotics).

Drugs that inhibit ganglionic nicotinic receptors such as curare, gallamine, and some general anesthetics, act directly to reduce both sympathetic and parasympathetic activity. General anesthetic inhibition of sympathetic activity contributes to reduced vascular tone and altered thermoregulation.

Neuronal nAChRs in various brain regions have also been linked to behaviors that are altered by anesthetics. The cholinergic basal forebrain regulates memory and arousal, while pontomesencephalic cholinergic neurons are involved with sleep, memory and locomotor activity (25). BTX-sensitive nAChRs directly mediate synaptic transmission in inhibitory interneurons in the hippocampus (26–28), and modulate pre-synaptic release of glutamate, GABA, serotonin, dopamine, and acetylcholine (29). The pre- and postsynaptic localization of nAChRs in the hippocampus raises the possibility that their inhibition may result in the amnesia caused by general anesthetics. Isoflurane and desflurane have an EC_{50} for amnesia of approx 20% their EC_{50} (MAC) for immobility (30,31), and significantly, inhibition of heteromeric neuronal nAChRs is observed at low concentrations of these agents (*see* Section on Anesthetic Effects on Neuronal nAChRs). Thus, modulation of neuronal nAChRs by general anesthetics may contribute to amnesia, sedation, and excitement during light planes of anesthesia.

CNS nAChRs in brain and spinal cord also modulate pain sensation, as demonstrated by the analgesia caused by direct agonism with nicotine or epibatidine and the indirect agonism caused by spinal neostigmine. Nicotine-associated analgesia is reduced in transgenic mice lacking the nAChR α_4 subunit gene, suggesting a role for heteromeric $\alpha_4\beta_2$ nAChRs in nociception (32). The increased spinal ACh caused by neostigmine could be acting through muscarinic or nicotinic targets. In studies on rats, muscarinic activation mediates a portion of the analgesic response to neostigmine in female and males (33). Nicotinic activation was important only in females. In addition to the analgesia associated with neuronal nAChR agonism, hyperalgesia in female mice is seen with isoflurane at low concentrations that inhibit neuronal nAChRs. This hyperalgesia is potentiated by mecamylamine, a nicotinic antagonist that acts additively with isoflurane, while nicotine reverses isoflurane-induced hyperalgesia (P. Flood, unpublished data).

ANESTHETIC DRUG INTERACTIONS WITH NICOTINIC RECEPTORS

A wide variety of anesthetic drugs alter the function of *Torpedo*, muscle, and neuronal nAChRs (*see* Table 1 and Fig. 3). Our discussion emphasizes studies on alcohols and volatile anesthetics, since these compounds have been investigated in the most detail and there is some structural data on where these compounds bind and act.

Anesthetic Effects on Torpedo nAChRs

In the absence of nicotinic agonists, high concentrations (over 3 MAC) of most volatile anesthetics (ethers, halogenated alkanes, and alcohols) shift the equilibrium between resting and desensitized (R/D in Fig. 2) *Torpedo* nAChRs towards the desensitized state (34). General anesthetic concentration-responses show Hill slopes over 4 and near saturating aqueous concentrations, up to 80% of *Torpedo* receptors are desensitized. This direct nAChR desensitization by general anesthetics displays a strong correlation between potencies and hydrophobicities, and little structural specificity. Barbiturates display a dual action on R/D equilibrium as they stabilize the resting state at low concentrations and the desensitized state at high concentrations.

At 1–2 MAC, many general anesthetics dose-dependently increase the apparent rate of desensitization induced by low concentrations of agonist, as measured by Dns-C_6-cho binding. Agonist concentration-dependent studies show that general anesthetics shift the agonist concentration-response curve for both agonist-induced ion flux and agonist-induced desensitization toward lower values (increased apparent agonist affinity). In the case of isoflurane, a clinically used inhalational anesthetic, the increase in apparent agonist affinity is thought to reflect tighter binding of agonist to

Table 1
Functional Effects of Anesthetic Agents on Nicotinic Receptors

Anesthetic agents	Torpedo nAChR	Muscle fetal nAChR	$\alpha_4\beta_{2-4}$ Neuronal nAChR
Volatile Anesthetics			
Halogenated alkanes	Desensitize / Inhibit current / Enhance ACh affinity	Inhibit current	Potently inhibit current
Halogenated ethers	"	Inhibit current / Enhance ACh affinity?	"
Non-Halogenated ether	"	"	"
Gaseous Anesthetics			
Xenon	ND	ND	Inhibit current
Nitrous Oxide	ND	ND	"
Non-Halogenated alkanes	Don't enhance ACh affinity	ND	Potently inhibit current
"Non-Immobilizers"	Don't enhance ACh affinity	Inhibit current	Inhibit current
Intravenous Anesthetics			
Barbiturates	Stabilize closed state / Inhibit current	Inhibit current	Inhibit current
Propofol	ND	"	Weakly inhibit
Benzodiazepines	ND	"	ND
Opiates	Inhibit current and acetylcholinesterase	"	Weakly inhibit
Etomidate	ND	"	Weakly inhibit
Ketamine	Desensitize / Inhibit current	"	Inhibit current
Alcohols			
Short-chain alcohols	Enhance ACh affinity (cut-off at pentanol) / ± Inhibit current	Enhance ACh affinity / ± Inhibit current	Enhance ACh affinity
Long-chain alcohols	Inhibit current	Inhibit current	Inhibit current
Local Anesthetics	Inhibit current	Inhibit current	Inhibit current
Muscle Relaxants			
Succinylcholine	Activate	Activate. Desensitize	Activate
Non-depolarizers	Comp. Inhibition	Comp. Inhibition	
Steroidals			Activation
Curariform			Comp. Inhibition
Cholinesterase Inhibitors	ND	Indirectly activate / Inhibit current	Indirectly activate

ND: No Data available.

nAChR's agonist site, although this affinity change could also be caused by altered equilibrium between open (A$_2$O) and pre-open (A$_2$R) states *(35)*. Notably, neither halogenated nonanesthetics, nor nonhalogenated alkane anesthetics induce this leftward shift, paralleling their lack of activity in GABA$_A$ receptors *(36,37)*.

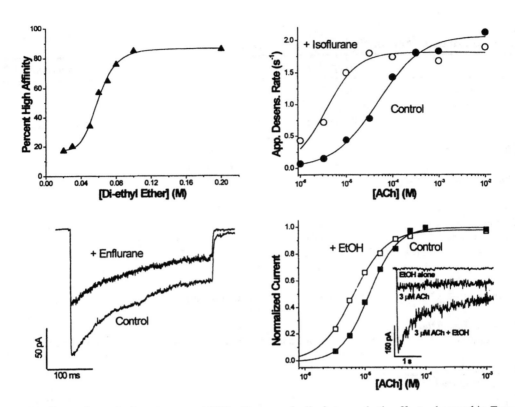

Fig. 3. Effects of anesthetic agents on nAChRs. Four panels display anesthetic effects observed in *Torpedo* and muscle nAChRs. The effects on muscle nAChR function are also found in some neuronal nAChRs. *Top left:* Anesthetics directly desensitize *Torpedo* nAChRs. Data derived from Firestone et al *(34)* shows the percentage of desensitized *Torpedo* nAChRs that bind ACh at nanomolar concentrations increasing as a function of [diethyl ether]. The EC_{50} is approx 60 mM and the Hill slope for the effect is near 6. *Top right:* Anesthetics increase the apparent ACh affinity of nAChRs. Data derived from Raines and Zachariah *(35)* shows the apparent rate of *Torpedo* nAChR desensitization (measured with a Dns-C_6-cho fluorescence binding assay) as a function of [ACh]. In the presence of isoflurane (1 m$M \approx$ 3.5 MAC) the rate vs [ACh] relationship is shifted leftward, but the maximal desensitization rate is not significantly altered. *Bottom left:* Anesthetics inhibit ACh-gated ionic currents through nAChRs. Data (Forman, S. A. unpublished data) shows maximal ACh-activated currents from a patch of membrane containing mouse muscle nAChRs. Enflurane (0.7 m$M \approx$ 2.5 MAC) inhibits the current, but does not alter the rate of desensitization at high ACh. *Bottom right:* Ethanol increases nAChR sensitivity to ACh without inhibiting ACh-activated currents. Electrophysiologic data are from studies of muscle type nAChRs expressed in *Xenopus* oocytes. Currents (*see* inset) were recorded from voltage-clamped outside-out oocyte membrane patches that were subjected to rapid ACh concentration jumps in the presence or absence of ethanol. Ethanol alone elicits no current, while 3 μM ACh (EC_5) elicits a small, slowly desensitizing current. Addition of 400 mM ethanol to 3 μM ACh results in a quadrupling of the peak current and acceleration of desensitization (inset). ACh concentration-response relationships normalized to a common control show that 300 mM ethanol causes a leftward shift without significantly altering the maximal currents (Zhou, Q. and Forman, S. A., unpublished results).

At 1–2 MAC, volatile anesthetics and long-chain normal alcohols, (but not methanol and ethanol) inhibit agonist-induced tracer ion flux in *Torpedo* nAChR-rich vesicles *(38)*. This concentration-dependent inhibition shows Hill slopes near 1.0 and is not surmountable with high agonist concentrations. Anesthetic potencies for flux inhibition also correlate with hydrophobicity. Unlike other general anesthetics, barbiturate inhibition of *Torpedo* nAChRs exhibits stereoselectivity, suggesting that barbiturates inhibit by binding to a discrete site on the nAChR *(39)*. Inhibition of *Torpedo* nAChR function by heptanol and octanol is mutually exclusive, also suggesting that a saturable site mediates this effect *(40)*.

Short-chain alcohols (methanol through pentanol) enhance *Torpedo* nAChR gating and ion flux at low agonist concentrations, resulting in leftward shifts of agonist concentration-response studies. Propanol through pentanol cause both gating enhancement at low agonist and inhibition of *Torpedo* nAChR flux at high agonist concentrations *(38)*.

A variety of other anesthetic compounds inhibit *Torpedo* nAChRs. Local anesthetics, both charged and amphiphilic, inhibit *Torpedo* nAChRs selectively in the opens state. Ketamine, phencyclidine, and propofol also inhibit *Torpedo* nAChR function. Phencyclidine allosterically stabilizes the desensitized nAChR.

Sites of Anesthetic Binding/Action on Torpedo nAChRs

Torpedo nAChR-rich membranes have proven a valuable system for studying anesthetic binding to ion channel protein, since this tissue is the only source of nAChRs that can be purified in milligram quantities with a high protein/lipid ratio. Indeed, despite the tendency for anesthetics to concentrate in lipids, radiolabeled barbiturates were shown to bind specifically to *Torpedo* nAChRs in an equilibrium assay *(41)*.

Another strategy to identify potentially relevant anesthetic binding sites on *Torpedo* nAChRs exploits anesthetic agents that covalently bind to proteins upon photoactivation. [^{14}C]-Halothane has been shown to photolabel a proteolytic fragment that contains TM1–TM3 *(42)*. Co-application of nonradioactive halothane (and to a lesser extent isoflurane) reduced incorporation of the [^{14}C]-halothane into nAChR protein, suggesting binding to a discrete site(s). Husain et al. *(43)* developed a radioactive photoactivatable analog of octanol (3-[^{3}H]-azi-octanol) that exhibits anesthetic activity in vivo and inhibits the nAChR. The advantage of this anesthetic is that it may be photoactivated using longer wavelengths that do not induce receptor photolysis. 3-[^{3}H]-Azi-octanol photolabels the nAChR α-subunit in an agonist-dependent manner (a 9-fold increase in labeling occurs in the desensitized state) and proteolytic/sequencing analysis identified the state-dependent incorporation site as α-Glu-262, an amino acid located at the carboxy-terminal end of the TM2 domain *(44)*. Other labeling occurred in TM4.

While binding and photolabeling of *Torpedo* nAChRs have unequivocally demonstrated that anesthetic binding sites exist on these receptors, these studies do not address whether the identified sites mediate the functional effects of anesthetics. Studies on recombinant muscle nAChRs (*see* Section on Detection on Sites of Anesthetic) have addressed this important issue.

Anesthetic Effects on Muscle nAChRs

Many of the anesthetic effects observed in *Torpedo* nAChRs are also observed in muscle nAChRs. Studies on muscle receptors have progressed from initial studies on spontaneous EPSCs in muscle tissue to single channel studies, and more recently to studies using recombinant nAChRs and "artificial synapse" experiments that allow study of state-dependent drug actions and the roles of nAChR molecular structures.

Early studies on muscle tissue showed that barbiturates, local anesthetics, volatile anesthetics and long-chain alcohols accelerated the decay of EPSCs, resulting in reduced current flow *(45,46)*. The rapid current decay caused by these compounds was consistent with an "open-channel-block" mechanism, whereby anesthetics waited until nAChR activation before inhibition occurred. As in *Torpedo* studies showing flux inhibition, the potency of EPSC inhibition by anesthetics correlated with their hydrophobicity.

Single-channel recordings from muscle showed that inhibition by volatiles, long-chain alcohols, many intravenous anesthetics, local anesthetics, and even cholinesterase inhibitors was associated with brief closures during channel openings *(47–49)*. For volatile anesthetics, the frequency of these closures (or blocking events) depends on the anesthetic concentration, as expected, but the overall open-channel time was also dependent on anesthetic concentration, ruling out a pure open-channel block mechanism *(50,51)*. Importantly, comparing nAChR inhibition by potent anesthetics with less potent compounds showed that the length of the "blockages" were longer with more potent inhibitors *(52)*. This observation rules out the possibility that an allosteric mechanism (such as a membrane perturbation) was inducing inhibition. Indeed, it suggests that more potent (hydrophobic) anesthetics occupy the inhibition site longer than less potent drugs.

Similar observations have also been made using "artificial synapse" experiments, wherein excised membrane patches from cells that contain nAChRs are subjected to rapid agonist and anesthetic concentration-jumps. These experiments were able to provide estimates of the binding and dissociation rates of isoflurane to open muscle nAChRs *(53)*. Furthermore, by enabling application of anesthetic exclusively to closed vs open nAChRs, this type of experiment confirmed that most of the inhibition caused by long-chain alcohols occurs *after* ACh activation of nAChRs, consistent with a dominant open-channel inhibition mechanism. Nonetheless, volatile anesthetics inhibit nAChRs both in the open and closed states. Volatile anesthetics and long-chain alcohols do not accelerate agonist-induced desensitization during long ACh pulses *(54)*.

Interestingly, "nonanesthetic" halogenated volatile compounds such as 1,2-dichlorohexafluoro-cyclobutane (F6) also inhibit muscle nAChRs, and display very strong open-channel selective block *(55)*. Thus, as steady-state inhibition is similar to that observed using volatile anesthetics, these compounds are much less potent when initial current inhibition is compared.

Again, reflecting their effects in *Torpedo* nAChRs, short-chain alcohols prolong EPSCs in muscle and enhance the frequency of single-channel openings *(56,57)*. Electrophysiological ACh concentration-responses in the presence of ethanol or methanol are shifted leftward, so that currents elicited with low agonist concentrations are actually increased. This enhancement of apparent agonist affinity is associated with longer open-channel bursts, indicating that channel closing rates are reduced by ethanol *(58)*. Ethanol also accelerates the rate of agonist-induced desensitization at both low and high ACh.

Sites of Anesthetic Action on Muscle nAChRs

Functional and kinetic studies on inhibition of both *Torpedo* and muscle nAChRs suggested that the nAChR pore may form an anesthetic site. To test this hypothesis, a "reverse pharmacology" approach was exploited, wherein the putative site of inhibition was mutated in recombinant receptors. The initial experiment focused on a hydrophilic serine (S) near the middle of the muscle α subunit TM2 domain (αS252). When this serine was mutated to a hydrophobic isoleucine (I) sidechain (αS252I), recombinant nAChRs were found to be nearly five times more sensitive to inhibition by long-chain alcohols and volatile anesthetics *(54)*. Receptors incorporating a range of different amino acids at this position showed sensitivities to alcohol inhibition that correlated with side-chain hydrophobicity, as predicted for a site where hydrophobic forces dominate binding. Furthermore, the mechanism of anesthetic inhibition was apparently unchanged by this mutation, because open-channel selective inhibition by long-chain alcohols was preserved. Subsequent studies have demonstrated that the homologous sidechain on the muscle β subunit also affects anesthetic sensitivity, whereas the side-chains on γ and δ subunits have a far smaller impact *(59)*. These mutations also alter sensitivity to "nonimmobilizers", indicating that this site cannot sterically discriminate between similar molecules *(55)*.

Recently, a series of hydrophobic mutations scanning from the inner to outer ends of TM2 on the α subunit identified a contiguous series of 6 amino acids (αL250–αV255) that appear to affect sensitivity to alcohol inhibition. This result suggests that the inhibition site within the nAChR pore is an extensive hydrophobic surface where a number of compounds interact and inhibit the passage of cations *(60)*. Mutations at the muscle nAChR αE262 site, homologous to the *Torpedo* residue photolabeled by azi-octanol, weakly alter sensitivity to anesthetic inhibition, but affect desensitization rates *(61)*. Thus, this site probably moves during desensitization, but does not represent the ultimate site of alcohol inhibition. A subset of α-TM2 mutations has also been examined to determine if they alter the ACh affinity enhancement ("leftward shift") associated with short-chain alcohols. A mutation at αL251 caused an increase in the sensitivity to ethanol-induced leftward shift, but no other mutations were associated with altered sensitivity to this action (62).

Other sites where anesthetics may act have also been examined using mutational analysis in nAChRs. Mutations within the agonist site do not alter sensitivity to volatile and alcohol inhibition, nor do they change sensitivity to ethanol-induced leftward shift. Propanol potently inhibits recombinant *Torpedo* nAChRs expressed in *Xenopus* oocytes in the resting state, possibly by inducing desensitization. A mutation in the α subunit TM4 domain, at the putative lipid-protein interface, eliminates propanol inhibition in this experiment (63).

Anesthetic Effects on Neuronal nAChRs

It has been known for many years that the volatile anesthetics and barbiturates inhibit synaptic transmission mediated by acetylcholine in the sympathetic nervous system (64,65). Ketamine inhibits nicotinic transmission at the renshaw synapse in the spinal cord (66). The optical isomers of isoflurane have been shown to inhibit neuronal nAChRs of the mollusk *Lymnea* in a stereospecific manner that mirrors their relative potencies in mice (67,68), suggesting that isoflurane may act at a protein site.

The general anesthetic sensitivities of different types of neuronal nAChRs have been explored electrophysiologically in *Xenopus* oocytes injected with mRNAs encoding selected subunits. The volatile anesthetics isoflurane, halothane, and sevoflurane potently inhibit the activity of heteromeric $\alpha_4\beta_2$, $\alpha_3\beta_4$, and $\alpha_2\beta_4$ nAChRs, while homomeric α_7 nAChRs are relatively unaffected (69,70). Indeed, for inhibition of heteromeric nAChRs by volatile anesthetics, IC_{50}s are near $0.2 \times MAC$. The intravenous anesthetics ketamine and thiopental inhibit both heteromeric and homomeric nAChRs (71–73). Neurosteroid based anesthetic drugs inhibit the activation of nAChRs composed of α_4 and β_2 subunits (74). However, the nAChRs certainly cannot be construed as a common receptor for general anesthetic drugs, since the intravenous anesthetics etomidate and propofol that potentiate the activity of GABA have little effect at nAChRs at clinically relevant concentrations (73,75). Inhibition of the nAChRs expressed in the central nervous system is thus common to many, but not all general anesthetic drugs.

Unlike muscle nAChRs, human neuronal nAChRs composed of $\alpha_2\beta_4$, $\alpha_3\beta_4$, and $\alpha_4\beta_2$ subunits (expressed in *Xenopus* oocytes) are apparently not inhibited by volatile "non-immobilizers" that disobey the Meyer-Overton rule (76). However, other data suggests that non-immobilizers that have amnestic actions may inhibit both ganglionic and central neuronal nAChRs (77).

As observed in both *Torpedo* and muscle nAChRs, ethanol actions in neuronal nAChRs differ from those of other anesthetics. Ethanol potentiates nAChR activation in neurons from septum, cortex and cerebellum (78–80). Ethanol (≥ 75 mM) also potentiates ACh-induced currents in heteromeric $\alpha_2\beta_4$, $\alpha_4\beta_4$, $\alpha_2\beta_2$, and $\alpha_4\beta_2$ receptors expressed in *Xenopus* oocytes (81). This effect was associated with an increase in maximal electrophysiological response, without a change in agonist EC_{50} or Hill coefficient. Neuronal $\alpha_2\beta_4$ nAChRs in *Xenopus* oocytes did not develop tolerance to repeated applications of ethanol or continuous exposure. The $\alpha_3\beta_2$ and $\alpha_3\beta_4$ subunit combinations were insensitive to ethanol. Low concentrations of ethanol (25 and 50 mM) significantly inhibit homomeric α_7 receptor function.

Sites of Anesthetic Actions on Neuronal nAChRs

In contrast to the detailed structural studies identifying binding sites and modulating sites on *Torpedo* and muscle nAChRs, relatively little is known about the sites where anesthetics act on neuronal nAChRs. Some information about possible location of anesthetic and ethanol actions on neuronal nAChRs has come from studies of chimeric subunits containing part of the α_7 nAChR subunit and part of the related 5HT3$_A$ receptor subunit. Volatile anesthetics at high concentrations inhibit oocyte expressed homomeric α_7 nAChRs, while these compounds potentiate of the response of homomeric 5HT3$_A$ receptors to low agonist *(82,83)*. A chimeric subunit constructed from the N-terminal extracellular portion of the nicotinic α$_7$ subunit and the C-terminal portion of the 5HT3$_A$ subunit formed receptors in *Xenopus* oocytes that were activated by ACh *(84)*. The chimeric protein, like α$_7$ nAChRs, was inhibited by both isoflurane and halothane, suggesting that the N-terminal domain of α$_7$ contains structural features that are associated with anesthetic actions. Similar experiments on this chimera also indicated a role for the N-terminal domain in ethanol actions *(85)*. Unfortunately the complementary chimera with N-terminus from 5HT$_{3A}$ and C-terminus from α$_7$ did not function, so the data cannot determine whether the N-terminal domain is both necessary and sufficient for determining anesthetic sensitivity. It is also difficult to extend these implications to heteromeric neuronal nAChRs, which are inhibited by much lower concentrations of volatile anesthetics and are also potentiated by ethanol.

More recently, Yamakura et al. *(86)* found that α$_4$β$_2$ and α$_4$β$_4$ nAChRs have differential sensitivity to some anesthetics. Using beta subunit chimeras, they identified homologous TM2 sites on both β$_2$ (V253) and β$_4$ (F255) subunits that affected sensitivity to isoflurane, pentobarbital, and hexanol, but not ketamine. Mutations at the homologous site on the α$_2$ subunit (V254) also affected anesthetic sensitivity. Furthermore, cysteine mutations at the α$_2$-V254 and β$_4$-F255 residues were irreversibly modified by a charged cysteine-specific reagent, methanethiosulfonate ethylammonium (MTSEA), but not by propyl methanethiosulfonate, a cysteine-modifying anesthetic. The authors suggested that these sites allosterically alter anesthetic actions in heteromeric nAChRs but are not involved directly in anesthetic binding.

SUMMARY

Nicotinic acetylcholine receptors comprise a subset of anesthetic-sensitive ligand-gated ion channels that are present in both muscle and neural tissue. Anesthetic-induced functional changes in nAChRs include both inhibition and gating enhancement, although the latter action is specific to short-chain alcohols. As anesthetic targets, nAChRs in muscle contribute to immobility, while those in autonomic and central nervous systems are very likely linked to behaviors observed at low anesthetic concentrations, such as amnesia, hyperalgesia, and excitation. Ongoing studies in transgenic animal models should provide tests for these hypotheses. Mechanistic studies in *Torpedo* and muscle models reveal that some inhibitory anesthetic actions are caused by binding to a site within the nAChR pore, which is formed by TM2 domains. It is uncertain whether a similar mechanism contributes to inhibition of neuronal nAChRs. Mechanistic studies on muscle and electroplaque nAChRs may also provide clues to how anesthetics interact with and affect other LGICs in the nicotinic superfamily, including GABA$_A$Rs, 5HT$_3$Rs, and GlyRs.

REFERENCES

1. Le Novere, N. and Changeux, J. P. (1995) Molecular evolution of the nicotinic acetylcholine receptor: an example of multigene family in excitable cells. *J. Mol. Evol.* **40**, 155–172.
2. Ortells, M. O. and Lunt, G.G. (1995) Evolutionary history of the ligand-gated ion-channel superfamily of receptors. *Trends Neurosci.* **18**, 121–127.
3. Galzi, J. L., Revah, F., Bessis, A., and Changeux, J. P. (1991) Functional architecture of the nicotinic acetylcholine receptor: from electric organ to brain. *Ann. Rev. Pharm. Tox.* **31**, 37–72.
4. Unwin, N. (1998) The nicotinic acetylcholine receptor of the Torpedo electric ray. *J. Struct. Biol.* **121**, 181–190.
5. Karlin, A. and Akabas, M. H. (1995) Toward a structural basis for the function of nicotinic acetylcholine receptors and their cousins. *Neuron* **15**, 1231–1244.
6. Finer-Moore, J. and Stroud, R. M. (1984) Amphipathic analysis and possible formation of the ion channel in an acetylcholine receptor. *Proc. Natl. Acad. Sci. USA* **81**, 155–159.
7. Damle, V. N., McLaughlin, M., and Karlin, A. (1978) Bromoacetylcholine as an affinity label of the acetylcholine receptor from Torpedo Califonica. *Biochem. Biophys. Res. Comm.* **84**, 845–851.
8. Kao, P. N., Dwork, A. J., Kaldany, R. J., et al. (1984) Identification of the alpha subunit half-cystine specifically labeled by an affinity reagent for the acetylcholine recepotr binding site. *J. Biol. Chem.* **259**, 11,662–11,665.
9. Dennis, M., Giraudat, J., Kotzyba-Hibert, F., et al. (1988) Amino acids of the Torpedo marmorata acetylcholine receptor alpha subunit labeled by a photoaffinity ligand for the acetylcholine binding site. *Biochemistry* **27**, 2346–2357.

10. Pedersen, S. E. and Cohen, J. B. (1990) d-Tubocurarine binding sites are located at alpha-gamma and alpha-delta subunit interfaces of the nicotinic acetylcholine receptor. *Proc. Natl. Acad. Sci. USA* **87,** 2785–2789.
11. Miyazawa, A., Fujiyoshi, Y., Stowell, M., and Unwin, N. (1999) Nicotinic acetylcholine receptor at 4.6 A resolution: transverse tunnels in the channel wall. *J. Mol. Biol.* **288,** 765–786.
12. Unwin, N. (1995) Acetylcholine receptor channel imaged in the open state. *Nature* **373,** 37–43.
13. Giraudat, J., Dennis, M., Heidmann, T., Chang, J. Y., and Changeux, J. P. (1986) Structure of the high-affinity binding site for noncompetitive blockers of the acetylcholine receptor: serine-262 of the delta subunit is labeled by [³H]-chlorpromazine. *Proc. Natl. Acad. Sci. USA* **83,** 2719–2723.
14. Changeux J. P., Heidmann T., and Oswald R. (1983) Multiple sites of action for noncompetitive nlockers on acetylcholine receptor rich membrane fragments from Torpedo Marmorata. *Biochemistry* **22,** 3112–3127.
15. Changeux, J. P., Devillers-Thiery, A., Galzi, J. L., Eisele, J. L., Bertrand, S., and Bertrand, D. (1993) Functional architecture of the nicotinic acetylcholine receptor: A prototype of ligand-gated ion channels. *J. Membr. Biol.* **136,** 97–112.
16. Akabas, M. H., Kaufmann, C., Archdeacon, P., and Karlin, A. (1994) Identification of acetylcholine receptor channel-lining residues in the entire M2 segment of the alpha subunit. *Neuron* **13,** 919–927.
17. Blanton, M. P. and Cohen, J. B. (1994) Identifying the lipid-protein interface of the Torpedo nicotinic acetylcholine receptor: secondary structure implications. *Biochemistry* **33,** 2859–2872.
18. Blanton, M. P. and Cohen, J. B. (1992) Mapping the lipid-exposed regions in the Torpedo californica nicotinic acetylcholine receptor. *Biochemistry* **31,** 3738–3750.
19. McGehee D. S. and Role L. W. (1995) Physiological diversity of nicotinic acetylcholine receptors expressed by vertebrate neurons. *Ann. Rev. Physiol.* **57,** 521–546.
20. Yu, C. R. and Role, L. W. (1998) Functional contribution of the alpha7 subunit to multiple subtypes of nicotinic receptors in embryonic chick sympathetic neurones. *J. Physiol.* **509,** 651–665.
21. Lingle, C. J., Maconochie, D., and Steinbach, J. H. (1992) Activation of skeletal muscle nicotinic acetylcholine receptors. *J. Mem. Biol.* **126,** 195–217.
22. Katz B. and Thesleff S. (1957) A study of the desensitization produced by acetylcholine at the motor endplate. *J. Physiol.* **138,** 63–80.
23. Colquhoun, D. and Hawkes, A. G. (1982) On the stochastic properties of bursts of singleton channel openings and of clusters of bursts. *Phil. Trans. Royal Soc. Lond. B.* **300,** 1–59.
24. Coggan, J. S., Paysan, J., Conroy, W. G., and Berg, D. K. (1997) Direct recording of nicotinic responses in presynaptic nerve terminals. *J. Neurosci.* **17,** 5798–5806.
25. Woolf, N. J. (1991) Cholinergic systems in mammalian brain and spinal cord. *Prog. Neurobiol.* **37,** 475–524.
26. Alkondon, M., Pereira, E. F., and Albuquerque, E. X. (1998) Alpha-bungarotoxin- and methyllycaconitine-sensitive nicotinic receptors mediate fast synaptic transmission in interneurons of rat hippocampal slices. *Brain Res.* **810,** 257–263.
27. Ji, D., and Dani, J. A. (2000) Inhibition and disinhibition of pyramidal neurons by activation of nicotinic receptors on hippocampal interneurons. *J. Neurophys.* **83,** 2682–2690.
28. Frazier, C. J., Rollins, Y. D., Breese, C. R., Leonard, S., Freedman, R., and Dunwiddie, T. V. (1998) Acetylcholine activates an alpha-bungarotoxin-sensitive nicotinic current in rat hippocampal interneurons, but not pyramidal cells. *J. Neurosci.* **18,** 1187–1195.
29. McGehee, D. S., Heath M. J., Gelber, S., Devay, P., and Role, L. W. (1995) Nicotine enhancement of fast excitatory synaptic transmission in CNS by presynaptic receptors. *Science* **269,** 1692–1696.
30. Chortkoff, B. S., Bennett, H. L., and Eger, E. I., 2nd (1993) Subanesthetic concentrations of isoflurane suppress learning as defined by the category-example task. *Anesthesiology* **79,** 16–22.
31. Dwyer R., Bennett, H. L., Eger, E. I., and Heilbron, D. (1992) Effects of isoflurane and nitrous oxide in subanesthetic concentrations on memory and responsiveness in volunteers. *Anesthesiology* **77,** 888–898.
32. Marubio, L. M., del Mar Arroyo-Jimenez, M., Cordero-Erausquin, M., et al. (1999) Reduced antinociception in mice lacking neuronal nicotinic receptor subunits. *Nature* **398,** 805–810.
33. Chiari, A., Tobin, J. R., Pan, H. L., Hood, D. D., and Eisenach, J. C. (1999) Sex differences in cholinergic analgesia I: a supplemental nicotinic mechanism in normal females. *Anesthesiology* **91,** 1447–1454.
34. Firestone, L. L., Alifimoff, J. K., and Miller, K. W. (1994) Does general anesthetic-induced desensitization of the Torpedo acetylcholine receptor correlate with lipid disordering? *Mol. Pharm.* **46,** 508–515.
35. Raines, D. E. and Zachariah, V. T. (1999) Isoflurane increases the apparent agonist affinity of the nicotinic acetylcholine receptor. *Anesthesiology* **90,** 135–146.
36. Raines, D. E. (1996) Anesthetic and nonanesthetic halogenated volatile compounds have dissimilar activities on nicotinic acetylcholine receptor desensitization kinetics. *Anesthesiology* **84,** 663–671.
37. Raines, D. E., Claycomb, R. J., Scheller, M., and Forman, S. A. (2001) Nonhalogenated alkane anesthetics fail to potentiate agonist actions on two ligand-gated ion channels. *Anesthesiology* **95,** 470–477.
38. Forman, S. A. and Miller, K. W. (1989) Molecular sites of anesthetic action in postsynaptic nicotinic membranes. *Trends. Pharm. Sci.* **10,** 447–452.
39. Roth, S. H., Forman, S. A., Braswell, L. M., and Miller, K. W. (1989) Actions of pentobarbital enantiomers on nicotinic cholinergic receptors. *Mol. Pharm.* **36,** 874–880.
40. Wood, S. C., Tonner, P. H., de Armendi, A. J., Bugge, B., and Miller, K. W. (1995) Channel inhibition by alkanols occurs at a binding site on the nicotinic acetylcholine receptor. *Mol. Pharm.* **47,** 121–130.
41. Dodson, B. A., Braswell, L. M., and Miller, K. W. (1987) Barbiturates bind to an allosteric regulatory site on nicotinic acetylcholine receptor-rich membranes. *Mol. Pharm.* **32,** 119–126.

42. Eckenhoff, R. G. (1996) An inhalational anesthetic binding domain in the nicotinic acetylcholine receptor. *Proc. Natl. Acad. Sci. USA* **93**, 2807–2810.

43. Husain, S. S., Forman, S. A., Kloczewiak, M. A., et al. (1999) Synthesis and properties of 3-(2-hydroxyethyl)-3-n-pentyldiazirine, a photoactivable general anesthetic. *J. Med. Chem.* **42**, 3300–3307.

44. Pratt, M. B., Husain, S. S., Miller, K. W., and Cohen, J. B. (2000) Identification of sites of incorporation in the nicotinic acetylcholine receptor of a photoactivatible general anesthetic. *J. Biol. Chem.* **275**, 29,441–29,451.

45. Gage, P. W. and Hamill, O. P. (1981) Effects of anaesthetics on ion channels in synapses, in *Neurophysiology IV* (Porter, R., ed.) University Park, Baltimore, MD, pp. 1–45.

46. McLarnon, J. G., Pennefather, P., and Quastel, D. M. J. (1988) Mechanisms of nicotinic channel blockade by anesthetics, in *Molecular and Cellular Mechanisms of Anesthetics* (Roth, S. H. and Miller, K. W., eds.) Plenum. New York, NY, pp. 155–164.

47. Lechleiter, J. and Gruener, R. (1984) Halothane shortens acetylcholine receptor channel kinetics without affecting conductance. *Proc. Natl. Acad. Sci. USA* **81**, 2929–2933.

48. Brett, R. S., Dilger, J. P., and Yland, K. F. (1988) Isoflurane causes "flickering" of the acetylcholine receptor channel: observations using the patch clamp. *Anesthesiology* **69**, 161–170.

49. Wachtel, R. E. and Wegrzynowicz, E. S. (1992) Kinetics of nicotinic acetylcholine ion channels in the presence of intravenous anaesthetics and induction agents. *Brit. J. Pharm.* **106**, 623–627.

50. Dilger, J. P. and Brett, R. S. (1991) Actions of volatile anesthetics and alcohols on cholinergic receptor channels. *Ann. N. Y. Acad. Sci.* **625**, 616–627.

51. Wachtel, R. E. and Wegrzynowicz, E. S. (1991) Mechanism of volatile anesthetic action on ion channels. *Ann. N. Y. Acad. Sci.* **625**, 116–128.

52. Dilger, J. P., Vidal, A. M., Mody, H. I., and Liu, Y. (1994) Evidence for direct actions of general anesthetics on an ion channel protein. A new look at a unified mechanism of action. *Anesthesiology* **81**, 431–442.

53. Dilger, J. P., Brett, R. S., and Mody, H. I. (1993) The effects of isoflurane on acetylcholine receptor channels: 2. Currents elicited by rapid perfusion of acetylcholine. *Mol. Pharm.* **44**, 1056–1063.

54. Forman, S. A., Miller, K. W., and Yellen, G. (1995) A discrete site for general anesthetics on a postsynaptic receptor. *Mol. Pharm.* **48**, 574–581.

55. Forman, S. A. and Raines, D. E. (1998) Nonanesthetic volatile drugs obey the Meyer-Overton correlation in two molecular protein site models. *Anesthesiology* **88**, 1535–1548.

56. Gage, P. W. (1965) The effects of methyl, ethyl, and n-propyl alcohol on neuromuscular transmission in the rat. *J. Pharm. Exp. Ther.* **150**, 236–243.

57. Bradley, R. J., Peper, K., and Sterz, R. (1980) Postsynaptic effects of ethanol at the frog neuromuscular junction. *Nature* **284**, 60–62.

58. Forman, S. A. and Zhou, Q. (1999) Novel modulation of a nicotinic receptor channel mutant reveals that the open state is stabilized by ethanol. *Mol. Pharm.* **55**, 102–108.

59. Forman, S. A. (1997) Homologous mutations on different subunits cause unequal but additive effects on n-alcohol block in the nicotinic receptor pore. *Biophys. J.* **72**, 2170–2179.

60. Zhou, Q. L., Zhou, Q., and Forman, S. A. (2000) The n-alcohol site in the nicotinic receptor pore is a hydrophobic patch. *Biochemistry* **39**, 14,920–14,926.

61. Forman, S. A. and Zhou, Q. L. (2000) Mutation of an anesthetic-photolabeled residue in the nAChR pore alters sensitivity to general anesthetics. *Anesthesiology* **93**, A-774.

62. Forman, S. A. and Zhou, Q. (1998) Leftward Shift of ACh concentration-response curves by ethanol is unaffected by nAChR pore mutations. *Alc. Clin. Exp. Res.* **22**, 47A.

63. Mercado, J. L., Cruz-Martin, A., Rojas, L. V., and Lasalde, J. A. (2001) Hydrophobic amino acid replacements in the M4 domain of the Torpedo Californica acetylcholine receptor dramatically reduce the inhibition by 1-propanol. *Biophys. J.* **80**, 461a.

64. Larrabee, M. G. and Posternak, J. M. (1952) Selective action of anesthetics on synapses and axons in mammalian sympathetic ganglia. *J. Neurophys.* **15**, 91–114.

65. Nicoll, R. A. (1998) Pentobarbital: differential postsynaptic actions on sympathetic ganglion cells. *Science* **199**, 451–452.

66. Anis, N. A., Berry, S. C., Burton, N. R., and Lodge D. (1983) The dissociative anaesthetics, ketamine and phencyclidine, selectively reduce excitation of central mammalian neurones by N-methyl-aspartate. *Brit. J. Pharm.* **79**, 565–575.

67. Franks, N. P. and Lieb, W. R. (1991) Stereospecific effects of inhalational general anesthetic optical isomers on nerve ion channels. *Science* **254**, 427–430.

68. McKenzie, D., Franks, N. P., and Lieb, W. R. (1995) Actions of general anaesthetics on a neuronal nicotinic acetylcholine receptor in isolated identified neurones of Lymnaea stagnalis. *Brit. J. Pharm.* **115**, 275–282.

69. Flood, P., Ramirez-Latorre, J., and Role, L. (1997) Alpha 4 beta 2 neuronal nicotinic acetylcholine receptors in the central nervous system are inhibited by isoflurane and propofol, but alpha 7-type nicotinic acetylcholine receptors are unaffected. *Anesthesiology* **86**, 859–865.

70. Violet, J. M., Downie, D. L., Nakisa, R. C., Lieb, W. R., and Franks, N. P. (1997) Differential sensitivities of mammalian neuronal and muscle nicotinic acetylcholine receptors to general anesthetics. *Anesthesiology* **86**, 866–874.

71. Downie, D. L., Franks N. P., and Lieb, W. R. (2000) Effects of thiopental and its optical isomers on nicotinic acetylcholine receptors. *Anesthesiology* **93**, 774–783.

72. Yamakura, T., Chavez-Noriega, L. E., and Harris, R. A. (2000) Subunit-dependent inhibition of human neuronal nicotinic acetylcholine receptors and other ligand-gated ion channels by dissociative anesthetics ketamine and dizocilpine. *Anesthesiology 2000* **92,** 1144–1153.

73. Flood, P. and Krasowski, M. D. (2000) Intravenous anesthetics differentially modulate ligand-gated ion channels. *Anesthesiology* **92,** 1418–1425.

74. Paradiso, K., Sabey, K., Evers, A. S., Zorumski, C. F., Covey, D. F., and Steinbach, J. H. (2000) Steroid inhibition of rat neuronal nicotinic alpha4beta2 receptors expressed in HEK 293 cells. *Mol. Pharm.* **58,** 341–351.

75. Flood, P. and Role, L. W. (1998) Neuronal nicotinic acetylcholine receptor modulation by general anesthetics. *Toxicol. Lett.* **100–101,** 149–153.

76. Cardoso, R. A., Yamakura, T., Brozowski, S. J., Chavez-Noriega, L. E., and Harris, R. A. (1999) Human neuronal nicotinic acetylcholine receptors expressed in *Xenopus* oocytes predict efficacy of halogenated compounds that disobey the Meyer-Overton rule. *Anesthesiology* **91,** 1370–1377.

77. Matsuura, T., Andoh, T., Kamiya, Y., Itoh, H., and Okumura, F. (2000) Inhibitory effects of isoflurane and nonimmobilizing halogenated compounds on neuronal nicotinic receptors. *Anesthesiology* **93,** A-763.

78. Nagata, K., Aistrup, G. L., Huang, C. S., et al. (1996) Potent modulation of neuronal nicotinic acetylcholine receptor-channel by ethanol. *Neurosci. Lett.* **217,** 189–193.

79. Aistrup, G. L., Marszalec, W., and Narahashi, T. (1999) Ethanol modulation of nicotinic acetylcholine receptor currents in cultured cortical neurons. *Mol. Pharml.* **55,** 39–49.

80. Yang, X., Criswell, H. E., and Breese, G. R. (1999) Action of ethanol on responses to nicotine from cerebellar interneurons and medial septal neurons: relationship to methyllycaconitine inhibition of nicotine responses. *Alc. Clin. Exp. Res.* **23,** 983–990.

81. Cardoso, R. A., Brozowski, S. J., Chavez-Noriega, L. E., Harpold, M., Valenzuela, C. F., and Harris, R. A. (1999) Effects of ethanol on recombinant human neuronal nicotinic acetylcholine receptors expressed in *Xenopus* oocytes. *J. Pharm. Exp. Ther.* **289,** 774–780.

82. Zhang, L., Oz M., Stewart, R. R., Peoples, R. W., and Weight, F. F. (1997) Volatile general anaesthetic actions on recombinant nAChalpha7, 5-HT3 and chimeric nAChalpha7-5-HT3 receptors expressed in *Xenopus* oocytes. *Brit. J. Pharm.* **120,** 353–355.

83. Jenkins, A., Franks, N. P., and Lieb, W. R. (1996) Actions of general anaesthetics on 5-HT3 receptors in N1E-115 neuroblastoma cells. *Brit. J. Pharm.* **117,** 1507–1515.

84. Eisele, J. L., Bertrand, S,. Galzi, J. L., Devillers-Thiery, A., Changeux, J. P., and Bertrand, D. (1993) Chimaeric nicotinic-serotonergic receptor combines distinct ligand binding and channel specificities. *Nature* **366,** 479–483.

85. Yu, D., Zhang, L., Eisele, J. L., Bertrand, D., Changeux, J. P., and Weight, F. F. (1996) Ethanol inhibition of nicotinic acetylcholine type alpha7 receptors involves the amino-terminal domain of the receptor. *Mol. Pharm.* **50,** 1010–1016.

86. Yamakura, T., Borghese, C., and Harris, R. A. (2000) A transmembrane site determines sensitivity of neuronal nicotinic acetylcholine receptors to general anesthetics. *J. Biol. Chem.* **275,** 40,879–40,886.

18
Actions of General Anesthetic
on Voltage-Gated Ion Channels

Norbert Topf, Esperanza Recio-Pinto,
Thomas J. J. Blanck, and Hugh C. Hemmings, Jr.

INTRODUCTION

Neuronal signaling depends on rapid changes in electrical fields across cell membranes mediated by ion channels. Three important properties of these transmembrane proteins facilitate the rapid changes in membrane potential: passive conduction of ions, ion selectivity, and open and closing (gating) in response to electrical, mechanical, or chemical signals.

Voltage-gated channels respond to changes in the plasma membrane potential by opening to allow the passive flux of ions down their electrochemical gradient into or out of the cell. This protein family consists of oligomeric integral membrane proteins with four internally homologous domains (Na^+ and Ca^{2+} channels) or four homologous subunits (K^+ channels). Each of the four homologous domains contains six potential transmembrane α-helical segments, which together form a central pore (Fig. 1). Three-dimensional structures of Na^+ and K^+ channels defined recently by either X-ray crystallography (1) or cryo-electron microscopy (2) have greatly expanded these structural models.

VOLTAGE-GATED SODIUM CHANNELS

Physiological and Pharmacological Classification

Voltage-gated Na^+ channels are responsible for the rapid depolarization phase of the action potential in electrically excitable cells such as nerve, muscle, and heart (3). Their modular architecture allows interactions between multiple regions of the channel to orchestrate gating, rapid channel opening and closure. A dynamic model of receptor gating has been developed to explain the pharmacological response of this channel and its ion selective conductance. A variety of drugs and toxins, including local anesthetics, class I antiarrhythmic drugs, and class I anti-epileptic drugs exhibit voltage-dependent (tonic) and frequency-dependent (phasic) block of Na^+ channels, as described by the modulated receptor hypothesis (4). According to this model, these properties are conferred by different drug affinities for the various functional states of the Na^+ channel: resting, open, and inactivated.

Voltage-dependent inhibition is explained by drug binding to the inactivated state of the channel. This impedes the voltage dependent transition of the channel from its inactivated state back to its resting state, which effectively reduces the number of resting channels available for activation in response to depolarization.

Frequency-dependent inhibition is explained by selective drug binding to the open state of the channel. Na^+ channels stimulated with increased frequency are statistically more likely to be in the

From: *Contemporary Clinical Neuroscience: Neural Mechanisms of Anesthesia*
Edited by: Joseph F. Antognini et al. © Humana Press Inc., Totowa, NJ

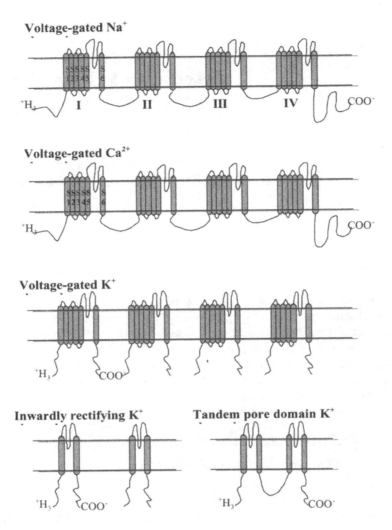

Fig. 1. Predicted topologies of prototypical voltage-gated ion channels illustrating their overall structural similarities, which is reflected in a high degree of amino acid sequence homology.

open state. This allows increased drug binding, but does not prevent subsequent channel inactivation. Local anesthetics that show frequency-dependent inhibition, enter from the intracellular side and bind to the inner pore of the Na$^+$ channel with high affinity. The binding site has been localized to transmembrane segment S6 of domain IV of the α-chain *(5)*.

Several potent toxins have been used to classify, purify and define functional domains of Na$^+$ channels *(6)*. The puffer fish poison tetrodotoxin (TTX) and the dinoflagellate toxin saxitoxin bind to an extracellular site (site 1) of the α-subunit. These toxins block Na$^+$ permeability with high potency (K_I = 1–10 nM), and have enabled the identification of outer pore structures and the selectivity filter. Tissue selectivity is evident in the 200-fold lower affinity of TTX for cardiac compared to brain Na$^+$ channels. Some peripheral nervous system Na$^+$ channels have even lower binding affinities for TTX *(7–9)*. Lipid soluble steroids such as the frog-skin toxin batrachotoxin and the plant alkaloids aconitine and veratridine bind to site 2. These toxins have a high affinity for the open state of the channel and lead to channel activation by slowing inactivation. Scorpion and anemone toxins specifically block the inactivation-gating step by binding to sites 3 and 4. Cadmium is a high affinity, nonspecific blocker of cardiac, but not of brain or skeletal Na$^+$ channels.

Structure, Function, and Regulation

The principle pore forming component of Na$^+$ channels in mammalian brain is the 260 kDa glycoprotein α-subunit *(10,11)*. It is a transmembrane protein with large intracellular N- and C-termini (Fig. 1). The subunit contains four internally homologous repeated domains (I–IV) with over 50% sequence identity. Each domain consists of six segments (S1–S6) that form transmembrane α-helices *(12)*.

Two additional integral membrane glycoprotein subunits have been identified *(10,11)*. The β1 (36 kDa) subunit interacts noncovalently with the α-subunit, while the β2 subunit (33 kDa) is attached via a disulfide bond. Both β-subunits have a single transmembrane segment, a large highly glycosylated N-terminal extracellular segment, and a short intracellular domain *(13)*. Both subunits contain immunoglobulin-like extracellular β-sheets which may be involved in intercellular interactions *(14)*. The binding of the β2-subunit to tenascins *(15)* suggests a possible role in regulation of local density of Na$^+$ channels, as in nodes of Ranvier.

The voltage-gated Na$^+$ channel family is large, with significant diversity in functional properties and tissue distribution *(3)* (Table 1). There are at least eight isoforms of the α-subunit, which vary in species and tissue expression. The TTX binding α-subunit appears to be the only component in eel electropax *(16)*. The α-subunit associates with β1 and β2 subunits in mammalian brain *(10)*. In skeletal muscle, the α-subunit associates only with the β1-subunit *(17)*. The α-subunit seems sufficient to carry out the basic function of the channel *(18,19)*. Coexpression of β-subunits accelerates inactivation and shifts voltage dependence toward more negative membrane potentials *(13,20)*.

Formation of the Pore

The four domains of the α-subunit form a central pore. Site-directed mutagenesis experiments have demonstrated that TTX binds to all four domains in the short hydrophobic segments between transmembrane α-helices S5 and S6 *(21)*. Cross-linking experiments suggest that the pore loops are asymmetrically organized and dynamic over the millisecond time scale of Na$^+$ channel gating *(22)*. Recent high resolution cryo-electron microscopic studies of the eel Na$^+$ channel demonstrate a bell shaped structure with several inner cavities, four small holes, and eight outer orifices *(2)*.

Na$^+$ Selectivity

The pore is lined by a highly conserved "P segment" comprised of the S5–S6 linker region. Mutations of these negatively charged regions in domain I–IV from DEKA to EEEE, as present in the homologous Ca^{2+} channels, confers Ca^{2+} selectivity to the Na$^+$ channel *(23)*. These residues interact to allow a specific flow of Na$^+$ (by a factor 100:1) over other cations with high throughput (>10^7 ions/s).

Gating

Voltage dependent gating of the Na$^+$ channel involves an outward movement of gating charges in response to changes in membrane potential *(24)*, which have been refined to ~12 positve charges moving outward during activation *(25)*. Mutagenesis experiments suggest the S4 α-helix as the voltage sensitive element *(26)*. A sliding helix *(27)* or helical screw model *(28)* proposes positive charges within the S4 segment are released on depolarization, moving the S4 segment outward along a spiral path and initiating a conformational change to open the pore. The recent finding that cysteine residues can be cross-linked upon gating suggests that the S4 segment emerges from the transmembrane region during gating *(29)*. Neurotoxins like β-scorpion toxin enhance Na$^+$ channel activation only once the channel is activated (i.e., they prevent inactivation), which is thought to be mediated by trapping the voltage sensor in its outward, activated position *(30)*.

Table 1
Voltage-Gated Na⁺ Channel Family

Names	New channel (α-subunit) names	Tissue expression	Modulators
Type I	Na$_V$ 1.1	CNS, PNS	Antagonists:
Type II/IIA	Na$_V$ 1.2	CNS	Tetrodotoxin (TTX)
Type III	Na$_V$ 1.3	CNS	Saxitoxin (STX)
μ1, Skm1	Na$_V$ 1.4	Skeletal muscle	μ-Conotoxin
h1, Skm2	Na$_V$ 1.5	Heart, skeletal muscle	Sea-anemone toxin Local anesthetics
TypeVI, SCN8a	Na$_V$ 1.6	CNS, PNS	Activators: Veratridine
PN-1, hNe, Nas	Na$_V$ 1.7	PNS, Swann cells	Batrachotoxin α/β-scorpion toxins
PN-3, SNS	Na$_V$ 1.8	PNS (dorsal root ganglion(DRG)	
PN-5, SCN12A	Na$_V$ 1.9	PNS	
SCL11, Na-G, Nav2.1	Na$_x$	Heart, uterus, skel.muscle, astrocytes, DRG	

Dorsal root ganglion, (DRG); Central nervous system, (CNS); Peripheral nervous system, PNS.

Inactivation

Na⁺ channel inactivation is an active process involving the intracellular mouth of the pore *(3)*. Proteolytic enzymes prevent inactivation *(31)*. Expression of Na⁺-channels in two distinct functional pieces with a cut between domains III and IV slows inactivation *(26)*. The phenylalanine residue within the IFM motif at position 1489 is critical for fast inactivation *(32,33)*. These data suggest that an intracellular structure functions as a "lid" to close the activated channel. According to the hinged lid hypothesis, the Na⁺-channel is inactivated within milliseconds of opening *(34)*. The outward movement of the S4 segment in domain IV initiates fast inactivation by closure of the intracellular inactivation gate *(35)*.

Phosphorylation

Na⁺ channels are modulated by several intracellular phosphorylation processes via multiple phosphorylation sites on the intracellular C-terminus, although their physiologic importance is still unclear. Activation of the D1 dopamine receptor via dopamine or cocaine decreases Na⁺ currents *(36,37)*. Phosphorylation by cAMP-dependent protein kinase *(38)*, a tyrosine kinase *(39)* or protein kinase C (PKC) *(40,41)* alters ion conductance and voltage dependent inactivation, and the transmembrane receptor tyrosine phosphatase RPTP-β causes a positive shift of the voltage dependence of channel inactivation *(42)*.

Anesthetic Effects on Na⁺ Channels

Early experiments rejected the role of Na⁺ channels as relevant anesthetic targets because of the high effective concentrations *(43)*. Invertebrate preparations such as the squid giant axon were insensitive to clinical concentrations of anesthetics. However, more recent experiments on mammalian preparations demonstrate significant sensitivity to intravenous and volatile anesthetics at clinically relevant concentrations (Table 2). Action potential propagation is relatively resistant to general anesthetics *(44)*, however branch points in small axons and action potential invasion of nerve terminals appear to be more sensitive *(45,46)*. Intravenous anesthetics (e.g., barbiturates *[47,48]*, propofol *[49]*) block human brain Na⁺ channels, volatile anesthetics at clinical concentrations inhibit rat brain Na⁺

Table 2
Summary of Anesthetic Effects on Voltage-Gated Ion Channels

Ion channel	General functions	Volatile anesthetics	Intravenous anesthetics
Na$^+$	• Axon potential propagation • Neurotransmitter release	• Reduction in peak Na$^+$ conductance • Depolarizing shift in activation • Hyperpolarizing shift in inactivation • Reduction in time constant for activation and inactivation • Axonal Na$^+$ channels require very high anesthetic concentration for inhibition • Synaptosomal Na$^+$ channels inhibited by 10% at clinical concentrations • Rat brain Na$^+$ channels are inhibited by 50% at clinical concentrations in transfected cells. • Presynaptic Na$^+$ influx inhibited by halothane	• Higher n-alkahols have potencies close to induction of anesthesia in animals • High concentrations of pentobarbital necessary for peak current inhibition • Voltage dependent hyperpolarizing shift of inactivation and voltage independent reduction of peak current by high concentrations of propofol • Ketamine decreases peak current at very high concentrations
Ca^{2+}	• Neurotransmitter release • Synaptic transmission • Excitation-contraction coupling	• Tissue dependent effects • HVA and LVA channels inhibited in hippocampal neurons • Decrease in peak and persistent L-type Ca^{2+} current • Peak N-type currents reduced and increasing rate of activation at clinical concentrations • Peak P/Q-type currents inhibited • Inhibition of late R-type currents (slowing rate of inactivation) • T-type current inhibition in DRG at clinical concentrations of isoflurane	• P-type relatively insensitive to thiopental, pentobarbital, and propofol • Inhibition of L-type peak current in tracheal smooth muscle thiopental, ketamine, and propofol at high concentrations
K$^+$	• Action potential conduction • Control of electrical excitability • Neurotransmitter release • Muscle contractility	K$_V$/K$_{Ca}$/K$_{ir}$: • Inhibition of peak K$^+$ current • Depolarizing shift in activation • Reduction in time constant for activation KCNK: • Activated by halothane (TASK1), chloroform (TREK1), and diethyl ether (TREK1)	K$_V$/K$_{Ca}$/K$_{ir}$: • Minimal K$_V$ current depression by opioids, thiopental, methohexital, propofol, ketamine, midazolam, droperidol • No SK channel inhibition by methohexital or ketamine at clinical concentrations • Inhibition of K$_{ir}$ channels by methohexital and pentobarbital at very high concentrations

303

channels by selectively interacting with the inactivated state of the channel *(50)*, and also inhibit Na$^+$ channel-dependent glutamate release from synaptosomes *(51)*. Because anesthetics have been shown to affect PKC activity *(52)* and intracellular Ca^{2+} concentration *(53)*, anesthetics may lead indirectly to altered Na$^+$-channel function.

Volatile anesthetics *(50)* and intravenous anesthetics (e.g., propofol) *(49)* inhibit rat brain type IIa Na$^+$ channels expressed in CHO cells by two mechanisms: voltage-independent block of peak currents and a concentration-dependent shift in steady-state inactivation to hyperpolarized potentials. This leads to a voltage dependence of current suppression, with greater blockade at less polarized potentials.

Neuroprotection

Inhibition of Na$^+$ channels may produce neuroprotective effects and may contribute to the neuroprotective properties of anesthetics. Down-regulation of Na$^+$ channels is a physiological neuroprotective mechanism that exists in reptiles able to survive prolonged periods of hypoxia *(54)*, in neonatal mammals *(55)*, and to a limited extent in anoxic human cerebral cortex *(55)*. Blockade of Na$^+$ channels may have neuroprotective effects in the early stages of ischemia by delaying or preventing anoxic depolarization and subsequent glutamate release by reversed uptake, or later after reperfusion, by reducing vesicular glutamate release, which can then activate potentially deleterious NMDA receptors *(56,57)*.

Effects on Myocardial Cells and Peripheral Neurons

The importance of Na$^+$ channels in the electric stability of the heart is illustrated by arrhythmias produced by Na$^+$ channel mutations in myocardial cells *(58)*. Recent data suggest the involvement of cardiac Na$^+$ channels in the dysrhythmic effects of volatile anesthetics. Isoflurane and halothane depress cardiac Na$^+$ currents directly and indirectly via G protein mediated pathways, and enhance the dysrhythmic effects of β-adrenergic agonists *(59,60)*. Other anesthetics in clinical use (e.g., meperidine *[61]* and ketamine *[62]*) block Na$^+$ currents of rat skeletal myocytes and peripheral nerve, respectively. The Na$^+$ channel blocking effect of local anesthetics is well described *(63)*. The tissue specific expression of TTX resistant, voltage-gated Na$^+$ channels, e.g., PN-1 in the PNS and PN-3 in the dorsal root ganglion (DRG), is of interest for the development of more selective drugs for specific treatment of pain syndromes *(64–67)*.

VOLTAGE-GATED CALCIUM CHANNELS

Physiological and Pharmacological Classification

Multiple cellular functions are determined by the concentration of intracellular free Ca^{2+} ([Ca^{2+}]$_i$), which is controlled by several important regulatory mechanisms. These include voltage-gated Ca^{2+} channels, capacitative Ca^{2+} channels, plasma membrane Ca^{2+}-ATPase (PMCA), endo/sarcoplasmic reticulum Ca^{2+}-ATPases (SERCA), Na$^+$/Ca^{2+} exchangers, and mitochondrial and cytosolic Ca^{2+} sequestration. Alteration of any of those mechanisms by anesthetics may lead to changes in synaptic transmission, gene expression, excitation-contraction coupling, and so on.

As a broad generalization, excitable cells translate their electricity into action by Ca^{2+} fluxes modulated by voltage sensitive Ca^{2+} channels" *(68)*. Ca^{2+} channels are localized to the plasma membrane; distinct isoforms are found in different, specialized locations in specific cell types. They are classified by the degree of depolarization required to gate the channel: low voltage activated (LVA) channels with an activation range that is positive to −70 mV and a peak current at about −30 mV, and high voltage activated (HVA) channels with an activation range positive to −30 mV and a peak current at about +10 mV. They are further classified by their rate and stimulus for inactivation, single channel conductance, sensitivities to specific pharmacologic blocking agents, and more recently by the molecular identity and homology of their α$_1$-subunits *(69,70)* (Table 3).

Table 3
Voltage-Gated Ca²⁺ Channel Family

Type	New channel (a-subunit) names	Tissue expression	Antagonists
L (HVA)	Cav1.1 (α_1S)	α1S-Skeletal muscle	• Dihydropyridines (DHP; e.g., nifedipine)
	Cav1.2 (α_1C)	α1C-Cardiac, CNS, aorta, lung, intestine, and uterus	• Phenylalkylamines (use-dependent; potency reduced by divalent cations; e.g., verapamil)
	Cav1.3 (α_1D)	α1D-CNS, pancreatic islets	• Benzothiazepines (use-dependent; e.g., diltiazem)
N (HVA)	Cav2.2 (α_1B)	Nervous system and neurosecretory cells, CNS and PNS	• ω-Conotoxin GVIA • Less sensitive to DHP
P (HVA)	Cav2.2 (α_1B) (β2a)	Purkinje cell dendrites, periglomerular cells of the olfactory bulb	• FTx (funnel web spider) • ω-Conotoxin MVIIC • ω-Agatoxin IVA
Q (HVA)	Cav2.1 (α_1A) (β1b/β3)	Cerebellar granule cells, hippocampus	• ω-conotoxin MVIIC • DHP-nimodipine *augments* currents containing α1A
R (IVA)	Cav2.3 (α_1E)	CNS most regions	• ω-Agatoxin IVA
T (LVA)	Cav3.1 (α_1G) Cav3.3 (α_1H)	Thalamic and hypothalamic neurons, DRG Cardiac SA & AV nodes, smooth muscle, endocrine cells, and sperm	• Less sensitive to DHP • ω-Agatoxin IVA • Mibefradil (μM) • Phenytoin (use and voltage-dependent, no effect on L-type) • Diphenylbutylpiperidine (DPBP)-based antipsychotic agents (penfluridol)

Location, Function, and Pharmacology

L-Type Ca²⁺ Channels

L-type channels are found mainly in cell bodies and proximal dendrites of neurons *(71)* and on the surface of cardiac myocytes, skeletal myocytes, and endocrine cells. They were the first Ca²⁺ channel subtype identified and have been extensively characterized in cardiac, skeletal, and neuronal tissue *(72)*. The L-type channel pore forming subunit in skeletal muscle is the $\alpha_1$1.1 subunit, in cardiac muscle the $\alpha_1$1.2, and in brain and endocrine cells the $\alpha_1$1.3. In skeletal and cardiac muscle, depolarization leads to channel opening and initiation of contraction. L-type channels can be blocked by 1,4-dihydropyridines (nifedipine, nimodipine) with affinities in the nanomolar range, and by phenylalkylamines (verapamil) and benzothiazepines (diltiazem) with slightly lower affinities.

The α_1-subunit found in L-, N-, P/Q-, and R-type Ca²⁺ channels is homologous to the pore forming α-subunit in Na⁺, and K⁺ channels (Fig. 1). The fourth segment (S4) in each homologous domain contains positively charged amino acids which sense depolarization of the plasma membrane and lead to a conformational change, pore opening (gating), and the selective movement of Ca²⁺ down its electrochemical gradient into the cell.

Inactivation, or the process of channel closing during a prolonged depolarization, occurs more slowly than activation. Inactivation of L-type Ca^{2+} channels occurs by two Ca^{2+}-dependent mechanisms: (1) Ca^{2+} that enters through the α_1-subunit elevates $[Ca^{2+}]_i$ within a few microns of the channel pore and leads to negative feedback *(73)*, and (2) calmodulin, a ubiquitous Ca^{2+} binding protein, is constitutively tethered to an isoleucine-glutamine (IQ) motif in the C-terminal domain of the $\alpha_1 1.2$ subunit, and mediates Ca^{2+}/calmodulin-dependent inactivation.

N-Type Channels

N-type channels ($\alpha_1 2.2$) are found only in neurons and neuroendocrine cells. They are widely distributed in the CNS *(74)* with high densities in striatum, hippocampus, frontal cortex, and cerebellar molecular and granular layers. The localizations of N- and L-type channels are complementary. L-type channels are localized to cell bodies and proximal dendrites, whereas N-type channels are found over all the dendritic surface and at nerve terminals. They are localized along the entire length of the dendrite in a wide range of neurons suggesting that they are important in the initiation of dendritic action potentials and the influx of Ca^{2+} into dendrites. N-type channels are characterized by a conductance of 10–20 pS, and are inhibited by the specific toxin ω-conotoxin GVIA (between 100 and 500 nM; Table 3). The localization of N-type channels to presynaptic terminals is supported by the finding that ω-conotoxin GVIA blocks hippocampal synaptic transmission *(75)*.

P/Q-Type Channels

P/Q-type channels ($\alpha_1 2.1$) were initially described in cerebellar Purkinje cells. They have conductances in the 10–20 pS range, are resistant to dihydropyridines and ω-conotoxin GVIA, and activate above −50 mV peaking at 10 mV. Inactivation is slow. P currents can be blocked by the funnael web spider venom toxin FTX or ω-agatoxin IVA.

P/Q-type channels are low in density in dendrites and high in density in nerve terminals. The α_1-subunit interacts with syntaxin 1A, a SNARE protein component of the protein machinery involved in synaptic vesicle docking and exocytosis. Compared to N-type channels, P/Q-type channels are more concentrated in nerve terminals and appear to be more closely related to neurotransmitter release *(76)*.

R-Type Channels

R-type channels ($\alpha_1 2.3$) are resistant to pharmacologic blockade. They are widely distributed in brain with greater concentration in deep midline structures such as caudate-putamen, thalamus, hypothalamus, amygdala, and cerebellum *(77)*. The $\alpha_1 2.3$ subunit is found in the soma, dendritic field of some neurons, and distal dendritic branches of cerebellar Purkinjie cells. R-type channels conduct transient Ca^{2+} currents and express rapid, voltage-dependent inactivation *(78)*. Activation occurs at relatively negative membrane potentials, resulting in the suggested classification as an intermediate voltage activated (IVA) channel.

T-Type Channels

T-type channels are responsible for pacemaker activity in the heart and for neuronal oscillatory activity. They have been studied in cerebellar Purkinjie cells, thalamic and hippocampal neurons, and in ventricular and atrial myocytes *(79)*. They are low voltage activated channels, with an activating threshold of −70 mV and a peak current at −30 mV. Activation and inactivation are both strongly voltage dependent and quite rapid. Inactivation has a time constant of ~20 ms. Deactivation, the rate at which channels close after a rapid return from a depolarizing pulse to a hyperpolarized potential, is slow *(80)*. T-type channels can be blocked by ω-agatoxin-IVA and by micromolar concentrations of mibefradil, a tetrol anti-hypertensive agent. The affinity of T-type channels for mibefradil is approx 12–13× greater than that of L-type channels. The exact pore-forming subunits have not been unambiguously identified, but appear to be $\alpha_1 3.1$, $\alpha_1 3.2$, and $\alpha_1 3.3$.

Anesthetic Effects on Ca^{2+} Channels

Volatile Anesthetics

CARDIAC L-TYPE CHANNELS

Volatile anesthetic effects on Ca^{2+} channels were first described in heart tissue, where halothane inhibited the slow Ca^{2+} current in kitten papillary muscle *(81)*. Subsequently, halothane, enflurane, and isoflurane were found to inhibit electrically evoked Ca^{2+} transients in guinea pig sinoatrial node *(82)*. Increasing extracellular Ca^{2+} overcame the inhibition, suggesting that the anesthetics inhibited Ca^{2+} entry through Ca^{2+} channels. Binding of radiolabeled nitrendipine was reversibly inhibited by halothane in isolated cardiac sarcolemmal membranes *(83)*, and in intact Langendorff-perfused rabbit hearts *(84)*. These data suggest that volatile anesthetics induce a conformational change in L-type Ca^{2+} channels, or alter accessibility of the binding site to the radiolabeled antagonist. Phenylalkylamine antagonist binding was also inhibited by halothane. These two antagonists bind at distinct sites on the L-type channel suggesting a major alteration in binding site exposure for the entire channel *(85)*.

NEURONAL Ca^{2+} CHANNELS

Owing to their central role in neuronal excitability and synaptic transmission, Ca^{2+} channels are potentially important targets for the action of volatile anesthetics. Blockade of Ca^{2+} channels has been shown to enhance anesthetic potency, suggesting a role for Ca^{2+} channels in anesthesia *(86)*. In spite of this, there is limited information regarding the anesthetic action on individual subtypes of "neuronal" Ca^{2+} channels.

LVA neuronal Ca^{2+} currents activate with small depolarizations and are primarily composed of T-type Ca^{2+} channels. HVA Ca^{2+} currents activate with large depolarizations and are composed of N, L-, P- and Q-type Ca^{2+} channels. Both types of Ca^{2+} currents also have toxin resistant R-type Ca^{2+} currents, which probably represent more than one subtype. Volatile anesthetics reduce peak Ca^{2+} currents in neuronal and neuro-secretory cells. Halothane blocked HVA-Ca^{2+} currents more strongly than LVA in clonal pituitary GH3 cells *(87)*, whereas halothane and isoflurane blocked HVA and LVA Ca^{2+} currents with similar potency in hippocampal pyramidal neurons *(88)*. The potency of halothane to reduce HVA peak Ca^{2+} currents was highest in GH3 cells (IC$_{50}$ = 0.85 mM) *(87)*, lower in rat dorsal root sensory neurons (IC$_{50}$ = 1.0–1.5 mM) *(89)*, and much lower in bovine adrenal chromaffin cells (~30% block at 1.4 mM) *(90)*. Halothane slows the rate of inactivation of HVA Ca^{2+} currents in dorsal root sensory neurons, while it accelerates inactivation in bovine adrenal chromaffin cells *(90)* and hippocampal CA1 neurons *(88)*. Halothane increases the rate of activation of HVA Ca^{2+} currents in dorsal root sensory neurons *(89)* and adrenal chromaffin cells *(91)*, but not in hippocampal CA1 neurons *(92)*. Such variability in anesthetic sensitivity and effects could result from the presence of different proportions of Ca^{2+} channel subtypes in different cells.

At clinically relevant concentrations, halothane decreased peak and persistent L-type Ca^{2+} currents, accelerated inactivation, and slowed activation in human neuroblastoma (SH-SY5Y) cells *(93)*. When expressed in *Xenopus* oocytes, the peak of various HVA neuronal Ca^{2+} currents (P/Q-, N-, L- and R- types, represented by $\alpha_1$2.1, $\alpha_1$2.2, $\alpha_1$1.3, and $\alpha_1$2.3 subunits, respectively, coexpressed with $\beta_{1/B}$ and α_2/δ subunits) were inhibited to a similar extent by halothane and isoflurane *(94)*. The late currents (reflecting the rate and/or level of inactivation) were more strongly inhibited in R- than in P/Q- and N-type channels. Interestingly, L-type currents did not display inactivation in the absence or presence of volatile anesthetics, as shown for L-type currents in muscle and neuronal cells *(95)*. Therefore, differences in volatile anesthetic actions on HVA Ca^{2+} currents observed in various neuronal cells may not be explained by the expression of different proportions of HVA Ca^{2+} channel subtypes. The data suggest that either subunit composition, regulatory mechanisms, and/or other environmental factors (neuronal vs *Xenopus* oocyte, different experimental conditions) contribute not only to baseline channel function but also to differences in anesthetic actions on HVA Ca^{2+} currents.

Volatile anesthetics may specifically affect neuronal intracellular Ca^{2+} by modulating the function of N-type Ca^{2+} channels. Isoflurane inhibited peak Ca^{2+} current (presumably N-type) and accelerated inactivation in parasympathetic neurons enzymatically isolated from bullfrog interatrial septum (96). G-protein signalling is affected by anesthetics (97–100), and G-protein activation lowers the potency of volatile anesthetics (99,100). In SH-SY5Y cells, 0.3 mM isoflurane reduced N-type currents by 50%, which was eliminated by G-protein activation with GTPγS (E. Recio-Pinto, unpublished observation). This suggests a novel mechanism of anesthetic effects on Ca^{2+} channel function that could underlie some of the cell type specific actions reported.

The effects of halothane, isoflurane, and enflurane on T-type Ca^{2+} currents were compared in four cell types from four different species: neonatal rat dorsal root gangion neurons, thyroid C cells derived from rat medullary thyroid carcinoma, calf adrenal glomerulosa cells, and guinea pig ventricular myocytes (80). The neonatal ventricular myocytes were least sensitive to inhibition (20% inhibition by high concentrations of isoflurane (1.2 mM) and halothane (1.4 mM). At a lower concentration (0.7 mM, ~2 MAC), isoflurane inhibited peak current between 30 and 50% in the three other cell types. In these three cell types, halothane was the least potent anesthetic. The differing sensitivities suggest several possibilities including different α_1-subunit isoforms modulatory accessory subunits, regulatory mechanisms and possibly membrane compositions. Isoflurane (1.5 MAC) and sevoflurane (1.5 MAC) dilate bronchial smooth muscle probably due to T-type channel inhibition (101).

Intravenous Anesthetics

Intravenous anesthetics also depress Ca^{2+} currents through in several systems. The overriding consideration in these studies is whether the concentrations studied encompass a clinically relevant range. The majority of studies have been performed on L-type Ca^{2+} channels in cardiac tissue or myocytes (102–106).

Ca^{2+} current in cultured canine myocytes was inhibited 33% by 60 μM propofol, and 16% by 60 μM etomidate (102), clearly supratherapeutic concentrations. In guinea pig myocytes (106), Ca^{2+} current was inhibited by propofol (K_D = 54 μM). In rat cardiac membranes, a significant decrease in the K_D for radiolabeled nitrendipine binding occurred at 6 μM propofol (103). In rat cerebral cortical membranes, binding of nitrendipine was inhibited by propofol, etomidate, and ketamine, while binding of verapamil was unaffected (107). This is different from the effects of halothane on cardiac L-type channels, where both binding sites were similarly altered (83,85). L-type Ca^{2+} channels in tracheal smooth muscle were much less sensitive to intravenous anesthetics; 50% depression of Ca^{2+} current occurred at 300 μM thiopental, 1000 μM ketamine, or 300 μM propofol, all clearly supratherapeutic concentrations. P-type channels in rat Purkinje cells were also relatively insensitive to thiopental, pentobarbital, and propofol (108). Propofol, ketamine, etomidate, and alphaxalone had negligible effects on ω-conotoxin MVII(A) binding to N-type channels in rat cerebrocortical membranes (104).

In summary, voltage-dependent Ca^{2+} channels may be important sites of volatile anesthetic action. Multiple types of Ca^{2+} channels have differing sensitivities to volatile anesthetics that are currently difficult to explain. The factors involved in determining Ca^{2+} channel sensitivity may include different subunit compositions, channel environments, and regulatory mechanisms. The findings for intravenous anesthetics also vary depending on the channel type, tissue source and anesthetic studied. In general, Ca^{2+} channels are less sensitive to intravenous than to volatile anesthetics.

POTASSIUM CHANNELS

Physiological and Pharmacological Classification

Potassium (K^+) channels are a large and diverse ion channel family; the *C. elegans* genome contains almost 100 unique K^+ channels (109). K^+ channels regulate multiple cellular function including electrical excitability, release of neurotransmitters, muscle contractility, and many other secretory and intracellular functions. Multiple subtypes of K$^+$ channels are distinguished by their activation properties (Table 4). K$^+$ channels can be controlled by a variety of important regulatory mechanisms (e.g., voltage, Ca^{2+}, ATP). The resting potential of most cells is -50 to -70 mV, whereas the Nernst equilibrium potential (E$_K$) for K$^+$ is approx -90 mV. Thus, K$^+$ channel opening allows K$^+$ to exit the cell (outward current), driving the membrane potential toward hyperpolarization (more negative potential). This moves the membrane potential away from the action potential threshold, thus decreasing excitability. Any drug or modulator that increases the probability of K$^+$ channel opening thus reduces excitability and vice versa. The discovery that certain diseases (e.g., long QT syndrome) are related to genetic mutations and malfunction of K$^+$ channels emphasizes their importance in the regulation of membrane potential.

Location, Function, and Pharmacology

Voltage-Gated K$^+$ Channels (K$_V$)

Nine families of voltage-gated K$^+$ channels have been described *(110)*. The structure of voltage-gated K$^+$ channels is similar with a large α-subunit (Fig. 1) whose structure is supported by the recent determination of the crystal structure of the K$_{CSA}$ channel from *Streptomyces lividans (1)*. In addition, an intracellular β-subunit has been described (Table 4).

The best described channels derive from the *Drosophila* K$^+$ channels Shaker, Shab, Shaw, and Shal. Structural and functional analysis of these channels has been possible with channel specific inhibitor peptides such as the peptide scorpion venoms that target the K$_V$1 family *(111)*. Charybdotoxin (ChTX) *(112)* blocks K$_V$1.2 and K$_V$1.3 channels by binding in the external vestibule of the pore. Many K$_V$1 blocking peptides are neurotoxic when administered intrathecally. K$_V$1 family members are widely distributed in the central and peripheral nervous system. K$_V$ 1.1 knockout mice develop spontaneous epileptic seizures because of altered electrical activity in the hippocampus *(113)*, hearing deficiencies *(114)*, and a lower pain threshold *(115)*. Mutations in the human K$_V$1.1 gene lead to episodic ataxia/myokymia *(116)*. Together, these data stress the importance of voltage-gated K$^+$-channels in electric stability in the CNS.

Voltage-gated K$^+$ channel opening (gating) occurs within 1 ms and the channel closes within 10 ms. Although the voltage threshold for each K$^+$-channel subtype is different, the basic molecular mechanism of channel opening is similar. Secondary to changes in V$_m$, conformational changes are thought to open the channel. Functional channels require the association of four subunits. Usually, only members of the same K$_V$ subfamily associate. Heterotetrameric channels are functional, with different biophysical and pharmacological properties *(117,118)*. Association of K$_V$ channels (e.g., K$_V$ 1) with the cytoplasmatic β-subunit alters channel inactivation kinetics *(119)*. The K$_V$8 and K$_V$9 subunits do not form functional channels alone, but associate with other channel subunits to form functional complexes *(120)*. Two distinct inactivation processes have been described for K$_V$ channels. Rapid inactivation (N-type inactivation) with Shaker type K$^+$ channels involves the N-terminus. Similar to the hinged lid mechanism in Na$^+$ channels, charged amino acids in the N-terminus move into the intracellular pore of the open channel and block further ion flow *(121)*. As the membrane recharges, the lid moves away from the pore opening, allowing new K$^+$ currents. Slow inactivation (C-type inactivation) involves the C-terminus and may be owing to a conformational change leading to narrowing of the mouth of the pore *(122)*.

Ca^{2+}-Activated K$^+$ Channels (K$_{Ca}$)

This large family of K$^+$ channels is characterized by the dependence of channel opening on intracellular Ca^{2+} concentration in the range of 1 μ*M*. They are further categorized by differences in single channel conductance as small (2–25 pS), intermediate (25–100 pS), and large (100–300 pS) conductance channels *(123)*. The best studied K$_{Ca}$ channel is the large conductance channel (BK) from rat brain (mSlo) with rapid activation (1–2 ms) and inactivation (~10 ms). BK channels can be activated by depolarization as well *(124)*.

Table 4
K$^+$ Channel Family

Names	New channel (a-subunit) names	Tissue expression	Antagonists
Voltage-gated (K$_V$)			
Shaker	K$_V$1.1-1.8	Brain, atrium,	• Charybdotoxin (CTX)
Shab	K$_V$2.1-2.2	ventricle, lung, islet	• Noxiustoxin (NxTX)
Shaw	K$_V$3.1-3.4	cells, kidney, retina,	• Margatoxin (MgTX)
Shal	K$_V$4.1-4.2	and liver	• Kaliotoxin (KTX)
LongQT (LQT)	K$_V$5		• Hongotoxin (HgTX)
Ether a-go-go/HERG	K$_V$6		• Agitoxin (AgTX)
Aplysia KV5.1	K$_V$7		• Dendrotoxin (DTX)
–	K$_V$8		
–	K$_V$9		
Calcium-activated (K$_{Ca}$)			
Large conductance, BK	BK$_{Ca}$	Brain, aorta, trachea,	BK:
Intermediate conductance	IK$_{Ca}$1	colon, coronary	• CTX
Small conductance	SK$_{Ca}$13–3	arteries	• Iberiotoxin (IbTX)
			• Limbatoxin (LbTX)
			• Tetraethylammonium (TEA)
			SK:
			• Apamin
			• Quinidine
Inward rectifier (K$_{ir}$)			
ROMK 1-2	K$_{ir}$ 1.1a/b	Cardiac, neuronal,	• TEA
IRK 1	K$_{ir}$ 2.1	endocrine cells,	• Cs$^+$, Rb$^+$, Na$^+$, Ba^{2+}, Mg^{2+}
IRK 2	K$_{ir}$ 2.2	atrial pacemaker cells,	
IRK 3	K$_{ir}$ 2.3	and smooth muscle	• Tolbutamide (K$_{ATP}$)
GIRK 1	K$_{ir}$ 3.1		• Glibenclamide (K$_{ATP}$)
GIRK 2/K$_{ATP}$-2	K$_{ir}$ 3.2		• Quinidine (K$_{ATP}$)
GIRK 3	K$_{ir}$ 3.3		• 4-Aminopyridine
GIRK 4/cK$_{ATP}$-1	K$_{ir}$ 3.4		(delayed rectifier)
BIR 10	K$_{ir}$ 4.1		
BIR 9	K$_{ir}$ 5.1		
u-K$_{ATP}$-1	K$_{ir}$ 6.1		
BIR/K$_{ATP}$	K$_{ir}$ 6.2		
Kir1.4	K$_{ir}$7.1		
Tandem pore domain (KCNK)			
TWIK-1		CNS, spinal cord	Resistant to TEA and
TASK		cerebellum, and	4-aminopyridine
TRAAK		myocuytes	

BK channels exist as a heterodimer of transmembrane α- and intracellular β-subunits. The α-subunit is somewhat different from voltage-gated K$^+$ channels as it possesses seven transmembrane domains rather than six. An extra transmembrane region (S$_0$) is located at the N-terminus

(125). The site of Ca^{2+} binding is located in the C-terminus *(126)*. A possible voltage sensor has been described in the S_4 region *(127)*.

The function of the α-subunit is altered by coexpression of auxiliary β-subunits. The β1 subunit is expressed mainly in aorta, trachea, colon, and coronary arteries, but not significantly in brain. A different subunit appears to be associated with BK channels in brain *(128)*. Coexpression of the β-subunit hyperpolarizes the membrane by shifting channel activation. The β2 subunit inactivates the BK channel rapidly and shifts the voltage dependence to hyperpolarized potentials *(129)*.

Inwardly Rectifying K⁺ Channels (K_Ir)

Inwardly rectifying K^+ channels regulate the resting membrane potential; they are therefore important for the regulation of cardiac, neuronal and endocrine cells *(130)*. Of the large family of K_{ir} channels, $K_{Ir}2$, 3, and 6 channels are important in brain. $K_{ir}2.x$ channels play a role in controlling the excitability of heart and brain. $K_{ir}3.x$ channels are G-protein activated and mediate the effects of G-protein-coupled receptors on electrical activity in cardiac, neuronal, and neurosecretory cells *(131)*. Of clinical importance is the K_{ATP} channel found in heart, pancreas, smooth muscle and CNS. This channel links cell metabolism to electrical activity. Clinically used sulphonylureas (glibenclamide, tolbutamide) bind to their receptor (SUR), which forms a functional complex with $K_{ir}6.2$ *(132,133)*. The resulting complex forms an active K^+ channel that is inhibited by intracellular ATP. At low metabolic states (low ATP), they open and hyperpolarize the cell membrane, preventing further energy consuming work of ion pumps. Different subunits of SUR and K_{ir} show tissue specific expression and function. Thus, the SUR1-$K_{ir}6.2$ complex is expressed in pancreatic β-cells, and plays a central role in insulin secretion. The SUR2a-$K_{ir}6.2$ isoform is expressed in cardiac cells and the SUR2b-$K_{IR}6.2$ complex forms channels in smooth muscle. K_{ATP} channels in cardiac cells play a role in the cardioprotection induced by ischemic preconditioning and possibly by anesthetic exposure *(134)*.

K_{ir} channels are tetramers of four identical (homomeric) or related (heteromeric) subunits. Each α-subunit consists of two transmembrane α-helices (TM1 and TM2), linked by a short stretch of ~30 amino acids that forms the helix for the pore and an extracellular loop *(130)*. These channels conduct higher currents at hyperpolarization. This is probably related to voltage-dependent block of outward current by cytoplasmatic cations (mainly Mg^{2+} and polyamines) that enter the pore under the influence of the membrane potential and impede K^+ efflux.

Rectification refers to the ability of K^+ channels to facilitate ion conduction more easily in one direction than the other, reflected in characteristic I/V relationships. This characteristic plays an important role in setting the membrane potential and regulating overall excitability *(135)*. The direction of current is defined by the reversal potential. At membrane potentials near the resting potential and below the reversal potential (~40 mV), they have a linear relationship between inward current and membrane potential. With small depolarizations they pass a small outward current, and with large depolarizations they are blocked, allowing action potential firing *(135)*.

K_{ir} channels are modulated by membrane potential and by intracellular ligands including the $G_{β/γ}$ subunits of heterotrimeric G-proteins, the membrane phospholipid PIP_2, ATP, and protons *(130)*. An example of G-protein mediated activation of K^+ channels is the muscarinic (M_2 subtype) receptor in atrial pacemaker cells. This receptor mobilizes G-proteins ($G_{β/γ}$) that activate inwardly rectifying K^+ channels (GIRK: G-protein linked inwardly rectifying K^+ channels). This hyperpolarizes the plama membrane in diastole and decreases the slope of spontaneous depolarization, slowing heart rate.

Tandem Pore Domain K⁺ Channels (KCNK)

The molecular structure of KCNK channels remained obscure until recently when a new family of background K^+ channels was cloned *(136)*. The original channel was cloned from yeast (TOK-1). Since then several mammalian channels with the functional properties of background K^+ channels have been described. They consist of the weak inward rectifiers TWIK-1/2, the outward rectifier (TREK-1/2, TRAAK, TASK) resembling the previously described "I_{kan}" and *Aplysia* K^+ channel, and the open rectifiers TASK-1/2 and TRAAK.

TRAAK and TREK-1/2 are directly opened by arachadonic acid and polyunsaturated fatty acids *(137,138)*, whereas TASK is pH sensitive. TWIK channels are Mg^{2+} dependent. Though all tandem pore channels are modified by multiple stimuli, they share resistance to traditional K^+ channel inhibitors (e.g., tetraethylammonium and 4-aminopyridine). Further investigation of their physiologic roles and tissue distributions is necessary to understand their impact in anesthesia.

KCNK channels are characterized by four transmembrane domains (TM1–4) flanking two pore regions (Fig. 1). The pore regions contain atypical selectivity filters and a large extracellular loop between TM1 and TM2. This extracellular loop (P1) is well conserved and forms the first pore. Subunits form heterodimers with four domains lining two ion channels *(139)*. Pore formation might involve disulfide bridges, since it is sensitive to reducing agents. The C-terminus of TRAK-1 participates in a number of fundamental properties, such as binding of phospholipids and mechanical or acid stimulation *(140,141)*. All channels are expressed in brain, and TRAAK expressed exclusively in the CNS. TASK-2 is mainly expressed in spinal cord *(142)*, TREK-2 in cerebellar tissue *(143)* and TASK-1 in myocardial cells and brainstem neurons.

Anesthetic Effects on K+ Channels

Given the important role of K^+ channels in the CNS, anesthetic effects on these channels would affect neuronal excitability, and K^+ channels have been proposed as possible targets for anesthetics. However, direct electrophysiologic measurements of most K^+ channels, with the notable exception of tandem pore channels, indicate minimal effects at relevant (clinical) anesthetic concentrations *(43)* (Table 2). The definition of clinically relevant concentrations of anesthetics in experimental settings is critical for the evaluation of the clinical relevance of in vitro data.

Central Nervous System

Many CNS receptors directly or indirectly activate the function of K_{ir} channels *(144)*. Stimulation of opioid receptors activates K^+ channels and produces neuronal hyperpolarization *(145)*. Early data suggested K^+ channels to be responsible for the hyperpolarization induced by volatile anesthetics. Diethyl ether and halothane hyperpolarized rat hippocampal neurons by increasing K^+ permeability *(146)*. Isoflurane (1.5–5 vol %) *(147,148)* and enflurane (1–5 vol %) *(149)* hyperpolarized rat and human cortical and hippocampal neurons. K^+ channels in invertebrate neurons were activated by volatile anesthetics in *Lymnae stagnalis (150)* and *Aplysia california (151,152)*. Rats infused at the locus ceruleus with several inhibitors of K_{Ca}, K_V and K_{ATP} channels showed reduction in the hypnotic effects of the α_{2a} agonist dexmedetomidine *(153)*.

VOLTAGE-GATED K+ CHANNELS (K_V)

Very high concentrations of halothane (5 mM, ~20 MAC), isoflurane, methoxyflurane (3 mM, ~10 MAC), or chloroform inhibit Shaker type K^+ channels in a receptor state dependent manner *(44,154)*.

Intravenous anesthetics (thiopental, propofol, ketamine, and midazolam) and opioids inhibited voltage-gated K^+ channels in a concentration-dependent manner. Nevertheless, K^+ current suppression at clinical concentrations is predicted to be less than 0.1% for opioids and approx 3% for intravenous anesthetics *(155)*.

CA2+-ACTIVATED K+ CHANNELS (K_{CA})

Volatile anesthetics failed to affect BK channels in hippocampal neurons *(156)*. K^+ channel blockers prevent the vasodilation in cerebrovascular smooth muscle cells of the rat *(157)* induced by halothane, suggesting the involvement of K_{Ca} channels in this effect.

Intravenous anesthetics inhibited SK-2 channels expressed in vitro while volatile anesthetics failed to produce significant effects at 1 MAC *(158)*.

INWARDLY RECTIFYING K+ CHANNELS (K_{IR})

Methohexital and pentobarbital reversibly inhibited K_{ir} channels in RBL-1 cells (IC_{50} of 145 μM and 218 μM, respectively), concentrations significantly above clinically relevant concentrations *(159)*.

Tandem Pore Domain K⁺ Channels (KCNK)

Evidence for volatile anesthetic sensitivity of tandem pore K⁺ channels came initially from the yeast channel TOK-1. This channel displays similarities to the *Aplysia* baseline K⁺ channel. Expression of this channel in *Xenopus* oocytes demonstrated potentiation and an increase in channel open probability at high concentrations of a series of volatile anesthetics (isoflurane, halothane, or desflurane) *(160)*. Initial data on mammalian tandem pore K⁺ channels demonstrated the activation of TASK-1 channels expressed in COS cells by isoflurane (2 mM) and halothane (0.1–0.3 mM) *(161)*. TREK-1 was also activated by chloroform (1 mM) and diethyl ether (0.6 mM). The activation was C-terminus dependent and occured at clinical concentrations. Further studies demonstrated sensitivity of hypoglossal nerve cells in rat brain slices to halothane and sevoflurane and linked it to the TASK-1 channel. Conductance of this channel increased after exposure to halothane in vitro *(162)*. Recently, the human baseline K⁺ channel KCNK5 (TASK-2) was reported to be potentiated by high concentrations of halothane and isoflurane *(142)*.

Cardiac Function

Most general anesthetics display cardiac side effects, which might be related to effects on cardiac K⁺ channels. Inhibition of cardiac K⁺ channels by volatile anesthetics overlaps their clinically relevant dose range *(163)*. Volatile anesthetics stimulate K$_{ATP}$ channels. The vasodilating effects of halothane *(164)* and isoflurane *(165)* were inhibited by glibenclamide suggesting the involvement of K$_{ATP}$ channels in myocardial preservation *(166–168)*. However, patch clamp experiments on isolated rabbit ventricular myocytes found isoflurane to inhibit K⁺ conductance *(169)*, suggesting possible indirect effects of volatile anesthetics on K⁺ channels *(170)* via G-protein coupled pathways. Thiopental inhibited inwardly rectifying K⁺ channels, possibly contributing to the arrhythmogenicity of other agents (halothane, epinephrine, CO_2).

SUMMARY

Voltage-gated ion channels are integral to multiple neuronal functions. Their function is significantly altered by a variety of general anesthetics, but their overall contribution to the clinical effects of general anesthesia is still unclear. Most channels are only sensitive to concentrations of anesthetics that are above clinical concentrations. Nevertheless, further investigation of these effects and their impact on neuronal networks should aid in the identification of ion channels relevant to the effects of general anesthetics. The ongoing characterization of ion channels and the increasing knowledge of their molecular and physiological properties may contribute to the development of drugs with greater tissue specificity and potentially fewer side effects.

REFERENCES

1. Doyle, D. A., Morais Cabral, J., Pfuetzner, R. A., et al. (1998) The structure of the potassium channel: molecular basis of K⁺ conduction and selectivity. *Science* **280,** 69–77.
2. Sato, C., Veno, Y., Asai, K., et al. (2001) The voltage-sensitive sodium channel is a bell-shaped molecule with several cavities. *Nature* **409,** 1047–1051.
3. Catterall, W. A. (2000) From ionic currents to molecular mechanisms: the structure and function of voltage-gated sodium channels. *Neuron* **26,** 13–25.
4. Ragsdale, D. S., McPhee, J. C., Scheuer, T., and Catterall, W. A. (1996) Common molecular determinants of local anesthetic, antiarrhythmic, and anticonvulsant block of voltage-gated Na⁺ channels. *Proc. Natl. Acad. Sci. USA* **93,** 9270–9275.
5. Ragsdale, D. S., McPhee, J. C., Scheuer, T., and Catterall, W. A. (1994) Molecular determinants of state-dependent block of Na⁺ channels by local anesthetics. *Science* **265,** 1724–1728.
6. Cestele, S. and Catterall, W. A. (2000) Molecular mechanisms of neurotoxin action on voltage-gated sodium channels. *Biochimie* **82,** 883–892.
7. Backx, P. H., Yue, D. T., Lawrence, J. H., Marban, E., and Tomaselli, G. F. (1992) Molecular localization of an ion-binding site within the pore of mammalian sodium channels. *Science* **257,** 248–251.
8. Satin, J., Kyle, J. W., Chen, M., et al. (1992) A mutant of TTX-resistant cardiac sodium channels with TTX-sensitive properties. *Science* **256,** 1202–1205.

9. Sivilotti, L., Okuse, K., Akopian, A. N., Noss, S., and Wood, J. N. (1997) A single serine residue confers tetrodotoxin insensitivity on the rat sensory-neuron-specific sodium channel SNS. *FEBS Lett.* **409,** 49–52.

10. Hartshorne, R. P. and Catterall, W. A. (1981) Purification of the saxitoxin receptor of the sodium channel from rat brain. *Proc. Natl. Acad. Sci. USA* **78,** 4620–4624.

11. Hartshorne, R. P., Messner, D. J., Coppersmith, J. C., and Catterall, W. A. (1982) The saxitoxin receptor of the sodium channel from rat brain. Evidence for two nonidentical beta subunits. *J. Biol. Chem.* **257,** 13,888–13,891.

12. Noda, M., Shimizu, S., Tanabe, T., et al. (1984) Primary structure of Electrophorus electricus sodium channel deduced from cDNA sequence. *Nature* **312,** 121–127.

13. Isom, L. L., De Jongh, K. S., Patton, D. E., et al. (1992) Primary structure and functional expression of the beta 1 subunit of the rat brain sodium channel. *Science* **256,** 839–842.

14. Isom, L. L., Ragsdale, D. S., De Jongh, K. S., et al. (1995) Structure and function of the beta 2 subunit of brain sodium channels, a transmembrane glycoprotein with a CAM motif. *Cell* **83,** 433–442.

15. Srinivasan, J., Schachner, M., and Catterall, W. A. (1998) Interaction of voltage-gated sodium channels with the extracellular matrix molecules tenascin-C and tenascin-R. *Proc. Natl. Acad. Sci. USA* **95,** 15,753–15,757.

16. Miller, J. A., Agnew, W. S., and Levinson, S. R. (1983) Principal glycopeptide of the tetrodotoxin/saxitoxin binding protein from Electrophorus electricus: isolation and partial chemical and physical characterization. *Biochemistry* **22,** 462–470.

17. Barchi, R. L. (1983) Protein components of the purified sodium channel from rat skeletal muscle sarcolemma. *J. Neurochem.* **40,** 1377–1385.

18. Noda, M., Ikeda, T., Suzuki, H., et al. (1986) Expression of functional sodium channels from cloned cDNA. *Nature* **322,** 826–828.

19. Goldin, A. L., Snutch, T., Lubbert, H., et al. (1986) Messenger RNA coding for only the alpha subunit of the rat brain Na channel is sufficient for expression of functional channels in *Xenopus* oocytes. *Proc. Natl. Acad. Sci. USA* **83,** 7503–7507.

20. Catterall, W. A. (1991) Functional subunit structure of voltage-gated calcium channels. *Science* **253,** 1499, 1500.

21. Terlau, H., Heinmann, S. H., Stuhmer, W., et al. (1991) Mapping the site of block by tetrodotoxin and saxitoxin of sodium channel II. *FEBS Lett.* **293,** 93–96.

22. Benitah, J. P., Chen, Z., Balser, J. R., Tomaselli, G. F., and Marban, E. (1999) Molecular dynamics of the sodium channel pore vary with gating: interactions between P-segment motions and inactivation. *J. Neurosci.* **19,** 1577–1585.

23. Heinemann, S. H., Terlau, H., Stuhmer, W., Imoto, K., and Numa, S. (1992) Calcium channel characteristics conferred on the sodium channel by single mutations. *Nature* **356,** 441–443.

24. Armstrong, C. M. (1981) Sodium channels and gating currents. *Physiol. Rev.* **61,** 644–683.

25. Hirschberg, B., Rovner, A., Liberman, M., and Patlak, J. (1995) Transfer of twelve charges is needed to open skeletal muscle Na$^+$ channels. *J. Gen. Physiol.* **106,** 1053–1068.

26. Stuhmer, W., Conti, F., Suzuki, H., et al. (1989) Structural parts involved in activation and inactivation of the sodium channel. *Nature* **339,** 597–603.

27. Catterall, W. A. (1986) Molecular properties of voltage-sensitive sodium channels. *Annu. Rev. Biochem.* **55,** 953–985.

28. Guy, H. R. and Seetharamulu, P. (1986) Molecular model of the action potential sodium channel. *Proc. Natl. Acad. Sci. USA* **83,** 508–512.

29. Wang, M. H., Yusaf, S. P., Elliott, D. J., Wray, D., and Sivaprasadaro, A. (1999) Effect of cysteine substitutions on the topology of the S4 segment of the Shaker potassium channel: implications for molecular models of gating. *J. Physiol. (Lond.)* **521 Pt 2,** 315–326.

30. Cestele, S., Qu, Y., Rogers, J. C., Rochat, H., Scheuer, T., and Catterall, W. A. (1998) Voltage sensor-trapping: enhanced activation of sodium channels by beta- scorpion toxin bound to the S3–S4 loop in domain II. *Neuron* **21,** 919–931.

31. Armstrong, C. M. (1975) Evidence for ionic pores in excitable membranes. *Biophys. J.* **15,** 932–933.

32. West, J. W., Patton, D. E., Scheuer, T., Wang, Y., Goldin, A. L., and Catterall, W. A. (1992) A cluster of hydrophobic amino acid residues required for fast Na(+)- channel inactivation. *Proc. Natl. Acad. Sci. USA* **89,** 10,910–10,914.

33. Kellenberger, S., West, J. W., Scheuer, T., and Catterall, W. A. (1997) Molecular analysis of the putative inactivation particle in the inactivation gate of brain type IIA Na$^+$ channels. *J. Gen. Physiol.* **109,** 589–605.

34. Kellenberger, S., West, J. W., Scheuer, T., and Catterall, W. A. (1997) Molecular analysis of potential hinge residues in the inactivation gate of brain type IIA Na$^+$ channels. *J. Gen. Physiol.* **109,** 607–617.

35. Cha, A., Ruben, P. C., George, A. L., Jr., Fujimoto, E., and Bezanilla, F. (1999) Voltage sensors in domains III and IV, but not I and II, are immobilized by Na$^+$ channel fast inactivation. *Neuron* **22,** 73–87.

36. Zhang, X. F., Hu, X. T., and White, F. J. (1998) Whole-cell plasticity in cocaine withdrawal: reduced sodium currents in nucleus accumbens neurons. *J. Neurosci.* **18,** 488–498.

37. Calabresi, P., Mercuri, N., Stanzione, P., Stefani, A., and Bernardi, G. (1987) Intracellular studies on the dopamine-induced firing inhibition of neostriatal neurons in vitro: evidence for D1 receptor involvement. *Neuroscience* **20,** 757–771.

38. Rossie, S. and Catterall, W. A. (1987) Cyclic-AMP-dependent phosphorylation of voltage-sensitive sodium channels in primary cultures of rat brain neurons. *J. Biol. Chem.* **262,** 12,735–12,744.

39. Hilborn, M. D., Vaillancourt, R. R., and Rane, S. G. (1998) Growth factor receptor tyrosine kinases acutely regulate neuronal sodium channels through the src signaling pathway. *J. Neurosci.* **18,** 590–600.

40. Costa, M. R. and Catterall, W. A. (1984) Phosphorylation of the alpha subunit of the sodium channel by protein kinase C. *Cell. Mol. Neurobiol.* **4,** 291–297.

41. Cantrell, A. R., Ma, J. Y., Scheuer, T., and Catterall, W. A. (1996) Muscarinic modulation of sodium current by activation of protein kinase C in rat hippocampal neurons. *Neuron* **16,** 1019–1026.

42. Ratcliffe, C. F., Qu, Y., Mc Cormick, K. A., et al. (2000) A sodium channel signaling complex: modulation by associated receptor protein tyrosine phosphatase beta. *Nat. Neurosci.* **3,** 437–444.

43. Franks, N. P. and Lieb, W. R. (1994) Molecular and cellular mechanisms of general anaesthesia. *Nature* **367,** 607–614.

44. Haydon, D. A. and Urban, B. W. (1986) The actions of some general anaesthetics on the potassium current of the squid giant axon. *J. Physiol.* **373,** 311–327.

45. Grossman, Y. and Kendig, J. J. (1982) General anesthetic block of a bifurcating axon. *Brain Res.* **245,** 148–153.

46. Langmoen, I. A., Larsen, M., and Berg-Johnsen, J. (1995) Volatile anaesthetics: cellular mechanisms of action. *Eur. J. Anaesthesiol.* **12,** 51–58.

47. Frenkel, C., Duch, D. S., and Urban, B. W. (1990) Molecular actions of pentobarbital isomers on sodium channels from human brain cortex. *Anesthesiology* **72,** 640–649.

48. Duch, D. S., Wartenberg, H. C., and Urban, B. W. (1995) Dissecting pentobarbitone actions on single voltage-gated sodium channels. *Eur. J. Anaesthesiol.* **12,** 71–81.

49. Rehberg, B. and Duch, D. S. (1999) Suppression of central nervous system sodium channels by propofol. *Anesthesiology* **91,** 512–520.

50. Rehberg, B., Xiao, Y. H., and Duch, D. S. (1996) Central nervous system sodium channels are significantly suppressed at clinical concentrations of volatile anesthetics. *Anesthesiology, discussion 27A* **84,** 1223–1233.

51. Schlame, M. and Hemmings, H. C., Jr. (1995) Inhibition by volatile anesthetics of endogenous glutamate release from synaptosomes by a presynaptic mechanism. *Anesthesiology* **82,** 1406–1416.

52. Hemmings, H. C. (1998) General anesthetic effects on protein kinase C. *Toxicol. Lett.* **100–101,** 89–95.

53. Kindler, C. H., Eilers, H., Donohoe, P., Ozer, S., and Bickler, P. E. (1999) Volatile anesthetics increase intracellular calcium in cerebrocortical and hippocampal neurons. *Anesthesiology* **90,** 1137–1145.

54. Perez-Pinzon, M. A., Rosenthal, M., Sick, T. J., Lutz, P. L., Pablo, J., and Mash, D. (1992) Downregulation of sodium channels during anoxia: a putative survival strategy of turtle brain. *Am. J. Physiol.* **262,** R712–R715.

55. Cummins, T. R., Jiang, C., and Haddad, G. G. (1993) Human neocortical excitability is decreased during anoxia via sodium channel modulation. *J. Clin. Invest.* **91,** 608–615.

56. Taylor, C. P. and Meldrum, B. S. (1995) Na$^+$ channels as targets for neuroprotective drugs. *Trends Pharmacol. Sci.* **16,** 309–316.

57. Hemmings, H. (1997) Neuroprotection by Sodium Channel Blockade and Inhibition of Glutamate Release, in *Neuroprotection,* T. Blanck, Editor, Williams & Wilkins: New York. pp. 23–46.

58. Tan, H. L., Bink-Boelkins, M. T., Bezzina, C. R., et al. (2001) A sodium-channel mutation causes isolated cardiac conduction disease. *Nature* **409,** 1043–1047.

59. Weigt, H. U., Kwok, W. M., Rehmert, G. C., and Bosnjak, Z. J. (1998) Sensitization of the cardiac Na channel to alpha1-adrenergic stimulation by inhalation anesthetics: evidence for distinct modulatory pathways. *Anesthesiology* **88,** 125–133.

60. Weigt, H. U., Kwok, W. M., Rehmert, G. C., and Bosnjak, Z. J. (1998) Modulation of the cardiac sodium current by inhalational anesthetics in the absence and presence of beta-stimulation. *Anesthesiology* **88,** 114–124.

61. Wagner, L. E., 2nd, Eaton, M., Sabnis, S. S., and Gingrich, K. J. (1999) Meperidine and lidocaine block of recombinant voltage-dependent Na$^+$ channels: evidence that meperidine is a local anesthetic. *Anesthesiology* **91,** 1481–1490.

62. Brau, M. E., Sander, F., Vogel, W., and Hempelmann, G. (1997) Blocking mechanisms of ketamine and its enantiomers in enzymatically demyelinated peripheral nerve as revealed by single-channel experiments. *Anesthesiology* **86,** 394–404.

63. Tetzlaff, J. E. (2000) The pharmacology of local anesthetics. *Anesthesiol. Clin. N. A.* **18,** 217–233.

64. Novakovic, S. D., Tzoumaka, E., McGivern, J. G., et al. (1998) Distribution of the tetrodotoxin-resistant sodium channel PN3 in rat sensory neurons in normal and neuropathic conditions. *J. Neurosci.* **18,** 2174–2187.

65. Sleeper, A. A., Cummins, T. R., Dib-Hajj, S. D., et al. (2000) Changes in expression of two tetrodotoxin-resistant sodium channels and their currents in dorsal root ganglion neurons after sciatic nerve injury but not rhizotomy. *J. Neurosci.* **20,** 7279–7289.

66. Akopian, A. N., Sivilotti, L., and Wood, J. N. (1996) A tetrodotoxin-resistant voltage-gated sodium channel expressed by sensory neurons. *Nature* **379,** 257–262.

67. Porreca, F., Lai, J., Bian, D., et al. (1999) A comparison of the potential role of the tetrodotoxin-insensitive sodium channels, PN3/SNS and NaN/SNS2, in rat models of chronic pain [published erratum appears in *Proc. Natl. Acad. Sci. USA* 1999 **96,** 10,548]. *Proc. Natl. Acad. Sci. USA* **96,** 7640–7644.

68. Hille, B. (1984) Ionic Channels of Excitable Membranes. Vol. First.: Sinauer Associates Incorporated, Sunderland, Mass.

69. Birnbaumer, L., Campbell, K. P., Catterall, W. A., et al. (1994) The naming of voltage-gated calcium channels. *Neuron* **13,** 505–506.

70. Ertel, E. A., Campbell, K. P., Harpold, M. M., et al. (2000) Nomenclature of voltage-gated calcium channels. *Neuron* **25,** 533–535.

71. Westenbroek, R. E., Ahlijanian, M. K., and Catterall, W. A. (1990) Clustering of L-type Ca^{2+} channels at the base of major dendrites in hippocampal pyramidal neurons. *Nature* **347,** 281–284.

72. Moreno, D. H. (1999) Molecular and functional diversity of voltage-gated calcium channels. *Ann. NY Acad. Sci.* **868,** 102–117.

73. Peterson, B. Z., Lee, J. S., Mulle, J. G., et al. (2000) Critical determinants of Ca(2+)-dependent inactivation within an EF- hand motif of L-type Ca(2+) channels. *Biophys. J.* **78,** 1906–1920.

74. Westenbroek, R. E., Hell, J. W., Warner, C., Dúbel, S. J., Snútch, T. P., and Catterall, W. A. (1992) Biochemical properties and subcellular distribution of an N-type calcium channel alpha 1 subunit. *Neuron* **9,** 1099–1115.

75. Wheeler, D. B., Randall, A., and Tsien, R. W. (1994) Roles of N-type and Q-type Ca^{2+} channels in supporting hippocampal synaptic transmission. *Science* **264**, 107–111.

76. Westenbroek, R. E., Sakurai, T., Elliott, E. M. et al. (1995) Immunochemical identification and subcellular distribution of the alpha 1A subunits of brain calcium channels. *J. Neurosci.* **15**, 6403–6418.

77. Yokoyama, C. T., Westenbroek, R. E., Hell, J. W., et al. (1995) Biochemical properties and subcellular distribution of the neuronal class E calcium channel alpha 1 subunit. *J. Neurosci.* **15**, 6419–6432.

78. Randall, A. and Tsien, R. W. (1997) Contrasting biophysical and pharmacological properties of T type and R type calcium channels. *Neuropharmacology* **36**, 879–893.

79. Westenbroek, R. E., Hoskins, L., and Catterall, W. A. (1998) Localization of Ca^{2+} channel subtypes on rat spinal motor neurons, interneurons, and nerve terminals. *J. Neurosci.* **18**, 6319–6330.

80. McDowell, T. S., Pancrazio, J. J., Barrett, P. Q., and Lynch, C., 3rd (1999) Volatile anesthetic sensitivity of T-type calcium currents in various cell types. *Anesth. Analg.* **88**, 168–173.

81. Lynch, C., 3rd, Vogel, S., and Sperelakis, N. (1981) Halothane depression of myocardial slow action potentials. *Anesthesiology* **55**, 360–368.

82. Bosnjak, Z. J. and Kampine, J. P. (1983) Effects of halothane, enflurane, and isoflurane on calcium currents in the SA node. *Anesthesiology* **58**, 314–321.

83. Drenger, B., Quigg, M., and Blanck, T. J. (1991) Volatile anesthetics depress calcium channel blocker binding to bovine cardiac sarcolemma. *Anesthesiology* **74**, 155–163.

84. Lee, D. L., Zhang, J., and Blanck, T. J. (1994) The effects of halothane on voltage-dependent calcium channels in isolated Langendorff-perfused rat heart. *Anesthesiology* **81**, 1212–1219.

85. Hoehner, P. and Blanck, T. J. (1991) Halothane depresses D600 binding to bovine heart sarcolemma. *Anesthesiology* **75**, 1019–1024.

86. Dolin, S. and Little, H. (1986) Augmentation by calcium channel antagonists of general anesthetic potency in mice. *Brit. J. Pharmacol.* **88**, 909–914.

87. Herrington, J., Stern, R. C., Evers, A. S., and Lingle, C. J. (1991) Halothane inhibits two components of calcium current in clonal (GH3) pituitary cells. *J. Neurosci.* **11**, 2226–2240.

88. Study, R. E. (1994) Isoflurane inhibits multiple voltage-gated calcium currents in hippocampal pyramidal neurons. *Anesthesiology* **81**, 104–116.

89. Takenoshita, M. and Steinbach, J. H. (1991) Halothane blocks low-voltage-activated calcium current in rat sensory neurons. *J. Neurosci.* **11**, 1404–1412.

90. Pancrazio, J. J., Park, W. K., and Lynch, C., 3rd (1993) Inhalational anesthetic actions on voltage-gated ion currents of bovine adrenal chromaffin cells. *Mol. Pharmacol.* **43**, 783–794.

91. Charlesworth, P., Pocock, G., and Richards, C. D. (1994) Calcium channel currents in bovine adrenal chromaffin cells and their modulation by anaesthetic agents. *J. Physiol.* **481** (Pt 3), 543–553.

92. Krnjevic, K. and Puil, E. (1988) Halothane suppresses slow inward currents in hippocampal slices. *Can. J. Physiol. Pharmacol.* **66**, 1570–1575.

93. Nikonorov, I. M., Blanck, T. J., and Recio-Pinto, E. (1998) The effects of halothane on single human neuronal L-type calcium channels. *Anesth. Analg.* **86**, 885–895.

94. Kamatchi, G. L., Chan, C. K., Snutch, T., Durieux, M. E., and Lynch, C., 3rd (1999) Volatile anesthetic inhibition of neuronal Ca channel currents expressed in *Xenopus* oocytes. *Brain Res.* **831**, 85–96.

95. Miller, R. J. (1987) Multiple calcium channels and neuronal function. *Science* **235**, 46–52.

96. Hirota, K., Fujimura, J., Wakasugi, M., and Ito, Y. (1996) Isoflurane and sevoflurane modulate inactivation kinetics of Ca^{2+} currents in single bullfrog atrial myocytes. *Anesthesiology* **84**, 377–383.

97. Bohm, M., Schmidt, U., Gierschik, P., Schwinger, R. H., Bohm, S., and Erdmann, E. (1994) Sensitization of adenylate cyclase by halothane in human myocardium and S49 lymphoma wild-type and cyc- cells: evidence for inactivation of the inhibitory G protein Gi alpha. *Mol. Pharmacol.* **45**, 380–389.

98. Rooney, T. A., Hager, R., Stubbs, C. D., and Thomas, A. P. (1993) Halothane regulates G-protein-dependent phospholipase C activity in turkey erythrocyte membranes. *J. Biol. Chem.* **268**, 15,550–15,556.

99. Puig, M. M., Turndorf, H., and Warner, W. (1990) Effect of pertussis toxin on the interaction of azepexole and halothane. *J. Pharmacol. Exp. Ther.* **252**, 1156–1159.

100. Puig, M. M., Turndorf, H., and Warner, W. (1990) Synergistic interaction of morphine and halothane in the guinea pig ileum: effects of pertussis toxin. *Anesthesiology* **72**, 699–703.

101. Yamakage (2001) Different Inhibitory Effects of Volatile Anesthetics on T- and L-type voltage dependent Ca channels. *Anesthesiology* **94**, 683.

102. Buljubasic, N., Marijic, J., Berczi, V., Supan, D. F., Kampine, J. P., and Bosnjak, Z. J. (1996) Differential effects of etomidate, propofol, and midazolam on calcium and potassium channel currents in canine myocardial cells. *Anesthesiology* **85**, 1092–1099.

103. Zhou, W., Fontenot, H. J., Liu, S., and Kennedy, R. H. (1997) Modulation of cardiac calcium channels by propofol. *Anesthesiology* **86**, 670–675.

104. Hirota, K. and Lambert, D. G. (2000) Effects of intravenous and local anesthetic agents on omega-conotoxin MVII(A) binding to rat cerebrocortex. *Can. J. Anaesth.* **47**, 467–470.

105. Xuan, Y. T. and Glass, P. S. (1996) Propofol regulation of calcium entry pathways in cultured A10 and rat aortic smooth muscle cells. *Brit. J. Pharmacol.* **117**, 5–12.

106. Luk, H. N., Yu, C. C., Lin, C. L., and Yang, C. Y. (1995) Electropharmacological actions of propofol on calcium current in guinea- pig ventricular myocytes. *J. Electrocardiol.* **28**, 332–333.

107. Hirota, K., Browne, T., Appadu, B. L., and Lambert, D. G. (1997) Do local anaesthetics interact with dihydropyridine binding sites on neuronal L-type Ca^{2+} channels? *Brit. J. Anaesth.* **78(2)**, 185–188.
108. Bence-Hanulec, K. K., Marshall, J., and Blair, L. A. (2000) Potentiation of neuronal L calcium channels by IGF-1 requires phosphorylation of the alpha1 subunit on a specific tyrosine residue. *Neuron* **27**, 121–131.
109. Bargmann, C. I. (1998) Neurobiology of the Caenorhabditis elegans genome. *Science* **282**, 2028–2033.
110. Robertson, B. (1997) The real life of voltage-gated K^+ channels: more than model behaviour. *Trends Pharmacol. Sci.* **18**, 474–483.
111. Garcia, M. L., Hanner, M., Knaus, H. G., et al. (1997) Pharmacology of potassium channels. *Adv. Pharmacol.* **39**, 425–471.
112. Miller, C. (1995) The charybdotoxin family of K^+ channel-blocking peptides. *Neuron* **15**, 5–10.
113. Smart, S. L., Lopantsev, V., Zhang, C. L., et al. (1998) Deletion of the K(V)1.1 potassium channel causes epilepsy in mice. *Neuron* **20(4)**, 809–819.
114. Meiri, N., Ghelardini, C., Tesco, G., et al. (1997) Reversible antisense inhibition of Shaker-like Kv1.1 potassium channel expression impairs associative memory in mouse and rat. *Proc. Natl. Acad. Sci. USA* **94**, 4430–4434.
115. Clark, J. D. and Tempel, B. L. (1998) Hyperalgesia in mice lacking the Kv1.1 potassium channel gene. *Neurosci. Lett.* **251**, 121–124.
116. Brandt, T. and Strupp, M. (1997) Episodic ataxia type 1 and 2 (familial periodic ataxia/vertigo). *Audiol. Neurootol.* **2**, 373–383.
117. Ruppersberg, J. P., Schroter, K. H., Sakmann, B., Stocker, M., Sewing, S., and Pongs., O. Z. (1990) Heteromultimeric channels formed by rat brain potassium-channel proteins. *Nature* **345**, 535–537.
118. Hopkins, W. F. (1998) Toxin and subunit specificity of blocking affinity of three peptide toxins for heteromultimeric, voltage-gated potassium channels expressed in Xenopus oocytes. *J. Pharmacol. Exp. Ther.* **285**, 1051–1060.
119. Rettig, J., Heinemann, S. H., Wunder, F., et al. (1994) Inactivation properties of voltage-gated K^+ channels altered by presence of beta-subunit. *Nature* **369**, 289–294.
120. Salinas, M., Duprat, F., Heurteaux, C., Hugnot, J. P., and Lazdunski, M. (1997) New modulatory alpha subunits for mammalian Shab K^+ channels. *J. Biol. Chem.* **272**, 24,371–24,379.
121. Isacoff, E. Y., Jan, Y. N. and Jan, L. Y. (1991) Putative receptor for the cytoplasmic inactivation gate in the Shaker K^+ channel. *Nature* **353**, 86–90.
122. Liu, Y., Jurman, M. E., and Yellen, G. (1996) Dynamic rearrangement of the outer mouth of a K^+ channel during gating. *Neuron* **16**, 859–867.
123. Kaczorowski, G. J. and Garcia, M. L. (1999) Pharmacology of voltage-gated and calcium-activated potassium channels. *Curr. Opin. Chem. Biol.* **3**, 448–458.
124. Cui, J., Cox, D. H., and Aldrich, R. W. (1997) Intrinsic voltage dependence and Ca^{2+} regulation of mslo large conductance Ca-activated K^+ channels. *J. Gen. Physiol.* **109**, 647–673.
125. Meera, P., Wallner, M., Song, M., and Toro, L. (1997) Large conductance voltage- and calcium-dependent K^+ channel, a distinct member of voltage-dependent ion channels with seven N-terminal transmembrane segments (S0–S6), an extracellular N terminus, and an intracellular (S9–6S10) C terminus. *Proc. Natl. Acad. Sci. USA* **94**, 14,066–14,071.
126. Schreiber, M. and Salkoff, L. (1997) A novel calcium-sensing domain in the BK channel. *Biophys. J.* **73**, 1355–1363.
127. Diaz, L., Meera, P, Amigo, J., et al. (1998) Role of the S4 segment in a voltage-dependent calcium-sensitive potassium (hSlo) channel. *J. Biol. Chem.* **273**, 32,430–32,436.
128. Wanner, S. G., Koch, R. O., Koschak, A., et al. (1999) High-conductance calcium-activated potassium channels in rat brain: pharmacology, distribution, and subunit composition. *Biochemistry* **38**, 5392–5400.
129. Wallner, M., Meera, P., and Toro, L. (1999) Molecular basis of fast inactivation in voltage and Ca^{2+}-activated K^+ channels: a transmembrane beta-subunit homolog. *Proc. Natl. Acad. Sci. USA* **96**, 4137–4142.
130. Reimann, F. and Ashcroft, F. M. (1999) Inwardly rectifying potassium channels. *Curr. Opin. Cell Biol.* **11**, 503–508.
131. Yamada, M., Inanobe, A., and Kurachi, Y. (1998) G protein regulation of potassium ion channels. *Pharmacol. Rev.* **50**, 723–760.
132. Inagaki, N., Gonoi, T., Clement, J. P., 4th, et al. (1995) Reconstitution of IKATP: an inward rectifier subunit plus the sulfonylurea receptor. *Science* **270**, 1166–1170.
133. Ammala, C., Moorhouse, A., Gribble, F., et al. (1996) Promiscuous coupling between the sulphonylurea receptor and inwardly rectifying potassium channels. *Nature* **379**, 545–548.
134. Kersten, J. R., Gross, G. J., Pagel, P. S., and Warltier, D. C. (1998) Activation of adenosine triphosphate-regulated potassium channels: mediation of cellular and organ protection. *Anesthesiology* **88**, 495–513.
135. Doupnik, C. A., Davidson, N., and Lester, H. A. (1995) The inward rectifier potassium channel family. *Curr. Opin. Neurobiol.* **5**, 268–277.
136. Ketchum, K. A., Joiner, W. J., Sellers, A. J., Kaczmarek, L. K., and Goldstein, S. A. (1995) A new family of outwardly rectifying potassium channel proteins with two pore domains in tandem. *Nature* **376**, 690–695.
137. Fink, M., Lesage, F., Duprat, F., et al. (1998) A neuronal two P domain K^+ channel stimulated by arachidonic acid and polyunsaturated fatty acids. *Embo. J.* **17**, 3297–3308.
138. Patel, A. J., Honore, E., Maingret, F., et al. (1998) A mammalian two pore domain mechano-gated S-like K^+ channel. *Embo J.* **17(15)**, 4283–4290.
139. Goldstein, S. A., Wang, K. W., Ilan, N., and Pausch, M. H. (1998) Sequence and function of the two P domain potassium channels: implications of an emerging superfamily. *J. Mol. Med.* **76**, 13–20.
140. Maingret, F., Patel, A. J., Lesage, F., Lazdunski, M., and Honore, E. (2000) Lysophospholipids open the two-pore domain mechano-gated $K^{(+)}$ channels TREK-1 and TRAAK. *J. Biol. Chem.* **275**, 10,128–10,133.
141. Maingret, F., Patel, A. J., Lesage, F., Lazdunski, M., and Honore, E. (1999) Mechano- or acid stimulation, two interactive modes of activation of the TREK-1 potassium channel. *J. Biol. Chem.* **274**, 26,691–26,696.

142. Gray, A. T., Zhao, B. B., Kindler, C. H., et al. (2000) Volatile anesthetics activate the human tandem pore domain baseline K$^+$ channel KCNK5. *Anesthesiology* **92,** 1722–1730.

143. Bang, H., Kim, Y., and Kim, D. (2000) TREK-2, a new member of the mechanosensitive tandem-pore K$^+$ channel family. *J. Biol. Chem.* **275,** 17,412–17,419.

144. Yost, C. S. (1999) Potassium channels: basic aspects, functional roles, and medical significance. *Anesthesiology* **90,** 1186–1203.

145. North, R. A. (1989) Twelfth Gaddum memorial lecture. Drug receptors and the inhibition of nerve cells. *Brit. J. Pharmacol.* **98,** 13–28.

146. Nicoll, R. A. and Madison, D. V. (1982) General anesthetics hyperpolarize neurons in the vertebrate central nervous system. *Science* **217,** 1055–1057.

147. Berg-Johnsen, J. and Langmoen, I. A. (1987) Isoflurane hyperpolarizes neurones in rat and human cerebral cortex. *Acta Physiol. Scand.* **130,** 679–685.

148. Berg-Johnsen, J. and Langmoen, I. A. (1990) Mechanisms concerned in the direct effect of isoflurane on rat hippocampal and human neocortical neurons. *Brain Res.* **507,** 28–34.

149. Southan, A. P. and Wann, K. T. (1989) Inhalation anaesthetics block accommodation of pyramidal cell discharge in the rat hippocampus. *Brit. J. Anaesth.* **63,** 581–586.

150. Franks, N. P. and Lieb, W. R. (1988) Volatile general anaesthetics activate a novel neuronal K$^+$ current. *Nature* **333,** 662–664.

151. Winegar, B. D., Owen, D. F., Yost, C. S., Forsayeth, J. R., and Mayeri, E. (1996) Volatile general anesthetics produce hyperpolarization of Aplysia neurons by activation of a discrete population of baseline potassium channels. *Anesthesiology* **85,** 889–900.

152. Winegar, B. D. and Yost, C. S. (1998) Volatile anesthetics directly activate baseline S K$^+$ channels in aplysia neurons. *Brain Res.* **807,** 255–262.

153. Nacif-Coelho, C., Correa-Sales, C., Chang, L. L., and Maze, M. (1994) Perturbation of ion channel conductance alters the hypnotic response to the alpha 2-adrenergic agonist dexmedetomidine in the locus coeruleus of the rat. *Anesthesiology* **81,** 1527–1534.

154. Correa, A. M. (1998) Gating kinetics of Shaker K$^+$ channels are differentially modified by general anesthetics. *Am. J. Physiol.* **275(4 Pt 1),** C1009–C1021.

155. Friederich, P. and Urban, B. W. (1999) Interaction of intravenous anesthetics with human neuronal potassium currents in relation to clinical concentrations. *Anesthesiology* **91,** 1853–1860.

156. McLarnon, J. and Sawyer, D. (1998) Effects of volatile anaesthetics on a high conductance calcium dependent potassium channel in cultured hippocampal neurons. *Toxicol. Lett.* **100–101,** 271–276.

157. Hong, Y., Puil, E., and Mathers, D. A. (1994) Effect of halothane on large-conductance calcium-dependent potassium channels in cerebrovascular smooth muscle cells of the rat. *Anesthesiology* **81,** 649–656.

158. Dreixler, J. C., Jenkins, A., Lao, Y. J., Roizen, J. D., and Houamed, K. M. (2000) Patch-clamp analysis of anesthetic interactions with recombinant SK2 subtype neuronal calcium-activated potassium channels. *Anesth. Analg.* **90,** 727–732.

159. Gibbons, S. J., Nuez-Hernandez, R., Maze, G., and Harrison, N. L. (1996) Inhibition of a fast inwardly rectifying potassium conductance by barbiturates. *Anesth. Analg.* **82,** 1242–1246.

160. Gray, A. T., Winegar, B. D., Leonoudakis, D. J., Forsayeth, J. R., and Yost, C. S. (1998) TOK1 is a volatile anesthetic stimulated K$^+$ channel. *Anesthesiology* **88,** 1076–1084.

161. Patel, A. J., Honore, E., Lesage, F., Fink, M., Romey, G., and Lazdunski, M. (1999) Inhalational anesthetics activate two-pore-domain background K$^+$ channels. *Nat. Neurosci.* **2,** 422–426.

162. Sirois, J. E., Lei, Q., Talley, E. M., Lynch, C., 3rd, and Bayliss, D. A. (2000) The TASK-1 two-pore domain K$^+$ channel is a molecular substrate for neuronal effects of inhalation anesthetics. *J. Neurosci.* **20,** 6347–6354.

163. Zorn, L., Kulkarni, R., Anantharam, V., Bayley, H., and Treistman, S. N. (1993) Halothane acts on many potassium channels, including a minimal potassium channel. *Neurosci. Lett.* **161,** 81–84.

164. Larach, D. R. and Schuler, H. G. (1993) Potassium channel blockade and halothane vasodilation in conducting and resistance coronary arteries. *J. Pharmacol. Exp. Ther.* **267,** 72–81.

165. Cason, B. A., Shubayev, I., and Hickey, R. F. (1994) Blockade of adenosine triphosphate-sensitive potassium channels eliminates isoflurane-induced coronary artery vasodilation. *Anesthesiology* **81,** 1245–1255; discussion 27A–28A.

166. Cason, B.A., Gordon, H. J., Avery, E. G., 4th, and Hickey, R. F. (1995) The role of ATP sensitive potassium channels in myocardial protection. *J. Card. Surg.* **10,** 441–444.

167. Kersten, J. R., Schmeling, T. J., Hettrick, D. A., Pagel, P. S., Gross, G. J., and Warltier, D. C. (1996) Mechanism of myocardial protection by isoflurane. Role of adenosine triphosphate-regulated potassium (KATP) channels. *Anesthesiology* **85,** 794–807.

168. Crystal, G. J., Gurevicius, J., Salem, M. R., and Zhous, X. (1997) Role of adenosine triphosphate-sensitive potassium channels in coronary vasodilation by halothane, isoflurane, and enflurane. *Anesthesiology* **86,** 448–458.

169. Han, J., Kim, E., Ho, W. K., and Earm, Y. E. (1996) Effects of volatile anesthetic isoflurane on ATP-sensitive K$^+$ channels in rabbit ventricular myocytes. *Biochem. Biophys. Res. Commun.* **229,** 852–856.

170. Kersten, J. R., Orth, K. G., Pagel, P. S., Mei, D. A., and Gross, G. J., (1997) Role of adenosine in isoflurane-induced cardioprotection. *Anesthesiology* **86,** 1128–1139.

19

Glutamate Receptors

Physiology and Anesthetic Pharmacology

Misha Perouansky and Joseph F. Antognini

GLUTAMATE —THE MOLECULE

Glutamic acid is found in very high levels in the CNS. As it does not cross the blood-brain barrier, it must originate from local metabolism. It participates in intermediary glucose metabolism, in addition to its role in intercellular communication and therefore shares with GABA the problem of dissociating neurotransmitter and metabolic roles. Glutamate is formed via two distinct pathways: either from glucose in the Krebs cycle and transamination of α-ketoglutarate or directly from glutamine. The latter is synthesized in glial cells by the enzyme glutaminase, which is localized to the mitochondria and possibly phosphate-activated. Inactivation of released glutamate is mainly through reuptake by dicarboxylic acid transporters. Enzymatic inactivation does not play a significant role. Glutamate is also the substrate for glutamic acid decarboxylase—the GABA synthesizing enzyme.

GLUTAMATE—THE TRANSMITTER

Half a century ago, following his discovery that L-glutamate can cause convulsions, Hayashi proposed that this amino acid could actually serve as a neurotransmitter in the central nervous system (CNS) *(1)*. Experimental support for this hypothesis was provided when it was found that glutamate excited individual neurons in the cat spinal cord *(2)*. In the decades since these early observations, glutamate has been firmly established as the major excitatory transmitter in the vertebrate CNS. Moreover, glutamate and its receptors provide an important molecular interface for neuron-glia interaction, as ionotropic and metabotropic glutamate receptors are widely expressed in various types of glial cells *(3)*. Glutamate released from neurons can activate these receptors and cause: (1) modulation of transmitter uptake into glial cells, thereby affecting synaptic transmission *(4)*, (2) modulation of K$^+$ conductances within glial cells and consequent changes in the extracellular ion composition, and (3) release of neuroactive substances from glia that can feedback and modulate synaptic transmission *(5)*.

GLUTAMATE—THE RECEPTORS

Glutamate receptors (GluRs) are currently classified into the ionotropic (ionic channel-linked) and metabotropic (G-protein-linked) receptor families (iGluRs vs mGluRs) (Fig. 1). The ionotropic family comprises three classes of receptors based on agonist specificities: AMPA (formerly quisqualate), kainate, and NMDA. The former two families were collectively referred to as non-NMDA receptors, as neither agonists nor, until recently, antagonists clearly distinguished between

From: *Contemporary Clinical Neuroscience: Neural Mechanisms of Anesthesia*
Edited by: Joseph F. Antognini et al. © Humana Press Inc., Totowa, NJ

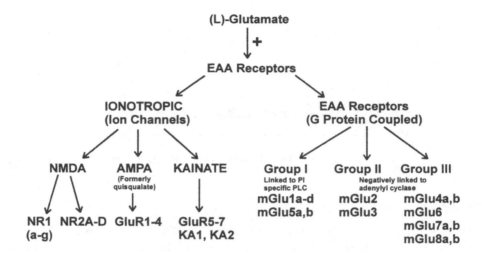

Fig. 1. Diagram of glutamate receptor classification (based on ref. *[120]*).

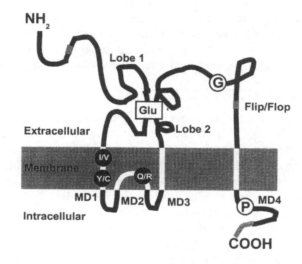

Fig. 2. Glutamate receptor structure. MD1, MD 3, and MD 4 are transmembrane domains, unlike MD2. The glutamate binding site is on lobes 1 and 2. The dark circles are sites of RNA editing; I/V and Y/C sites for GluR6 transcripts, Q/R site for GluR2, GluR5, and GluR6. Glycosylation occurs at the circled G (based on Ref. *[121]*).

them. Cloning studies have demonstrated, however, that AMPA and kainate activate distinct receptor complexes. Only the ionotropic glutamate receptors will be discussed in this chapter.

Ionotropic Receptors

The ionotropic glutamate receptors are tetra- or pentameric proteins: four (or five) subunits assemble to form a functional receptor-channel complex. Each subunit consists of a large extracellular N-terminal domain, three hydrophobic transmembrane segments (M1, M3, and M4) and an intracellular C-terminus. The pore region is formed by the amphipathic reentrant hairpin loop M2, similar in structure to the pore-forming region of K⁺ channels (Fig. 2). The ligand binds to two regions, one before M1, the other between M3 and M4 *(6)*.

AMPA Receptors

AMPA receptors mediate fast excitatory transmission at most synapses in the CNS. The four subunits, GluR1–GluR4, are encoded by four closely related genes. AMPA receptors are either homomeric or heteromeric tetramers composed of these multiple subunits, which results in a marked functional diversity of the native receptors.

Channel Properties

AMPA receptor channels pass cations. Originally thought to be permeable only to the monovalent ions, it was later discovered that this selectivity was conferred by a single amino acid residue in the M2 segment of the GluR2 subunit. This residue is the positively charged amino acid arginine in GluR2 as opposed to the neutral glutamine in GluR1, GluR3, GluR4. Co-expression of the GluR2 subunit with either combination of the other subunits results in the formation of receptors with little Ca^{2+} permeability, while receptors composed without GluR2 are Ca^{2+} permeable *(7)*. Glutamate and AMPA elicit rapidly desensitizing responses, while AMPA receptor-mediated responses to kainate do not desensitize *(8,9)*. The speed of desensitization depends on the subunit composition and on the splice variant (flip or flop), and can vary by more than an order of magnitude *(10,11)*. The single-channel properties of non-NMDA receptor channels are not well described, mostly due to technical difficulties in resolving the small conductance levels. Some experimental evidence supports the existence of three conductance levels that can all be activated by AMPA, glutamate and kainate. The mean open time was only 0.5 ms, and most channel activations were composed of single openings *(12)*. Not unexpectedly, single-channel properties were influenced by the subunit composition and their editing-state *(13)*. Experiments combining whole-cell patch-clamp recording with reverse-transcription, followed by PCR amplification confirmed that AMPA receptor properties in native neurons (i.e., Ca^{2+} permeability, desensitization) are in accordance with the findings in expression systems *(14–16)*.

Pharmacology

At least three binding sites can be identified on AMPA receptors. In addition to the agonist-binding site, there is a site influencing receptor desensitization and a binding site within the channel. The binding site for glutamate and competitive antagonists, e.g., GYKI52466 *(17)*, is formed by two discontiguous segments located between the N-terminal and M1 and between M3 and M4, respectively *(18)*. Desensitization can be slowed and AMPA responses potentiated by drugs binding at or near the flip-flop domain. The flip form carries a serine in position 750 and is strongly susceptible to removal of desensitization. Exchange of the serine for glutamine (flop-variant) makes the receptor insensitive to removal of desensitization by both aniracetam (a pyrrolidinone) and CTZ (cyclothiazide, a benzothiadiazine) *(19–21)*.

Physiology

The AMPA receptor-mediated component of the glutamatergic (EPSC) excitatory postsynaptic current is characterized by its fast time course. That, in turn, is determined by two factors: the time-concentration profile of glutamate in the synaptic cleft and the properties of the postsynaptic receptors. The release of transmitter into the synaptic cleft causes a sudden increase in glutamate concentration to approx 1.1 mM *(22)*. Diffusion of transmitter away from the synaptic cleft appears to be very rapid (estimated time constant 1.2 ms *[22]*) and deactivation rather than desensitization of receptors determines the time constant of EPSC decay *(23,24)*. At certain synapses, however, desensitization may be the determining factor *(25)*. Typically, postsynaptic Ca^{2+} entry at a glutamatergic synapse takes place through NMDA receptor channels, with AMPA receptor-mediated depolarization of the postsynaptic membrane relieving the voltage-dependent block of NMDA receptor channels by Mg^{2+}. However, native AMPA receptors with high Ca^{2+} permeability (i.e., lacking the edited GluR2 subunit) have been observed in a variety of cells, most of which are

GABAergic and express the Ca^{2+} binding protein parvalbumin *(15,26)*. Recently, mice lacking the GluR2 subunit have been produced by gene targeting *(27)*. Despite the increased Ca^{2+} permeability, and the ensuing physiologic changes in vitro, these mice survived into adulthood without obvious deficits except for reduced anesthetic drug requirements for certain anesthetic end-points *(28,29)*.

Kainate Receptors

The kainate receptor family comprises five subunits: GluR5, GluR6, GluR7 (the low affinity kainate binding sites, K_D of ~50 n*M*), and KA1, KA2 (high affinity kainate binding sites, K_D ~5 n*M*). GluR5–GluR7 are of similar size (~900 amino acids), share 75–80% sequence identity with each other and ~40% with GluR1–GluR4. KA1–KA2 are larger (~970 amino acids), share 70% sequence identity with each other and ~40% with GluR1–GluR7. When expressed in host cells, KA1–KA2 and GluR7 do not form functional ion channels without GluR5–6 *(30)*. RNA editing of GluR5 and GluR6, but not GluR7, occurs at the same site as in GluR2. The editing is, however, incomplete and both edited and unedited variants are found in the adult brain. Receptor diversity is achieved by editing at two additional sites (GluR6) and alternative splicing (GluR5) *(31)*. Both high and low affinity kainate binding sites, imaged with radioligand binding, are abundant throughout the CNS with some areas (e.g., hippocampal CA3) showing particularly high levels *(32)*. *In situ* hybridization and immunohistochemistry have revealed that kainate receptor subunits are differentially distributed in the CNS *(33)*. While AMPA and kainate receptor subunits can coexist in the same neuron *(34)*, they do not co-assemble with each other *(35)*.

Channel Properties

Kainate, the agonist most widely used to activate kainate receptors, elicits large nondesensitizing currents at AMPA receptors, thereby obscuring kainate channel activity in native preparations. When expressed in isolation, homomeric channels formed by GluR5 and GluR6 show rapid desensitization. Co-expression of KA2 changes the time course of desensitization and the current-voltage relationship, and makes the receptor activatable by AMPA *(30)*. Native kainate receptors are likely to be heteromers composed of different combinations of these subunits *(36)*. Because of the pharmacologic overlap with AMPA receptors, the properties of kainate receptors were, until the recent development of selective antagonists, difficult to define (hence the encompassing term "non-NMDA" receptors). GluR5 and GluR6 receptors are subject to editing at the glutamine/arginine site. Introduction of arginine in the M2 loop is thought to create a ring of positive charges within the putative pore-lining hydrophobic domain with a number of functional consequences *(37)*: (1) edited homomeric receptors have a significantly reduced Ca^{2+} permeability *(38)*, analogous to the edited GluR2 in AMPA receptors; (2) a single low conductance state (femtosiemens) instead of multiple conductance states (picosiemens); (3) an approximately linear current-voltage relationship, instead of the inward or double rectifying properties of the unedited variants *(39)*; and (4) an increased permeability to Cl^- *(40)*. Co-expression of GluR5 and GluR6 with the unedited KA2 gives rise to channels with a significantly higher unitary conductance than homomeric channels *(41,39)*.

Pharmacology

Three types of drugs assist in the pharmacologic separation of AMPA and kainate receptors: drugs that affect desensitization, selective agonists, and selective antagonists. Concanavalin A is a lectin that selectively removes desensitization of kainate receptor-mediated responses *(42,43)*. It is, however, technically difficult to use in brain slice preparations. The selective agonists and antagonists available so far affect primarily GluR5-containing receptors, which have a limited distribution in the CNS when assessed by GluR5 mRNA expression *(36)*. (*S*)-5-iodowillardiine is an agonist with a more than 100-fold selectivity for kainate receptors compared to AMPA receptors (EC_{50} 0.14 μ*M* vs 19 μ*M*), *(44)*, activating preferentially GluR5 homomers *(45)*. Similarly, ATPA ([rs]-2-amino-3[3-hydroxy-5-*tert*-butylisoxazol-4yl]propanoic acid) displaces kainate bound to GluR5 containing receptors with a 1000-fold higher potency than AMPA bound to GluR1–4 and kainate bound to

GluR7 and KA2, with no activity at GluR6 *(46)*. The only selective kainate antagonist also targets preferentially GluR5 containing receptors: LY294486 does not affect binding to recombinant GluR6, GluR7, and KA2 receptors *(46)*.

Physiology

Functional native kainate receptors have been originally demonstrated in dorsal root ganglion (DRG) neurons *(47)*. In this location, the receptors probably contain GluR5 and KA2 subunits *(48,30)*. Functional receptors could also be demonstrated in cultured hippocampal neurons, expressing mostly GluR6 mRNA *(49)*. In the hippocampus, fast synaptic transmission onto pyramidal cells does not seem to involve postsynaptic kainate receptors *(50)*, except under conditions of high-frequency stimulation of the mossy fiber pathway *(51,52)*. Kainate receptors, however, are involved in synaptic transmission onto hippocampal interneurons *(53)* and retinal bipolar cells *(54)*. Kainate receptors are also intricately involved in the modulation of transmitter release *(55)*. In the hippocampus, release of GABA onto pyramidal cells and interneurons appears to be differentially regulated by kainate receptors. In pyramidal cells, GABAergic inhibitory postsynaptic currents (IPSCs) were suppressed by activation of presynaptic kainate receptors both by exogenous *(46,56–58)* and by synaptically released glutamate *(59)*. In contrast, GABA release onto hippocampal interneurons is enhanced by activation of kainate receptors *(60)*. Even though the precise location of kainate receptors on interneurons is subject to debate *(61,62)*, this example of differential and selective distribution of kainate receptors illustrates the complexity of the regulation of excitation and inhibition in neuronal networks.

NMDA Receptors

The NMDA receptor family comprises five subunits: the "fundamental," NR1, and the modulatory, NR2A–NR2D. The NR1 subunit is composed of 938 amino acids and can form homomeric receptor channels with the basic NMDA receptor channel properties, but small amplitude current responses *(63)*. NR1 shows 25–28% sequence homology with other iGluR subunits and shares a similar hydrophobicity profile, while the sequence identity with the NR2 subunits is lower—only ~18%. NR2 subunits do not form functional receptors on their own, but their coexpression with NR1 amplifies the current responses through the heteromeric receptors by several orders *(64)*. The NR2A–NR2D subunits are larger than NR1 (1250–1482 amino acids) and share 40–50% of sequence identity *(65)*. As for the other glutamate receptors, diversity is increased with alternative splicing: eight splice vaiants have been reported for the NR1 subunit *(64)*. *In situ* hybridization and immuno-histochemistry have determined that the NR1 subunit is ubiquitous in the rodent brain. The NR2 subunits show distinct regional patterns and developmental changes in subunit expression *(66,67)*.

Channel Properties

NMDA receptor channels mediate excitatory neurotransmission in a way that is different from, and complimentary to, frequently co-localized AMPA receptors. AMPA receptors have a low affinity to glutamate, as well as the fast binding and unbinding kinetics. NMDA receptors, by contrast, have high affinity to glutamate, prolonged binding, and repeated channel openings. The 10–90% rise time of NMDA receptor-gated currents is ~10 ms, meaning the AMPA receptor-mediated component of the synaptic current has largely decayed before the NMDA component reaches its peak. The decay is typically bi-exponential (determined by repeated channel openings and desensitization), with time constants of tens and hundreds of milliseconds *(68)*. The desensitization of NMDA receptors varies depending on the experimental conditions, but is always significantly slower than the desensitization of AMPA receptors *(69,70)*. In contrast to AMPA receptors, a high permeability for Ca^{2+} is the rule rather than the exception for NMDA receptor channels. The fractional Ca^{2+} currents through recombinant NMDA receptors ranged from 8.2–11% *(71)*. The Ca^{2+} permeability is characteristically combined with a voltage-dependent block of the channel by Mg^{2+}, which provides the NMDA receptor with its signature current-voltage relationship: in the presence of extracellular Mg^{2+}, current through NMDA receptors is maximal between -20 and -30 mV. At more negative potentials, it gradually decays despite the increasing driving force, thereby exhibiting an area of negative slope conductance between -30 and -80 mV *(72,73)* (Fig.3).

Single-channel studies have shown that the NMDA recptor channel has a conductance of 40–50 pS in salines containing no Mg^{2+}. Addition of Mg^{2+} causes the single-channel currents to occur in bursts of short-lasting openings separated by brief closures, implicating a block of the open channel *(72,74)*. Both Ca^{2+} permeability and block by Mg^{2+} are determined by the presence of an asparagine at a position analogous to the Q/R site that governs Ca^{2+} permeability in the AMPA receptor *(71)*. In addition, the degree of sensitivity to block by Mg^{2+} is determined by the type of NR2 subunit that forms the receptor-channel complex *(75,76)*.

Pharmacology

Glycine is an essential co-agonist of glutamate at the NMDA receptor. It binds to the NR1 subunit at a region that corresponds to the glutamate recognition site at the NR2 subunits and has been termed the "strychnine-insensitive" glycine binding site. The ED_{50} of glycine is 0.1–0.7 μM *(77)*. D-serine and D-alanine are naturally occurring agonists at the glycine site. In expression systems, the ED_{50} of D-serine as an NMDA co-agonist, is three to four times lower than that of glycine *(78)*. Considering that the extracellular concentration of D-serine in rodent frontal cortex is 6.5 μM, enough to saturate the glycine-binding site of the NMDA receptor, D-serine may also act as an endogenous co-agonist *(78)*. The glycine recognition site on NR1 and the glutamate recognition site on NR2 are homologous to the glutamate binding site of the AMPA receptor *(79,80)*. In addition to these two sites, drugs affecting the NMDA receptor can bind at the intra-ion channel binding site and at multiple modulatory sites, such as the redox, the H^+, the Zn^{2+} and the polyamine binding sites *(81)*.

Physiology

Three characteristic features endow the NMDA receptor with a special role in synaptic transmission: (1) At resting membrane potential the channel is blocked by Mg^{2+} and current flows only if the neuronal membrane is depolarized. This depolarization is typically provided in the postnatal brain by AMPA receptors, which have been shown to colocalize at the same synapses *(82)*. In the prenatal brain, glutamatergic synapses may lack AMPA receptors. Glutamatergic synaptic transmission is mediated purely by NMDA receptors *(83,84)*. The depolarization necessary to overcome the voltage-dependent block by Mg^{2+} may be provided by activation of $GABA_A$ receptors that have a depolarizing effect during early postnatal development due to a more depolarized reversal potential for Cl^- *(85)*. (2) Once current flows, extracellular Ca^{2+} enters the cell through the NMDA receptor channel. (3) The synaptic currents last for prolonged periods of time. Taken together, these properties enable the NMDA receptor channel to function as a "coincidence detector" of presynaptic activity and postsynaptic depolarization, and, via the injection of Ca^{2+}, to play a critical role in synaptogenesis and to initiate plastic changes in the strength of synaptic connections. Long-term potentiation (LTP, the strengthening of synaptic connections) *(86–88)*, and long-term depression (LTD, the weakening of synaptic connections) *(89,90)* are such changes that depend on the temporal pattern of synaptic activity and are mediated via glutamate receptors.

ANESTHETIC EFFECTS ON GLUTAMATE RECEPTORS AND GLUTAMATE PHYSIOLOGY

A significant amount of research has established the glutamate receptor as a potentially important target for anesthetic molecules. Several research techniques have been exploited to further our understanding of anesthetic effects on glutamate and its receptors. These techniques include patch clamping, molecular biology, and genetic manipulations, as well as classical pharmacology (e.g., use of agonists and antagonists). In general, most anesthetics alter GluR function, although there are notable exceptions. Propofol and etomidate have little effect on GluRs at clinically relevant

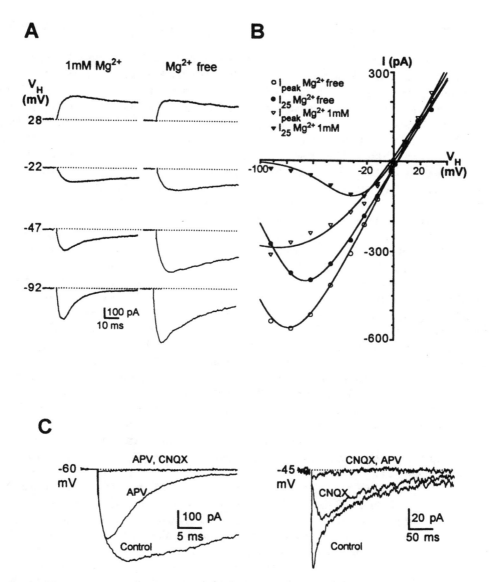

Fig. 3. Basic physiology and pharmacology of glutamate receptor-mediated excitatory postsynaptic currents (glu-EPSCs). Glu-EPSCs consist typically of a non-NMDA and an NMDA receptor-mediated component. (**A**) In Mg^{2+} containing solution, glu-EPSCs have a fast time course at negative holding potentials, determined mainly by the non-NMDA receptor-mediated component. Depolarization of the holding potential removes the voltage-dependent block of the NMDA receptor-channels by Mg^{2+} and recruits a slow glu-EPSC component. In Mg^{2+}-free saline, the slow, NMDA receptor-mediated component, is present at all holding potentials. (**B**) The current-voltage relationship graphically illustrates these issues. The non-NMDA receptor-mediated component of the EPSC shows a linear current-voltage relationship across a wide range of voltages in the presence (open triangles) and absence (open circles) of Mg^{2+}. The NMDA receptor-mediated component, by contrast, displays a nonlinear behavior at voltages more negative than -20 mV in the presence of Mg^{2+} (closed triangles— negative slope conductance) that is rectified in nominally Mg^{2+}-free saline (closed circles). The nonlinearities of the I/V relationships in Mg^{2+}-free saline at negative holding potentials are probably due to residual Mg^{2+}. (**C**) Selective antagonists were instrumental in delineating the physiological roles of the glu-EPSC components. The slow, NMDA-receptor mediated component can be blocked by aminophosphonovaleric acid (APV), leaving the non-NMDA receptor mediated component that is sensitive to 6-nitro-7-cyano-quinoxaline-2,3-dione (CNQX), which does not distinguish between AMPA and kainate receptors. Conversely, application of CNQX leaves a slow APV-sensitive component (from ref. *[97]*).

concentrations, while other anesthetics (ketamine, xenon, N_2O) appear to exert effects primarily at GluRs (*see* ref. *[91]* for review).

Volatile anesthetic effects at different GluRs (AMPA, kainate, NMDA) have not been extensively studied, but sufficient data exist to make basic conclusions *(91)*. For example, enflurane, halothane, and isoflurane do not appear to have major effects on the NMDA type of GluRs *(92,93)*, but these anesthetics potentiate kainate receptors and depress AMPA-sensitive GluRs *(94,95)*. Kainate-induced currents (using voltage clamping) were examined in frog oocytes that expressed different subunits of the GluRs. These authors found that diverse anesthetics (halothane, isoflurane, pentobarbital) had differential effects on GluRs. They also determined that nonanesthetics, such as 2,3-chlorooctofluorobutane (F8) did not have effects on GluRs. In another study, these investigators determined that the transmembrane (TM4) region of GluR6 (kainate sensitive) was critical for the effects of volatile anesthetics. Site-directed mutagenesis subsequently showed that a specific amino acid, glycine 819 in TM4, is important for enhancement of receptor function by halothane, isoflurane, enflurane, and 1-chloro-1,2,2-trifluorocyclobutane *(94)*. Native neuronal glutamate receptors are inhibited by volatile anesthetics at high concentrations. In the hippocampus, responses of CA-1 pyramidal cells to exogenously applied AMPA and NMDA were inhibited by halothane with EC_{50}s of 1.7 mM and 5.9 mM, respectively *(96)*. Glutamatergic synaptic currents in the same preparation were far more sensitive (EC_{50} of 0.66 mM and 0.57 mM for non-NMDA and NMDA receptor-mediated components) *(97,98)* (Fig. 4., top). These results indicate that halothane affects glutamatergic synaptic transmission predominantly by a presynaptic mechanism. This was further investigated by analyzing halothane's effect on paired-pulse facilitation (PPF). In the disinhibited hippocampus, application of two consecutive stimuli to afferent pathways results in facilitation of the second EPSC, a phenomenon termed PPF *(99)*. PPF, presumably, is inversely related to the magnitude of the presynaptic Ca^{2+} entry during depolarization of the terminal *(100)*. Halothane increased PPF, indicating a reduction of presynaptic Ca^{2+} inflow *(96,101)* (Fig. 4., bottom). Other experiments provided evidence for presynaptic actions of isoflurane on excitatory synapses. This effect was partially mediated by inhibition of axonal action potential conduction *(102)*, consistent with the notion that inhibitory effects of volatile anesthetics on glutamatergic synaptic transmission are mostly presynaptic in nature (*see* also Chapter 21).

Xenon, a noble gas, has been found to have few effects at $GABA_A$ receptors, but depressed NMDA sensitive GluRs *(103,104)*. De Sousa et al. examined isoflurane and xenon effects on total charge transfer (glutamatergic and GABAergic) at synapses of autaptic cultures of rat hippocampal neurons *(104)*. Xenon did not exert any GABAergic effects, but did alter total charge transfer related to NMDA. Isoflurane, on the other hand, had significant GABAergic effects. Others have had similar findings. Xenon, N_2O and isoflurane effects were determined using voltage clamping of oocytes expressing GABA, glycine, NMDA, AMPA, and acetylcholine receptors; NMDA and AchR were likely targets for xenon and N_2O *(105)*.

Current evidence suggests that N_2O exerts its effects via GluRs, specifically the NMDA sensitive GluR. *(106,107)*. For example, Mennerick et al. investigated N_2O effects on excitatory and inhibitory synaptic transmission in rat hippocampal neurons. N_2O (80%) depressed excitatory currents evoked by NMDA, and to a lesser extent, AMPA *(106)*. Ketamine also has significant action at GluRs. In lamprey, a parasitic fish, fictive locomotion can be induced by NMDA; this is blocked by ketamine *(108)*. In oocytes expressing NMDA sensitive GluRs, ketamine depressed ionic currents (voltage clamping) and this effect was potentiated by volatile anesthetics *(109)*. Orser et al. examined ketamine effects on NMDA GluR kinetics and determined that ketamine blocked the open channel, which decreased the time that the channel was open, and it also decreased the frequency of channel opening *(110)*. Other intravenous agents at clinically relevant concentrations, such as barbiturates and propofol, do not appear to have significant effects on NMDA sensitive GluRs *(111,112)*. Barbiturates, however, depress AMPA and kainate sensitive GluRs (94,95), whereas propofol does not have similar depressant effects on AMPA and kainate GluRs *(111)*. Because motoneurons express GluRs,

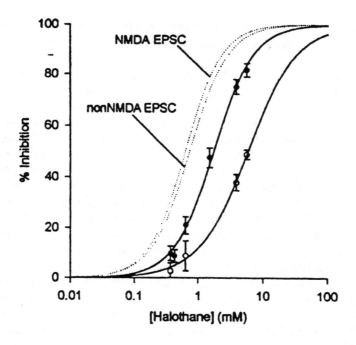

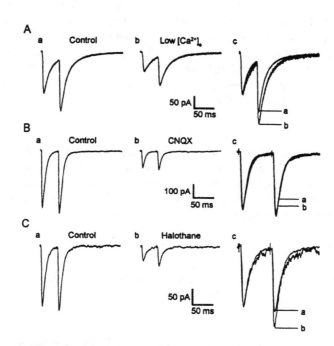

Fig. 4. Volatile anesthetics affect glutamatergic transmission mainly presynaptically. Block of synaptically vs exogenously evoked responses. The *upper panel:* shows the dose-response relationship of halothane's block of synaptic responses (*dotted lines*), is shown together with its effect on responses to exogenously applied AMPA and NMDA (*solid lines*). Note that synaptic currents are more sensitive. The *lower panel:* Halothane enhances paired pulse facilitation. Reducing extracellular Ca^{2+} depresses the first of two consecutively evoked synaptic currents more than the second (traces Aa to Ac). The competitive antagonist CNQX inhibits both responses to a similar degree (traces Ba to Bc). Halothane (traces Ca to Cc) mimics low extracellular $[Ca^{2+}]$ and enhances paired-pulse facilitation, pointing to a presynaptic site of action, e.g., reduced Ca^{2+} + influx (from ref. *[96]*).

and in fact, glutamate is the major excitatory neurotransmitter on motoneurons, some investigators have examined the role of glutamatergic transmission on motoneurons. Motoneuronal activity can be documented by recording activity of ionic currents and EPSPs in whole motoneurons of neonatal rats. Enflurane depressed glutamate evoked currents; GABA and glycine were not involved as blockade with appropriate GABA and glycine antagonists did not alter the enflurane effect *(113)*. Ethanol effects were similar *(114)*. As mentioned in the Section on Pharmacologoy of NMDA receptors, glycine is important for GluR function as it is a coligand with glutamate. ACEA-1021 is an antagonist at the glycine recognition site on the NMDA receptor. When administered systemically at doses that do not cause sedation or motor effects in the awake rat, ACEA-1021 decreases MAC by about 50% *(115)*. Several studies have documented the anesthetic sparing effect of NMDA antagonists. NBQX, an AMPA antagonist, decreased halothane MAC by 75% at the highest dose studied *(116)*. The NMDA antagonist MK-801 likewise causes significant MAC reduction *(117)*. Genetic engineering techniques have been developed to alter GluR composition in intact mice as well as oocytes expressing GluRs. This has permitted comparison of receptor function to behavioral end-points. Joo et al. examined anesthetic sensitivity in mice lacking the GluR2 sub-unit. Behaviorally, these mice are more sensitive to pentobarbital and volatile anesthetics, as demonstrated by increased sleep time (with pentobarbital), increased hind-paw withdrawal latency (with volatile anesthetics), and decreased threshold for loss of righting reflex and pinch reflex *(28,29)*, although MAC was not affected. However, in vitro, the mutant GluRs were less sensitive to these anesthetics. This paradox, as explained by the authors, underscores the difficulty in extrapolating in vitro data to whole animal behavior and physiology. The authors speculate that global depression of glutamatergic excitatory transmission might explain the sensitivity to anesthetics, and caution that clinical disease states associated with down-regulation of the GluR2 sub-unit (Alzheimer disease, cerebral palsy, stroke, amyotrophic lateral sclerosis) will have increased sensitivity to anesthetics on that basis. Finally, volatile anesthetics also affect the handling of extracellular glutamate. Isoflurane enhanced glutamate uptake by presynaptic terminals *(118)* and most potent inhalational anesthetics enhanced the uptake of [^{3}H]-glutamate by astrocytes *(119)*. It is unclear how these actions affect physiologic function and whether they contribute to any aspect of the anesthetic.

SUMMARY

Glutamate is a major neurotransmitter in the mammalian CNS. Because it is the primary excitatory neurotransmitter, anesthetics might exert their effects via glutamatergic actions. This could result in production of each of the three anesthetic end-points: amnesia, unconsciousness, and immobility. Further work is required to determine how each anesthetic affects glutamatergic neurotransmission (relative to other receptor systems), and how these actions contribute to anesthesia.

REFERENCES

1. Hayashi, T. (1954) Effects of sodium glutamate on the nervous system. *Keio J. Med.* **3**, 183–192.
2. Curtis, D. R., Phillis, J. W., and Watkins, J. C. (1959) Chemical Excitation of Spinal Neurones. *Nature* **183**, 611–612.
3. Gallo, V. and Ghiani, C. A. (2000) Glutamate receptors in glia: new cells, new inputs and new functions. *Trends Pharmacol. Sci.* **21**, 252–258.
4. Bergles, D. E. and Jahr, C. E. (1997) Synaptic activation of glutamate transporters in hippocampal astrocytes. *Neuron* **19**, 1297–1308.
5. Araque, A., Parpura, V., Sanzgiri, R. P., and Haydon, P. G. (1999) Tripartite synapses: glia, the unacknowledged partner. *Trends Neurosci.* **22**, 208–215.
6. Wo, Z. G. and Oswald, R. E. (1995) Unraveling the modular design of glutamate-gated ion channels. *Trends Neurosci.* **18**, 161–168.
7. Jonas, P. and Burnashev, N. (1995) Molecular mechanisms controlling calcium entry through AMPA-type glutamate receptor channels. *Neuron* **15**, 987–990.
8. Kiskin, N. I., Krishtal, O. A., Tsyndrenko, A. Y., and Akaike, N. (1986) Are sulfhydryl groups essential for function of the glutamate-operated receptor-ionophore complex? *Neurosci. Lett.* **66**, 305–310.
9. Trussell, L. O., Thio, L. L., Zorumski, C. F., and Fischbach, G. D. (1988) Rapid desensitization of glutamate receptors in vertebrate central neurons. *Proc. Natl. Acad. Sci. USA* **85**, 4562–4566.

10. Mosbacher, J., Schoepfer, R., Monyer, H., Burnashev, N., Seeburg, P. H., and Ruppersberg, J. P. (1994) A molecular determinant for submillisecond desensitization in glutamate receptors. *Science* **266,** 1059–1062.

11. Ozawa, S., Kamiya, H., and Tsuzuki, K. (1998) Glutamate receptors in the mammalian central nervous system. *Prog. Neurobiol.* **54,** 581–618.

12. Wyllie, D. J., Traynelis, S. F., and Cull-Candy, S. G. (1993) Evidence for more than one type of non-NMDA receptor in outside-out patches from cerebellar granule cells of the rat. *J. Physiol.* **463,** 193–226.

13. Swanson, G. T., Kamboj, S. K., and Cull-Candy, S. G. (1997) Single-channel properties of recombinant AMPA receptors depend on RNA editing, splice variation, and subunit composition. *J. Neurosci.* **17,** 58–69.

14. Lambolez, B., Audinat, E., Bochet, P., Crepel, F., and Rossier, J. (1992) AMPA receptor subunits expressed by single Purkinje cells. *Neuron* **9,** 247–258.

15. Bochet, P., Audinat, E., Lambolez, B., et al. (1994) Subunit composition at the single-cell level explains functional properties of a glutamate-gated channel. *Neuron* **12,** 383–388.

16. Lambolez, B., Ropert, N., Perrais, D., Rossier, J., and Hestrin, S. (1996) Correlation between kinetics and RNA splicing of alpha-amino-3-hydroxy-5-methylisoxazole-4-propionic acid receptors in neocortical neurons. *Proc. Natl. Acad. Sci. USA* **93,** 1797–1802.

17. Stern-Bach, Y., Bettler, B., Hartley, M., Sheppard, P. O., O'Hara, P. J., and Heinemann, S. F. (1994) Agonist selectivity of glutamate receptors is specified by two domains structurally related to bacterial amino acid-binding proteins. *Neuron* **13,** 1345–1357.

18. Lerma, J., Paternain, A. V., Naranjo, J. R., and Mellstrom, B. (1993) Functional kainate-selective glutamate receptors in cultured hippocampal neurons. *Proc. Natl. Acad. Sci. USA* **90,** 11,688–11,692.

19. Partin, K. M., Bowie, D., and Mayer, M. L. (1995) Structural determinants of allosteric regulation in alternatively spliced AMPA receptors. *Neuron* **14,** 833–843.

20. Partin, K. M., Fleck, M. W., and Mayer, M. L. (1996) AMPA receptor flip/flop mutants affecting deactivation, desensitization, and modulation by cyclothiazide, aniracetam, and thiocyanate. *J. Neurosci.* **16,** 6634–6647.

21. Partin, K. M., Patneau, D. K., and Mayer, M. L. (1994) Cyclothiazide differentially modulates desensitization of alpha-amino-3-hydroxy-5-methyl-4-isoxazolepropionic acid receptor splice variants. *Mol. Pharmacol.* **46,** 129–138.

22. Clements, J. D., Lester, R. A., Tong, G., Jahr, C. E., and Westbrook, G. L. (1992) The time course of glutamate in the synaptic cleft. *Science* **258,** 1498–1501.

23. Hestrin, S. (1992) Activation and desensitization of glutamate-activated channels mediating fast excitatory synaptic currents in the visual cortex. *Neuron* **9,** 991–999.

24. Hestrin, S. (1993) Different glutamate receptor channels mediate fast excitatory synaptic currents in inhibitory and excitatory cortical neurons. *Neuron* **11,** 1083–1091.

25. Barbour, B., Keller, B. U., Llano, I., and Marty, A. (1994) Prolonged presence of glutamate during excitatory synaptic transmission to cerebellar Purkinje cells. *Neuron* **12,** 1331–1343.

26. Leranth, C., Szeidemann, Z., Hsu, M., and Buzsaki, G. (1996) AMPA receptors in the rat and primate hippocampus: a possible absence of GluR2/3 subunits in most interneurons. *Neuroscience* **70,** 631–652.

27. Jia, Z., Agopyan, N., Miu, P., et al. (1996) Enhanced LTP in mice deficient in the AMPA receptor GluR2. *Neuron* **17,** 945–956.

28. Joo, D. T., Gong, D., Sonner, J. M., et al. (2001) Blockade of AMPA receptors and volatile anesthetics—Reduced anesthetic requirements in GluR2 null mutant mice for loss of the righting reflex and antinociception but not minimum alveolar concentration. *Anesthesiology* **94,** 478–488.

29. Joo, D. T., Xiong, Z., MacDonald, J. F., et al. (1999) Blockade of Glutamate Receptors and Barbiturate Anesthesia: Increased Sensitivity to Pentobarbital-induced Anesthesia Despite Reduced Inhibition of AMPA Receptors in GluR2 Null Mutant Mice. *Anesthesiology* **91,** 1329–1341.

30. Herb, A., Burnashev, N., Werner, P., Sakmann, B., Wisden, W., and Seeburg, P. H. (1992) The KA-2 subunit of excitatory amino acid receptors shows widespread expression in brain and forms ion channels with distantly related subunits. *Neuron* **8,** 775–785.

31. Seeburg, P. H. (1993) The TINS/TiPS Lecture. The molecular biology of mammalian glutamate receptor channels. *Trends Neurosci.* **16,** 359–365.

32. Monaghan, D. T. and Cotman, C. W. (1982) The distribution of [³H]kainic acid binding sites in rat CNS as determined by autoradiography. *Brain Res.* **252,** 91–100.

33. Schoepfer, R., Monyer, H., Sommer, B., et al. (1994) Molecular biology of glutamate receptors. *Prog. Neurobiol.* **42,** 353–357.

34. Mackler, S. A. and Eberwine, J. H. (1993) Diversity of glutamate receptor subunit mRNA expression within live hippocampal CA1 neurons. *Mol. Pharmacol.* **44,** 308–315.

35. Wenthold, R. J., Trumpy, V. A., Zhu, W. S., and Petralia, R. S. (1994) Biochemical and assembly properties of GluR6 and KA2, two members of the kainate receptor family, determined with subunit-specific antibodies. *J. Biol. Chem.* **269,** 1332–1339.

36. Wisden, W. and Seeburg, P. H. (1993) A complex mosaic of high-affinity kainate receptors in rat brain. *J. Neurosci.* **13,** 3582–3598.

37. Burnashev, N. (1996) Calcium permeability of glutamate-gated channels in the central nervous system. *Curr. Opin. Neurobiol.* **6,** 311–317.

38. Kohler, M., Burnashev, N., Sakmann, B., and Seeburg, P. H. (1993) Determinants of Ca²⁺ permeability in both TM1 and TM2 of high affinity kainate receptor channels: diversity by RNA editing. *Neuron* **10,** 491–500.

39. Swanson, G. T., Feldmeyer, D., Kaneda, M., and Cull-Candy, S. G. (1996) Effect of RNA editing and subunit co-assembly single-channel properties of recombinant kainate receptors. *J. Physiol.* **492,** 129–142.

40. Burnashev, N., Villarroel, A., and Sakmann, B. (1996) Dimensions and ion selectivity of recombinant AMPA and kainate receptor channels and their dependence on Q/R site residues. *J. Physiol.* **496,** 165–173.

41. Howe, J. R. (1996) Homomeric and heteromeric ion channels formed from the kainate-type subunits GluR6 and KA2 have very small, but different, unitary conductances. *J. Neurophysiol.* **76,** 510–519.

42. Partin, K. M., Patneau, D. K., Winters, C. A., Mayer, M. L., and Buonanno, A. (1993) Selective modulation of desensitization at AMPA versus kainate receptors by cyclothiazide and concanavalin A. *Neuron* **11,** 1069–1082.

43. Wong, L. A. and Mayer, M. L. (1993) Differential modulation by cyclothiazide and concanavalin A of desensitization at native alpha-amino-3-hydroxy-5-methyl-4-isoxazolepropionic acid- and kainate-preferring glutamate receptors. *Mol. Pharmacol.* **44,** 504–510.

44. Wong, L. A., Mayer, M. L., Jane, D. E., and Watkins, J. C. (1994) Willardiines differentiate agonist binding sites for kainate- versus AMPA-preferring glutamate receptors in DRG and hippocampal neurons. *J. Neurosci.* **14,** 3881–3897.

45. Swanson, G. T., Green, T., and Heinemann, S. F. (1998) Kainate receptors exhibit differential sensitivities to (S)-5-iodowillardiine. *Mol. Pharmacol.* **53,** 942–949.

46. Clarke, V. R., Ballyk, B. A., Hoo, K. H., et al. (1997) A hippocampal GluR5 kainate receptor regulating inhibitory synaptic transmission. *Nature* **389,** 599–603.

47. Huettner, J. E. (1990) Glutamate receptor channels in rat DRG neurons: activation by kainate and quisqualate and blockade of desensitization by Con A. *Neuron* **5,** 255–266.

48. Bettler, B., Boulter, J., Hermans-Borgmeyer, I., et al. (1990) Cloning of a novel glutamate receptor subunit, GluR5: expression in the nervous system during development. *Neuron* **5,** 583–595.

49. Ruano, D., Lambolez, B., Rossier, J., Paternain, A. V., and Lerma, J. (1995) Kainate receptor subunits expressed in single cultured hippocampal neurons: molecular and functional variants by RNA editing. *Neuron* **14,** 1009–1017.

50. Lerma, J., Morales, M., Vicente, M. A., and Herreras, O. (1997) Glutamate receptors of the kainate type and synaptic transmission. *Trends Neurosci.* **20,** 9–12.

51. Castillo, P. E., Malenka, R. C., and Nicoll, R. A. (1997) Kainate receptors mediate a slow postsynaptic current in hippocampal CA3 neurons. *Nature* **388,** 182–186.

52. Vignes, M. and Collingridge, G. L. (1997) The synaptic activation of kainate receptors. *Nature* **388,** 179–182.

53. Frerking, M., Malenka, R. C., and Nicoll, R. A. (1998) Synaptic activation of kainate receptors on hippocampal interneurons. *Nat. Neurosci.* **1,** 479–486.

54. DeVries, S. H. and Schwartz, E. A. (1999) Kainate receptors mediate synaptic transmission between cones and 'Off' bipolar cells in a mammalian retina. *Nature* **397,** 157–160.

55. Frerking, M. and Nicoll, R. A. (2000) Synaptic kainate receptors. *Curr. Opin. Neurobiol.* **10,** 342–351.

56. Rodriguez-Moreno, A., Herreras, O., and Lerma, J. (1997) Kainate receptors presynaptically downregulate GABAergic inhibition in the rat hippocampus. *Neuron* **19,** 893–901.

57. Cossart, R., Esclapez, M., Hirsch, J. C., Bernard, C., and Ben-Ari, Y. (1998) GluR5 kainate receptor activation in interneurons increases tonic inhibition of pyramidal cells. *Nat. Neurosci.* **1,** 470–478.

58. Bureau, I., Bischoff, S., Heinemann, S. F., and Mulle, C. (1999) Kainate receptor-mediated responses in the CA1 field of wild-type and GluR6-deficient mice. *J. Neurosci.* **19,** 653–663.

59. Min, M. Y., Melyan, Z., and Kullmann, D. M. (1999) Synaptically released glutamate reduces gamma-aminobutyric acid (GABA) ergic inhibition in the hippocampus via kainate receptors. *Proc. Natl. Acad. Sci. USA* **96,** 9932–9937.

60. Cossart, R., Dinocourt, C., Hirsch, J. C., et al. (2001) Dendritic but not somatic GABAergic inhibition is decreased in experimental epilepsy. *Nat. Neurosci.* **4,** 52–62.

61. Frerking, M., Petersen, C. C. H., and Nicoll, R. A. (1999) Mechanisms underlying kainate receptor-mediated disinhibition in the hippocampus. *Proc. Natl. Acad. Sci. USA* **96,** 12,917–12,922.

62. Rodriguez-Moreno, A., Lopez-Garcia, J. C., and Lerma, J. (2000) Two populations of kainate receptors with separate signaling mechanisms in hippocampal interneurons. *Proc. Natl. Acad. Sci. USA* **97,** 1293–1298.

63. Moriyoshi, K., Masu, M., Ishii, T., Shigemoto, R., Mizuno, N., and Nakanishi, S. (1991) Molecular cloning and characterization of the rat NMDA receptor. *Nature* **354,** 31–37.

64. Mori, H. and Mishina, M. (1995) Structure and function of the NMDA receptor channel. *Neuropharmacology* **34,** 1219–1237.

65. Hollmann, M. and Heinemann, S. (1994) Cloned glutamate receptors. *Ann. Rev. Neurosci.* **17,** 31–108.

66. Monyer, H., Burnashev, N., Laurie, D. J., Sakmann, B., and Seeburg, P. H. (1994) Developmental and regional expression in the rat brain and functional properties of four NMDA receptors. *Neuron* **12,** 529–540.

67. Petralia, R. S., Wang, Y. X., and Wenthold, R. J. (1994) Histological and ultrastructural localization of the kainate receptor subunits, KA2 and GluR6/7, in the rat nervous system using selective antipeptide antibodies. *J. Comp. Neurol.* **349,** 85–110.

68. Lester, R. A., Clements, J. D., Westbrook, G. L., and Jahr, C. E. (1990) Channel kinetics determine the time course of NMDA receptor-mediated synaptic currents. *Nature* **346,** 565–567.

69. Benveniste, M., Clements, J., Vyklicky, L., Jr., and Mayer, M. L. (1990) A kinetic analysis of the modulation of N-methyl-D-aspartic acid receptors by glycine in mouse cultured hippocampal neurones. *J. Physiol.(Lond.)* **428,** 333–357.

70. Sather, W., Johnson, J. W., Henderson, G., and Ascher, P. (1990) Glycine-insensitive desensitization of NMDA responses in cultured mouse embryonic neurons. *Neuron* **4,** 725–731.

71. Burnashev, N., Zhou, Z., Neher, E., and Sakmann, B. (1995) Fractional calcium currents through recombinant GluR channels of the NMDA, AMPA and kainate receptor subtypes. *J. Physiol.* **485,** 403–418.

72. Nowak, L., Bregestovski, P., Ascher, P., Herbet, A., and Prochiantz, A. (1984) Magnesium gates glutamate-activated channels in mouse central neurones. *Nature* **307,** 462–465.

73. MacDermott, A. B., Mayer, M. L., Westbrook, G. L., Smith, S. J., and Barker, J. L. (1986) NMDA-receptor activation increases cytoplasmic calcium concentration in cultured spinal cord neurones. *Nature* **321,** 519–522.

74. Ascher, P. and Nowak, L. (1988) The role of divalent cations in the *N*-methyl-D-aspartate responses of mouse central neurones in culture. *J. Physiol.* **399,** 247–266.

75. Kutsuwada, T., Kashiwabuchi, N., Mori, H., et al. (1992) Molecular diversity of the NMDA receptor channel. *Nature* **358,** 36–41.

76. Monyer, H., Sprengel, R., Schoepfer, R., et al. (1992) Heteromeric NMDA receptors: molecular and functional distinction of subtypes. *Science* **256,** 1217–1221.

77. Johnson, J. W. and Ascher, P. (1987) Glycine potentiates the NMDA response in cultured mouse brain neurons. *Nature* **325,** 529–531.

78. Matsui, T., Sekiguchi, M., Hashimoto, A., Tomita, U., Nishikawa, T., and Wada, K. (1995) Functional comparison of D-serine and glycine in rodents: the effect on cloned NMDA receptors and the extracellular concentration. *J. Neurochem.* **65,** 454–458.

79. Kuryatov, A., Laube, B., Betz, H., and Kuhse, J. (1997) Mutational analysis of the glycine-binding site of the NMDA receptor: structural similarity with bacterial amino acid-binding proteins. *Neuron* **12,** 1291–1300.

80. Laube, B., Hirai, H., Sturgess, M., Betz, H., and Kuhse, J. (1997) Molecular determinants of agonist discrimination by NMDA receptor subunits: analysis of the glutamate binding site on the NR2B subunit. *Neuron* **18,** 493–503.

81. Sucher, N. J., Awobuluyi, M., Choi, Y. B., and Lipton, S. A. (1996) NMDA receptors: from genes to channels. *Trends Pharmacol. Sci.* **17,** 348–355.

82. Jones, K. A. and Baughman, R. W. (1991) Both NMDA and non-NMDA subtypes of glutamate receptors are concentrated at synapses on cerebral cortical neurons in culture. *Neuron* **7,** 593–603.

83. Durand, G. M., Kovalchuk, Y., and Konnerth, A. (1996) Long-term potentiation and functional synapse induction in developing hippocampus. *Nature* **381,** 71–75.

84. Wu, G., Malinow, R., and Cline, H. T. (1996) Maturation of a central glutamatergic synapse. *Science* **274,** 972–976.

85. Ben-Ari, Y., Khazipov, R., Leinekugel, X., Caillard, O., and Gaiarsa, J. L. (1997) GABAA, NMDA and AMPA receptors: a developmentally regulated "menage a trois." *Trends Neurosci.* **20,** 523–529.

86. Tsien, J. Z. (2000) Linking Hebb's coincidence-detection to memory formation. *Curr. Opin. Neurobiol.* **10,** 266–273.

87. Feldman, D. E., Nicoll, R. A., and Malenka, R. C. (1999) Synaptic plasticity at thalamocortical synapses in developing rat somatosensory cortex: LTP, LTD, and silent synapses. *J. Neurobiol.* **41,** 92–101.

88. Nicoll, R. A. and Malenka, R. C. (1999) Expression mechanisms underlying NMDA receptor-dependent long-term potentiation. *Ann. NY Acad. Sci.* **868,** 515–525.

89. Kullmann, D. M., Asztely, F., and Walker, M. C. (2000) The role of mammalian ionotropic receptors in synaptic plasticity: LTP, LTD and epilepsy. *Cell. Mol. Life Sci.* **57,** 1551–1561.

90. Manabe, T. (1997) Two forms of hippocampal long-term depression, the counterpart of long-term potentiation. *Rev. Neurosci.* **8,** 179–193.

91. Krasowski, M. D. and Harrison, N. L. (1999) General anesthetic actions on ligand-gated ion channels. *Cell Mol. Life Sci.* **55,** 1278–1303.

92. Carl, V. and Moroni, F. (1992) General anaesthetics inhibit the responses induced by glutamate receptor agonists in the mouse cortex. *Neurosci. Lett.* **146,** 21–24.

93. Wakamori, M., Ikemoto, Y., and Akaike, N. (1991) Effects of two volatile anesthetics and a volatile convulsant on the excitatory and inhibitory amino acid responses in dissociated CNS neurons of the rat. *J. Neurophysiol.* **66,** 2014–2021.

94. Minami, K., Wick, M. J., Stern-Bach, Y., et al. (1998) Sites of volatile anesthetic action on kainate (Glutamate receptor 6) receptors. *J. Biol. Chem.* **273,** 8248–8255.

95. Dildy-Mayfield, J. E., Eger, E. I., 2nd, and Harris, R. A. (1996) Anesthetics produce subunit-selective actions on glutamate receptors. *J. Pharmacol. Exper. Ther.* **276,** 1058–1065.

96. Kirson, E. D., Yaari, Y., and Perouansky, M. (1998) Presynaptic and postsynaptic actions of halothane at glutamatergic synapses in the mouse hippocampus. *Brit. J. Pharmacol.* **124,** 1607–1614.

97. Perouansky, M., Baranov, D., Salman, M., and Yaari, Y. (1995) Effects of halothane on glutamate receptor-mediated excitatory postsynaptic currents. *Anesthesiology* **83,** 109–119.

98. Perouansky, M., Kirson, E. D., and Yaari, Y. (1996) Halothane blocks synaptic excitation of inhibitory interneurons. *Anesthesiology* **85,** 1431–1438.

99. Creager, R., Dunwiddie, T., and Lynch, G. (1980) Paired-pulse and frequency facilitation in the CA1 region of the in vitro rat hippocampus. *J. Physiol.* **299,** 409–424.

100. Manabe, T., Wyllie, D. J., Perkel, D. J., and Nicoll, R. A. (1993) Modulation of synaptic transmission and long-term potentiation: effects on paired pulse facilitation and EPSC variance in the CA1 region of the hippocampus. *J. Neurophysiol.* **70,** 1451–1459.

101. Perouansky, M., Kirson, E. D., and Yaari, Y. (1998) Mechanism of action of volatile anesthetics: effects of halothane on glutamate receptors in vitro. *Toxicol. Lett.* **100–101,** 65–69.

102. Mikulec, A. A., Pittson, S., Amagasu, S. M., Monroe, F. A., and MacIver, M. B. (1998) Halothane depresses action potential conduction in hippocampal axons. *Brain Res.* **796,** 231–238.

103. Franks, N. P., Dickinson, R., de Sousa, S. L., Hall, A. C., and Lieb, W. R. (1998) How does xenon produce anaesthesia? *Nature* **396,** 324.

104. de Sousa, S. L., Dickinson, R., Lieb, W. R., and Franks, N. P. (2000) Contrasting synaptic actions of the inhalational general anesthetics isoflurane and xenon. *Anesthesiology* **92,** 1055–1066.

105. Yamakura, T. and Harris, R. A. (2000) Effects of gaseous anesthetics nitrous oxide and xenon on ligand-gated ion channels. Comparison with isoflurane and ethanol. *Anesthesiology* **93,** 1095–1101.

106. Mennerick, S., Jevtovic-Todorovic, V., Todorovic, S. M., Shen, W., Olney, J. W., and Zorumski, C. F. (1998) Effect of nitrous oxide on excitatory and inhibitory synaptic transmission in hippocampal cultures. *J. Neurosci.* **18,** 9716–9726.

107. Jevtovic-Todorovic, V., Todorovic, S. M., Mennerick, S., et al. (1998) Nitrous oxide (laughing gas) is an NMDA antagonist, neuroprotectant and neurotoxin. *Nat. Med.* **4,** 460–463.

108. Yamamura, T., Harada, K., Okamura, A., and Kemmotsu, O. (1990) Is the site of action of ketamine anesthesia the *N*-methyl-D-aspartate receptor? *Anesthesiology* **72,** 704–710.

109. Hollmann, M. W., Liu, H. T., Hoenemann, C. W., Liu, W. H., and Durieux, M. E. (2001) Modulation of NMDA receptor function by ketamine and magnesium. Part II: Interactions with volatile anesthetics. *Anesth. Analg.* **92,** 1182–1191.

110. Orser, B. A., Pennefather, P. S., and MacDonald, J. F. (1997) Multiple mechanisms of ketamine blockade of *N*-methyl-D-aspartate receptors. *Anesthesiology* **86,** 903–917.

111. Yamakura, T., Sakimura, K., Shimoji, K., and Mishina, M. (1995) Effects of propofol on various AMPA-, kainate- and NMDA-selective glutamate receptor channels expressed in *Xenopus* oocytes. *Neurosci. Lett.* **188,** 187–190.

112. Orser, B. A, Bertlik, M., Wang, L. Y., and MacDonald, J. F. (1995) Inhibition by propofol (2,6 di-isopropylphenol) of the *N*-methyl-D-aspartate subtype of glutamate receptor in cultured hippocampal neurones. *Brit. J. Pharmacol.* **116,** 1761–1768.

113. Cheng, G. and Kendig, J. J. (2000) Enflurane directly depresses glutamate AMPA and NMDA currents in mouse spinal cord motor neurons independent of actions on GABA$_A$ or glycine receptors. *Anesthesiology* **93,** 1075–1084.

114. Wang, M. Y., Rampil, I. J., and Kendig, J. J. (1999) Ethanol directly depresses AMPA and NMDA glutamate currents in spinal cord motor neurons independent of actions on GABA$_A$ or glycine receptors. *J. Pharmacol. Exper. Thera.* **290,** 362–367.

115. McFarlane, C., Warner, D. S., Nader, A., and Dexter, F. (1995) Glycine receptor antagonism Effects of ACEA-1021 on the minimum alveolar concentration for halothane in the rat. *Anesthesiology* **82,** 963–968.

116. McFarlane, C., Warner, D. S., Todd, M. M., and Nordholm, L. (1992) AMPA receptor competitive antagonism reduces halothane MAC in rats. *Anesthesiology* **77,** 1165–1170.

117. Scheller, M. S., Zornow, M. H., Fleischer, J. E., Shearman, G. T., and Greber, T. F. (1989) The noncompetitive *N*-methyl-D-aspartate receptor antagonist, MK-801 profoundly reduces volatile anesthetic requirements in rabbits. *Neuropharmacology* **28,** 677–681.

118. Miyazaki, H., Nakamura, Y., Arai, T., and Kataoka, K. (1997) Increase of glutamate uptake in astrocytes: a possible mechanism of action of volatile anesthetics. *Anesthesiology* **86,** 1359–1366.

119. Larsen, M. and Langmoen, I. A. (1998) The effect of volatile anaesthetics on synaptic release and uptake of glutamate. *Toxicol. Lett.* **100–101,** 59–64.

120. Watkins, J. C. (2000) L-Glutamate as a central neurotransmitter: looking back. *Biochem. Soc. Trans.* **28,** 297–310.

121. Bettler, B. and Mulle, C. (1995) Review: Neurotransmitter Receptors II AMPA and Kainate Receptors. *Neuropharmacology* **34,** 123–139.

20

General Anesthetic Effects on Glycine Receptors

Stephen Daniels

INTRODUCTION

Glycine was first identified as an inhibitory neurotransmitter in a paper by Aprison and Werman *(1)*. This role was subsequently confirmed in two papers detailing a combined neurochemical and neurophysiological approach, which led to a general acceptance of this role for glycine *(2,3)*. Subsequently, it was established that strychnine was a selective antagonist at the glycine receptor *(4)*. The identification and characterization of the glycine receptor as a transmembrane protein composed of two subunits, α and β, followed over a decade later *(5–9)*.

The glycine receptor is now accepted to be a member of one of the two superfamilies of postsynaptic ligand-gated ion channels that mediate fast synaptic transmission in the mammalian central nervous system *(10)*. The first of these families includes the nicotinic acetylcholine (nACh), γ-aminobutyric acid-A (GABA$_A$), glycine (Gly), and 5-hydroxytryptamine-3 (5-HT$_3$) receptors. The second comprises the glutamate receptors; those that are sensitive to N-methyl-D-aspartate (Glu^{NMDA}), and those sensitive to kainate and α-amino-3-hydroxy-5-methyl-4-isoxazoleproprionic acid, collectively referred to as the nonNMDA receptors (Glu^{KA} and Glu^{AMPA}). In the first superfamily, the nACh and 5-HT$_3$ receptors mediate excitatory synaptic transmission by regulating the passage of Na$^+$ and K$^+$ across the neuronal membrane. The GABA$_A$ and Gly receptors mediate inhibitory neurotransmission by regulating the passage of Cl$^-$ across the neuronal membrane. The glutamate receptors mediate excitatory neurotransmission.

GLYCINE RECEPTOR STRUCTURE, FUNCTION, LOCATION

Members of the first receptor superfamily share a common architecture, being composed of five subunits that span the cell membrane, arranged in a cylindrical fashion to form a central ion-conducting pore. The individual subunits each possess a large N-terminal extracellular domain, containing the ligand binding sites, and four transmembrane regions, the second of which forms the ion-channel lining (for reviews *see* refs. *11–13*). Two of the members of this family of receptors, the nACh and GABA$_A$ receptors, possess a rich diversity of subunits with, respectively, five and seven different subunits identified, and with multiple isoforms of these different subunits. In contrast, the Gly and 5-HT$_3$ receptors appear to have only two different subunits each with relatively few isoforms. In the case of the Gly receptor, there are two glycosylated membrane-spanning subunits, the ligand-binding α (48 kDa) and the structural β (58 kDa) *(14)*. To date, four α-subunit genes and a single β-subunit gene have been identified *(15)*. All α-subunits will assemble into functional homomeric receptors, and the $\alpha 1$ and $\alpha 2$ subunits will co-assemble with variable stoichiometry *(16)*. The β-subunit will only form functional heteromers with an invariant $\alpha_3\beta_2$ stoichiometry *(16)*. Native Gly receptors in

From: *Contemporary Clinical Neuroscience: Neural Mechanisms of Anesthesia*
Edited by: Joseph F. Antognini et al. © Humana Press Inc., Totowa, NJ

adult spinal cord are $\alpha1_3\beta_2$ heteromers, whereas in embryonic spinal cord, the receptors are likely to be $\alpha2_5$ homomers *(17–19)*.

It has been widely held that glycine receptors are found predominantly in the spinal cord and brain stem *(20)*. However, there is now considerable evidence from immunocytochemistry and *in situ* hybridization studies that glycine receptors are present in many higher brain regions, including the olfactory bulb, midbrain, and cerebellum (for review *see* ref. *21*). Spinal cord, brain stem, and colliculi are reported to contain $\alpha1$ subunits; hippocampus, cerebral cortex and thalamus contain $\alpha2$ subunits; and olfactory bulb, hippocampus, and cerebellum contain $\alpha3$ subunits. The β-subunit was found throughout the brain. It would appear, therefore, that glycine receptors play an important role in both motor and sensory processing and, as such, represent a potentially important target for general anesthetics.

Detailed structural information on the glycine receptor has been elucidated from a wide variety of studies on mutated receptors expressed in *Xenopus* oocytes or human embryonic kidney cells (HEK293). The ligand binding sites for glycine and strychnine lie within the N-terminal domain with residues 190–202 important for glycine binding and residues 144, 149, 159 and 160 for strychnine binding (*see* Fig. 1, *[21,22]*). The intracellular loop M1–M2 (residues 243–252), and the extracellular loop M2–M3 (residues 271–284) appear to function as "hinges," which control the rotation of M2 following glycine binding that is essential for channel-opening *(23,24)*. In particular, the proline at residue 250 in the intracellular M1–M2 loop *(25)*, and the lysine at residue 276 in the extracellular M2–M3 loop *(24)* appear important (*see* Fig. 1).

It has been suggested that the extracellular M2–M3 loop interacts with the glycine binding site on the N-terminal region because mutations in this region (271–284) are associated with larger increases in glycine K_i values than mutations elsewhere *(23)*. In contrast, mutations to two of the residues in the intracellular M1–M2 loop (W243A and I244A) partially disrupt channel gating *(23)*. Finally, it has been suggested that phosphorylation sites on the intracellular M3–M4 loop (*see* Fig. 1) might interact with channel gating residues in the M1–M2 loop *(23)*.

Further evidence that the M2–M3 extracellular loop is implicated in the gating mechanism of the glycine receptor comes from experiments in which the residues 271–277 of human homomeric $\alpha1$ receptors, expressed in human embryonic kidney cells (HEK293), were covalently modified by positively charged methanethiosulphonate ethyltrimethylammonium and negatively charged methanethiosulphonate ethylsulphonate. These modifications were faster in the glycine-bound state implying that the surface accessibility of the M2–M3 loop increased as the channel transitions from closed to open state. This suggests that the loop moves during channel activation *(26)*.

Finally, exchanging histamine for glutamine at residue 266 (Q266H), some 2/3 into the M2 domain (*see* Fig. 1), reduces channel open time with little change in closed times *(27)*. This implies that the open state is destabilized. The passage of Cl^- through the channel would not be affected because the histidine residue points to the interior of the protein. Therefore, the rotation of M2, necessary for opening the channel, may be hindered.

The general picture of the structure and function of the glycine receptor is therefore a collection of five subunits arranged in a cylindrical fashion in which the α-subunits possess long extracellular N-terminal domains that contain the ligand binding sites. Four transmembrane domains, linked by intra- and extracellular loops, follow this domain. The second transmembrane domain is a kinked α-helix that forms the ion-channel lining. When the ligand binds, there is an interaction with the extracellular loop between M2 and M3 that allows M2 to rotate, thus opening the channel. Interaction with this loop or with the intracellular loop joining M1 and M2 would allosterically modulate channel activation. This general model is supported by electron density data from nACh receptors *(13)* and molecular modelling *(22)*, and might represent a general structural and functional arrangement for all the ligand-gated ion-channels in this superfamily (nACh, $GABA_A$, Gly, and $5-HT_3$).

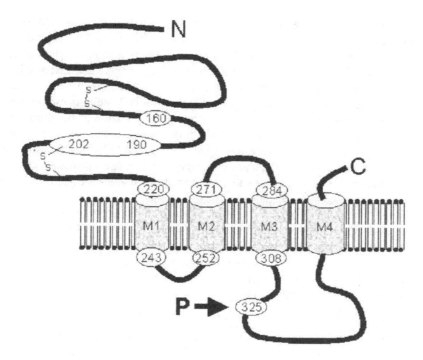

Fig. 1. Illustration of the structural organization of the $\alpha1$ subunit of the human glycine receptor. The numbers refer to the residue numbers and 'P' indicates a site for phosphorylation.

EFFECTS OF ANESTHETICS ON RECOMBINANT RECEPTORS IN EXPRESSION SYSTEMS

Early studies on the effects of anesthetics were made on acutely dissociated mammalian neurons. Whole-cell patch clamp studies were used to observe the effect of halothane and enflurane on glycine-elicited currents from acutely dissociated neurons from rat nucleus tractus solitarius *(28)*. Both halothane (1 mM) and enflurane (1 mM) potentiated the response to glycine, producing a leftward shift in the equilibrium concentration response curves. The K_d for glycine was reduced by 50 and 35% by halothane and enflurane, respectively, with no effect on E_{max} or Hill coefficent (1.8). Interestingly, the volatile convulsant, hexafluoro-diethyl ether had no effect on the glycine-evoked current. Whole-cell patch clamp recordings of neurons were also used to study the effects of propofol and pentobarbitone on glycine-elicited currents from acutely dissociated embryonic mouse spinal neurons *(29)*. The amplitude of strychnine-sensitive currents elicited by glycine (100 μM) were potentiated (120–180%) by propofol (8.4–16.8 μM), but not by pentobarbitone (10 and 100 μM).

These early studies clearly established that the strychnine-sensitive glycine receptor could be potentiated by general anesthetic substances in a manner similar to the GABA$_A$ receptor.

The Effect of General Anesthetics on Recombinant Glycine Receptors Expressed in Xenopus *Oocytes*

The experiments described below have employed the *Xenopus* oocyte expression technique to examine the effects of a wide variety of anesthetics on recombinant human glycine receptors. The majority of experiments have involved expression of homomeric $\alpha1_5$ receptors, but some have looked at heteromeric $\alpha1/\beta$ receptors and homomeric $\alpha2_5$ receptors. Glycine-activated currents recorded from *Xenopus* oocytes expressing glycine receptors are somewhat different from those recorded from native receptors in acutely dissociated cells (*see* for example *30*). They are less sensitive to glycine, with the EC_{50} concentration typically an order of magnitude greater in oocytes, although the Hill coefficients are similar. This is also the case when comparing oocytes and mammalian cell expression systems (e.g., HEK293). It is possible that this apparent reduction in glycine affinity for receptors expressed in oocytes is an artifact of cell size and consequent difficulty in establishing equilibrium conditions, or alternatively, arises from differences in phosphorylation of the intracellular loops of the receptor protein that in turn affect the channel-gating properties. However, it is more likely that differences in receptor clustering that are known to affect function *(31–33)*, are responsible for these differences as co-expression of gephyrin, a protein that anchors receptor proteins to the plasma membrane and enables cluster formation, causes a leftward shift in the glycine equilibrium concentration-response curve *(31)*.

Currents elicited from oocytes also differ from those from mammalian cells in that the currents from oocytes tend to exhibit outward rectification and a reversal potential of −23 mV. Whereas in mammalian cells, the current-voltage relationship is linear with a reversal potential of 0 mV. The different reversal potentials simply reflect the different intracellular ionic composition in amphibian and mammalian cells. However, it remains unclear as to why the current-voltage relationship in the oocyte should exhibit outward rectification.

Simple Gases, Alcohols, and Volatile Anesthetics

The simplest possible anesthetic gas, xenon, potentiated the response of human homomeric $\alpha 1_5$ receptors to glycine (EC_{10}) by approx 50% at clinically relevant concentrations (1–2 m*M*). Nitrous oxide, also at a clinically relevant concentration (20–30 m*M*), potentiated the response to bath applied glycine (EC_{10}) by 75% *(34)*. Although the potentiation by these gases is modest, it should be noted that the degree of potentiation increased markedly at higher doses, exemplified by nitrous oxide which, at a calculated aqueous concentration of 300 m*M*, produced a potentiation of 1400%. In contrast to other anesthetics, nitrous oxide also potentiated the response when using maximal concentrations (EC_{100}) of applied glycine (1 m*M*) *(34)*.

Although not considered conventional anesthetics, alcohols can induce anesthesia in vivo and exhibit a "cut-off" in effect for alcohols above a certain chain length. This cut-off has been taken as one of the cornerstones of the argument that anesthetics act at specific sites within proteins, and not via some physicochemical interaction with a bulk phase *(35)*. The cut-off has been observed in tadpoles *(36)*, with the luminescent protein luciferase *(35)*, and more recently, in $GABA_A$ receptors *(37)*.

Glycine (EC_2) responses were potentiated by *n*-alcohols (chain length 2–12) in a dose dependent fashion, with homomeric $\alpha 1_5$ and $\alpha 2_5$ receptors affected equally *(38)*. The degree of potentiation increased with increasing chain length, from 100% with ethanol (C2) to 300% with decanol (C10). Dodecanol (C12) produced almost no potentiation. This cut-off at C10/12 agrees closely with that found for $GABA_A$ receptors *(37)* and tadpoles *(36)*.

Trichloroethanol, the principal active metabolite of choral hydrate, potentiated glycine responses at both $\alpha 1_5$ and $\alpha 1\beta$ receptors by some 80–90% *(39)*. This was considerably more than was observed at $GABA_A$ receptors (50%).

In HEK293 cells expressing $\alpha 1_5$ receptors the tertiary alcohols t-butanol, 1,1,1-trichloro-2-methyl-2-propanol and 1,1,1-tribromo-2-methyl-2-propanol all potentiated the response to glycine, by 57, 146, and 196%, respectively *(40)*.

The potency of the alcohols at potentiating the response to glycine is broadly in agreement with the predictions, on the basis of lipid solubility (Fig. 2). Tertiary butanol appears somewhat less, and butanol and hexanol, somewhat more potent than expected. Although the results for the *n*-alcohols and tertiary alcohols were obtained using different expression systems, oocytes, and HEK293 cells, respectively. The calculated molar volumes for decanol and dodecanol are 614 cm^3/mol and 726 cm^3/mol, suggesting that molecules larger than ~700 cm^3/mol would either not affect the glycine receptor, or

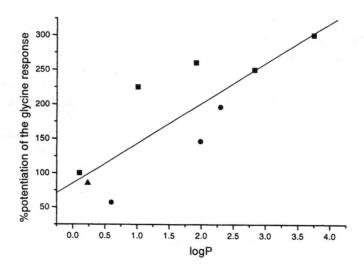

Fig. 2. The potentation by alcohols of the glycine-elicited current responses from *Xenopus* oocytes and HEK293 cells expressing homomeric α1 glycine receptors plotted against the logP values for the alcohols. Data represented by squares are for ethanol, butanol, hexanol, octanol, and decanol (oocytes: ref. *38*). Data represented by circles are for *t*-butanol; 1,1,1-trichloro-2methyl-2-propanol and 1,1,1-tribromo-2-methyl-2-propanol (HEK293 cells: ref. *40*). Data represented by upward facing triangle are for trichloroethanol (oocytes: ref. *39*). LogP values are the logarithm of the partition coefficient for *n*-Octanol/Water calculated by fragmentation methods (CS Chemdraw Ultra).

would do so at a different site. The calculated molar volumes for the tertiary alcohols were 267 cm³/ mol, 403cm³/mol and 442 cm³/mol for *t*-butanol, 1,1,1-trichloro-2-methyl-2-propanol and 1,1,1-tribromo-2-methyl-2-propanol, respectively.

Volatile Anesthetics

The volatile anesthetics all potentiate the response to glycine (EC_{10}) at homomeric α1$_5$ receptors. Halothane is the most potent, potentiating the response by over 200% at clinically relevant concentrations *(30,34,41,42)*. Isoflurane, enflurane, methoxyflurane, and sevoflurane produced progressively less potentiation; 177, 163, 100, and 63%, respectively *(30)*. Chloroform (100%) and diethyl ether (200%), also potentiate the response to glycine *(34)*. Isoflurane produced a parallel leftward shift in the glycine equilibrium concentration response curve *(30)* similar to that observed in nulceus tractus solitarius neurons *(28)*. Halothane, chloroform, and diethyl ether had no effect on the response to saturating concentrations of glycine (EC_{100}) *(34)*.

Diethyl ether, enflurane, isoflurane, methoxyflurane, and sevoflurane all potentiated the response to glycine (EC_{20}) at homomeric α1$_5$ receptors expressed in HEK293 cells *(40)*. The degree of potentiation was similar to that observed in oocytes, with the exception of sevoflurane, which effected a considerably greater potentiation to the response in HEK293 cells, 142% compared to 63% in oocytes. Interestingly, the degree of potentiation by these anesthetics to glycine responses from acutely dissociated medullary neurons was uniformly less (approximately half) than that observed in oocytes *(30)*.

In vivo and in vitro anesthetics have been observed to exhibit stereoselectivity *(35)*. However, at the α1$_5$ glycine receptor, no stereoselectivity for *S*-(+)- or *R*-(−)-isoflurane was observed *(30)*. This does not rule out a role for the glycine receptor in anesthesia, but does suggest that it cannot be an exclusive role.

Isoflurane (305 µ*M*) reduced the EC_{50} of the endogenous partial agonist taurine at homomeric α1$_5$ glycine receptors by 44% (1.6–0.9 m*M*). This was similar to the reduction in EC_{50} observed for glycine at the same receptors, 215–113 µ*M* (47%) *(30)*. However, for taurine in the presence of isoflurane, E_{max} increased 25%. This implies that the effect of isoflurane at the glycine receptor is not solely to reduce the affinity of the receptor for glycine. The anesthetic must be affecting partially or even solely, the gating mechanism by which glycine binding leads to channel activation.

Further evidence that anesthetics exert their action via specific interactions with neuroactive proteins is that compounds exist that, on the basis of their lipid solubility, are predicted to be anesthetic, but are not *(43)*. Chloro-1,2,2-trifluorocyclobutane and 1,2-dichlorohexafluorocyclobutane are both predicted to be anesthetics on the basis of their lipid solubility. However, only chloro-1,2,2-trifluorocyclobutane is anesthetic in vivo. Chloro-1,2,2-trifluorocyclobutane potentiated homomeric $\alpha 1_5$ glycine receptors by up to 700%, whereas 1,2-dichlorohexafluorocyclobutane had no effect *(38)*. The lack of effect of 1,2-dichlorohexafluorocyclobutane is not simply a size exclusion, since its calculated molar volume is 403 cm³/mol, well below the cut-off size predicted by the *n*-alcohols.

Barbiturates

The barbiturates form a structurally coherent group of anesthetics. The four barbiturates considered here: pentobarbitone, thiopentone, methohexitone, and phenobarbitone, all have calculated molar volumes greater than 700 cm³/mol. The initial report on the effect of pentobarbitone indicated that it only weakly potentiated $\alpha 1_5$ receptors *(38)*. Subsequent studies have reported that pentobarbitone, at a concentration of approx 800 μM, potentiates the response of $\alpha 1_5$ glycine receptors by approx 70% *(39,44)*. However, a separate study reported that using concentrations between 100 μM and 400 μM, pentobarbitone potentiated $\alpha 1_5$ receptors by 200% *(34)*. Thiopentone is more potent than pentobarbitone. In the clinical range of concentration (10–40 μM), it potentiates $\alpha 1_5$ glycine receptors by approx 300%, and at higher concentrations (200 μM) by 1300% *(34)*. Methohexitone and phenobarbitone were without effect on this receptor.

Pentobarbitone, thiopentone, methohexitone, and phenobarbitone all acted as noncompetitive antagonists at the $\alpha 1_5$ glycine receptors when the receptors were activated with a saturating concentration of glycine (EC_{100}) *(34)*.

Propofol, Etomidate, and Ketamine

The initial report of the effect of propofol on $\alpha 1_5$ glycine receptors indicated that the response to glycine was only weakly potentiated *(38)*. Subsequently, Pistis and colleagues *(39)* reported concentration dependent enhancement of glycine responses of approx 100% using either $\alpha 1_5$ or $\alpha 1\beta$ receptors. These findings were in agreement with experiments in which glycine receptors were expressed in oocytes following injection of mRNA extracted from rat brain *(45)*. Subsequently, potentiation of the glycine response at $\alpha 1_5$ receptors of 200% *(34)* and 100% *(44)* have been reported for propofol concentrations between 10 and 20 μM. Propofol had no effect on $\alpha 1_5$ glycine receptors when the receptors were activated with a saturating concentration of glycine (EC_{100}) *(34)*.

Etomidate has been reported to have no effect on glycine receptors *(38)*, or to potentiate the current response by less than 30% at both $\alpha 1_5$ and $\alpha 1\beta$ receptors *(34,39,44)*. Etomidate acts as a noncompetitive antagonist at $\alpha 1_5$ receptors activated with concentrations of glycine greater than the EC_{50} *(34)*. Ketamine has been reported to have no effect at $\alpha 1_5$ receptors *(38)*.

Steroids

The anesthetic steroid 5α-pregnan-3α-ol-20-one potentiates the $GABA_A$ receptor in a concentration dependent manner *(44,46)*. In contrast, it has no effect on glycine $\alpha 1_5$ or $\alpha 1\beta$ receptors *(44)*. It has also been reported to be without effect on chick spinal neurons *(47)*. However, alphaxalone has been reported to weakly potentiate $\alpha 1_5$ glycine receptors *(38)*, and minaxolone positively modulates glycine receptors expressed in oocytes following injection of rat brain mRNA *(45)*. Furthermore, 20-α hydrocortisone, α-corticol, and hydrocortisone all positively modulate the glycine receptor, but have no effect at the $GABA_A$ receptor *(48)*.

Anesthetic Additivity

Anesthetics act additively in vivo, a fact that is recognized and exploited in clinical anesthesia. If binary combinations of anesthetics act in an additive manner, then this can be taken as evidence that they might share a common site of action.

Experiments have been performed on *Xenopus* oocytes expressing homomeric $\alpha 1_5$ glycine receptors in which equilibrium concentration-response curves were established for pentobarbitone, thiopentone, and a mixture of pentobarbitone and thiopentone, using an EC_{10} concentration of glycine to elicit a response. Glycine elicited an inward, desensitizing current that was potentiated by both thiopentone and pentobarbitone. The potentiation by the binary mixture of thiopentone and pentobarbitone was in all cases, equal to the sum of the potentiation by the individual anesthetics (*see* Fig. 3, *[49]*).

It is not surprising that two such similar anesthetics would exhibit additivity in this way. However, similar experiments using *Xenopus* oocytes expressing homomeric $\alpha 1_5$ glycine receptors have revealed that pentobarbitone and propofol also act additively. Equilibrium concentration-response curves for propofol and pentobarbitone indicated that the EC_{33} and EC_{66} concentrations were 30 and 60 μM for propofol and 500 and 1000 μM for pentobarbitone. In these experiments, pentobarbitone was observed to have a glycine mimetic effect, in addition to its effect of potentiating the current elicited by glycine (Fig. 4). Propofol had no such glycine mimetic effect. When propofol and pentobarbitone were applied together, at their respective EC_{33} concentrations, the glycine mimetic effect was of the same amplitude as that elicited by pentobarbitone alone. However, the potentiating effect on the response to glycine was of an amplitude equivalent to that elicited by an EC_{66} concentration of either anesthetic alone (*see* Fig. 4, *[49]*). This suggests that propofol and pentobarbitone may be acting at the same site to allosterically modulate the response of the receptor to its agonist, glycine. However, it would appear that this site is distinct from that at which pentobarbitone acts to elicit a response in the absence of glycine.

Pistis and colleagues *(39)* have also reported an additive mode of action of pentobarbitone and propofol. In experiments using *Xenopus* oocytes expressing homomeric $\alpha 1_5$ glycine receptors, glycine equilibrium concentration-response curves were established alone, and in the presence of pentobarbitone (3 mM), propofol (100 μM), and a mixture of pentobarbitone and propofol. Both pentobarbitone and propofol produced a leftward shift in the dose-response curve, by 2.4- and 4.7-fold, respectively. The binary mixture of anesthetics produced a leftward shift in the dose-response curve of 4.7-fold (equivalent to that by propofol alone). This was taken as evidence that these two anesthetics act via a common saturable site, or mechanism, at the glycine receptor.

High Pressure and Anesthetic Interactions

High pressure and anesthetics interact in vivo to produce the well-established pressure-reversal of anesthesia *(50)*. Until this phenomenon could be exploited to probe the mechanism of anesthesia, it was necessary to understand the mechanism by which pressure affects the central nervous system. It has since been established that pressure has a selective effect on the glycine receptor, such that the glycine EC_{50} is shifted rightwards by increasing pressure, with no change in E_{max} *(51–54)*. The effect of pressure on a chemical processes, such as ligand binding to a receptor protein that leads to a structural rearrangement necessary for function, is given by the standard thermodynamic equation $(\partial \ln K / \partial P)_T = -\Delta V / RT$. The equilibrium constant for the process in this context is the EC_{50} for receptor activation by the ligand. Applying this analysis indicated that the volume change associated with glycine binding at the glycine $\alpha 1_5$ receptor was approx 150 cm^3/mol. This is a large change in volume for a bimolecular reaction, and considerably greater than that observed for the activation of other ligand-gated ion channels or the voltage-dependent ion channels *(51,53,55)*.

In initial experiments, a concentration of nitrous oxide approx 10-fold higher than the anesthetic concentration (300 mM) was applied to oocytes expressing homomeric $\alpha 1_5$ glycine receptors. The

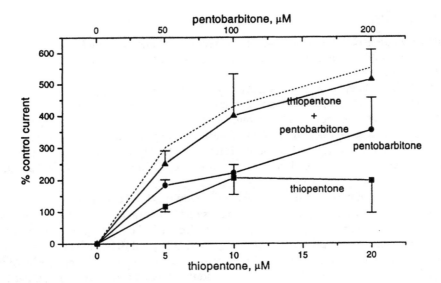

Fig. 3. Currents elicited by 50 µ*M* glycine in the presence of thiopentone (squares), pentobarbitone (circles), and thiopentone and pentobarbitone togther (upward facing triangle). All currents are expressed as a percentage of the current elicited by 50 µ*M* glycine alone. The results are the mean from four different oocytes and the error bars represent the standard error of the mean. The anesthetic concentrations used in the mixture of thiopentone and pentobarbitone were 5 + 50 µ*M*, 10 + 100 µ*M*, and 20 + 200 µ*M*; thiopentone + pentobarbitone, respectively. The dashed line represents the result that would have been expected on the basis of simple additivity.

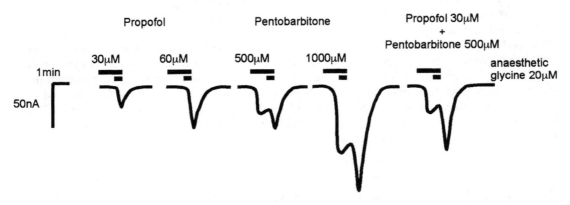

Fig. 4. Inward currents recorded from a *Xenopus* oocyte expressing the homomeric human α1 glycine receptor elicited using 20 µ*M* glycine in the presence of propofol (30 µ*M* and 60 µ*M*), pentobarbitone (500 µ*M* and 1000 µ*M*), and propofol (30 µ*M*) plus pentobarbitone (500 µ*M*).

current elicited by glycine (EC_{10}) was potentiated about 15-fold. At an ambient pressure of 10 MPa (using helium), the current was only potentiated 2.3-fold *(56,57)*. A pressure of 10 MPa, in the absence of anesthetic, would have been expected to reduce the current response by 60% *(54)*. If there were no interaction between pressure and nitrous oxide, the expected potentiation would have been 6.1. The mechanism by which nitrous oxide interacts with the glycine receptor must involve, therefore, a large increase in volume that is opposed by increased pressure.

The potentiation of the glycine response by pentobarbitone was not affected by pressure *(53)* suggesting that pentobarbitone acts at a different site or via a different mechanism, to nitrous oxide.

Glycine equilibrium concentration-response curves for the $α1_5$ receptor have been established in the presence of xenon (2 m*M*) and propofol (40 µ*M*) at atmospheric pressure (0.1 MPa), and at 10 MPa

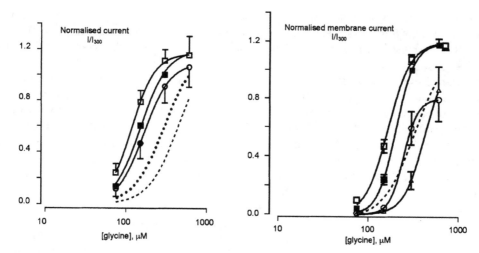

Fig. 5. Dose-response curves for currents elicited by glycine from *Xenopus* oocytes expressing homomeric human α1 glycine receptors. In all cases currents are shown as the mean (*n* = 6), +/– SEM) current normalized with respect to the current elicited by 300 μM glycine. *Left panel:* Dose-response curve for glycine (filled squares), glycine in the presence of 2 m*M* xenon (open squares) and glycine in the presence of xenon but at a total ambient pressure of 10 MPa (applied using helium) (open circles). The dashed line represents the expected position of the dose-response curve for glycine alone at 10 MPa pressure and the dotted line represents the expected position of the glycine dose-response curve at pressure and in the presence xenon. *Right panel:* Dose-response curve for glycine (filled squares), glycine in the presence of 40 μM propofol (open squares), glycine alone at 10 MPa (applied using helium) (upward facing triangles), and glycine in the presence of propofol and at a total ambient pressure of 10 MPa (open circles). The dashed line represents the expected position of the glycine dose-reponse curve at pressure and in the presence of propofol.

(helium) (Fig. 5, *[56]*). Xenon alone produced a parallel leftward shift in the glycine dose-response curve. At the elevated pressure of 10 MPa, the dose-response curve was shifted rightward, but not by as much as expected, indicating at interaction between pressure and xenon. Propofol alone produced a parallel leftward shift in the dose-response curve for glycine, and pressure alone produced a rightward shift in the glycine dose-response curve. At pressure, the glycine dose-response in the presence of propofol fell exactly where expected, but indicated that propofol does not act as a simple allosteric modulator of the receptor. Thus, the site at which propofol acts is not particularly pressure labile, unlike that at which nitrous oxide and xenon act. This taken together with the evidence that the modulation by pentobarbitone also shows little effect of pressure *(53)*, and that pentobarbitone and propofol act additively, suggests that propofol and pentobarbitone may act at a common site, or via a common mechanism, at the α1$_5$ glycine receptor.

Chimeric and Mutated Glycine Receptors

Our increased knowledge of the structure and functional elements of the glycine receptor, together with the ability to selectively alter particular amino acids within the receptor protein by mutating the DNA or to construct chimeric receptors, has enormously progressed our understanding of the molecular basis of the interaction between anesthetics and the receptor.

Although the homomeric GABAρ receptor is closely related to the homomeric glycine α1$_5$ receptor, it is negatively, not positively, modulated by a number of anesthetics. This difference was exploited in experiments aimed at deducing the elements of the glycine receptor critical for anesthetic interaction *(58)*. The interaction of enflurane and ethanol with chimeric constructs containing various domains from the α1 glycine and GABAρ receptor subunits, expressed in *Xenopus* oocytes, led to the conclusion that the critical region of the glycine receptor was the M2 and M3 domains (*see* Fig. 1). More detailed analysis revealed that, if the serine residue located at position 267 (halfway up the M2 transmembrane domain) was changed to an isoleucine, then sensitivity to ethanol, but not enflurane, was lost. However, if S267 was changed to an even bulkier tyrosine, then sensitivity to enflurane also was lost. It is possible that this region of the protein forms a hydrophobic pocket, in which some anesthetics might bind.

An additional site of interaction for ethanol with the $\alpha 1_5$ glycine receptor has been identified to be the alanine residue at position 52 in the N-terminal domain (*see* Fig. 1). Whereas substituting this residue with serine reduced the sensitivity to ethanol, it did not affect the sensitivity to propofol *(42)*.

Krasowski and Harrison *(40)* found that substituting the serine at position 267 with isoleucine had little effect on the potentiation of the mutant receptor by enflurane, isoflurane, methoxyflurane, and sevoflurane, but markedly affected the sensitivity to diethyl ether and abolished the effect of the tertiary alcohols, trichloroethanol, tribromoethanol, and trichloroethylene. They also found that substituting the alanine at residue 288 with tryptophan completely abolished the sensitivity to all the anesthetics.

These results are consistent with the suggestion that an M2 domain residue and an M3 domain residue combine to form a water accessible alcohol and anesthetic binding site *(59)*. Thus, the evidence appears to favor the hypothesis that anesthetics affect channel gating, rather than ligand binding. The precise mechanism by which anesthetics achieve this must await more detailed knowledge of receptor structure. However, it is entirely plausible that within the M2/M3 domains, there are hydrophobic pockets that can accommodate the different anesthetics to enable them to bring about their common effect.

SUMMARY

The importance of the spinal cord and brain stem in anesthesia is often overlooked *(60,61)*. Though glycine receptors have a major inhibitory role in these neuronal areas, the effects of anesthetics on these receptors is likely to play a significant part in contributing to general anesthesia. However, as described previously, not all general anesthetics affect glycine receptors and for many, the effects are only seen at relatively high doses. It is likely therefore, that anesthesia is brought about by a combined action of anesthetics on a number of different ligand-gated ion channels from both superfamilies of receptor. The importance of the glycine receptor may lie in its relatively simple structural architecture, which makes it easier to identify the critical regions at which anesthetics act. The central questions concerning the molecular mechanism of anesthesia remain: (1) do all anesthetics act via a common mechanism; and (2), is there a single site or mechanism responsible for anesthesia? Research involving the interactions of anesthetics with the glycine receptor and between anesthetics and high pressure has progressed in addressing these questions.

REFERENCES

1. Aprison, M. H. and Werman, R. (1965) The distribution of glycine in cat spinal cord and roots. *Life Sci.* **4**, 2075–2083.
2. Davidoff, R. A., Shank, R. P., Graham, L. T., Jr., Aprison, M. H., and Werman, R. (1967) Association of glycine with spinal interneurons. *Nature* **214**, 680–681.
3. Aprison, M. H. and Werman, R. (1968) A combined neurochemical and neurophysiological approach to the identification of central nervous system neurotransmitters. In: *Neurosciences Research* (vol. 1, Ehrenpreis, S. and Solnitzky, O.C., eds.), 143–174. Academic Press: New York.
4. Young, A. B. and Snyder, S. H. (1974) The glycine receptor: Evidence that strychnine binding is associated with the ionic conductance mechanism. *Proc. Natl. Acad. Sci. USA* **71**, 4002–4005.
5. Pfeiffer, F., Graham, D., and Betz, H. (1982) Purification by affinity chromotography of the glycine receptor of rat spinal cord. *J. Biol. Chem.* **257**, 9389–9393.
6. Graham, D., Pfeiffer, F., Simler, R., and Betz, H. (1985) Purification and characterisation of the glycine receptor of pig spinal cord. *Biochem.* **24**, 990–994.
7. Schmieden, V., Grenningloh, G., Schofield, P., and Betz, H. (1989) Functional expression in *Xenopus* oocytes of the strychnine binding 48 kd subunit of the glycine receptor. *EMBO J.* **8**, 695–700.
8. Sontheimer, H., Becker, C.-M., Pritchett, D. B., et al. (1989) Functional chloride channels by mammalian cell expression of rat glycine receptor subunit. *Neuron* **2**, 1491–1497.

9. Grenningloh, G., Schmieden, V., Schofield, P. R., Seeburg, P. H., Siddique, T., Mohandas, T. K., et al. (1990) Alpha subunit variants of the human glycine receptor: primary structures, functional expression and chromosomal localisation of the corresponding genes. *EMBO J.* **9**, 771–776.
10. Ortells, M. O. and Lunt, G. G. (1995) Evolutionary history of the ligand-gated ion-channel superfamily of receptors. *TINS* **18**, 121–127.
11. Devilliers-Thiery, A., Galzi, J. L., Eisele, J. L., Bertrand, S., Bertrand, D., and Changeux, J. P. (1993) Functional architecture of the nicotinic acetylcholine receptor: a prototype of ligand-gated ion channels. *J. Membr. Biol.* **136**, 97–112.
12. Karlin, A. and Akabas, M. H. (1995) Toward a structural basis for the function of nicotinic acetylcholine receptors and their cousins. *Neuron* **15**, 1231–1244.
13. Unwin, N. (1995) Acetylcholine receptor channel imaged in the open state. *Nature* **373**, 37–43.
14. Betz, H. (1992) Structure and function of inhibitory glycine receptors. *Q. Rev. Biophys.* **25**, 381–394.
15. Kuhse, J., Betz, H., and Kirsch, J. (1995) The inhibitory glycine receptor: architecture, synaptic localisation and molecular pathology of a postsynaptic ion-channel complex. *Curr. Opin. Neurobiol.* **5**, 318–323.
16. Griffon, N., Buttner, C., Nicke, A., Kuhse, J., Schmalzing, G., and Betz, H. (1999) Molecular determinants of glycine subunit assembly. *EMBO J.* **18**, 4711–4721.
17. Langosch, D., Thomas, L., and Betz, H. (1988) Conserved quaternary structure of ligand-gated ion channels: the postsynaptic glycine receptor is a pentamer. *Proc. Natl. Acad. Sci. USA* **85**, 7394–7398.
18. Hoch, W., Betz, H., and Becker, C.-M. (1989) Primary cultures of mouse spinal cord express the neonatal isoform of the inhibitory glycine receptor. *Neuron* **3**, 339–348.
19. Takahashi, T., Momiyama, A., Hirai, K., Hishinuma, B., and Akagi, H. (1992) Functional correlation of fetal and adult forms of glycine receptors with developmental changes in inhibitory synaptic receptor channels. *Neuron* **9**, 115–1161.
20. Snyder, S. H. (2000) The glycine synaptic receptor in the mammalian central nervous system. *Brit. J. Pharmacol.* **131(Special Edition)**, 103–114.
21. Betz, H. (1991) Glycine receptors: hetergeneous and widespread in the mammalian brain. *TINS* **14**, 458–461.
22. Gready, J. E., Ranganathan, S., Schofield, P. R., Matsuo, Y., and Nishikawa, K. (1997) Predicated structure of the extracellular region of ligand-gated ion-channel receptors shows SH2-like and SH3-like domains forming the ligand-binding site. *Protein Sci.* **6**, 983–998.
23. Lynch, J. W., Rajendra, S., Pierce, K. D., Handford, C. A., Barry, P. H., and Schofield, P. R. (1997) Identification of intracellular and extracellular domains mediating signal transduction in the inhibitory glycine receptor chloride channel. *EMBO J.* **16**, 110–120.
24. Lewis, T. M., Sivilotti, L. G., Colquhoun, D., Gardiner, R. M., Schoepfer, R., and Rees, M. (1998) Properties of human glycine receptors cotaining the hyperekplexia mutation α1(K276E) expressed in *Xenopus* oocytes. *J. Physiol.* **507**, 25–40.
25. Saul, B., Kuner, T., Sobetzko, D., et al. (1999) Novel GLRA1 missense mutation (P250T) in dominant hyperekplexia defines an intracellular determinant of glycine receptor channel gating. *J. Neurosci.* **19**, 869–877.
26. Lynch, J. W., Reena Han, N.-L., Haddrill, J., Pierce, K. D., and Schofield, P. R. (2001) The surface accessibility of the glycine receptor M2–M3 loop is increased in the channel open state. *J. Neurosci.* **21**, 2589–2599.
27. Moorhouse, A. J., Jacques, P., Barry, P. H., and Schofield, P. R. (1999) The Startle Disease mutation Q266H, in the second transmembrane domain of the human glycine receptor, impairs channel gating. *Mol. Pharmacol.* **55**, 386–395.
28. Wakamori, M., Ikemoto, Y., and Akaike, N. (1991) Effects of 2 Volatile Anesthetics and a Volatile Convulsant On the Excitatory and Inhibitory Amino-Acid Responses in Dissociated CNS Neurons of the Rat. *J. Neurophysiol.* **66**, 2014–2021.
29. Hales, T. G. and Lambert, J. J. (1991) The actions of propofol on inhibitory amino acid receptors of bovine adrenomedullary chromaffin cells and rodent central neurons. *Brit. J. Pharmacol.* **104**, 619–628.
30. Downie, D. L., Hall, A. C., Lieb, W. R., and Franks, N. P. (1996) Effects of inhalational general anaesthetics on native glycine receptors in rat medullary neurones and recombinant glycine receptors in *Xenopus* oocytes. *Brit. J. Pharmacol.* **118**, 493–502.
31. Takagi, T., Pribilla, I., Kirsch, J., and Betz, H. (1992) Coexpression of the receptor-associated protein gephyrin changes the ligand binding affinities of α2 glycine receptors. *FEBS Letts.* **303**, 178–180.
32. Taleb, O. and Betz, H. Expression of the human glycine receptor α1 subunit in *Xenopus* oocytes: apparent affinities of agonists increase at high receptor density. *EMBO J.* **13**, 1318–1324.
33. Lévi, S., Vannier, C., and Triller, A. (1998) Strychnine-sensitive stabilisation of postsynaptic receptor clusters. *J. Cell Science* **111**, 335–345.
34. Daniels, S. and Roberts, R. J. (1998) Post-synaptic inhibitory mechanisms of anaesthesia; glycine receptors. *Toxicol. Lett.* **100–101**, 71–76.
35. Franks, N. P. and Lieb, W. R. (1994) Molecular and cellular mechanisms of general anaesthesia. *Nature* **367**, 607–614.
36. Alifimoff, J. K., Firestone, L. L., and Miller, K. W. (1989) Anaesthetic potencies of primary alkanols: implications for the molecular dimension of the anaesthetic site. *Brit. J. Pharmacol.* **96**, 9–16.
37. Dildy-Mayfield, J. E., Mihic, S. J., Liu, Y., Deitrich, R. A., and Harris, R. A. (1996) Actions of long chain alcohols on GABA$_A$ but not glutamate receptors correlate with their in vivo effects. *Brit. J. Pharmacol.* **118**, 378–384.
38. Mascia, M. P., Machu, T. K., and Harris, R. A. (1996) Enhancement of homomeric glycine receptor function by long-chain alcohols and anesthetics. *Brit. J. Pharmacol.* **119**, 1331–1336.
39. Pistis, M., Belelli, D., Peters, J. A., and Lambert, J. J. (1997) The interaction of general anaesthetics with recombinant GABA$_A$ and glycine receptors expressed in *Xenopus laevis* oocytes: a comparative study. *Brit. J. Pharmacol.* **122**, 1707–1719.

40. Krasowski, M. D. and Harrison, N. L. (2000) The actions of ether, alcohol and alkane general anesthetics on GABA$_A$ and glycine receptors and the effects of TM2 and TM3 mutations. *Brit. J. Pharmacol.* **129,** 731–743.

41. Machu, T. K. and Harris, R. A. (1994) Alcohols and anaesthetics potentiate glycine receptor responses. *Alcohol Clin. Exp. Res.* **18,** 517.

42. Mascia, M. P., Mihic, S. J., Valenzuela, C. F., Schofield, P. R., and Harris, R. A. (1996) A single amino acid determines differences in ethanol actions on strychnine-sensitive glycine receptors. *Mol. Pharmacol.* **50,** 402–406.

43. Koblin, D. D., Chortkoff, B. S., Laster, M. J., Eger, E.I. 2nd, Halsey, M. J., and Jonescu, P. (1994) Polyhalogenated and perfluorinated compounds that disobey the Meyer-Overton hypothesis. *Anesth. Analg.* **79,** 1043–1048.

44. Belelli, D., Pistis, M., Peters, J. A., and Lambert, J. J. (1999) The interaction of general anesthetics and neurosteroids with GABA$_A$ and glycine receptors. *Neurochem. Int.* **34,** 447–452.

45. Shepherd, S. E., Peters, J. A., and Lambert, J. J. (1996) The interaction of intravenous anaesthetics with rat inhibitory and excitatory receptors expressed in *Xenopus laevis* oocytes. *Brit. J. Pharmacol.* **119,** 346P.

46. Pistis, M., Belelli, D., McGurk, K., Peters, J. A., and Lambert, J. J. (1999) Complementary regulation of anesthetic activation of human ($\alpha6\beta3\gamma2L$) and *Drosophila* (RDL) GABA receptors by a single amino acid residue. *J. Physiol.* **515,** 3–18.

47. Wu, F. S., Gibbs, T. T., and Farb, D. H. (1990) Inverse modulation of gamma-aminobutyric acid and glycine–induced currents by progesterone. *Mol. Pharmacol.* **37,** 597–602.

48. Prince, R. J. and Simmonds, M. A. (1992) Steroid modulation of the strychnine-sensitive glycine receptor. *Neuropharmacol.* **31,** 201–205.

49. Daniels, S., Wittmann, S., and Fraser, C. S. (1999) General anesthetics can act additively at a single neurotransmitter receptor protein. *J. Pharmacy Pharmacol.* **51S,** 16.

50. Lever, M. J., Miller, K. W., Paton, W. D. M., and Smith, E. B. (1971) Pressure reversal of anesthesia. *Nature* **231,** 368–371.

51. Daniels, S., Zhao, D. M., Inman, N., Price, D. J., Shelton, C. J., and Smith, E. B. (1991) Effects of general anesthetics and pressure on mammalian excitatory receptors expressed in *Xenopus* oocytes. *Ann. N.Y. Acad. Sci.* **625,** 108–115.

52. Shelton, C. J., Doyle, M. G., Price, D. J., Daniels, S., and Smith, E. B. (1993) The effect of high pressure on glycine and kainate sensitive receptor channels expressed in *Xenopus* oocytes. *Proc. Roy. Soc. Lond.* **B254,** 131–137.

53. Shelton, C. J., Daniels, S., and Smith, E. B. (1996) Rat brain GABA$_A$ receptors expressed in *Xenopus* oocytes are insensitive to high pressure. *Pharmacol. Comm.* **7,** 215–220.

54. Roberts, R. J., Shelton, C. J., Daniels, S., and Smith, E. B. (1996) Glycine activation of human homomeric $\alpha1$ glycine receptors is sensitive to pressure in the range of the high pressure nervous syndrome. *Neurosci. Lett.* **208,** 125–128.

55. Heinemann, S. H., Stuhmer, W., and Conti, F. (1987) Single acetylcholine receptor channel currents recorded at high hydrostatic pressures. *Proc. Natl. Acad. Sci. USA* **84,** 3229–3233.

56. Daniels, S. (2000) Pressure reversal of anesthesia at a molecular level. *Progress in anesthetic mechanism* **6,** 590–596.

57. Daniels, S. (2000) Pressure and anesthesia, In *Molecular bases of anesthesia* (Moody, E. and Skolnick, P., eds.) CRC Press: Boca Raton.

58. Mihic, S. J., Qing, Y., Wick, M. J., Koltchines, V. V., Krasowski, M. D., Finn, S. E., et al. (1997) Sites of alcohol and volatile anesthetic action on GABA$_A$ and glycine receptors. *Nature* **389,** 385–389.

59. Mascia, M. P., Trudell, J. R., and Harris, R. A. (2000) Specific binding sites for alcohols and anesthetics on ligand-gated channels. *Proc. Natl. Acad. Sci. USA* **97,** 9305–9310.

60. Antognini, J. F. and Schwartz, K. (1993) Exaggerated anesthetic requirements in the preferentially anesthetized brain. *Anesthesiolology* **79,** 1244–1249.

61. Rampil, I. J., Mason, P., and Singh, H. (1993) Anesthetic potency (MAC) is independent of forebrain structures in the rat. *Anesthesiology* **78,** 707–712.

21

Presynaptic Actions of General Anesthetics

Misha Perouansky and Hugh C. Hemmings, Jr.

HISTORICAL PERSPECTIVE

Early in the 20th century, Sowton and Sherrington identified the synapse as a likely target of general anesthetic action (1). Brooks and Eccles (2) and Bremer and Bonnet (3) later demonstrated depression of synaptic transmission in the central nervous system (CNS), by concentrations of general anesthetics that did not affect axonal conduction. Larrabee and Pasternak (4) showed that impulse conduction in myelinated and unmyelinated axons of the autonomic nervous system was resistant to a variety of intravenous and volatile anesthetics, whereas excitatory synaptic transmission was significantly suppressed. This important paper firmly established the synapse as a major site of action of general anesthetics.

Subsequent research focused on whether the principal target of general anesthetics is pre- or postsynaptic. Quilliam and co-workers (5) combined physiology (retraction of the nictating membrane) with neurochemistry (a bioassay) to show that acetylcholine release was depressed by concentrations of intravenous agents in the range of those achieved under anesthesia. Synaptic transmission was affected more than the release of acetylcholine *per se*, by all agents except chloral hydrate. These findings indicated that anesthetics act at multiple pre- and postsynaptic sites, and that anesthetics differ in their activity profiles. These general conclusions are supported by most subsequent investigations.

Improved understanding of synaptic physiology and refined electrophysiological techniques have permitted more direct analysis of anesthetic effects. Extracellular and intracellular recordings (6–8) provided more data on the presumptive sites of anesthetic action, although interpretations varied. Løyning (7) suggested that anesthetics acted principally on presynaptic elements (e.g., Na^+ current), whereas Somjen and Gill (6) favored postsynaptic targets. These interpretations were biased by the generally accepted notion that anesthetics acted through a common mechanism, loosely understood as modification of membrane excitability (9). The following sections review those experiments that have contributed significantly to our current understanding of the diverse presynaptic actions of general anesthetics.

BASIC PHYSIOLOGY OF TRANSMITTER RELEASE

The nervous system uses a variety of mechanisms to facilitate information flow and processing among a large collection of individual cells. One of the most elegant forms of this communication occurs at chemical synapses, where the exocytosis of synaptic vesicles is regulated to provide rapid secretion of a few thousand molecules of neurotransmitter on demand. The orchestration of this cellular process is initiated by a rise in intracellular Ca^{2+} and is critically dependent on the correct

From: *Contemporary Clinical Neuroscience: Neural Mechanisms of Anesthesia*
Edited by: Joseph F. Antognini et al. © Humana Press Inc., Totowa, NJ

functioning of specific proteins on both the synaptic vesicle and plasma membranes. Modulation of the release of neurotransmitter is thus a fundamental property critical to nervous system function. Notably, the synaptic machinery is a major target of most therapies for neuropsychiatric disease, further underscoring the importance of this specialized subcellular compartment. A detailed understanding of the molecular and cellular processes responsible for synaptic transmission is essential for determining the way in which synaptic function is altered by anesthetics to produce the characteristic triad of amnesia, unconsciousness, and immobility.

No other aspect of the presynaptic terminal is so tightly linked to the release process as the concentration of cytoplasmic calcium ion. The relationship between extracellular Ca^{2+} and neurotransmitter release was described by Dodge and Rahamimoff *(10)*, who demonstrated the exponential relationship between the release of transmitter and extracellular Ca^{2+} concentration ($[Ca^{2+}]_e$). This is not caused by a high-order dependence of presynaptic Ca^{2+} entry upon $[Ca^{2+}]_e$, but reflects a steep dependence of release upon cytoplasmic $[Ca^{2+}]$ in the presynaptic nerve terminal *(11)*. Thus, Ca^{2+} entering through presynaptic voltage-gated Ca^{2+} channels acts in a highly cooperative manner to evoke exocytosis. The degree of cooperativity should directly reflect the number of calcium ions participating in the process leading to fusion of a synaptic vesicle with the plasma membrane: from 2.7 in some synapses of the mammalian CNS *(12)*, to 4 at the neuromuscular junction of amphibia and invertebrates *(10,11)*. A maximum of one vesicle is released by each action potential from a single release site, although this point is under debate. The presynaptic features that have a profound influence on the modulation of neurotransmitter release are the amount of Ca^{2+} entering the presynaptic terminal, the efficiency with which Ca^{2+} controls exocytosis, the cooperativity of the Ca^{2+} action, and the maximum amount of release.

Recent progress in defining the molecular details of transmitter release and its regulation, provides a useful framework within which to analyze the mechanisms of general anesthetic effects on synaptic transmission. The basic mechanisms underlying release are conserved among different neurotransmitters, although transmitter-specific specializations exist, as in the specific Ca^{2+} channel types coupled to release and modulation of release by presynaptic receptors *(13–15)*. In fact, the general similarities between the temporally, spatially, and quantitatively highly regulated neurotransmitter release and other, relatively less regulated (constitutive), forms of cellular secretion have facilitated the biochemical and genetic analysis of the protein components involved in mediating the underlying membrane fusion and exocytosis *(16,17)*. This explosion in knowledge has allowed the formation of detailed models of the supramolecular complexes involved. These recent advances make this process accessible to genetic and pharmacological analysis of general anesthetic effects on specific steps in the synaptic vesicle exocytosis/endocytosis pathway. The prevailing model of the release process is outlined in Fig. 1. Depolarization and Ca^{2+} entry, which determine the amount of transmitter released, can be varied by regulation of ion channel function (i.e., Na^+, Ca^{2+}, and K^+ channels), and by modulation via second messenger/protein phosphorylation mechanisms. Potential targets for general anesthetic effects on transmitter release include: nerve terminal depolarization and Ca^{2+} influx (by effects on ion channels), modulation of synaptic vesicle availability and mobilization (by effects on the cytoskeleton and/or synaptic vesicle-associated proteins), the coupling between Ca^{2+} and exocytosis, exocytosis mediated by SNARE and associated proteins, and the endocytosis process. Our current knowledge of anesthetic actions on these processes, an emerging area of investigation, is reviewed here.

EFFECTS ON NEUROTRANSMITTER RELEASE

The relative contributions of presynaptic vs postsynaptic general anesthetic effects on synaptic transmission have been difficult to determine. The small size of most nerve terminals in the CNS (<1 μm diameter) hampers direct electrophysiological analysis of presynaptic events, and direct measurement of action potential-evoked transmitter release from single CNS synapses, is not possible.

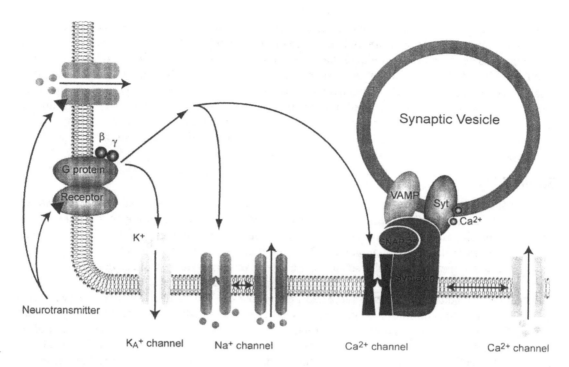

Fig. 1. Presynaptic nerve terminal showing basic mechanisms involved in neurotransmitter release and potential targets for general anesthetic effects. *Ion channel loci*: The action potential invades and leads to depolarization mediated by voltage-gated Na^+ channels, which can be activated directly by veratridine. Blockade of K_A^+ channels by 4-aminopyridine in synaptosomes results in repetitive depolarizations akin to action potential invasion in vivo. Depolarization opens noninactivating voltage-gated Ca^{2+} channels that allow localized Ca^{2+} influx. Interaction of N-type Ca^{2+} channels with syntaxin 1 inhibits channels activation. The specific Ca^{2+} channels involved in transmitter release are clustered near release sites for amino acid transmitters, but are diffusely distributed for peptide and catecholamine transmitters. Na^+ and Ca^{2+} channels are also modulated via intracellular signalling pathways involving phosphorylation. *Intrasynaptosomal loci*: the increase in Ca^{2+} is coupled to transmitter release through the fusion pore from available (readily releasable) small synaptic vesicles by a Ca^{2+}-sensitive release trigger, possibly synaptotagmin (Syt) that promotes vesicle fusion/exocytosis mediated by the SNARE complex (SNAP-25, syntaxin and VAMP). In synaptosomes, release can also be activated by unlocalized Ca^{2+} entry with a Ca^{2+} ionophore (such as ionomycin), which bypasses the ion channels involved in the physiological activation of transmitter release. Presynaptic receptors modulate transmitter release, either positively or negatively depending on the receptor, the transmitter and the specific synapse. This modulation occurs via effects on vesicle availability, ionotropic and metabotropic receptors. Ionotropic receptors mediate cation (depolarizing; e.g., Na^+, Ca^{2+}) or anion (hyperpolarizing; e.g., Cl^-) influx through the coupled ligand-gated ion channels. Metabotropic receptors exert indirect effects on ion channels via second messenger mediated signaling pathways (indicated by *arrows*).

Attempts to overcome this limitation by fusing synaptosomes to create larger structures have been unsuccessful (Tzan, C. J. and Hemmings, H. C., Jr., unpublished observations). Alternate approaches such as quantitative fluorescence confocal microscopy of cultured rat hippocampal neurons labeled with FM1–43 to monitor synaptic vesicle exocytosis, may provide an independent method for probing the presynaptic actions of general anesthetics *(18,19)*. However, the recent development of specialized preparations aimed at accessing the presynaptic terminal with electrophysiological techniques may soon improve our understanding in this area.

The complex regulatory mechanisms involved in neurotransmitter release, which have only recently begun to be identified, have further impeded mechanistic studies of presynaptic anesthetic actions, particularly at the molecular level. A variety of approaches have attempted to overcome these obstacles, each with intrinsic limitations, as outlined in this section. Experiments also differ in the brain areas used, and the techniques used to stimulate and measure transmitter release. Chemical stimulation is not physiological in its persistence, and electrical stimulation, though also not physiological, is perhaps more so than chemical stimulation in being transient and of variable frequency and intensity. Early studies employed biological assays of transmitter release. Current techniques most often involve either neurochemical analysis of endogenous transmitter or prelabeling with radiolabeled transmitter or precursor. Overall, a convincing body of evidence suggests that general anesthetics affect the release of some, if not all, neurotransmitters.

Brain Slices

Brain slices have been used extensively to study the effects of general anesthetics on transmitter release. In fact, most earlier studies of the effects of general anesthetics on transmitter release have employed this preparation. General anesthetics consistently decrease depolarization-induced release of the excitatory transmitter glutamate (20–23) from brain slices. Glutamate is the major excitatory transmitter in the mammalian CNS, so anesthetic effects on this system would have significant functional implications. A wide variety of anesthetics inhibit glutamate release evoked by elevated KCl from brain slices including isoflurane (20,22,23), enflurane (22), and barbiturates (21). Liachenko et al. (24) described similar inhibition of glutamate release by the experimental anesthetic F3 (1-chloro-1,2,2-trifluorocyclobutane) and by a high (relative to its predicted anesthetic) concentration of the nonanesthetic ("nonimmobilizer") F6 (dichlorohexafluorocyclobutane). However, Eilers et al. (22) found that F6 had no effect at predicted anesthetic concentrations, and actually stimulated release at 70 μM (~3× predicted MAC). The latter finding is consistent with a role for inhibition of glutamate release in the production of anesthesia, while stimulation of glutamate release may underlie the proconvulsant actions of certain nonanesthetic analogs of anesthetic compounds (25). In contrast, the effects of general anesthetics on release of the inhibitory transmitter GABA in brain slices are inconsistent: both inhibition (21,23) and stimulation (26) have been reported.

General anesthetics inhibit acetylcholine release in several preparations. In vivo, halothane (1–1.5 vol%) inhibited acetylcholine release, detected on the surface of rabbit brain (27) and in the pontine reticular formation of cats (28). Halothane (1 MAC), also inhibited KCl-evoked acetylcholine release from rat cortical slices (IC$_{50}$ = 0.38 vol%), detected as choline using a chemiluminescent assay in the absence or presence of an acetylcholinesterase inhibitor (29). In rat midbrain slices, a variety of barbiturate anesthetics and chloral hydrate inhibited acetylcholine release induced by a prolonged (30 min) incubation with high [KCl] (30). In contrast, Bazil and Minneman (31) failed to detect any effect of halothane, enflurane, or methoxyflurane on release using [³H]choline to prelabel transmitter pools, possibly owing to the absence of a cholinesterase inhibitor in their assays to distinguish choline from acetylcholine release. The mechanism for halothane inhibition of acetylcholine release appears to be direct because there was no effect on synthesis or choline uptake.

The physiological and biochemical mechanisms of these interactions are poorly understood. Interpretation of results obtained using intact brain tissue preparations such as brain slices, is complicated by the involvement of multiple synapses, cellular interactions, and postsynaptic actions owing to the presence of intact neuronal circuits and glia. The resulting transmitter efflux depends on the complex interplay of vesicular release, nonvesicular release, reuptake, synthesis, metabolism, and diffusion within the slice. Inhibition of glutamate efflux from brain slices evoked by depolarization with elevated KCl concentrations, appears to result primarily from enhanced inhibition owing to potentiation of postsynaptic GABA$_A$ receptors on glutamatergic neurons by thiopental (IC$_{50}$ = 11 μM) and propofol (32). Thus, the GABA$_A$ receptor antagonist bicuculline reversed the inhibitory effects of thiopental and propofol, but not of ketamine, on glutamate release. This is consistent with electrophysiological studies in hippocampal slices, where inhibition of electrically evoked population spikes by pentobarbital and propofol was also reversed by bicuculline *(33)*. In contrast, the effects of volatile anesthetics on glutamatergic transmission were relatively resistant to bicuculline, consistent with a direct mechanism of inhibition *(34,35)*. These electrophysiological methods overcome some of the limitations inherent in the analysis of transmitter efflux, though they rely on recordings of postsynaptic events, which may themselves be affected by anesthetics, to assess presynaptic effects.

Direct measurements of anesthetic effects on glutamate or GABA uptake indicated that thiopental, pentobarbital, methohexital, halothane, ketamine, and urethane had no significant effects *(36,21,37)*. However, indirect measurements using inhibitors of reuptake have shown that isoflurane inhibited glutamate ($IC_{50} = 0.8$ mM) and GABA reuptake ($IC_{50} = 0.5$ mM) in mouse cortical brain slices *(23)*. This suggested that the net effects of isoflurane on synaptic GABA concentrations may depend on competition between inhibition of release ($IC_{50} = 0.23$ mM) and reuptake, because both effects occurred at clinical concentrations, whereas effects on synaptic glutamate are determined primarily by inhibition of release ($IC_{50} = 0.3$ mM).

SYNAPTOSOMES

The release of glutamate and other transmitters is coupled to changes in the activity of various ion channels, presynaptic receptors, and second messenger pathways, many of which are potential targets for anesthetics *(38)*. Synaptosomes have been widely used to study these presynaptic mechanisms regulating transmitter release *(39)*. Synaptosomes are isolated nerve terminals prepared by gentle homogenation and differential centrifugation, often involving a density gradient step to remove contaminating mitochondria and myelin. They are distinct from synaptoneurosomes; a crude preparation containing resealed postsynaptic elements, nuclei, and cellular debris. The resealed nerve terminals contain mitochondria, synaptic vesicles, and the cellular machinery necessary for the generation and maintenance of ionic gradients, and the synthesis, uptake, storage, and release of transmitters. Synaptosomes are depleted of glial and postsynaptic neuronal cell body elements, and are devoid of cellular interactions that may confound the effects of the studied drugs on the release process in tissue slices. Thus, pharmacological effects observed in synaptosomes are indicative of a presynaptic site of action.

Synaptosomes are too small for electrical field stimulation. Transmitter release must be stimulated pharmacologically. Typically, one of the following four secretagogues, each of which involves distinct components of the endogenous release mechanisms *(39)* is used: (1) Step elevations of extracellular KCl induce a "clamped" depolarization of the synaptosomal plasma membrane, above the threshold for activation of voltage-gated Ca^{2+} channels present in the presynaptic terminal. KCl-evoked release is sensitive to Ca^{2+} channel blockade, but persists even if Na^+ channels are blocked, e.g., with tetrodotoxin (TTX); (2) Inhibition of presynaptic K_A^+-channels by 4-aminopyridine produces transient depolarizations. This leads to activation of voltage-gated Na^+ channels that potentiate the depolarization, and allow activation of voltage-gated Ca^{2+} channels. The consequent release of transmitter is sensitive to inhibition of Na^+ channels with TTX, similar to evoked transmitter release in more intact preparations; (3) Indirect Na^+ channel activation by veratridine, a neurotoxin that inhibits channel inactivation, leads to prolonged synaptosome depolarization and influx of Ca^{2+}. Because Na^+ channel activation is required, release is TTX-sensitive; (4) Ca^{2+} ionophores (e.g., ionomycin, calcimycin) evoke glutamate release by promoting direct Ca^{2+} entry independent of Na^+ or Ca^{2+} channel activation. Hence, ionophore-evoked release is insensitive to ion channel blockers.

The interpretation of release data obtained with each of these secretagogues is fraught with caveats. All pharmacological stimuli are long lasting and usually supramaximal in intensity, compared to action potential invasion and activation of terminals. In addition, interpretation of KCl-evoked release can be complicated by depolarization induced reversal of electrogenic transporters normally involved in transmitter reuptake *(39)*. Moreover, for a given increase in intracellular Ca^{2+} ($[Ca^{2+}]i$), ionomycin is considerably less effective than Ca^{2+} channel activation by KCl, 4-aminopyridine, or veratridine in evoking release of fast neurotransmitters (e.g., glutamate). This suggests an important difference between Ca^{2+} entry through Ca^{2+} channels vs diffuse Ca^{2+} entry through artificial pores. The specific Ca^{2+} channels coupled to release are contiguous with the synaptic vesicle exocytotic machinery. The latter, therefore, is influenced by the high local Ca2+ concentration at the mouth of the channel pore *(40)*.

The effects of anesthetics on transmitter release have been studied in the greatest depth for the excitatory transmitter glutamate. This transmitter is highly concentrated in synaptosomes prepared from the cerebral cortex, an abundant and accessible source for their preparation. In general, anesthetics inhibit glutamate release from both brain slices and synaptosomes. In synaptosomes from multiple species and brain regions, volatile anesthetics (e.g., isoflurane) are more potent than intravenous agents (e.g., propofol) at "equi-anesthetic" concentrations *(see ref. 41)*. The effects in synaptosomes clearly implicate a presynaptic site of action, in contrast to the ambiguous results obtained using brain slices. Whether this effect, which appears to be present at glutamatergic terminals throughout the CNS, is mediated primarily via inhibition of presynaptic Na^+ *(42–44)*, Ca^{2+} channels *(45)*, and/or other presynaptic targets is controversial. Reduced glutamate release from synaptosomes, also has been attributed to increased glutamate uptake *(46)* and actions on other steps in the transmitter release pathway *(47)*.

Attempts have been made to determine whether primary inhibition of Na^+ or Ca^{2+} channels mediates anesthetic inhibition of evoked glutamate release by quantitative comparisons of their effects on KCl (Na^+ channel independent) vs 4-aminopyridine- or veratridine-induced (Na^+ channel dependent) release. Isoflurane, halothane, and enflurane dose-dependently inhibited KCl-evoked glutamate release, and Ca^{2+} entry (measured with the Ca^{2+} sensitive fluorescent probe fura 2) with an IC_{50} of ~0.69 mM for isoflurane, which suggested blockade of neuronal Ca^{2+} channels as a likely target *(45)*. The IC_{50} of isoflurane for inhibition of glutamate release was significantly higher (~1.6 mM) in a subsequent study *(48)*. Halothane *(49)*, isoflurane *(48)*, and propofol *(42)* inhibited Na^+ channel-dependent release more potently than Na^+ channel-independent release. These findings do not support a major role for blockade of the presynaptic Ca^{2+} channels coupled to glutamate release in the actions of these agents. Such selectivity may be a general property of anesthetic drugs as it was shared by the model anesthetic F3 (1-chloro-1,2,2-trifluorocyclobutane), but not the structurally similar nonanesthetic F6 (1,2-dichlorohexafluorocyclobutane) *(44)*. Thus, presynaptic Na^+ channels are apparently more sensitive to these anesthetics than the particular Ca^{2+} channels coupled to glutamate release. This conclusion is supported by findings that halothane and propofol potently and specifically antagonize radioligand binding to synaptosomal Na^+ channels *(50,43)*. Taken together with independent electrophysiological evidence of anesthetic blockade of neuronal voltage-dependent Na^+ channels at clinical concentrations *(51,52)*, these findings suggest that anesthetic block of presynaptic Na^+ channels, and the ensuing inhibition of nerve terminal depolarization, contribute to depression of glutamate release *(53)*.

Reduction of transmitter release from glutamatergic terminals also has been ascribed to stimulation of glutamate re-uptake by anesthetics. Larsen et al. *(46)* reported that isoflurane increased glutamate uptake into rat cerebrocortical synaptosomes by a dose-dependent increase in the maximal velocity of high affinity glutamate uptake. Activation of glutamate transporters by protein kinase C that is stimulated by volatile anesthetics in synaptosomes *(54)*, was proposed as a potential mechanism for this effect. However, Nicol et al. *(55)* reported no effect of isoflurane, halothane, propofol, thiopental, or ketamine on glutamate uptake into rat cortical synaptosomes at clinical concentrations, whereas Bianchi et al. *(56)*, using the same model, reported that high concentrations of propofol inhibited glutamate uptake (probably vesicular uptake) and release. These findings provide evidence against facilitation of neuronal glutamate transport as an important mechanism for reductions in glutamate release.

The effects of anesthetics on basal transmitter release also have been studied in synaptosomes. High concentrations of halothane and enflurane increased basal glutamate release from mouse cortical synaptosomes, by unknown mechanisms *(57)*. However, most investigators have not detected substantial anesthetic effects on basal glutamate release in brain slices *(22)*, despite the enhancement of glutamate uptake by volatile anesthetics observed in cultured astrocytes, or synaptosomes *(45,49)*. Propofol increased basal release of GABA from rat cortical synaptosomes, an effect that appears to involve presynaptic GABA$_A$ receptors *(58)*.

The effects of anesthetic on the release of transmitters other than glutamate have not been investigated as extensively. Halothane inhibited KCl-evoked acetylcholine release from rat cortical slices (IC$_{50}$ = 0.38 vol%) *(29)*. This effect was not primarily owing to an inhibition of choline uptake, as this effect occurred at higher concentrations, nor was it owing to an inhibition of acetylcholinesterase *(59)*. Similarly, in synaptosomes, halothane reduced choline uptake via an increase in K$_m$ *(60)*. Halothane (3 vol%) inhibited acetylcholine release directly, as evidenced by a 50% inhibition of KCl-evoked release by 50%.

The effects of general anesthetics on release of the inhibitory transmitter GABA are similarly unclear. Isoflurane (1.5 and 3 vol%) had no effect on total KCl (30 mM)-evoked release of endogenous GABA or [^{3}H]GABA uptake in rat cortical synaptosomes, but was reported to increase Ca^{2+}-dependent release by virtue of an inhibitory effect on Ca^{2+}-independent release *(61)*. A lower concentration (0.5%) inhibited release. The mechanism of this biphasic effect remains to be elucidated. Other studies have employed radiolabeled GABA to prelabel synaptosomal GABA. Using rat striatal synaptosomes, propofol, etomidate, thiopental, ketamine, halothane, enflurane, and isoflurane had no effect on spontaneous or KCl (15 mM)-evoked [^{3}H]GABA release *(62)*. In contrast, the same group reported that thiopental inhibited veratridine- or KCl-evoked release in the same preparation *(63)*. This study agrees with the early report of Haycock et al. *(64)* that a relatively high concentration of pentobarbital inhibited KCl (50 mM)- or veratridine-evoked [^{14}C]GABA release from mouse forebrain syanptosomes. Ionophore (A23187) evoked release was not affected, suggesting an effect upstream of Ca^{2+}-release coupling or exocytosis. The intravenous agents inhibited GABA uptake, but only at supraclinical concentrations. In contrast, propofol, etomidate, pentobarbital, and alphaxalone, but not ketamine, enhanced KCl (15 or 30 mM)-evoked [^{3}H]GABA release from rat cortical synaptosomes at clinical concentrations *(58)*. Propofol also enhanced spontaneous release that was Ca^{2+} and bicuculline sensitive.

Several studies have analyzed the effects of anesthetics on catecholamine release from synaptosomes. Halothane inhibited KCl-evoked [^{3}H]norepinephrine release from rat cortical synaptosomes *(31)*, and pentobarbital (200 µM) inhibited KCl- or veratridine-evoked [^{3}H]norepinephrine release from mouse forebrain synaptosomes *(64)*. In a systematic study of multiple agents on [^{3}H]dopamine release from rat striatal synaptosomes, volatile anesthetics (halothane, enflurane, isoflurane) enhanced spontaneous release, inhibited KCl (15 mM)-evoked release, but did not affect KCl (50 mM)-evoked release *(62)*. Thiopental and ketamine did not affect spontaneous release, but had similar effects on evoked release. Release evoked by glutamate agonists was also sensitive. Halothane, isoflurane, ketamine, and thiopental inhibited glutamate- and NMDA-evoked release, whereas enflurane inhibited glutamate-evoked release but enhanced NMDA-evoked release. In contrast, halothane and isoflurane had no effect on [^{3}H]dopamine release from whole brain synaptosomes in another study *(65)*, though both agents inhibited dopamine uptake.

Taken together, these findings indicate that there are complex transmitter-, brain region-, sectretagogue- and agent-specific effects on the release process. Differences in presynaptic receptors, voltage-gated Ca^{2+} channel subtypes coupled to release, and/or Ca^{2+}-release coupling may contribute to these differences *inter alia*. Given the current state of knowledge in this area, it is clear that further studies are necessary to clarify the presynaptic actions of general anesthetics on transmitter release and their mechanisms.

Neurosecretory Cells

Early studies showed that general anesthetics suppressed spontaneous release of catecholamines from the adrenal gland as well as release in response to splanchnic nerve stimulation *(66–68)*. This preparation became an early and widely used model system for research in anesthetic mechanisms. It is technically easier for many experiments than neuronal models, the released transmitters have been unambiguously identified, tools for their measurement are available, and many basic steps in the mechanism of transmitter release are similar to those in neurons. Therefore, insights obtained from this preparation were able to guide research on anesthetic mechanisms in the CNS.

Initial studies were conducted on whole adrenal glands. Barbiturates and volatile anesthetics had a similar action profile. Pentobarbital *(69)* competitively inhibited catecholamine secretion evoked by activation of nicotinic acetylcholine receptors (nAChR; IC_{50} ~50 μM). In contrast, release evoked by elevated KCl-induced depolarization or activation of histamine receptors was far less sensitive (IC_{50} ~155 μM) *(69)*. Halothane was more selective: 1.4 mM completely inhibited nAChR-mediated catecholamine secretion, while muscarinic and histamine receptor-mediated secretion or KCl depolarization-induced release were unaffected by up to 4.3 mM *(70)*. The effects of enflurane were similar but not identical: KCl-induced secretion was inhibited by 39% at 3.7 mM *(71)*. These studies indicate that barbiturates and volatile anesthetics do not inhibit evoked catecholamine secretion primarily by inhibition of Ca^{2+} entry.

Further insight into the mechanism of anesthetic modulation of neurosecretion was obtained from experiments on isolated bovine adrenal chromaffin cells, in which anesthetic effects on Ca^{2+} uptake were measured in parallel with the effects on catecholamine secretion *(72)*. The results confirmed that nAChR mediated secretion of catecholamines was about twice as sensitive to inhibition by pentobarbital as KCl-evoked secretion. Corroborating the results obtained in whole glands, pentobarbital inhibited $^{45}Ca^{2+}$ influx in response to nAChR stimulation with an IC_{50} three times lower than that for inhibition of KCl-induced Ca^{2+} influx. To further delineate effects on Ca^{2+} influx vs effects downstream in the stimulus-secretion process, the effect of pentobarbital was studied in electropermeabilized cells. Pentobarbital (up to 500 μM) had no effect on catecholamine secretion induced by varying extracellular Ca^{2+} concentrations (which, in this model, are in equilibrium with intracellular Ca^{2+} concentrations). Inhibition of catecholamine secretion by barbiturates was due to noncompetitive inhibition of the nAChR, though at higher concentrations, barbiturates also blocked depolarization-induced Ca^{2+} entry.

Similar experiments probing the mechanism of volatile anesthetic-induced inhibition of catecholamine secretion showed that methoxyflurane, halothane, isoflurane, and enflurane inhibited nAChR-induced catecholamine secretion (IC_{50} values of 250, 300, 400, and 450 μM, respectively) *(73)*. The concentrations required to inhibit KCl-evoked release by a similar amount were 5–8-fold higher. Experiments measuring the effect of volatile anesthetics on $^{45}Ca^{2+}$ entry into and catecholamine release from electropermeabilized cells indicated that, like pentobarbital, they had no major effect on voltage-gated Ca^{2+} channels (VGCC) and exocytotic mechanisms.

In clonal rat pheochromocytoma (PC12) cells, the Ca^{2+} trigger for catecholamine release involves two different pathways. Depolarization activates primarily dihydropyridine sensitive L-type VGCCs, while nAChR-activation involves Ca^{2+} influx through nAChRs and dihydropyridine insensitive VGCCs. In contrast to their effects on chromaffin cells, volatile anesthetics inhibited increases in intracellular Ca^{2+} and catecholamine secretion in response to both stimuli equipotently *(74)*. Differences in the regulation of VGCCs by second messenger-activated protein kinases may explain this discrepancy. Muscarinic receptor-induced release of Ca^{2+} from intracellular stores was insensitive to volatile anesthetics, explaining the lack of effect of anesthetics on pilocarpine-induced secretion of catecholamines observed in the intact adrenal gland *(70)*.

Experiments in GH_3 clonal pituitary cells offer insights into anesthetic interactions with additional secretory pathways *(75,76)*. Increases in intracellular Ca^{2+} and secretion of prolactin after stimulation by TRH occurs in two phases: an initial, rapid phase occurs due to IP_3-mediated Ca^{2+} release from intracellular stores followed by a sustained elevation in intracellular Ca^{2+} and continued release of prolactin due to influx of extracellular Ca^{2+} through VGCCs. Similar to its effects in PC12 cells, halothane inhibited the sustained increase in Ca^{2+} and the concomitant secretion of prolactin more effectively ($IC_{50} = 0.4$ mM) than the IP_3-mediated phase. Activation of prolactin secretion with 10 mM KCl, a concentration that depolarized GH_3 cells to a similar degree as the TRH dose employed (but a much lower concentration than that used in the chromaffin and PC12 cells experiments), was also effectively inhibited by halothane. Release of prolactin involves activation of high voltage activated L-type Ca^{2+} channels, which are moderately sensitive to halothane (IC_{50} of 0.5 and 0.8 mM for peak and "steady-state" components, respectively, [76]). It is therefore likely that inhibition of L-type VGCCs by halothane inhibits prolactin release.

In summary, barbiturates and volatile anesthetics inhibit nAChR-mediated release in native neurosecretory (chromaffin) cells more potently than release evoked by KCl-induced depolarization. In a neurosecretory cell line, this difference between nAChR and KCl-evoked release is diminished for volatile anesthetics. The results from PC12 and GH cells indicate that VGCC coupled to transmitter release are sensitive to volatile agents. Muscarinic receptor- or TRH-induced release of Ca^{2+} from intracellular stores, mediated by IP_3, is insensitive to volatile anesthetics.

Quantal Analysis

The quantal nature of transmitter release has made it possible to probe the synaptic sites of anesthetic action by quantal analysis. Early studies examined the effects of barbiturates, halothane, and diethyl ether on the excitatory group Ia afferent synapses onto cat lumbosacral motoneurons, where the neurotransmitter is likely glutamate. Thiopental and pentobarbital depressed the excitatory postsynaptic potentials (EPSPs) in a dose dependent manner. Either drug reduced the quantal content of the EPSPs by ~24%, the quantal size remained unchanged, and there was no change in the input resistance (77). Similar results were obtained for halothane (78) and ether (79). Ether depressed monosynaptic and polysynaptic spinal reflexes by 44–90% at concentrations of 15–25 mM, with no significant effect on input resistance, resting membrane potential, or quantal size. In contrast, ether reduced mean quantal content by 68%.

Interpretation of these results assumed a simple binomial distribution of the amplitudes of group Ia EPSPs, which was later shown to be incorrect for this synapse (80). However, an independent study which made no assumptions about the underlying distribution of neurotransmitter release probabilities reached similar conclusions: thiopental (20–100 μM free plasma concentration) and halothane (0.7–1.2 vol% end-tidal concentration) depressed EPSPs by shifting the probability towards the occurrence of smaller amplitude EPSPs without any appreciable effect on quantal size (81).

Therefore, it is likely that barbiturates and volatile anesthetics depress the release of glutamate from Ia afferents of motoneurons. Whether this conclusion can be generalized to other CNS synapses depends on its mechanism. If either one or both drugs act principally by potentiating or mimicking presynaptic inhibition, which can decrease quantal content (82), depression of release will be confined to synapses with a similar architecture (81). However, if general anesthetics affect stimulus-secretion coupling and/or the release process itself, depression of release should be a generalized phenomenon.

EFFECTS ON SPECIFIC COMPONENTS OF THE RELEASE PROCESS

Axonal Conduction

Larrabee and Pasternak (4) showed that axonal conduction in peripheral ganglia was about one order of magnitude less sensitive to general anesthetics than synaptic transmission. Nevertheless, depression of synaptic transmission by virtue of partial blockade of impulse conduction by anesthetics in small diameter terminal branches of nerve fibers seemed likely (83). To test this possibility, the effect of pentobarbital on synaptic transmission in the lateral olfactory tract was compared to the effects of the selective sodium channel blocker TTX. Depression of excitatory postsynaptic potentials (EPSPs) by TTX was characteristically proportional to the reduction of the compound action potential amplitude and accompanied by an increase in the latency of EPSP onset. By contrast, most general anesthetics reduced the amplitude of field EPSPs before they affected their latency of onset *(84)*. Isoflurane appeared to represent an exception: in hippocampus, it decreased the amplitude of the compound action potential recorded from small diameter (0.1–0.2 microns) unmyelinated fibers but not from larger (1 micron) myelinated fibers *(85)*. This depression contributed significantly to the depression of excitatory synaptic transmission, and suggested Na^+ channel block as a possible mechanism. The latter interpretation seems unlikely, however, as the decline in compound action potential amplitude was not accompanied by an increase in latency, which is expected if isoflurane acts directly on the inward Na^+ current. It is more likely that isoflurane decreased the number of recruited axons either by a change in threshold for action potential generation or by hyperpolarization of the axon membrane *(86)*. Halothane had a similar effect on action potential conduction in hippocampal axons *(53)*. In these experiments, glutamate receptor antagonists were used to isolate the presynaptic fiber volley as an indicator of presynaptic Na^+ channel activity. Halothane dose-dependently suppressed the fiber volley amplitude (18% block at 1.2 mM, ~3 MAC) without changing the time between stimulus onset and peak volley negativity. This indicates that halothane, in accordance with the findings of Richards *(87)*, decreased the number of discharging axons (an effect that could be simulated by decreasing stimulus intensity) and not action potential amplitude in an individual axon (as does TTX). By analyzing the relationship between fiber volley and EPSP amplitude, ~30% of the depression of the excitatory synaptic response recorded in the hippocampal CA1 region could be attributed to anesthetic-induced depression of the fiber volley *(53)*.

The effects of anesthetics on dendritic action potential initiation and back propagation have not been investigated to date. In addition to effects on action potential initiation, which presumably account for the depression of axonal conduction described in this section, general anesthetics also exert direct effects on Na^+ channels.

Voltage-Gated Na^+ Channels

Voltage-gated Na^+ channels are found on nerve terminals in numerous preparations *(88)*. They generate the action potential, which depolarizes the nerve terminal and activates presynaptic Ca^{2+} channels coupled to transmitter release. The amount of Ca^{2+} entering the nerve terminal, and hence the amount of transmitter released, depends on the amplitude and duration of the action potential *inter alia (89)*. There is no evidence to suggest that the pharmacological properties of presynaptic Na^+ channels differ from those of channels found elsewhere in the neuron, though this is difficult to study. The effects of general anesthetics on presynaptic Na^+ channels may therefore conditionally be assumed to be similar to their effects on Na^+ channels in general. It is also not known whether persistent, TTX-sensitive Na^+ channels are expressed in nerve terminals. Persistent Na^+ channels activate at more negative potentials than transient Na^+ channels and their activity persists for long time periods *(90)*. They may be more sensitive to volatile anesthetics than the transient Na^+ channels (Perouansky, M. unpublished observations).

Early studies of anesthetic effects on voltage-gated Na^+ channels in invertebrate preparations indicated that they were relatively insensitive to general anesthetics (Topf et al., Chapter 18). Re-examination of this issue using vertebrate Na^+ channels indicated that they are more sensitive than previously appreciated, and can be blocked by clinical concentrations of several anesthetics, particularly volatile agents. This is consistent with indirect evidence for a role of Na^+ channel blockade in the inhibitory effects of volatile anesthetics and propofol on glutamate release discussed above.

Voltage-Gated Ca^{2+} Channels (VGCCs)

The principal route of Ca^{2+} entry into nerve terminals is through VGCCs. Some transmitter activated channels are also permeable to Ca^{2+} (e.g., nACh and NMDA receptors), and Ca^{2+} is also released from intracellular stores. The VGCC most influential in the release of neurotransmitter appears to be the N- and P/Q-types associated with the $\alpha_1 2.2$ (α_{1B}) and $\alpha_1 2.1$ (α_{1A}) subunits, respectively *(91,92)*. In some cases, other VGCC types contribute significantly to release *(93,94)* including the recently characterized R-type *(95)*. The various VGCC controlling Ca^{2+} entry and the release process can differ between neuronal types in the same brain area *(94)*, and probably between species in the same brain region *(96)*. Even when release is controlled by N- and P/Q-type channels, the ratio between the two channels may differ between terminals *(97)*, and may change with development *(98)*. Although the relationship between Ca^{2+} influx and transmitter release is complex, a reduction in Ca^{2+} influx ultimately reduces transmitter release. VGCC are subject to inhibition by various neuromodulators, which often act via G-protein β/γ subunits.

General anesthetics can inhibit VGCC. However, the sensitivity of individual channel types, and whether presynaptic VGCC represent an important target for anesthetics is not clear. Functionally, halothane augmented paired pulse facilitation in the CA1 area of the hippocampus using both extracellular *(35)* and intracellular recordings *(99)*, an action indicative of presynaptic depression of Ca^{2+} influx. Most studies of the direct interactions between anesthetics and VGCCs have employed electrophysiological recordings from the cell body of cultured cells or acutely dissociated neurons. Although there is a large body of literature dealing with this issue in general, few papers specifically address the interaction of general anesthetics with N- and P/Q-type Ca^{2+} channels, and even fewer deal specifically with presynaptic Ca^{2+} channels (*see* Topf et al., Chapter 18).

N-Type Channels

N-type channels [($\alpha_1 2.2$ (α_{1B})-containing] are defined pharmacologically by sensitivity to ω-conotoxin GVIA and resistance to dihydropyridines *(100)*. N-type channels are prominent in neurons of the peripheral sympathetic nervous system and in presynaptic terminals and dendrites of many CNS neurons *(101–103,91)*. The release of GABA from some hippocampal interneurons relies mainly on N-type Ca^{2+} channels *(104)*.

N-type currents are moderately sensitive to volatile anesthetics. Isoflurane (0.68–1 mM) reduced peak and sustained currents by 30–50% and 50–70%, respectively, in hippocampal pyramidal cells *(105)*, dorsal root ganglion neurons *(106)*, and in the *Xenopus* expression system *(107)*. In contrast, N-type channels expressed in *Xenopus* oocytes were quite insensitive to barbiturates *(108,109)*.

P/Q-Type Channels

The P/Q type ($Ca_v 2.1$) channels contain the $\alpha_1 2.1$ (α_{1A}) α subunit. Originally discovered in cerebellar Purkinje cells, P-type channels are blocked by nanomolar concentrations of the funnel spider toxin agatoxin-IVA (IC_{50} 1–3 nM), but not by the *Conus* snail toxin ω-conotoxin GVIA *(110)*. In some experiments, agatoxin-IVA is used at concentrations that also inhibit Q-type channels (IC_{50} 90 nM), thus blurring the distinction *(103)*. P-type channels have been anatomically localized to the molecular layer of the cerebellar cortex, olfactory bulb, habenula, inferior olive, and trapezoid nucleus by immunocytochemistry *(111)*. Moderate to high levels can also be detected by in situ hybridization of $\alpha_1 2.1$ mRNA in the olfactory bulb, dentate gyrus and the CA fields of the hippocampus, areas that are not particularly rich in agatoxin-IVA sensitive Ca^{2+} channels. In the cerebellum, labeling was also present in granule cells *(112)*.

In addition to the conspicuous dendritic localization *(111,113)*, P-type channels are also present in presynaptic terminals of the mammalian neuromuscular junction and in synaptosomes derived from whole brain *(114)*. Glutamate release from synaptosomes derived from rat frontal cortex was partially inhibited by 30 nM agatoxin-IVA *(115)*. Other excitatory pathways where neurotransmitter release is sensitive in part to agatoxin-IVA include: the cerebellar climbing fiber to Purkinje synapse *(116)*, the mossy fiber *(117)*, and Schaffer collateral synapses in the CA1 and the CA3 areas of the hippocampus *(118)*. As release of glutamate appears to be under the control of multiple types of Ca^{2+} channels at any single synapse, the Ca^{2+} channels controlling the release of the inhibitory transmitter GABA exhibit less heterogeneity. In certain synapses of the cerebellum and the spinal cord, inhibitory synaptic transmission relies heavily on P-type channels *(118)*. In cultured hippocampal slices, single toxins (either the N-type selective ω-conotoxin MVIIA or the P/Q-type selective agatoxin-IVA) almost completely suppressed inhibitory postsynaptic currents elicited from certain populations of interneurons. These results, obtained using paired recordings, indicate that in a majority of CA3 interneurons, one channel type (either N or P/Q) predominantly controls transmitter release. In the same preparation however, full suppression of excitatory synaptic transmission always required simultaneous use of more than two toxins *(104)*. It has been suggested that Q-type channels also regulate glutamate release from hippocampal pyramidal cells *(91)*. Greater sensitivity to ω-conotoxin-MVIIC together with lower sensitivity to agatoxin-IVA compared to P-type channels has been used to identify their contribution to the release-triggering Ca^{2+} inflow in cortical synaptosomes *(119,96)* and bovine chromaffin cells *(120)*.

The effects of anesthetics on P/Q-type channels have been investigated in very few studies. Cerebellar P-type channels were insensitive to a variety of intravenous and volatile general anesthetics in the clinically relevant concentration range *(121)*. Approximately 1 mM isoflurane inhibited peak and sustained components of the residual, inactivating Ca^{2+} current in the presence of ω-conotoxin-VIA and nitrendipine (i.e., a combination of P/ Q- and R-type) by 44 and 71%, respectively *(105)*. The P/Q-type current was inhibited by isoflurane in dorsal root ganglion neurons (IC$_{50}$ = 0.68 mM; *[106]*). Currents through isolated recombinant α_{1A} subunits expressed in *Xenopus* oocytes were also found to be modestly sensitive to 0.59 mM halothane and 0.7 mM isoflurane (~45 and ~40% block, respectively, *[107]*).

R-Type Channels

R-type (Ca$_v$2.3) Ca^{2+} channel $\alpha_1$2.3 (α_{1E}) mRNA is most prominent in hippocampus, hypothalamus and thalamus in rat brain *(112)*. R-type channels are characterized pharmacologically by resistance to the Ca^{2+} channel toxins mentioned above and by sensitivity to low micromolar Cd^{2+}, hence their characterization as "residual" current *(122)*. The absence of Ca^{2+}-dependent inactivation distinguishes them biophysically from P/Q-type channels. Due to unavailability of selective antagonists, direct investigation of volatile anesthetic effects on this channel in central neurons is lacking; even less is known about the effects of other general anesthetics on P/Q- and R- type Ca^{2+} channels. The toxin resistant current in dorsal root ganglion neurons was also resistant to isoflurane *(106)*. Halothane (0.59 vol%) and isoflurane (0.70 vol%) blocked currents through isolated recombinant $\alpha_1$2.3 subunits expressed in *Xenopus* oocytes to a similar degree: peak and late components were blocked by 30 and 60%, respectively *(107)*.

K$^+$ Channels

Potassium (K$^+$) channels are probably the channel type exhibiting the largest heterogeneity amongst all channels present in presynaptic nerve terminals. Functionally, K$^+$ channels can be broadly classified into four families *(123)*: voltage-gated (K$_V$: delayed rectifier, fast transient A, slowly activating K$_S$), Ca^{2+}-activated (K$_{Ca}$: BK, IK, SK), inwardly rectifying (K$_{IR}$, including K$_{ATP}$), and the tandem pore domain (TPD). In rat synaptosomes, multiple classes of K$^+$ conductances have been identified, including a resting (background) conductance, fast and slowly inactivating voltage-gated channels and Ca^{2+}-activated K$^+$ channels *(124)*. To date, one or more members of each family of K$^+$ channels have been identified in any nerve terminal that has been investigated *(88)*. The effects of volatile anesthetics on this channel class have been recently reviewed *(125)*.

Voltage-Gated K$^+$ Channels (Kv)

Delayed rectifier, fast transient and slowly activating K$^+$ channels have been found in nerve endings in a variety of invertebrate and vertebrate preparations. In rodents, members of this family have been identified in motor nerve endings *(126–128)*, in the calyx of Held *(129)*, posterior pituitary terminals *(130–132)* presynaptic terminals of cerebellar basket cells *(133)*, and in hippocampal mossy fiber boutons *(134)*. In the latter location, K$_V$ channels contribute to the modulation of activity-dependent changes in transmitter release.

The influence of anesthetics on voltage-gated K$^+$ channels has been investigated in the squid giant axon and in expressed channels. A high concentration of halothane (5 m*M*), shifted steady-state activation in the depolarizing direction by ~27 mV, reduced the maximum conductance by ~50%, and shortened the time constant of activation of the delayed rectifier conductance *(135)*. Much lower halothane concentrations (0.5 m*M*) reduced K$^+$ conductances other than the delayed *(136)*, leading to axonal depolarization by ~2 mV and a transient reduction of the threshold for action potential generation. Cloned mammalian voltage-activated K$^+$ channels expressed in *Xenopus* oocytes were inhibited by halothane with an IC$_{50}$ of 0.8 m*M*, as was a representative of the min K$^+$ channel family *(137,138)*. The latter currents were also mildly sensitive to the intravenous anesthetic ketamine (~28% depression by 75 μ*M*).

Ca^{2+}-Activated K$^+$ Channels (K$_{Ca}$)

Members of this family have been found in almost every nerve terminal preparation that has been investigated for their presence. They can be divided into two groups: MaxiK or BK (large-conductance) and SK (small conductance) Ca^{2+}-activated K$^+$ channels. K$_{Ca}$ channels are strategically located close to sites of neurotransmitter release and activate rapidly in response to a rise in intracellular Ca^{2+} *(139)* suggestive of a role in the regulation of neurotransmitter release *(140)*. However, selective inhibition of I$_{K\ Ca2+}$ has not affected transmitter release in a consistent manner *(88)*. In nonneuronal cells, these channels are inhibited by volatile anesthetics. Halothane and halogenated ethers depressed ^{86}Rb flux through K$_{Ca2+}$ channels in rat glioma cells, with an IC$_{50}$ of 200 μ*M* for halothane *(141)*. Similarly, enflurane inhibited BK channels isolated from the Australian green algae *Chara australis* *(142)* In bovine adrenal chromaffin cells, halothane (0.9 m*M*), isoflurane (0.78 m*M*) and enflurane (1.7 m*M*) reduced K$_{Ca}$ by 52, 40, and 60%, respectively. Halothane and enflurane reduced the opening probability of BK channels without affecting their conductance. Ca^{2+} independent K$^+$ currents were less sensitive to inhibition *(143,144)*.

Indirect, functional experiments in mammalian CNS slices support the impression of a predominantly inhibitory effect of volatile anesthetics on K$_{Ca}$. Halothane, isoflurane, and enflurane (0.3–0.9 m*M*) blocked the posttetanic hyperpolariation mediated by these channels and the fast afterhyperpolarization after single action potentials in hippocampal CA1 and CA3 pyramidal cells *(145)*. The same anesthetics depressed accommodation of action potential firing in hippocampal CA1 pyramidal cells, evidence for an inhibitory action on K$_{Ca}$ or on the muscarinic receptor-coupled K$^+$ current *(146)*. However, direct investigations failed to identify the susceptible channels: unitary properties of high conductance K$_{Ca}$ channels recorded from patches excised from cultured hippocampal neurons were not affected by either halothane or isoflurane *(147)*.

SK channels are small conductance, voltage-insensitive K$^+$ channels with a high sensitivity to intracellular Ca^{2+}. The SK channel group underlies the slow after-hyperpolarization in central neurons. In contrast to the large-conductance channels, rat-brain SK2 channels expressed in HEK 293 cells were largely insensitive to inhibition by halothane, isoflurane or enflurane *(148)*.

K$_{IR}$ Channels

This family includes G protein-gated inward rectifiers and K$_{ATP}$ channels, which are important mediators of transmitter action in various tissues *(149)*. Anatomical studies support a presynaptic localization of K$_{ATP}$ channels *(150)*. However, there is no electrophysiological evidence for the presence of these channels in nerve terminals.

TPD Channels

This is a recently discovered, probably very abundant family of K[+] channels *(151)*. Inhibition of one member of this family, the serotonin-sensitive current (K_S), facilitated neurotransmitter release from *Aplysia* sensory neurons *(152)*, whereas activation of K_S led to synaptic depression *(153)*. Some channels in this family are activated by volatile anesthetics, which causes hyperpolarization and reduced excitability *(154–157)*. Whether TPD channels are located on presynaptic terminals is unknown. A volatile anesthetic-insensitive member of this family, rTASK, was found to be associated with a PDZ domain suggesting a postsynaptic localization *(158)*. However, because some of the TPD channels are activated by volatile anesthetics, they could contribute to anesthetic-mediated inhibition of transmitter release.

Presynaptic Transmitter-Activated Receptors: Ionotropic and Metabotropic

Receptors for a vast array of neurotransmitters exist on presynaptic terminals (*see* refs. *14* and *18* for a review). For GABA$_A$ receptors, a physiological role in the homo- and heterosynaptic regulation of transmitter release has been convincingly demonstrated *(159)*. For glutamate and acetylcholine, substantial evidence exists for such roles. The functional significance of other receptor types is less understood. The interactions of anesthetics with the postsynaptic and/or somatic counterparts of these receptors have been investigated and are discussed elsewhere in this volume. Presynaptic receptors merit a separate discussion for a number of reasons. In recent years, multiple subtypes for each subunit comprising these multimeric receptors have been identified, some of which confer distinct physiological and pharmacological properties to the assembled receptor. Most of the anesthetic effects have been described without knowing the precise subunit composition and most electrophysiological experiments have not been conducted on nerve terminals. Therefore, it cannot be assumed that conclusions about anesthetic-receptor interactions can be extrapolated from the somatodendritic domain to the presynaptic terminal.

GABA, Acetylcholine, and Serotonin

Ionotropic and metabotropic receptors activated by these transmitters exist on presynaptic terminals. The ionotropic receptors belong to the same gene superfamily of fast-acting ligand-gated ion channels, (which also includes the glycine receptor), that have emerged as strong candidates for anesthetic targets.

Virtually any general anesthetic enhances the action of GABA$_A$ receptors at clinically relevant concentrations. A similar action on presynaptic receptors could decrease the release of various transmitters. Activation of presynaptic GABA$_A$ receptors depresses the release of excitatory transmitter at the crayfish neuromuscular junction and in the mammalian spinal cord, as well as the release of neuropeptides from the pituitary gland *(160,161)*. Indeed, barbiturates do enhance presynaptic inhibition *(162)* and this mechanism could also underlie the depressant effect of halothane and ether on glutamate release in the spinal cord. However, these findings may not be generalizable to all synapses; the interaction between volatile anesthetics and GABA$_A$ receptors depends on its subunit composition *(163)* and has been shown to be different for postsynaptic receptors vs receptors present on the somatic membrane *(164,165)*.

Metabotropic GABA$_B$ receptors, coupled to inhibition of VGCC, are colocalized on some of these terminals *(166)* but may require selective patterns of presynaptic activation for recruitment *(167)*. This indicates that multiple pathways for the regulation of transmitter release by the same transmitter coexist on certain synapses. As for other metabotropic receptors, anesthetic effects on GABA$_B$ receptors are not well defined (*see* ref. *168* for muscarinic receptors). This is owing in part to difficulties in differentiating between effects on metabotropic receptors and effects further downstream in the transduction pathway that may be shared with other receptors. However, 3% halothane did not reduce paired-pulse depression of monosynaptic GABA$_A$ responses, which is mediated by presynaptic GABA$_B$ receptors. Notably, halothane did depress the late GABA$_B$ receptor-mediated IPSP *(169)*.

Anatomical and neurochemical studies demonstrated the presence of nAChRs on cholinergic, glutamatergic, GABAergic, dopaminergic, and serotoninergic nerve endings in various parts of CNS and PNS. Presynaptic nAChRs are likely to be as varied as their postsynaptic counterparts. Differences between certain subtype combinations that are particularly important include affinity for acetylcholine (reduced in $\alpha 7$- or $\alpha 5$-containing receptors), rapid desensitization ($\alpha 7$- or $\alpha 5$-containing receptors), sensitivity to blockers (e.g., α-bungarotoxin blocks homomeric receptors formed from $\alpha 7$, $\alpha 8$ or $\alpha 9$ subunits), and Ca^{2+} permeability (highest in $\alpha 7$ homomers; [170]). Activation of presynaptic nAChRs can stimulate release of transmitters. Inhibition of this stimulating effect by anesthetics would be consistent with depressed CNS function. Indeed, intravenous and volatile anesthetics depress neuronal nAChRs [171,172]. The heteromeric $\alpha 4\beta 2$ receptor may contribute to modulation of the release of GABA [173,174], glutamate [174], and acetylcholine (*see* ref. 175 for review); therefore anesthetic effects on this receptor may be relevant. When expressed in *Xenopus* oocytes, inhibition of the $\alpha 4\beta 2$ receptor by ketamine, propofol, and isoflurane occurred at such low concentrations that the relevance of this effect for the mechanisms of anesthesia was questioned [176,177]. Inhibition was selective for the $\alpha 4\beta 2$ subunit combination, since $\alpha 7$ homomers were insensitive [176]. In contrast to heterologously expressed receptors, $\alpha 4\beta 2$ and $\alpha 7$ receptors in cultured cortical neurons were blocked by halothane at higher, i.e., clinically relevant concentrations (IC_{50} values of 105 μM and 552 μM, respectively) [178]. This emphasizes the necessity for testing anesthetic interactions with receptors in their native cellular environment.

In the CNS, a significant portion of 5-HT$_3$ receptors (the ionotropic receptor for serotonin) appears to be localized presynaptically [179]. Presynaptic 5-HT$_3$ receptors have slower kinetics and higher Ca^{2+} permeability than somatic receptors in various parts of the rodent brain [180]. Drugs acting at 5-HT3 receptors have widespread clinical uses [181] including the modulation of substance-induced emesis. Striking differences exist between volatile vs intravenous anesthetic effects on ion fluxes mediated by 5-HT$_3$ receptors. In mouse NIE-115 neuroblastoma cells, volatile anesthetics potentiated currents evoked by application of serotonin while thiopental suppressed them [182]. In excised patches obtained from the same type of cells, propofol was shown to be a more potent inhibitor of 5-HT$_3$ receptor-mediated currents than pentobarbital (IC_{50} values of 10.5 μM and 131 μM, respectively) [183]. The effects of general anesthetics on presynaptic metabotropic 5-HT$_3$ receptors are unknown.

Glutamate

Three classes of ionotropic glutamate receptors have been defined pharmacologically: AMPA, kainate, and NMDA (*see* Chapter 19). All three are expressed homo- and heterosynaptically on presynaptic terminals. Transmitters whose release may be regulated by presynaptic glutamate receptors include glutamate [184], substance P [185], monoamine transmitters [186], GABA [187–189], and acetylcholine [190–191].

With the exception of the block of NMDA receptors by ketamine [192,193], nitrous oxide [194,195], and xenon [196], postsynaptic AMPA and NMDA receptors are only moderately sensitive to anesthetics [38]. However, it would be, premature to conclude that anesthetic effects on presynaptic glutamate receptors are irrelevant. NMDA, AMPA, and kainate receptors are encoded by at least six gene families, and are subject to posttranscriptional alterations, resulting in extensive structural and functional diversity [197], which may affect anesthetic sensitivity. Subunit-selective actions of anesthetics on expressed glutamate receptors have been reported [198]. Subunit-dependent changes in anesthetic sensitivity have also been observed *in situ*: AMPA receptors lacking the GluR2 subunit are far less sensitive to block by barbiturates than are GluR2 containing receptors [199], but are equally insensitive to block by volatile anesthetics [200].

Kainate receptors are intricately involved in the modulation of transmitter release [201]. In the hippocampus, release of GABA onto pyramidal cells and interneurons appears to be differentially regulated by kainate receptors. In pyramidal cells, GABAergic IPSCs were suppressed by activation of presynaptic kainate receptors both by exogenous *(202–206)* and by synaptically released glutamate *(207)*. In contrast, GABA release onto hippocampal interneurons is enhanced by activation of kainate receptors *(208)*. Even though the precise location of kainate receptors on interneurons is subject to debate *(209,210)*, this example illustrates just how complicated the regulation of excitation and inhibition in neuronal networks appears to be.

Modulation of kainate receptors by general anesthetics is least well defined of all the glutamate receptors. Earlier studies reported modest inhibition of presumably kainate receptor mediated responses *(211,212)*. In contrast, responses mediated by expressed GluR6-containing receptors (one of the kainate receptor-specific subunits) were enhanced by 2 mM halothane *(198)*. Recently developed selective AMPA receptor blockers *(197)* should help clarify the effects of anesthetics on native kainate receptors.

It is conceivable that presynaptic glutamate receptors differ from postsynaptic receptors in their sensitivity to anesthetics. It is also unclear how much of an effect constitutes a "significant" effect. Presynaptic kainate receptors in the hippocampus may contribute to the maintenance of a very fine balance between excitation and inhibition necessary for optimal functioning and even slight alterations, e.g., by anesthetics, may have functional consequences.

ATP

The two main types of receptors for extracellular ATP identified in the nervous system are broadly classified into ionotropic P_{2X} and metabotropic P_{2Y} purinoceptors. ATP activates nonselective cation channels on neurons via P_{2x} receptors, which are ubiquitous in the nervous system. Recent data suggest a role for P_{2X} receptors in the modulation of transmitter release. In spinal pain pathways, ATP activates both somatic P_{2X} receptors and heterosynaptic prejunctional receptors that modulate the release of glutamate *(213)* and GABA *(214,215)*. ATP activates P_{2X} receptor-mediated currents in synaptosomes *(216)* and is coreleased with noradrenaline from chromaffin cells where it autoregulates transmitter release *(217)*. Pressure application of ATP directly to calyx-type presynaptic terminals in the chick ciliary ganglion evoked currents that were blocked by suramin, indicating the presence of P_{2x} receptors on cholinergic terminals *(216)*. As ATP regulates the release of a wide variety of transmitters, anesthetic effects on purinergic receptors are of interest and may be of relevance for their mechanism of action. In PC12 cells, thiopental, propofol, and ketamine did not affect currents evoked by ATP *(218,219)*. Interestingly, intracerebroventricular administration of P_{2x} receptor antagonists reduced the MAC of volatile anesthetics *(220)*.

SNARE Proteins

One of the major goals of synaptic physiology is to determine the molecular basis of synaptic vesicle mobilization, exocytosis and endocytosis. Sustained synaptic transmission requires the efficient delivery of vesicles to the active zone to repopulate the "readily-releasable" pool once it has been consumed (mobilization), as well as recycling of synaptic vesicle components via endocytic recapture from the plasma membrane. Subtle modulation of these steps by agents such as general anesthetics might lead to profound effects on synaptic transmission. Previous studies in brain slices, isolated cells, and synaptosomes have focussed on general anesthetic effects on presynaptic ion channels and their impact on transmitter release. Anesthetic effects on other aspects of presynaptic function, such as the endocytosis/exocytosis cycle and Ca^{2+}-secretion coupling, are not easily accessible by measuring transmitter release from intact preparations, and therefore have not been adequately investigated. The difficulty in pinpointing the mechanism of any pharmacological modulator of synaptic transmission with great precision stems from the fact that electrophysiological measures report only successful exocytotic events. These events must be detected by postsynaptic recordings, which themselves are affected by anesthetic actions on postsynaptic receptors. Recent advances, such as quantitative confocal microscopy using fluorescent probes to monitor exocytosis, provide novel methods for studying the effects of general anesthetics on synaptic vesicle exocytosis and endocytosis independent of postsynaptic effects *(19)*.

A specific aspect of presynaptic physiology that may be a potential target for anesthetic actions is the protein machinery underlying the process of synaptic vesicle fusion and exocytosis. The molecular analysis of this special form of exocytosis has been greatly facilitated by the observation that the key molecules in intracellular vesicular transport, including neurotransmitter release, are conserved from yeast to man *(16)*. This led Rothman and colleagues *(221,222)* to develop the SNARE (soluble NSF attachment protein receptor) hypothesis of a universal vesicle docking and fusion complex. This model consists of four key components: (1) a vesicle membrane protein or v-SNARE; (2) a target membrane protein or t-SNARE which specifically binds its cognate v-SNARE; (3) a cytosolic N-ethylmaleimide-sensitive fusion protein (NSF); and (4), adapters for NSF termed SNAPs (soluble NSF attachment proteins). In nerve terminals, VAMP (vesicle-associated membrane protein; also known as synaptobrevin) is the v-SNARE, and syntaxin and SNAP (synaptosome-associated protein)-25 interact as t-SNARES. Homologous proteins exist on other secretory and endocytic pathways. VAMP, syntaxin and SNAP-25 assemble spontaneously in vitro to form a very stable SDS-resistant 7S ternary complex *(221,223,224)*. Although the precise function of v- and t-SNARE pairing is unknown, it could act at an early step to determine specificity of docking or act at a late step to mediate lipid bilayer fusion, *inter alia*. When two membranes fuse, the v-SNARE may grab the t-SNAREs in the target membrane and intertwine to form a *trans* complex, which is thought to cause fusion by pulling the two membranes together. This complex is so stable that energy in the form of ATP is required by NSF to catalyze its disassembly. Fusion cannot occur without SNARE proteins (eliminated genetically or by proteolytic cleavage by specific clostridial neurotoxins), whereas purified SNARE proteins can mediate fusion when reconstituted into liposomes *(17)*. The SNARE hypothesis is but a general model of the protein machinery regulating vesicle fusion, and the precise mechanisms underlying synaptic vesicle docking and Ca^{2+}-dependent membrane fusion remain to be characterized in detail.

Current electrophysiological and neurochemical approaches have not been successful in directly probing the effects of general anesthetics on the exocytosis machinery. However, a recent screening of existing mutants of the nematode *C. elegans* for alterations in sensitivity to volatile anesthetics identified mutations in all 3 components of the core fusion complex *(225)*. A mutation in the neuronal syntaxin gene dominantly conferred resistance to isoflurane and halothane, while other mutations in syntaxin, VAMP and SNAP-25 produced hypersensitivity. Mutations in rab3, a synaptic vesicle-associated protein not essential for docking or fusion, had no effect. The X-ray crystal structure of a core SNARE complex containing syntaxin-1A, synaptobrevin II and SNAP-25B reveals a twisted and parallel four helix bundle (coiled coil) with central leucine zipper-like layers forming a hydrophobic core *(226)*. These findings suggest the interesting possibility that the hydrophobic core of this complex, which is thought to mediate vesicle fusion, may form an anesthetic binding site. Indirect support of this possibility is provided by the finding that a synthetic peptide forming a four helical bundle binds halothane with reasonable affinity *(227)*. Thus, the potential exists for anesthetics to alter transmitter release via interactions with the SNARE complex.

SUMMARY

In many respects, our understanding of presynaptic physiology lags behind our grasp on the postsynaptic events. The complexity of the presynaptic terminal is evident in the multiple molecular interactions involved in the docking of vesicles at release sites and the assembly of the exocytotic machinery. This complexity paired with the small size and inaccessibility of nerve terminals creates formidable challenges for researchers. Recently, new techniques have emerged which allow scientists to gain access to a variety of mammalian presynaptic terminals facilitating rapid progress in this field *(228)*. Paralleling the progress in neuroscience, the postsynaptic effects of anesthetics have been defined in reasonable detail, if not necessarily fully understood on the mechanistic level. The future will clarify the presynaptic effects of general anesthetics and hopefully a complete understanding of the sensitivity of synaptic transmission to anesthetics discovered by Sherrington almost a century ago *(1)*.

REFERENCES

1. Sowton, S. and Sherrington, C. (1905) On the relative effects of chloroform upon the heart and other muscular organs. *BMJ* **2,** 181, 182.
2. Brooks, C. and Eccles, J. C. (1947) A study of the effects of anaesthesia and asphyxia on the monosynaptic pathway through the spinal cord. *J. Neurophysiol.* **10,** 349–360.
3. Bremer, F. and Bonnet, V. (1948) Action particuliere des barbituriques sur la transmission synaptique centrale. *Arch. Int. Physiol.* **56,** 100–102.
4. Larrabee, M. G. and Posternak, J. M. (1952) Selective action of anesthetics on synapses and axons in mammalian sympathetic ganglia. *J. Neurophysiol.* **15,** 91–114.
5. Matthews, E. K. and Quilliam J. P. (1964) Effects of central depressant drugs upon acetylcholine release. *Brit. J. Pharmacol.* **22,** 415–440.
6. Somjen, G. G. and Gill, M. (1963) The mechanism ofthe blockade of synaptic transmission in the mammalian spinal cord by diethyl ether and by thiopental. *J. Pharmacol. Exp. Ther.* **140,** 19–30.
7. Loyning, Y., Oshima, T., and Yokota, T. (1964) Site of action of thiamylal sodium on the monosynaptic spinal reflex pathway in cats. *J. Neurophysiol.* **27,** 408–428.
8. Shapovalov, A. I. (1963) Intracellular microelectrode investigation of effect of anesthetics on transmission of excitation in the spinal cord. *Farmakologiya i Toksikologiya* **26,** T113–T116.
9. Frank, G. and Sanders, H. D. (1963) A proposed common mechanism of action for general and local anaesthetics in the central nervous system. *Brit. J. Pharm. Chemoth.* **21,** 1–9.
10. Dodge, F. A. J. and Rahamimoff, R. (1967) On the relationship between calcium concentration and the amplitude of the end-plate potential. *J. Physiol.* **189,** 90P–92P.
11. Lando, L. and Zucker, R. S. (1994) Ca^{2+} cooperativity in neurosecretion measured using photolabile Ca^{2+} chelators. *J. Neurophysiol.* **72,** 825–830.
12. Wu, L. G., Westenbroek, R. E., Borst, J. G. G., Catterall, W. A., and Sakmann, B. (1999) Calcium channel types with distinct presynaptic localization couple differentially to transmitter release in single calyx-type synapses. *J. Neurosci.* **19,** 726–736.
13. Wu, L. G. and Saggau, P. (1997) Presynaptic inhibition of elicited neurotransmitter release. *Trends Neurosci.* **20,** 204–212.
14. MacDermott, A. B., Role, L. W., and Siegelbaum, S. A. (1999) Presynaptic ionotropic receptors and the control of transmitter release. *Annu. Rev. Neurosci.* **22,** 443–485.
15. Rahamimoff, R., Butkevich, A., Duridanova, D., Ahdut, R., Harari, and Kachalsky, S. G. (1999) Multitude of ion channels in the regulation of transmitter release. Philosophical Transactions of the Royal Society of London - Series B: Biological Sciences **354,** 281–288.
16. Scheller, R. H. (1995) Membrane trafficking in the presynaptic nerve terminal. *Neuron* **14,** 893–897.
17. Jahn, R. and Sudhof, T. C. (1999) Membrane fusion and exocytosis. *Annu. Rev. Biochem.* **68,** 863–911.
18. Ryan, T. A., Reuter, H., and Smith, S. J. (1997) Optical detection of a quantal presynaptic membrane turnover. *Nature* **388,** 478–482.
19. Sankaranarayanan, S. and Ryan, T. A. (2000) Real-time measurements of vesicle-SNARE recycling in synapses of the central nervous system. *Nat. Cell Biol.* **2,** 197–204.
20. Larsen, M., Grondahl, T. O., Haugstad, T. S., and Langmoen, I. A. (1994) The effect of the volatile anesthetic isoflurane on Ca(2+)- dependent glutamate release from rat cerebral cortex. *Brain Res.* **663,** 335–337.
21. Kendall, T. J. and Minchin, M. C. (1982) The effects of anaesthetics on the uptake and release of amino acid neurotransmitters in thalamic slices. *Brit. J. Pharmacol.* **1982,** 219–27219–277.
22. Eilers, H., Kindler, C. H., and Bickler, P. E. (1999) Different effects of volatile anesthetics and polyhalogenated alkanes on depolarization-evoked glutamate release in rat cortical brain slices. *Anesth. Analg.* **88,** 1168–1174.
23. Liachenko, S., Tang, P., Somogyi, G. T., and Xu, Y. (1999) Concentration-dependent isoflurane effects on depolarization-evoked glutamate and GABA outflows from mouse brain slices. *Brit. J. Pharmacol.* **127,** 131–138.
24. Liachenko, S., Tang, P., Somogyi, G. T., and Xu, Y. (1998) Comparison of anaesthetic and non-anaesthetic effects on depolarization-evoked glutamate and GABA release from mouse cerebrocortical slices. *Brit. J. Pharmacol.* **123,** 1274–1280.
25. Wei, L., Schlame, M., Downes, H., and Hemmings, H. C. (1996) CHEB, a convulsant barbiturate, evokes calcium-dependent spontaneous glutamate release from rat cerebrocortical synaptosomes. *Neuropharmacology* **35,** 695–701.
26. Collins, G. G. (1980) Release of endogenous amino acid neurotransmitter candidates from rat olfactory cortex slices: possible regulatory mechanisms and the effects of pentobarbitone. *Brain Res.* **190,** 517–528.
27. Kanai, T. and Szerb, J. C. (1965) Mesencephalic reticular activating system and cortical acetylcholine output. *Nature* **205,** 80–82.
28. Keifer, J. C., Baghdoyan, H. A., Becker, L., and Lydic, R. (1994) Halothane decreases pontine acetylcholine release and increases EEG spindles. *Neuroreport* **5,** 577–580.
29. Griffiths, R., Greiff, J. M., Haycock, J., Elton, C. D., Rowbotham, D. J., and Norman, R. I. (1995) Inhibition by halothane of potassium-stimulated acetylcholine release from rat cortical slices. *Brit. J. Pharmacol.* **116,** 2310–2314.
30. Richter, J. A. and Werling, L. L. (1979) K-Stimulated acetylcholine release: inhibition by several barbiturates and chloral hydrate but not by ethanol, chlordiazepoxide or 11-OH- delta9-tetrahydrocannabinol. *J. Neurochem.* **32,** 935–941.

31. Brazil, C. W. and Minneman, K. P. (1989) Clinical concentrations of volatile anesthetics reduce depolarization-evoked release of [³H]norepinephrine, but not [³H]acetylcholine, from rat cerebral cortex. *J. Neurochem.* **53,** 962–965.

32. Buggy, D. J., Nicol, B., Rowbotham, D. J., and Lambert, D. G. (2000) Effects of intravenous anesthetic agents on glutamate release: a role for GABAA receptor-mediated inhibition. *Anesthesiology* **92,** 1067–1073.

33. Wakasugi, M., Hirota, K., Roth, S., and Ito, Y. (1999) The effects of general anesthestics on excitatory and inhibitor synaptic transmission in area CA1 of the rat hippocampus in vitro. *Anesth. Analg.* **88,** 676–680.

34. Perouansky, M., Baranov, D., Salman, M., and Yaari, Y. (1995) Effects of halothane on glutamate receptor-mediated excitatory postsynaptic currents. a patch-clamp study in adult mouse hippocampal slices. *Anesthesiology* **83,** 109–119.

35. MacIver, M. B., Mikulec, A. A., Amagasu, S. M., and Monroe, F. A. (1996) Volatile Anesthetics Depress Glutamate Transmission via Presynaptic Actions. *Anesthesiology* **85,** 823–834.

36. Minchin, M. C. (1981) The effect of anaesthetics on the uptake and release of gamma-aminobutyrate and D-aspartate in rat brain slices. *Brit. J. Pharmacol.* Jul;**73(3),** 681–699.

37. Griffiths, R. and Norman, R. I. (1993) Effects of anaesthetics on uptake, synthesis and release of transmitters. *Brit. J. Anesth.* **71,** 96–107.

38. Franks, N. P. and Lieb, W. R. (1994) Molecular and cellular mechanisms of general anesthesia. *Nature* **367,** 607–614.

39. Nicholls, D. G. (1993) The glutamatergic nerve terminal. *Eur. J. Biochem.* **212,** 613–631.

40. Sihra, T. S., Bogonez, E., and Nicholls, D. G. (1992) Localized Ca²⁺ entry preferentially effects protein dephosphory-lation, phosphorylation, and glutamate release. *J. Biol. Chem.* **267,** 1983–1989

41. Lingamaneni, R., Krasowski, M. D., Jenkins, A., Pashkov, V. N., Truong T, MacIver, M. B., Harrison, N. L., and Hemmings, H. C., Jr. (2001) Anesthetic properties of 4-iodopropofol: Implications for mechanisms of anesthesia. *Anesthesiology* **94,** 1050–1057.

42. Ratnakumari, L. and Hemmings, H. C., Jr. (1997) Effects of propofol on sodium channel-dependent sodium influx and glutamate release in rat cerebrocortical synaptosomes. *Anesthesiology* **86,** 428–439.

43. Ratnakumari, L. and Hemmings, H. C. (1998) Inhibition of presynaptic sodium channels by halothane. *Anesthesiology* **88,** 1043–1054.

44. Ratnakumari, L., Vysotskaya, T. N., Duch, D. S., and Hemmings, H. C., Jr. (2000) Differential effects of anesthetic and nonanesthetic cyclobutanes on neuronal voltage-gated sodium channels. *Anesthesiology* **92,** 529–541.

45. Miao, N., Frazer, M. J., and Lynch, C. 3rd. (1995) Volatile anesthetics depress Ca²⁺ transients and glutamate release in isolated cerebral synaptosomes. *Anesthesiology* **83,** 593–603.

46. Larsen, M., Hegstad, E., Berg-Johnsen, J., and Langmoen, I. A. (1997) Isoflurane increases the uptake of glutamate in synaptosomes from rat cerebral cortex. *Brit. J. Anesth.* **78,** 55–59.

47. Larsen, M., Valo, E. T., Berg-Johnsen, J., and Langmoen, I. A. (1998) Isoflurane reduces synaptic glutamate release without changing cytosolic free calcium in isolated nerve terminals. *Eur. J. Anaesth.* **15,** 224–229.

48. Lingamaneni, R. and Hemmings, H. C., Jr. (2001) Widespread inhibition of sodium channel-dependent glutamate release from isolated nerve terminals by isoflurane and propofol. *Anesthesiology* **95,** 1460–1466.

49. Schlame, M. and Hemmings, H. C., Jr. (1995) Inhibition by volatile anesthetics of endogenous glutamate release from synaptosomes by a presynaptic mechanism. *Anesthesiology* **82,** 1406–1416.

50. Ratnakumari, L. and Hemmings, H.C., Jr. (1996) Inhibition by propofol of [³H]-batrachotoxinin-A 20-alpha-benzoate binding to voltage-dependent sodium channels in rat cortical synaptosomes. *Brit. J. Pharmacol.* **119,** 1498–1504.

51. Rehberg, B., Xiao, Y. H., and Duch, D. S. (1996) Central nervous system sodium channels are significantly suppressed at clinical concentrations of volatile anesthetics. *Anesthesiology* **84,** 1223–1233.

52. Rehberg, B. and Duch, D. S. (1999) Suppression of central nervous system sodium channels by propofol. *Anesthesiology* **91,** 512–520.

53. Mikulec, A. A., Pittson, S., Amagasu, S. M., Monroe, F. A., and MacIver, M. B. (1998) Halothane depresses action potential conduction in hippocampal axons. *Brain Res.* **796,** 231–238.

54. Hemmings, H. C., Jr. and Adamo, A. I. (1996) Activation of endogenous protein kinase C by halothane in synapto-somes. *Anesthesiology* **84,** 652–662.

55. Nicol, B., Rowbotham, D. J., and Lambert, D. G. (1995) Glutamate uptake is not a major target site for anaesthetic agents. *Brit. J. Anaesth.* **75,** 61–65.

56. Alger, B. E., Jahr, C. E., and Nicoll, R. A. (1981) Electrophysiological analysis of GABAergic local circuit neurons in the central nervous system. *Adv. Biochem. Psychopharmacol.* **26,** 77–91.

57. Hirose, T., Inoue, M., Uchida, M., and Inagaki, C. (1992) Enflurane-induced release of an excitatory amino acid, glutamate, from mouse brain synaptosomes. *Anesthesiology* **77,** 109–113.

58. Murugaiah, K. D. and Hemmings, H. C., Jr. (1998) Effects of intravenous general anesthetics on [³H]GABA release from rat cortical synaptosomes. *Anesthesiology* **89,** 919–928.

59. Griffiths, R., Greiff, J. M., Boyle, E., Rowbotham, D. J., and Norman, R. I. (1994) Volatile anesthetic agents inhibit choline uptake into rat synaptosomes. *Anesthesiology* **81,** 953–958.

60. Johnson, G. V. and Hartzell, C. R. (1985) Choline uptake, acetylcholine synthesis and release, and halothane effects in synaptosomes. *Anesth. Analg.* **64,** 395–399.

61. Larsen, M., Haugstad, T. S., Berg-Johnsen, J., and Langmoen, I. A. (1998) Effect of isoflurane on release and uptake of gamma-aminobutyric acid from rat cortical synaptosomes. *Brit. J. Anesth.* **80,** 634–638.

62. Mantz, J., Lecharny, J. B., Laudenbach, V., Henzel, D., Peytavin, G., and Desmonts, J. M. (1995) Anesthetics affect the uptake but not the depolarization-evoked release of GABA in rat striatal synaptosomes. *Anesthesiology* **82,** 502–511.

63. Lecharny, J. B., Salord, F., Henzel, D., Desmonts, J. M., and Mantz, J. (1995) Effects of thiopental, halothane and isoflurane on the calcium-dependent and -independent release of gaba from striatal synaptosomes in the rat. *Brain Res.* **670,** 308–312.

64. Haycock, J. W., Levy, W. B., and Cotman, C. W. (1977) Pentobarbital depression of stimulus-secretion coupling in brain–selective inhibition of depolarization-induced calcium-dependent release. *Biochem. Pharmacol.* **26,** 159–161.

65. el Maghrabi, E. A. and Eckenhoff, R. G. (1993) Inhibition of dopamine transport in rat brain synaptosomes by volatile anesthetics. *Anesthesiology* **78,** 750–756.

66. Li, T. H., Shaul, M. S., and Etsten, B. E. (1968) Decreased adrenal venous catecholamine concentrations during methoxyflurane anesthesia. *Anesthesiology* **29,** 1145–1152.

67. Gothert, M. and Dreyer, C. (1973) Inhibitory effect of halothane anesthesia on catecholamine release from the adrenal medulla. Naunyn-Schmiedebergs *Arch. Pharmacol* **277,** 253–266.

68. Gothert, M. and Wendt, J. (1977) Inhibition of adrenal medullary catecholamine secretion by enflurane: I. Investigations in vivo. *Anesthesiology* **46,** 400–403.

69. Holmes, J. C. and Schneider, F. H. (1973) Pentobarbitone inhibition of catecholamine secretion. *Brit. J. Pharmacol.* **49,** 205–213.

70. Gothert, M., Dorn, W., and Loewenstein, I. (1976) Inhibition of catecholamine release from the adrenal medulla by halothane. Site and mechanism of action. Naunyn-Schmiedebergs *Arch. Pharmacol* **294,** 239–249.

71. Gothert, M. and Wendt, J. (1977) Inhibition of adrenal medullary catecholamine secretion by enflurane: II. Investigations in isolated bovine adrenals–site and mechanism of action. *Anesthesiology* **46,** 404–410.

72. Pocock, G. and Richards, C. D. (1987) The action of pentobarbitone on stimulus-secretion coupling in adrenal chromaffin cells. *Brit. J. Pharmacol.* **90,** 71–80.

73. Pocock, G. and Richards, C. D. (1988) The action of volatile anaesthetics on stimulus-secretion coupling in bovine adrenal chromaffin cells. *Brit. J. Pharmacol.* **95,** 209–217.

74. Kress, H. G., Muller, J., Eisert, A., Gilge, U., Tas, P. W., and Koschel, K. (1991) Effects of volatile anesthetics on cytoplasmic Ca^{2+} signaling and transmitter release in a neural cell line. *Anesthesiology* **74,** 309–319.

75. Stern, R. C., Herrington, J., Lingle, C. J., and Evers, A. S. (1991) The action of halothane on stimulus-secretion coupling in clonal (gh3) pituitary cells. *J. Neurosci.* **11,** 2217–2225.

76. Herrington, J., Stern, R. C., Evers, A. S., and Lingle, C. J. (1991) Halothane inhibits two components of calcium current in clonal (GH3) pituitary cells. *J. Neurosci.* **11,** 2226–2240.

77. Weakly, J. N. (1969) Effect of barbiturates on "quantal" synaptic transmission in spinal motoneurones. *J. Physiol.* **204,** 63–77.

78. Zorychta, E., Esplin D. W., and Capek, R. (1975) Action of halothane on transmitter release in the spinal monosynaptic pathway. *Feder. Proceed.* **34,** 2999–2999.

79. Zorychta, E. and Capek, R. (1978) Depression of spinal monosynaptic transmission by diethyl ether: quantal analysis of unitary synaptic potentials. *J. Pharmacol. Exp. Ther.* **207,** 825–836.

80. Jack, J. J., Redman, S. J., and Wong, K. (1981) The components of synaptic potentials evoked in cat spinal motoneurones by impulses in single group Ia afferents. *J. Physiol.* **321,** 65–96.

81. Kullmann, D. M., Martin, R. L., and Redman, S. J. (1989) Reduction by general anaesthetics of group Ia excitatory postsynaptic potentials and currents in the cat spinal cord. *J. Physiol. (Lond.)* **412,** 277–296.

82. Clements, J. D., Forsythe, I. D., and Redman, S. J. (1987) Presynaptic inhibition of synaptic potentials evoked in cat spinal motoneurones by impulses in single group Ia axons. *J. Physiol.* **383,** 153–169.

83. Seeman, P. (1972) The membrane actions of anesthetics and tranquilizers. *Pharmacol. Rev.* **24,** 583–655.

84. Richards, C. D. (1982) The actions of pentobarbitone, procaine and tetrodotoxin on synaptic transmission in the olfactory cortex of the guinea-pig. *Brit. J. Pharmacol.* **75,** 639–646.

85. Berg-Johnsen, J. and Langmoen, I. A. (1986) The effect of isoflurane on unmyelinated and myelinated fibres in the rat brain. *Acta Physiol. Scand.* **127,** 87–93.

86. Richards, C. D. (1995) The synaptic basis of general anaesthesia. *Eur. J. Anaesth.* **12,** 5–19.

87. Richards, C. D. (1982) The actions of pentobarbitone, procaine and tetrodotoxin on synaptic transmission in the olfactory cortex of the guinea-pig. *Brit. J. Pharmacol.* **75,** 639–646.

88. Meir, A., Ginsburg, S., Butkevich, A., et al. (1999) Ion channels in presynaptic nerve terminals and control of transmitter release. *Physiol. Rev.* **79,** 1019–1088.

89. Katz, B. and Miledi, R. (1965) Release of acetylcholine from a nerve terminal by electric pulses of variable strength and duration. *Nature* **207,** 1097–1098.

90. Crill, W. E. (1996) Persistent sodium current in mammalian central neurons. *Annu. Rev. Physiol.* **58,** 349–362.

91. Wheeler, D. B., Randall, A., and Tsien, R. W. (1994) Roles of N-type and Q-type Ca^{2+} channels in supporting hippocampal synaptic transmission. *Science* **264,** 107–111.

92. Wu, L. G. and Saggau, P. (1994) Pharmacological identification of two types of presynaptic voltage-dependent calcium channels at CA3-CA1 synapses of the hippocampus. *J. Neurosci.* **14,** 5613–5622.

93. Heidelberger, R. and Matthews, G. (1992) Calcium influx and calcium current in single synaptic terminals of goldfish retinal bipolar neurons. *J. Physiol.* **447,** 235–256.

94. Doroshenko, P. A., Woppmann, A., Miljanich, G., and Augustine, G. J. (1997) Pharmacologically distinct presynaptic calcium channels in cerebellar excitatory and inhibitory synapses. *Neuropharmacology* **36,** 865–872.

95. Wu, L. G., Borst, J. G., and Sakmann, B. (1998) R-type Ca^{2+} currents evoke transmitter release at a rat central synapse. *Proc. Nat. Acad. Sci. USA* **95,** 4720–4725.

96. Bowman, D., Alexander, S., and Lodge, D. (1993) Pharmacological characterisation of the calcium channels coupled to the plateau phase of KCl-induced intracellular free Ca^{2+} elevation in chicken and rat synaptosomes. *Neuropharmacology* **32**, 1195–1202.

97. Reuter, H. (1995) Measurements of exocytosis from single presynaptic nerve terminals reveal heterogeneous inhibition by Ca(2+)-channel blockers. *Neuron* **14**, 773–779.

98. Iwasaki, S., Momiyama, A., Uchitel, O. D., and Takahashi, T. (2000) Developmental changes in calcium channel types mediating central synaptic transmission. *J. Neurosci.* **20**, 59–65.

99. Kirson, E. D., Yaari, Y., and Perouansky, M. (1998) Presynaptic and postsynaptic actions of halothane at glutamatergic synapses in the mouse hippocampus. *Brit. J. Pharmacol.* **124**, 1607–1614.

100. Fox, A. P., Hirning, L. D., Madison, D. V., et al. (1986) Physiology of multiple calcium channels. (None Specified) 63–74.

101. Regan, L. J., Sah, D. W., and Bean, B. P. (1991) Ca^{2+} channels in rat central and peripheral neurons: high-threshold current resistant to dihydropyridine blockers and omega-conotoxin. *Neuron* **6**, 269–280.

102. Umemiya, M. and Berger, A. J. (1994) Properties and function of low- and high-voltage-activated Ca^{2+} channels in hypoglossal motoneurons. *J. Neurosci.* **14**, 5652–5660.

103. Randall, A. and Tsien, R. W. (1995) Pharmacological dissection of multiple types of Ca^{2+} channel currents in rat cerebellar granule neurons. *J. Neurosci.* **15**, 2995–3012.

104. Poncer, J. C., McKinney, R. A., Gahwiler, B. H., and Thompson, S. M. (1997) Either N- or P-type calcium channels mediate GABA release at distinct hippocampal inhibitory synapses. *Neuron* **18**, 463–472.

105. Study, R. E. (1994) Isoflurane inhibits multiple voltage-gated calcium currents in hippocampal pyramidal neurons. *Anesthesiology* **81**, 104–116.

106. Kameyama, K., Aono, K., and Kitamura, K. (1999) Isoflurane inhibits neuronal Ca^{2+} channels through enhancement of current inactivation. *Brit. J. Anesth.* **82**, 402–411.

107. Kamatchi, G. L., Chan, C. K., Snutch, T., Durieux, M. E., and Lynch, C. (1999) Volatile anesthetic inhibition of neuronal Ca channel currents expressed in *Xenopus* oocytes. *Brain Res.* **831**, 85–96.

108. Gundersen, C. B., Umbach, J. A., and Swartz, B. E. (1988) Barbiturates depress currents through human brain calcium channels studied in *Xenopus* oocytes. *J. Pharmacol. Exp. Ther.* **247**, 824–829.

109. Gross, R. A. and Macdonald, R. L. (1988) Differential actions of pentobarbitone on calcium current components of mouse sensory neurones in culture. *J. Physiol.* **405**, 187–203.

110. Llinas, R., Sugimori, M., Lin, J. W., and Cherksey, B. (1989) Blocking and isolation of a calcium channel from neurons in mammals and cephalopods utilizing a toxin fraction (FTX) from funnel-web spider poison. *Proc. Nat. Acad. Sci. USA* **86**, 1689–1693.

111. Hillman, D., Chen, S., Aung, T. T., Cherksey, B., Sugimori, M., and Llinas, R. R. (1991) Localization of P-type calcium channels in the central nervous system. *Proc. Nat. Acad. Sci. USA* **88**, 7076–7080.

112. Stea, A., Tomlinson, W. J., Soong, T. W., Bourinet, E., Dubel, S. J., Vincent, S. R., and Snutch, T. P. (1994) Localization and functional properties of a rat brain alpha 1A calcium channel reflect similarities to neuronal Q- and P-type channels. *Proc. Nat. Acad. Sci. USA* **91**, 10,576–10,580.

113. Hell, J. W., Westenbroek, R. E., Elliott, E. M., and Catterall, W. A. (1994) Differential phosphorylation, localization, and function of distinct alpha 1 subunits of neuronal calcium channels. Two size forms for class B, C, and D alpha 1 subunits with different COOH-termini. *Ann. NY Acad. Sci.* **747**, 282–293.

114. Uchitel, O. D., Protti, D. A., Sanchez, V., Cherksey, B. D., Sugimori, and Llinas, R. (1992) P-type voltage-dependent calcium channel mediates presynaptic calcium influx and transmitter release in mammalian synapses. *Proc. Nat. Acad. Sci. USA* **89**, 3330–3333.

115. Turner, T. J., Adams, M. E., and Dunlap, K. (1992) Calcium channels coupled to glutamate release identified by omega-Aga-IVA. *Science* **258**, 310–313.

116. Regehr, W. G. and Mintz, I. M. (1994) Participation of multiple calcium channel types in transmission at single climbing fiber to Purkinje cell synapses. *Neuron* **12**, 605–613.

117. Castillo, P. E., Weisskopf, M. G., and Nicoll, R.A. (1994) The role of Ca^{2+} channels in hippocampal mossy fiber synaptic transmission and long-term potentiation. *Neuron* **12**, 261–269.

118. Takahashi, T. and Momiyama, A. (1993) Different types of calcium channels mediate central synaptic transmission. *Nature* **366**, 156–158.

119. Adams, M. E., Myers, R. A., Imperial, J. S., and Olivera, B. M. (1993) Toxityping rat brain calcium channels with omega-toxins from spider and cone snail venoms. *Biochemistry* **32**, 12,566–12,570.

120. Lopez, M. G., Villarroya, M., Lara, B., et al. (1994) Q- and L-type Ca^{2+} channels dominate the control of secretion in bovine chromaffin cells. *FEBS Lett.* **349**, 331–337.

121. Hall, A. C., Lieb, W. R., and Franks, N. P. (1994) Insensitivity of P-type calcium channels to inhalational and intravenous general anesthetics. *Anesthesiology* **81**, 117–123.

122. Dunlap, K., Luebke, J. I., and Turner, T. J. (1995) Exocytotic Ca^{2+} channels in mammalian central neurons. *Trends Neurosci.* **18**, 89–98.

123. Yost, C. S. (1999) Potassium channels: basic aspects, functional roles, and medical significance. *Anesthesiology* **90**, 1186–1203.

124. Bartschat, D. K. and Blaustein, M. P. (1985) Potassium channels in isolated presynaptic nerve terminals from rat brain. *J. Physiol.* **361**, 419–440.

125. Perouansky, M. and Pearce, R. A. (2000) Is anesthesia caused by potentiation of synaptic or intrinsic inhibition? Recent insights into the mechanisms of volatile anesthetics. *J. Basic Clin. Physiol. Pharmacol.* **11,** 83–107.

126. Brigant, J. L. and Mallart, A. (1982) Presynaptic currents in mouse motor endings. *J. Physiol.* **333,** 619–636.

127. Dreyer, F. and Penner, R. (1987) The actions of presynaptic snake toxins on membrane currents of mouse motor nerve terminals. *J. Physiol.* **386,** 455–463.

128. Mallart, A. (1985) A calcium-activated potassium current in motor nerve terminals of the mouse. *J. Physiol. (Lond.)* **368,** 577–591.

129. Forsythe, I. D. (1994) Direct patch recording from identified presynaptic terminals mediating glutamatergic EPSCs in the rat CNS, in vitro. *J. Physiol.* **479,** 381–387.

130. Bielefeldt, K., Rotter, J. L., and Jackson, M. B. (1992) Three potassium channels in rat posterior pituitary nerve terminals. *J. Physiol. (Lond.)* **458,** 41–67.

131. Jackson, M. B., Konnerth, A., and Augustine, G. J. (1991) Action potential broadening and frequency-dependent facilitation of calcium signals in pituitary nerve terminals. *Proc. Nat. Acad. Sci. USA* **88,** 380–384.

132. Thorn, P. J., Wang, X. M., and Lemos, J. R. (1991) A fast, transient K^+ current in neurohypophysial nerve terminals of the rat. *J. Physiol.* **432,** 313–326.

133. Southan, A. P. and Robertson, B. (1998) Patch-clamp recordings from cerebellar basket cell bodies and their presynaptic terminals reveal an asymmetric distribution of voltage-gated potassium channels. *J. Neurosci.* **18,** 948–955.

134. Geiger, J. R. P. and Jonas, P. (2000) Dynamic control of presynaptic Ca^{2+} inflow by fast-inactivating K^+ channels in hippocampal mossy fiber boutons. *Neuron* **28,** 927–939.

135. Haydon, D. A. and Urban, B. W. (1986) The actions of some general anesthetics on the potassium current of the squid giant axon. *J. Physiol.* **373,** 311–327.

136. Haydon, D. A., Requena, J., and Simon, A. J. (1988) The potassium conductance of the resting squid axon and its blockage by clinical concentrations of general anesthetics. *J. Physiol.* **402,** 363–374.

137. Kulkarni, R. S., Zorn, L. J., Anantharam, V., Bayley, H., and Treistman, S. N. (1996) Inhibitory effects of ketamine and halothane on recombinant potassium channels from mammalian brain. *Anesthesiology* **84,** 900–909.

138. Zorn, L., Kulkarni, R., Anantharam, V., Bayley, H., and Treistman, S. N. (1993) Halothane acts on many potassium channels, including a minimal potassium channel. *Neurosci. Lett.* **161,** 81–84.

139. Robitaille, R., Garcia, M. L., Kaczorowski, G. J., and Charlton, M. P. (1993) Functional colocalization of calcium and calcium-gated potassium channels in control of transmitter release. *Neuron* **11,** 645–655.

140. Robitaille, R., Adler, E. M., and Charlton, M. P. (1993) Calcium channels and calcium-gated potassium channels at the frog neuromuscular junction. *J. Physiol. (Paris)* **87,** 15–24.

141. Tas, P. W., Kress, H. G., and Koschel, K. (1989) Volatile anesthetics inhibit the ion flux through Ca^{2+}-activated K^+ channels of rat glioma C6 cells. *Biochim. Biophys. Acta.* **983,** 264–268.

142. Antkowiak, B. and Kirschfeld, K. (1992) Enflurane is a potent inhibitor of high conductance Ca(2+)-activated K^+ channels of Chara australis. *FEBS Lett.* **313,** 281–284.

143. Pancrazio, J. J., Park, W. K., and Lynch, C. (1992) Effects of enflurane on the voltage-gated membrane currents of bovine adrenal chromaffin cells. *Neurosci. Lett.* **146,** 147–151.

144. Pancrazio, J. J., Park, W. K., and Lynch, C. (1993) Inhalational anesthetic actions on voltage-gated ion currents of bovine adrenal chromaffin cells. *Mol. Pharmacol.* **43,** 783–794.

145. Fujiwara, N., Higashi, H., Nishi, S., Shimoji, K., Sugita, S., and Yoshimura, M. (1988) Changes in spontaneous firing patterns of rat hippocampal neurones induced by volatile anaesthetics. *J. Physiol. (Lond.)* **402,** 155–175.

146. Southan, A. P. and Wann, K. T. (1989) Inhalation anaesthetics block accommodation of pyramidal cell discharge in the rat hippocampus. *Brit. J. Anesth.* **63,** 581–586.

147. McLarnon, J. and Sawyer, D. (1998) Effects of volatile anaesthetics on a high conductance calcium dependent potassium channel in cultured hippocampal neurons. *Toxicol. Lett.* **100–101,** 271–276.

148. Dreixler, J. C., Jenkins, A., Cao, Y. J., Roizen, J. D., and Houamed, K. M. (2000) Patch-clamp analysis of anesthetic interactions with recombinant SK2 subtype neuronal calcium-activated potassium channels. *Anesth. Analg.* **90,** 727–732.

149. Hille, B. (2001) Ionic Channels of Excitable Membranes. 3rd ed., Sinauer, Sunderland, MA.

150. Ponce, A., Bueno, E., Kentros, C., et al. (1996) G-protein-gated inward rectifier K^+ channel proteins (GIRK1) are present in the soma and dendrites as well as in nerve terminals of specific neurons in the brain. *J. Neurosci.* **16,** 1990–2001.

151. Goldstein, S. A., Bockenhauer, D., O'Kelly, I., and Zilberberg, N. (2001) Potassium leak channels and the KCNK family of two-P-domain subunits. *Nat. Rev. Neurosci.* **2,** 175–184.

152. Siegelbaum, S. A., Camardo, J. S., and Kandel, E. R. (1982) Serotonin and cyclic amp close single K^+ channels in aplysia sensory neurones. *Nature* **299,** 413–417.

153. Piomelli, D., Volterra, A., Dale, N., et al. (1987) Lipoxygenase metabolites of arachidonic acid as second messengers for presynaptic inhibition of Aplysia sensory cells. *Nature* **328,** 38–43.

154. Franks, N. P. and Lieb, W. R. (1988) Volatile general anaesthetics activate a novel neuronal K^+ current. *Nature* **333,** 662–664.

155. Ries, C. R. and Puil, E. (1999) Ionic mechanism of isoflurane's actions on thalamocortical neurons. *J. Neurophysiol.* **81,** 1802–1809.

156. Ries, C. R. and Puil, E. (1999) Mechanism of anesthesia revealed by shunting actions of isoflurane on thalamocortical neurons. *J. Neurophysiol.* **81,** 1795–1801.

157. Sirois, J. E., Lei, Q., Talley, E. M., Lynch, C., and Bayliss, D. A. (2000) The TASK-1 two-pore domain K$^+$ channel is a molecular substrate for neuronal effects of inhalation anesthetics. *J. Neurosci.* **20,** 6347–6354.

158. Leonoudakis, D., Gray, A. T., Winegar, B. D., et al. (1998) An open rectifier potassium channel with two pore domains in tandem cloned from rat cerebellum. *J. Neurosci.* **18,** 868–877.

159. Rudomin, P. and Schmidt, R. F. (1999) Presynaptic inhibition in the vertebrate spinal cord revisited. *Exp. Brit. Res.* **129,** 1–37.

160. Oertel, W. H., Mugnaini, E., Tappaz, M. L., et al. (1982) Central GABAergic innervation of neurointermediate pituitary lobe: biochemical and immunocytochemical study in the rat. *Proc. Nat. Acad. Sci. USA* **79,** 675–679.

161. Jackson, M. B. and Zhang, S. L. J. (1995) Action potential propagation and propagation block by gaba in rat posterior pituitary nerve terminals. *J. Physiol. (Lond.)* **483,** 597–611.

162. Eccles, J. C., Schmidt, R., and Willis, W. D. (1963) Pharmacological studies on presynaptic inhibition. *J. Physiol. (Lond.)* **168,** 500–530.

163. Banks, M. I., Saad, A. A., and Pearce, R. A. (2000) Subunit-specific modulation of recombinant GABA$_A$ receptors by isoflurane. *Soc. Neurosci. Abstr.* **26,** 629.

164. Banks, M. I., Li, T. B., and Pearce, R. A. (1997) Effects of isoflurane on mIPSCs and excised neuronal GABA$_A$ receptors. *Soc. Neurosci. Abstr.* **23,** 104.

165. Bai, D., Zhu, G., Pennefather, P., Jackson, M. F., MacDonald, J. F., and Orser, B. A. (2001) Distinct functional and pharmacological properties of tonic and quantal inhibitory postsynaptic currents mediated by γ-aminobutyric acid$_A$ receptors in hippocampal neurons. *Mol. Pharmacol.* **59,** 814–824.

166. Mathews, G. C., Bolos-Sy, A. M., Holland, K. D., et al. (1994) Developmental alteration in GABA$_A$ receptor structure and physiological properties in cultured cerebellar granule neurons. *Neuron* **13,** 149–158.

167. Fischer, Y. and Parnas, I. (1996) Differential activation of two distinct mechanisms for presynaptic inhibition by a single inhibitory axon. *J. Neurophysiol.* **76,** 3807–3816.

168. Durieux, M. E. (1996) Muscarinic signaling in the central nervous system - recent developments and anesthetic implications. *Anesthesiology* **84,** 173–189.

169. Pearce, R. A. (1996) Volatile anesthetic enhancement of paired-pulse depression investigated in the rat hippocampus in vitro. *J. Physiol.* (Lond.) **492.3,** 823–840.

170. Wonnacott, S. (1997) Presynaptic nicotinic ACh receptors. *Trends Neurosci.* **20,** 92–98.

171. Nicoll, R. A. (1978) Pentobarbital: differential postsynaptic actions on sympathetic ganglion cells. *Science* **199,** 451–452.

172. Flood, P. and Role, L. W. (1998) Neuronal nicotinic acetylcholine receptor modulation by general anesthetics. *Toxicol. Lett.* **100–101,** 149–153.

173. Lena, C., Changeux, J. P., and Mulle, C. (1993) Evidence for "preterminal" nicotinic receptors on GABAergic axons in the rat interpeduncular nucleus. *J. Neurosci.* **13,** 2680–2688.

174. Guo, J. Z., Tredway, T. L., and Chiappinelli, V. A. (1998) Glutamate and GABA release are enhanced by different subtypes of presynaptic nicotinic receptors in the lateral geniculate nucleus. *J. Neurosci.* **18,** 1963–1969.

175. Vizi, E. S., Sershen, H., Balla, A., et al. (1995) Neurochemical evidence of heterogeneity of presynaptic and somatodendritic nicotinic acetylcholine receptors. *Ann. NY Acad. Sci.* **757,** 84–99.

176. Flood, P., Ramirez-Latorre, J., and Role, L. (1997) Alpha 4 beta 2 neuronal nicotinic acetylcholine receptors in the central nervous system are inhibited by isoflurane and propofol, but alpha 7-type nicotinic acetylcholine receptors are unaffected [see comments]. *Anesthesiology* **86,** 859–865.

177. Violet, J. M., Downie, D. L., Nakisa, R. C., Lieb, W. R., and Franks, N. P. (1997) Differential sensitivities of mammalian neuronal and muscle nicotinic acetylcholine receptors to general anesthetics. *Anesthesiology* **86,** 866–874.

178. Mori, T., Zhao, X., Zuo, Y., et al. (2001) Modulation of neuronal nicotinic acetylcholine receptors by halothane in rat cortical neurons. *Mol. Pharmacol.* **59,** 732–743.

179. Kidd, E. J., Laporte, A. M., Langlois, X., et al. (1993) 5-HT3 receptors in the rat central nervous system are mainly located on nerve fibres and terminals. *Brain Res.* **612,** 289–298.

180. Nayak, S. V., Ronde, P., Spier, A. D., Lummis, S. C., and Nichols, R. A. (1999) Calcium changes induced by presynaptic 5-hydroxytryptamine-3 serotonin receptors on isolated terminals from various regions of the rat brain. *Neuroscience* **91,** 107–117.

181. Peroutka, S. J. and Mahler, E. (1999) Serotonin (5-hydroxytryptamine) receptor subtypes: clinical relevance.2nd, 1842–1845.

182. Jenkins, A., Franks, N. P., and Lieb, W. R. (1996) Actions of general anaesthetics on 5-HT3 receptors in N1E-115 neuroblastoma cells. *Brit. J. Pharmacol.* **117,** 1507–1515.

183. Barann, M., Dilger, J. P., Bonisch, H., Gothert, M., Dybek, A., and Urban, B. W. (2000) Inhibition of 5-HT(3) receptors by propofol: equilibrium and kinetic measurements. *Neuropharmacology* **39,** 1064–1074.

184. Berretta, N. and Jones, R. S. (1996) Tonic facilitation of glutamate release by presynaptic N-methyl-D-aspartate autoreceptors in the entorhinal cortex. *Neuroscience* **75,** 339–344.

185. Liu, H., Mantyh, P. W., and Basbaum, A. I. (1997) NMDA-receptor regulation of substance P release from primary afferent nociceptors. *Nature* **386,** 721–724.

186. Pittaluga, A., Bonfanti, A., and Raiteri, M. (1997) Differential desensitization of ionotropic non-NMDA receptors having distinct neuronal location and function. Naunyn-Schmiedebergs *Arch. Pharmacol* **356,** 29–38.

187. Bureau, I. and Mulle, C. (1998) Potentiation of GABAergic synaptic transmission by AMPA receptors in mouse cerebellar stellate cells: changes during development. *J. Physiol.* **509,** 817–831.

188. Glitsch, M. and Marty, A. (1999) Presynaptic effects of NMDA in cerebellar Purkinje cells and interneurons. *J. Neurosci.* **19,** 511–519.

189. Satake, S., Saitow, F., Yamada, J., and Konishi, S. (2000) Synaptic activation of AMPA receptors inhibits GABA release from cerebellar interneurons. *Nat. Neurosci.* **3,** 551–558.

190. Fu, W. M., Liou, J. C., Lee, Y. H., and Liou, H. C. (1995) Potentiation of neurotransmitter release by activation of presynaptic glutamate receptors at developing neuromuscular synapses of *Xenopus. J. Physiol.* **489,** 813–823.

191. Liou, H. C., Yang, R. S., and Fu, W. M. (1996) Potentiation of spontaneous acetylcholine release from motor nerve terminals by glutamate in *Xenopus* tadpoles. *Neuroscience* **75,** 325–331.

192. Anis, N. A., Berry, S. C., Burton, N. R., and Lodge, D. (1983) The dissociative anaesthetics, ketamine and phencyclidine, selectively reduce excitation of central mammalian neurones by *N*-methyl-aspartate. *Brit. J. Pharmacol.* **79,** 565–575.

193. Thomson, A. M., West, D. C., and Lodge, D. (1985) An N-methylaspartate receptor-mediated synapse in rat cerebral cortex: a site of action of ketamine? *Nature* **313,** 479–481.

194. Jevtovic-Todorovic, V., Todorovic, S. M., Mennerick, S., et al. (1998) Nitrous oxide (laughing gas) is an NMDA antagonist, neuroprotectant and neurotoxin. *Nat. Med.* 460–463.

195. Mennerick, S., Jevtovic-Todorovic, V., Todorovic, S. M., Shen, W., Olney, J. W., and Zorumski, C. F. (1998) Effect of nitrous oxide on excitatory and inhibitory synaptic transmission in hippocampal cultures. *J. Neurosci.* **18,** 9716–9726.

196. Franks, N. P., Dickinson, R., de Sousa, S. L., Hall, A. C., and Lieb, W. R. (1998) How does xenon produce anaesthesia? *Nature* **396,** 324.

197. Dingledine, R., Borges, K., Bowie, D., and Traynelis, S. F. (1999) The glutamate receptor ion channels. *Pharmacol. Rev.* **51,** 7–61.

198. Dildy-Mayfield, J. E., Eger, E. I., and Harris, R. A. (1996) Anesthetics produce subunit-selective actions on glutamate receptors. *J. Pharmacol. Exp. Ther.* **276,** 1058–1065.

199. Joo, D. T., Xiong, Z., MacDonald, J. F., et al. (1999) Blockade of Glutamate Receptors and Barbiturate Anesthesia: Increased Sensitivity to Pentobarbital-induced Anesthesia Despite Reduced Inhibition of AMPA Receptors in GluR2 Null Mutant Mice. *Anesthesiology* **91,** 1329–1341.

200. Joo, D. T., Gong, D., Sonner, J. M., Jia, Z. P., MacDonald, J. F., Eger, E. I., and Orser, B. A. (2001) Blockade of AMPA receptors and volatile anesthetics - Reduced anesthetic requirements in GluR2 null mutant mice for loss of the righting reflex and antinociception but not minimum alveolar concentration. *Anesthesiology* **94,** 478–488.

201. Frerking, M. and Nicoll, R. A. (2000) Synaptic kainate receptors. *Curr. Opin. Neurobiol.* **10,** 342–351.

202. Clarke, V. R., Ballyk, B. A., Hoo, K. H., et al. (1997) A hippocampal GluR5 kainate receptor regulating inhibitory synaptic transmission. *Nature* **389,** 599–603.

203. Rodriguez-Moreno, A., Herreras, O., and Lerma, J. (1997) Kainate receptors presynaptically downregulate GABAergic inhibition in the rat hippocampus. *Neuron* **19,** 893–901.

204. Frerking, M., Malenka, R. C., and Nicoll, R. A. (1998) Synaptic activation of kainate receptors on hippocampal interneurons. *Nature Neuroscience* **1,** 479–486.

205. Cossart, R., Esclapez, M., Hirsch, J. C., Bernard, C., and Ben-Ari, Y. (1998) GluR5 kainate receptor activation in interneurons increases tonic inhibition of pyramidal cells. *Nature Neuroscience* **1,** 470–478.

206. Bureau, I., Bischoff, S., Heinemann, S. F., and Mulle, C. (1999) Kainate receptor-mediated responses in the CA1 field of wild-type and GluR6-deficient mice. *J. Neurosci.* **19,** 653–663.

207. Min, M. Y., Melyan, Z., and Kullmann, D. M. (1999) Synaptically released glutamate reduces gamma-aminobutyric acid (GABA)ergic inhibition in the hippocampus via kainate receptors. *Proc. Nat. Acad. Sci. USA* **96,** 9932–9937.

208. Cossart, R., Dinocourt, C., Hirsch, J. C., et al. (2001) Dendritic but not somatic GABAergic inhibition is decreased in experimental epilepsy. *Nat. Neurosci.* **4,** 52–62.

209. Frerking, M., Petersen, C. C. H., and Nicoll, R. A. (1999) Mechanisms underlying kainate receptor-mediated disinhibition in the hippocampus. *Proc. Nat. Acad. Sci. USA* **96,** 12,917–12,922.

210. Rodriguez-Moreno, A., Lopez-Garcia, J. C., and Lerma, J. (2000) Two populations of kainate receptors with separate signaling mechanisms in hippocampal interneurons. *Proc. Nat. Acad. Sci. USA* **97,** 1293–1298.

211. Wakamori, M., Ikemoto, Y., and Akaike, N. (1991) Effects of two volatile anesthetics and a volatile convulsant on the excitatory and inhibitory amino acid responses in dissociated CNS neurons of the rat. *J. Neurophysiol.* **66,** 2014–2021.

212. Lin, L. H., Chen, L. L., and Harris, R. A. (1993) Enflurane inhibits nmda, ampa, and kainate-induced currents in xenopus oocytes expressing mouse and human brain mrna. *FASEB J.* **7,** 479–485.

213. Gu, J. G. and MacDermott, A. B. (1997) Activation of ATP P2X receptors elicits glutamate release from sensory neuron synapses. *Nature* **389,** 749–753.

214. Hugel, S. and Schlichter, R. (2000) Presynaptic P2X receptors facilitate inhibitory GABAergic transmission between cultured rat spinal cord dorsal horn neurons. *J. Neurosci.* **20,** 2121–2130.

215. Khakh, B. S. (2001) Molecular physiology of P2X receptors and ATP signalling at synapses. *Nat. Rev. Neurosci.* **2,** 165–174.

216. Sun, X. P. and Stanley, E. F. (1996) An ATP-activated, ligand-gated ion channel on a cholinergic presynaptic nerve terminal. *Proc. Nat. Acad. Sci. USA* **93,** 1859–1863.

217. Hollins, B. and Ikeda, S. R. (1997) Heterologous expression of a P2x-purinoceptor in rat chromaffin cells detects vesicular ATP release. *J. Neurophysiol.* **78,** 3069–3076.

218. Andoh, T., Furuya, R., Oka, K., et al. (1997) Differential effects of thiopental on neuronal nicotinic acetylcholine receptors and P2X purinergic receptors in PC12 cells. *Anesthesiology* **87,** 1199–1209.

219. Furuya, R., Oka, K., Watanabe, I., Kamiya, Y., Itoh, H., and Andoh, T. (1999) The effects of ketamine and propofol on neuronal nicotinic acetylcholine receptors and P2x purinoceptors in PC12 cells. *Anesth. Analg.* **88,** 174–180.

220. Masaki, E., Ebisawa, T., Kondo, I., Hayashida, K., Matsumoto, Y., and Kawamura, M. (2000) P2-purinergic receptor antagonists reduce the minimum alveolar concentration of inhaled volatile anesthetics. *Brain Res.* **864,** 130–133.

221. Sollner, T., Bennett, M. K., Whiteheart, S. W., Scheller, R. H., and Rothman, J. E. (1993) A protein assembly-disassembly pathway in vitro that may correspond to sequential steps of synaptic vesicle docking, activation, and fusion. *Cell* **75,** 409–418.

222. Sollner, T., Whiteheart, S. W., Brunner, M., et al. (1993) SNAP receptors implicated in vesicle targeting and fusion. *Nature* **362,** 318–324.

223. Andrade, R. and Nicoll, R. A. (1987) Pharmacologically distinct actions of serotonin on single pyramidal neurones of the rat hippocampus recorded in vitro. *J. Physiol. (Lond.)* **394,** 99–124.

224. Hayashi, T., McMahon, H., Yamasaki, S., et al. (1994) Synaptic vesicle membrane fusion complex: action of clostridial neurotoxins on assembly. *EMBO J.* **13,** 5051–5061.

225. van Swinderen, B., Saifee, O., Shebester, L., Roberson, R., Nonet, M. L., and Crowder, C. M. (1999) A neomorphic syntaxin mutation blocks volatile-anesthetic action in Caenorhabditis elegans. *Proc. Nat. Acad. Sci. USA* **96,** 2479–2484.

226. Sutton, R. B., Fasshauer, D., Jahn, R., and Brunger, A. T. (1998) Crystal structure of a SNARE complex involved in synaptic exocytosis at 2.4 Å resolution. *Nature* **395,** 347–353.

227. Johansson, J. S., Scharf, D., Davies, L. A., Reddy, K. S., and Eckenhoff, R. G. (2000) A designed four-alpha-helix bundle that binds the volatile general anesthetic halothane with high affinity. *Biophys. J.* **78,** 982–993.

228. Neher, E. (1998) Vesicle pools and Ca^{2+} microdomains: new tools for understanding their roles in neurotransmitter release. *Neuron* **20,** 389–399.

22

The Meyer-Overton Relationship and Its Exceptions

Warren S. Sandberg and Keith W. Miller

INTRODUCTION

General anesthesia is induced by a large group of structurally unrelated compounds. Hans Meyer and Ernest Overton, working independently, observed at the end of the 19th century that the potencies of general anesthetics are directly proportional to their hydrophobicities (Fig. 1). This seminal observation became known as the Meyer-Overton rule, and it has influenced all subsequent research into the mechanisms of general anesthesia. Early theories of anesthesia postulated that general anesthetics interacted with membrane lipids and embraced the notion that anesthesia might result from indirect effects on membrane protein. Lipid-based theories of anesthesia fail because anesthetic induced effects are small, and modern work focuses on interactions between anesthetics and proteins. Despite the change in proposed targets of anesthetic action, the Meyer-Overton correlation still holds true, and any theory of anesthetic action, whether membrane- or protein-based, must account for it.

Historical Perspective

Bernard, in 1875 had proposed that all general anesthetics worked through a common target (1), and this proposal became known as the 'unitary hypothesis' of anesthesia. At the time, protein structure was viewed as rigid, each protein permitting interaction with a specific substrate or effector in a 'lock-and key' manner. The lipid component of cells was thought to be a more amorphous substance. The observation that anesthetic potency is correlated with solubility in oil led to the logical presumption that anesthetics acted on cellular lipids. In the early 20th century, as cellular architecture became known, and with the discovery of excitable membranes, the lipid bilayer seemed certain to be the site of anesthetic action. It was conceptually simpler to propose the lipid bilayer as the target (thereby conceiving of a single target for all anesthetics) than to suppose that each anesthetic had a unique protein target. The bilayer's hydrocarbon interior provided the lipid site of anesthetic action predicted by the Meyer-Overton rule, while its deformable structure appeared accommodating to the many diverse structural compounds capable of producing the anesthetic state (Fig. 2). Consequently, decades of effort were devoted to testing theories of anesthetic action arising from the Meyer-Overton correlation and the prediction that the membrane was the site of action.

The Meyer-Overton correlation persists as a backdrop for current investigation of the mechanisms of anesthesia. Theories of anesthetic action based upon the interaction between anesthetics and proteins have dominated the last two decades of research. Focus on protein sites of anesthesia has been accompanied by a diminution or outright rejection of the potential role of the membrane in anesthetic action, an apparent reaction to the previously dominant theories.

From: *Contemporary Clinical Neuroscience: Neural Mechanisms of Anesthesia*
Edited by: Joseph F. Antognini et al. © Humana Press Inc., Totowa, NJ

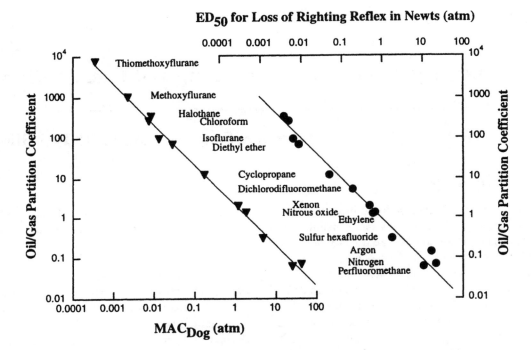

Fig. 1. The Meyer-Overton correlation. Oil/gas partition coefficients for volatile and gaseous anesthetic agents plotted against two measures of anesthetic potency in vivo. The left plot, indicated by triangles, uses MAC, (here determined in dogs), while the right plot, indicated by circles, uses the anesthetic ablating the righting reflex in 50% of newts (ED_{50}). Data are from ref. *(120)*. All axes use logarithmic scales. Potencies of some compounds have not been determined in both species; in such cases only one data point is shown. Unit lines are drawn through the data. Unrestrained least-squares regression of each data set gives a correlation coefficient greater than 0.95.

The Classical Meyer-Overton Relationship

In general terms, the Meyer-Overton relationship describes the close correlation between an anesthetic's potency in vivo and its hydrophobicity. The correlation is insensitive to the method used to assess anesthetic potency (Fig. 1). For example, potency in vivo can be expressed in terms of the concentration of agent required to ablate the righting reflex, or as MAC, the minimum alveolar concentration of agent required to suppress response to noxious stimuli. The partitioning of the solute of interest from either the gas or aqueous phase into an apolar solvent is used as a general measure of hydrophobicity. Initially, olive oil was used as the apolar phase. However, olive oil is an undefined mixture of lipids, and it might more appropriately be supplanted in hydrophobicity estimates by more defined apolar solvents such as benzene, octanol or lecithin. The choice of apolar phase has some influence on the strength of the correlation between in vivo potency and partitioning, with slightly polar or polarizable solvents such as alcohols or benzene yielding a tighter correlation than completely apolar solvents such as hexane.

Theories of Anesthetic Action Inspired by the Meyer-Overton Relationship

The observation that anesthetic potency is correlated with lipid solubility for a wide range of anesthetics led to the supposition that anesthetics acted on the lecithin component of cells. That the cellular lecithin later proved to comprise the lipid bilayer of the cell membrane lent additional plausibility to such a notion, as the membrane was clearly a critical component in the cellular signaling evidently interrupted by anesthetics. A number of theories were advanced to explain exactly how

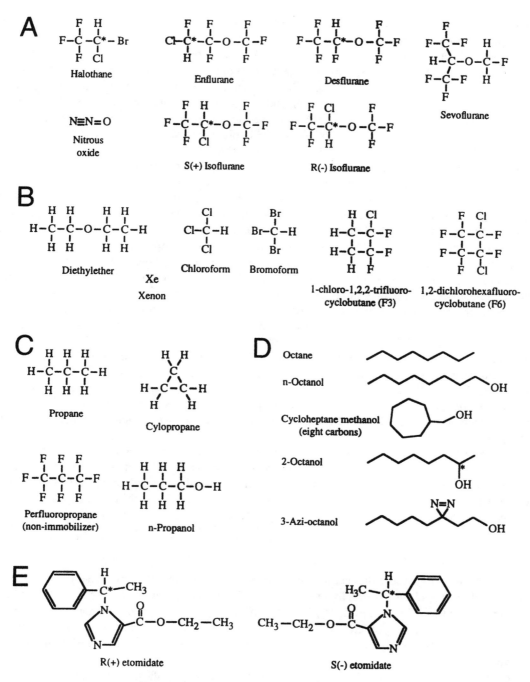

Fig. 2. Structures of the anesthetics mentioned in the text. The term anesthetic is used loosely here, as some of the compounds shown are actually non-immobilizers. Note the many of these structures have chiral carbon atoms, denoted by the *. (**A**) Some common clinically used volatile and gaseous anesthetics. Both stereoisomers of isoflurane are shown. (**B**) Anesthetics of historical and experimental interest. Note that F3 (anesthetic) and F6 (non-immobilizer) are considered to be structural homologs. (**C**) Examples of 3-carbon anesthetics, including cyclopropane (an agent used clinically in the past), n-propanol (a potent short chain alcohol anesthetic) and perfluoropropane (a non-immobilizer). (**D**) A series of 8-carbon anesthetics, including 3-azi-octanol. This agent can be photoactivated at non-destructive wavelengths, leading to covalent labeling of the site occupied during irradiation. (**E**) Stereoisomers of etomidate, an injectable anesthetic displaying strong chirality effects.

anesthetics might exert their effects in the membrane. These are now known collectively as 'membrane perturbation' theories.

One such theory came to be known as the critical volume hypothesis, stating that as anesthetics dissolve in the membrane they increase the total volume of the system until some critical threshold is reached, beyond which anesthesia ensues. Clinical concentrations of anesthetics do expand membrane volume by a few tenths of a percent (2), and this accounts for the pressure reversal of anesthesia (3). However, such effects are readily mimicked by small changes in temperature. Increasing temperature by 1°C increases membrane area (4) and volume (5), while thickness decreases (6), (all by about 0.1% per degree) without causing anesthesia. Theories of anesthetic action based solely on changes in membrane dimensions could not account for these observations.

If the dimensional changes in membranes were small, what about the changes in other physical properties? Anesthetics were observed to increase membrane fluidity (7), leading to the hypothesis that changes in lipid fluidity affected membrane proteins and produced anesthesia. Similarly, it was proposed that nerve membrane lipids might undergo a phase transition, based on the observation that most anesthetics depress the gel to liquid crystal phase transition temperature for pure lipid systems (8–10). Both theories ultimately fail because the effects produced by anesthetics can be reproduced by increases in temperature of a few tenths of a °C (11,12) and because they both predict anesthetic potency to increase with temperature, which is not the case (13–15).

Anesthetics, at clinically relevant concentrations, raise liposomal membrane permeability to cations (16–18). Cation permeability mediated by simple ionophores, such as the carrier valinomycin and the channel gramicidin, was also influenced by anesthetics (17), showing that lipid perturbation could be sensed by these model "proteins." Such effects are up to one hundred fold larger than the underlying structural changes discussed above. These observations were developed into a theory suggesting that anesthetics worked by collapsing pH gradients across cell membranes (19). This theory has not been borne out in practice, largely because the effects were shown in subsequent measurements to be small (20), and because not all anesthetics change membrane permeability to ions (21).

Lipid-membrane theories account for both the structural diversity of compounds capable of producing anesthesia, and for our inability to find a chemical antagonist of the anesthetic state. However, all of these theories have failed because bulk membrane physical properties are changed very little at clinically relevant anesthetic concentrations. Consequently, research has shifted to focusing on lipid microenvironments, such as at the lipid-protein interface, and on direct anesthetic-protein interactions.

Objective of the Chapter

The vast majority of anesthetics have in vivo potencies that are close to those predicted from measures of their lipid solubilities. In other words, the Meyer-Overton rule still serves as a useful test for potential theories of anesthetic action. Theories of anesthesia must account for the Meyer-Overton correlation. Similarly, the biological systems used in vitro to investigate and develop new theories of anesthetic action approximate to a greater or lesser degree the Meyer-Overton correlation observed in vivo.

This chapter will review new developments in mechanisms of anesthesia research in the context of the Meyer-Overton correlation, with emphasis on three questions:

1. Is it reasonable to expect a liquid solvent to accurately model the properties of the site(s) of anesthetic action? In other words: Is the Meyer-Overton correlation relevant?
2. Can the Meyer-Overton correlation be reconciled with protein sites of anesthesia?
3. Is there a renewed role for the lipid bilayer in theories of anesthetic action?

We begin by examining several areas where the Meyer-Overton correlation fails to explain the observed behaviors of anesthetics and related compounds. These failures are important because they either call into question the usefulness of the Meyer-Overton correlation as an aid to understanding anesthetic action or the explanation of such behaviors will refine our theories.

"PROBLEMS" WITH THE M-O RELATIONSHIP

Since Meyer and Overton's original observations, a variety of exceptions to the Meyer-Overton correlation have been observed. In other words, many compounds turn out to be less potent (or sometimes more potent) as anesthetics than predicted based on their solubilities in apolar solvents. These deviations in potency have been ascribed to various properties of the anesthetics, or to the properties of the apolar solvents used to demonstrate the Meyer-Overton correlation, or they have been used to make predictions about the nature of the anesthetic binding site. In many cases, valuable insights have been gained, some of which are elaborated below.

The Cutoff Effect

Historically, one of the most important exceptions to the Meyer-Overton correlation has been the observation that as one ascended a homologous series of hydrophobic compounds, the largest members, predicted to be potent anesthetics, were in fact non-anesthetic in animals (i.e., the "cutoff" effect). To produce anesthesia a compound must achieve sufficient concentration at its target and it must possess suitable efficacy (22). Cutoff in anesthetic action may result from failure of either property, or both. Thus the term "cutoff" can be defined several ways. As used above, cutoff is purely a descriptive term applied to the observation that potency suddenly vanishes for large compounds predicted by the Meyer-Overton correlation to very potent. Used as a descriptor for potential mechanisms whereby potency is lost, one may consider "efficacy limited cutoff" and "solubility limited cutoff." Anesthetics are hydrophobic molecules acting in aqueous systems, and it is often the case that the largest (and most hydrophobic) members of a homologous series simply cannot achieve a sufficient concentration at the target site to elicit an effect. This would be an example of solubility limited cutoff. Drugs that bind to their targets but fail to affect function, or that are precluded by their large size from binding a target of fixed dimensions would be subject to efficacy limited cutoff. Typically, the cutoff effect has been interpreted to mean that the size of the anesthetic site is constrained.

The ability (or lack thereof) to explain cutoff has been useful in the evaluation of various theories of anesthesia. For example, a cutoff in in vivo potency is observed with n-alcohols (23), cycloalkanemethanols (24), perfluoroalkanes (25), and possibly the n-alkanes (26). Long chain alcohols, such as tetradecanol and hexadecanol, do not cause anesthesia but are nonetheless freely soluble in the bilayer (27, 28), and indeed cause membrane expansion (29). Thus, membrane theories of anesthesia based on changes in membrane dimensions do not explain the cutoff effect.

In contrast, membrane fluidization theories did partly account for the cutoff phenomenon, because small alcohols were found to decrease membrane order measured on the twelfth acyl carbon (favoring anesthesia), while larger alcohols actually enhanced membrane order (28). To explain cutoff on the basis of changing membrane order, long chain alcohols should be anesthetic antagonists (not the case). However, subsequent studies showed that when probed at the fifth acyl carbon, short chain alcohols still disordered but long chain ones now failed to change order in any direction (Firestone and Miller, unpublished data). Thus, the membrane fluidity model only correctly accounts for cutoff when shallow regions of the bilayer are probed.

Unlike membrane based theories, a protein site theory of anesthesia could readily explain the cutoff effect. A ligand binding site on a protein has defined dimensions, beyond which exogenous ligands are sterically precluded from effectively binding. Thus, the cutoff effect in protein systems has been conceptualized in terms of steric hindrance. For example, the cutoff in inhibitory action of alcohols on firefly luciferase has been rationalized in terms of binding site dimensions. In luciferase, alcohols compete for the luciferin binding pocket. The alcohol concentration required to achieve

50% inhibition (IC_{50}) increases linearly with chain length up to dodecanol and then remains approximately constant until hexadecanol. Above this, the alcohols are too insoluble in water to achieve an IC_{50} concentration and no inhibition is observed. The explanation put forward is that only the first 12 carbons fit in the substrate binding site, additional carbons remaining in the aqueous phase and contributing no binding energy *(30)*. As a model for anesthesia, this particular site is inexact because the in vivo cutoff at dodecanol is approached smoothly *(31)*.

Additionally, it has been pointed out that the cutoff effect does not imply that steric hindrance is at work in protein models in the absence of evidence for specific binding *(32)*. Alcohols of increasing chain length increase the stability of bovine serum albumin (BSA) but destabilize myoglobin. These results are interpreted in terms of specific and non-specific binding of the alcohols to the protein targets. Alcohol binding destabilizes myoglobin, implying that a non-specific binding interaction with the relatively unstructured, unfolded state predominates. For myoglobin, the unfolded protein is proposed to be the alcohol binding target, and increasing alcohol concentrations shift the conformational equilibrium towards the unfolded (disordered) state by recruiting nonspecific binding sites. In such a situation, steric constraints to ligand binding should not occur. On the other hand, alcohols stabilize BSA, and this is interpreted in terms of favorable ligand-protein interactions stabilizing the folded conformation. However, in both cases a cutoff in the ability to alter stability was observed at alkanol chain lengths of about 10 carbons *(32)*. Larger alkanols could not achieve sufficient aqueous concentrations and a cutoff was observed for both protein systems, but specific binding was observed only to BSA. These results suggest that the simple observation of a cutoff in anesthetic effect can only be interpreted in steric terms when direct evidence for specific anesthetic binding to the target has been obtained and anesthetic concentration is not limited by solubility *(32)*.

Chirality Effects

Many anesthetics are racemic mixtures, and the differential potencies of enantiomeric pairs have been interpreted as evidence that anesthetics act at binding sites able to make specific interactions, e.g., proteins. There are striking potency differences between stereoisomers of some, but not all anesthetics *(see* Fig. 2 for examples of enantiomeric pairs). For example, no potency differences were found between secondary alcohol enantiomers for production of anesthesia in tadpoles *(33)*. On the other hand, experiments with isoflurane on anesthetic sensitive mulluscan ion channels showed that the (+) isomer was more potent than the (−) isomer *(34)*. The two isoflurane isomers had identical effects on membrane melting temperatures *(34)*, and the partition coefficients between water and lipid bilayers for the two isomers are identical *(35)*, suggesting that they do not interact stereoselectively with membrane phospholipids. It is currently unclear whether isoflurane stereoisomers have different potencies in whole animals. Some workers have found (+)-isoflurane to be about 50% more potent than (−)-isoflurane *(36,37)* while others find minimal differences *(38)*.

Stereoisomerism reveals potency differences in other protein-based systems as well. For example, stereoisomers of volatile anesthetics also show modest potency differences on the GABA receptor. In this system, (+) isoflurane was about 2-fold more effective than (−) isoflurane in stimulating GABA receptor agonist binding and in retarding GABA receptor antagonist binding to mouse neuronal membranes *(39,40)*. Similar modest differences for enhancing agonist binding were seen between enantiomers of barbiturates ([−]-pentobarbital was about 1.5× as potent as (+)-pentobarbital) *(41)*. Pentobarbital also directly induces chloride currents in the GABA receptor, with (−)-pentobarbital being several fold more potent than (+)-pentobarbital *(42,43)*.

The nAChR also shows stereoselectivity of anesthetic binding *(44,45)*. For example, (−)-pentobarbital binds the receptor, but with a fourfold lower affinity than (+)-pentobarbital (the potency differences are opposite those seen for pentobarbital-GABA receptor interactions). On the other hand, inhibition of agonist induced cation flux showed no stereoselectivity *(44)*.

Etomidate stereoisomers show the most dramatic differences in potency. In in vitro studies with the GABA receptor, (+)-etomidate, but not (−)-etomidate potentiated GABA-ergic inhibitory firing in hippocampal slices *(46)*. More recently, (+)-etomidate was found to be 16 fold more potent than (−)-etomidate in producing anesthesia in tadpoles, and was more potent at potentiating GABA induced currents in cells expressing bovine $\alpha 1\beta 2\gamma 2L$ receptors *(47)*. Such large potency differences implicate a protein site, although interaction with chiral lipids such as cholesterol has not been experimentally ruled out.

Exploration of the stereoselective effects of anesthetics on their potential targets is an active area of endeavor, with the potential to add much to our knowledge of the mechanism of action of anesthetics. Stereoselectivity of anesthesia is regarded as strong evidence in favor of a protein site of anesthetic action, because proteins can most readily provide the structural basis for stereoselectivity. Demonstration of stereospecific anesthetic effects on ligand gated ion channels is an important test of their plausible involvement in anesthesia in vivo. However, the effects of chirality are generally rather small compared to systems in which the ligand binds to its target with higher affinity.

Compounds Whose Potency Differs From that Predicted by Solubility

One of the most important experimental developments in the search for the mechanism of general anesthesia has been the discovery of volatile agents that are far less potent anesthetics than predicted by their solubilities in apolar solvents. As volatile agents, they are much easier to give to mammals and to apply to in vitro systems than the sparingly soluble larger members of homologous series used to study cutoff effects. This has the advantage that more detailed behavioral work is possible in mammals. Their structural similarity to conventional volatile anesthetics holds out the promise of being able to identify structural themes that distinguish between the two types of compounds. From these differences, it may be possible to make useful inferences about the site of anesthetic action.

The "non-anesthetic" volatile agents fall into two groups. The first group consists of agents that: (1) have no ability to eliminate movement in response to noxious stimulus, (2) do not reduce the requirement (MAC, i.e., suppression of movement response to noxious stimulus) for conventional anesthetics, and (3) frequently cause convulsions at partial pressures predicted to be anesthetic based on their apolar solubilities. These compounds appeared at first to be devoid of any anesthetic properties as measured by MAC and were thus called "nonanesthetics." It was soon appreciated that the "nonanesthetics" suppressed learning (i.e., they were amnestic) and so they are more properly called "nonimmobilizers." A second group of compounds that are not well described by the Meyer-Overton correlation have: (1) some potency to ablate movement in response to noxious stimuli (either alone or based on their ability reduce the MAC of a known conventional anesthetic), but (2) are far less potent than predicted based on their solubilities in apolar solvents. These agents have been called "transitional" compounds to denote their apparent place somewhere between conventional anesthetics (which suppress learning and movement) and the nonimmobilizers.

Over the past decade, Eger and coworkers have characterized so many agents that are far less potent than predicted by their hydrophobicities that one is led to ask if the Meyer-Overton correlation exists at all *(48–58)*. To answer this rather simplistic question, we have gathered together the published data for these anesthetic and transitional compounds and re-plotted the Meyer-Overton correlation (Fig. 3). Compounds were included in the analysis if their apolar solubilities and in vivo potencies had been determined using methods that allowed useful comparisons between compounds. In other words, compounds were included if the determinations of hydrophobicities and in vivo potencies were each carried out in internally consistent manners. By far, the largest data set has been accumulated in rats, measuring MAC to prevent movement in response to painful stimulus (mechanical or electrical) applied to the tail. Eger and coworkers determined MAC directly when compounds were sufficiently potent, or as a function of the ability to reduce the requirement for the conventional

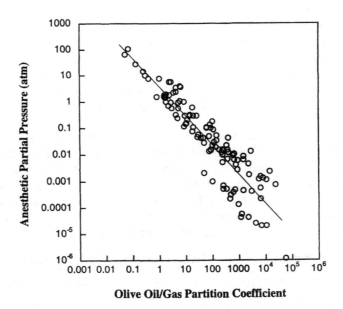

Olive Oil/Gas Partition Coefficient

Fig. 3. Potency vs hydrophobicity for a large number of inhaled anesthetics. These agents include current and former clinically used compounds, non-halogenated, halogenated, and perfluorinated alkanes, halogenated, and unhalogenated alkanols, halogenated methylethyl ethers, cyclic and aromatic hydrocarbons, noble gases and alkanethiols. Data are from refs. *(48–58)*. Potency is expressed as MAC, determined in rats, either for the pure anesthetic or as a function of the compound's ability to reduce the requirement for desflurane. Hydrophobicity is expressed as the olive oil/gas partition coefficient. Both axes use logarithmic scales. Sixteen agents were completely devoid of anesthetic potency and are not shown in the figure. Unrestrained least-squares regression of the data set plotted in the figure gives a correlation coefficient of 0.91.

anesthetic desflurane. Anesthetic hydrophobicity was most frequently measured as the partition coefficient between gas and olive oil, so the oil/gas partition coefficients have been used here. The choice of solvent used to model the apolar phase in the Meyer-Overton correlation will be discussed in the next section.

Examination of Fig. 3 reveals that when all of the compounds are considered together, the correlation between potency and oil solubility is quite strong, despite numerous large individual deviations between predicted and measured potencies. Not included in this analysis are the 16 compounds that are completely devoid of anesthetic potency. As with all correlations, the Meyer-Overton rule describes the properties of a large number of compounds quite well, but cannot reliably predict the potency of individual agents.

Degree of Correlation Influenced by Choice of Apolar Phase

A long-standing question in the history of the Meyer-Overton correlation concerns what organic liquid (taken to model the site of anesthetic action) should be used to derive the partition coefficients used to develop the correlation. Olive oil was originally used, but this solvent is actually an inhomogeneous and undefined mixture of apolar molecules. Various alternative systems have been proposed as appropriate apolar phases, most notably octanol and lecithin. Octanol was proposed as a solvent because the *n*-alkanols deviated systematically from other compounds in a Meyer-Overton correlation based on olive oil but gave a good correlation when octanol-water partition coefficients were used *(59)*. Based on this result, it was proposed that anesthetics acted at a protein site rather than a purely hydrophobic one, because octanol and protein interiors had roughly the same polarity and the more polar solvent gave the best correlation when n-alkanol anesthetics were included. This improved

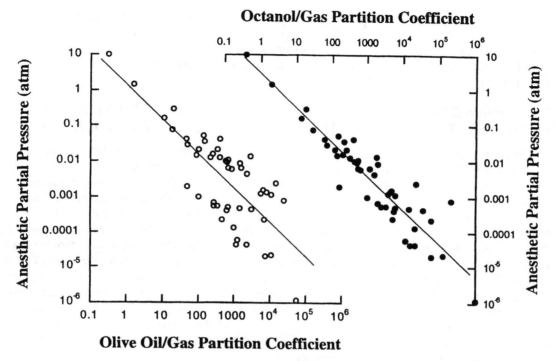

Fig. 4. Potency vs hydrophobicity of inhaled agents for which solubility has been measured in both octanol and olive oil. The agents are a subset of those shown in Fig. 3, and include current and former clinically used compounds, nonhalogenated and halogenated alkanes, halogenated and unhalogenated alkanols, cyclic and aromatic hydrocarbons. Data are from refs. *(48–52,54,56,58)*. Potency is measured as in Fig. 3. Hydrophobicity is expressed as the olive oil/gas or the octanol/gas partition coefficient. Both axes use logarithmic scales. Unrestrained least-squares regression lines are shown. For the same agents, potency vs olive oil solubility gives a correlation coefficient of 0.77, while the correlation coefficient for potency vs octanol solubility was 0.93.

correlation is still observed when an expanded set of anesthetics is studied. Figure 4 shows correlations between potency (MAC) and partition coefficients between the gas phase and either octanol or olive oil for the compounds where both solubility measurements have been published refs. *(48–52,54,56,58)*. It can be seen that the correlation is much tighter when octanol is used as the apolar solvent, although large deviations between predicted and measured potency are frequent. Clearly, both solvents fail to fully describe the nature of the anesthetic site of action, but octanol still appears to be a better descriptive model system than olive oil.

It is clear that lipid bilayers possess polar regions as well. For example, the polar headgroup of a phosphatidylcholine molecule contributes about 40% of its mass. Not surprisingly, good correlations between partitioning and anesthetic potency are found when phosphatidylcholine bilayers *(60)* and bulk lecithin *(48)* are used as the apolar phase.

The observation that weakly polar solvents give a better solubility-potency correlation now underlies the general hypothesis that anesthetics act at a site possessing some polar character. Suitable candidate sites include the polar portion of the lipid membrane, proteins and regions of the lipid protein interface. As discussed previously, sites involving a protein component are currently thought to be the most likely relevant targets. When apolar solvents that model buried protein side chains are used as the apolar phase in solubility determinations of anesthetics (enflurane, halothane, isoflurane, sevoflurane), modest enhancements of gas to apolar liquid partitioning are observed relative to partitioning into hexane *(61)*. This result is taken as evidence that anesthetics are likely to interact preferentially with target sites in microenvironments possessing more polar character than the aliphatic region of the lipid bilayer. However, different anesthetics dissolved preferentially into different solvents. For example, enflurane and isoflurane partitioned best into methanol, a solvent model of serine side chains, while sevoflurane partitioned best into ethanol, an analog of the threonine side chain *(61)*.

HOW WELL DOES BULK SOLVENT ACCURATELY MODEL CELLULAR COMPONENTS THAT ARE POTENTIAL SITES OF ANESTHETIC ACTION?

The use of partition coefficients between aqueous and apolar phases to estimate anesthetic potency is predicated on the notion that the apolar phase accurately represents the environment of the anesthetic bound to its effector site. This assumption cannot be strictly correct in the case of highly ordered systems such as proteins. For example, folded proteins are very tightly packed molecules, with interiors better described by semicrystalline solids than apolar liquids. For example, mutations of interior residues frequently lead to changes in stability that are much larger than those predicted from estimates of the hydrophobicity change *(62–66)*. The deformability of the protein interior varies from site to site within a given protein in a non-predictable way, reflecting a heterogeneous balance of forces from site to site *(63,64,67)*. On the other hand, solution studies of proteins reveal that the average protein structure is actually a constellation of tiny variations arising from minute concerted movements of protein atoms with respect to each other. This phenomenon is frequently described as 'breathing' and explains how solutes gain access to completely buried interior cavities where they are sometimes found bound in structural studies of proteins *(68)*. Thus, folded proteins appear to behave as inhomogeneous elastic solids rather than liquids.

Consistent with this notion, most protein-ligand interactions are of high affinity and frequently manifest high structural specificity resulting from ordered arrangements of binding site atoms from the protein side chains and backbone. Ligand binding is usually stabilized by attractive van der Waals interactions, the hydrophobic effect, hydrogen bonds and electrostatic interactions, all of which offset the loss of entropy accompanying formation of the ligand-protein complex, incompletely relieved steric clashes, and unsatisfied potential hydrogen bond and electrostatic interactions. Ligand binding is usually accompanied by subtle shifts in the protein structure to optimize favorable contacts. Unfavorable van der Waals interactions due to steric clashes rise quite sharply when the protein is not freely deformable, explaining in part the observed structural specificity of ligand binding.

Domain and subunit interfaces in multidomain and multisubunit proteins are as tightly and efficiently packed as the interiors of monomeric proteins. Cavities, whether in interfacial or interior regions of proteins, are rare and generally are either smaller than a water molecule or are occupied by bound water.

In addition to their high order and consequent low deformability, proteins differ from completely apolar liquids in two other aspects. First, their interiors contain many polar atoms from the main chain and side chains. The dielectric constant of the protein interior (to the extent that it is possible to describe an inhomogeneous solid by a bulk parameter) appears to approximate that of octanol. Additionally, proteins include an interface between their hydrophobic core and the surrounding water. This region contains many polar atoms from the main and side chains, as well as many ordered water molecules. Thus the polarity of the protein is higher than most apolar solvents and is not evenly distributed.

In summary, proteins contain many features that are not well modeled by the apolar solvents used to construct the partition coefficient-potency curves revealing the Meyer-Overton correlation. Instead, they are tightly packed, highly ordered, elastic structures with variable deformability and polarity throughout the structure, and cavities are quite rare. In light of these observations, it is somewhat surprising that any proteins have been found which behave according to the Meyer-Overton relationship.

The lipid bilayer represents a somewhat less ordered structure than folded proteins, but it still contains considerable structure and heterogeneity that is not well modeled by apolar liquids. For example, lipid bilayers are heterogeneous with respect to distribution of polarity. The bilayer can be divided into three regions: (1) the headgroups facing the aqueous phase and invariably bearing charges (for example the zwitterionic phosphatidylcholine headgroup), (2) the shallow part of the hydrocarbon layer, including the glycerol backbone and, usually, ester carbonyls, having moderate polarity, and (3) the central portions consisting of the hydrocarbon tails which are almost completely non-polar. Each leaflet of the bilayer thus possesses a dipole moment, each of opposite direction to the other. The bilayer has no net dipole, but large canceling internal dipole potentials due to the ordered orientations of their lipids. The bilamellar structure of lipid bilayers in biological membranes gives them the properties of a fluid, in which molecules are free to move in only two dimensions. Additionally, there is considerable evidence to suggest that bilayers containing mixtures of lipids can support lateral heterogeneity (i.e., microdomains enriched for specific lipids).

Biological membranes consist of lipid bilayers with transmembrane and membrane associated proteins. It thus encompasses all of the structural complexity of protein structure and bilayer organization, with the additional complication of the membrane protein interface. At this interface, densely packed hydrophobic side chains from proteins contact the two dimensional fluid of the bilayer. The bilayer varies throughout its depth with respect to polarity, and so does the lipid protein interface. Relatively more aromatic residues, notably Trp, are found at the polar headgroup level of the bilayer. Proteins residing in the bilayer induce changes in membrane thickness to achieve a match between hydrophobic regions of the protein and the bilayer core. This in turn can be expected to alter properties such as viscosity and chain order in the hydrocarbon region of the bilayer. Furthermore, membrane proteins induce heterogeneity in the bilayer by ordering the lipids in their surrounding annulus. Thus, given the structural heterogeneity within biological membranes, it is hard to imagine that such a complex system could be completely modeled by a simple apolar liquid.

HOW TO RECONCILE THE M-O RELATIONSHIP WITH PROTEIN-BASED THEORIES OF ANESTHETIC ACTION?

Dissatisfaction with lipid theories of anesthesia led to a search for protein sites whose behavior was described by the Meyer-Overton correlation. Proteins are distributed ubiquitously in cells and can be broadly classified into those that are soluble (i.e., aqueously dissolved), proteins that are membrane associated, and membrane dissolved (transmembrane) proteins. Studying anesthetic interactions with soluble proteins generally involves a multi-component but relatively simple system comprised of the protein, (± ligands), the aqueous solvent and the anesthetic. The significant interactions are assumed to occur between the protein (or the protein-ligand complex) and the anesthetic. Experimental systems that involve membrane lipids add an extra level of complexity due to significant interactions between the anesthetic and the membrane. Of the soluble proteins that have been used to study anesthetic mechanisms, a few display anesthetic interactions consistent with the Meyer-Overton correlation *(30,69,70)*.

Each of the protein systems used to study anesthetic mechanisms only partly explains the Meyer-Overton correlation. A ligand binding site on a protein has defined dimensions, beyond which exogenous ligands are sterically precluded from effectively binding. This could provide a natural explanation based on steric hindrance for the cutoff effect. Conversely, the small potency differences typically observed between stereoisomers of some, but not all anesthetics probably speaks of low affinity interactions, rather than a lack of site structural specificity. General anesthetics encompass a huge range of dissimilar chemical structures, yet the Meyer-Overton rule (i.e., potency predicted almost purely by hydrophobicity) describes the behavior of the overwhelming majority of them. A seeming conundrum thus arises: membrane-only theories cannot explain how anesthesia occurs, but it is hard to imagine a single protein site capable of accommodating such a diverse range of compounds. In the following sections, we discuss in general terms the probable characteristics of "protein-only" sites of anesthesia, and then expand the discussion to include a role for membrane lipids in protein theories of anesthetic action. Two obvious solutions present themselves: a protein binding site (or a few sites) with relatively lax specificity requirements, or a constellation of protein sites, each capable of producing anesthesia and each binding a small subset of anesthetics.

Promiscuous Protein Binding Sites

Several characteristics of a potential single protein site of anesthesia can be predicted. These include: (1) a large and/or distensible binding site, (2) (a) lax specificity, i.e., almost no specificity, implying primarily non-specific attractive interactions and repulsive forces, but (b) sufficient specificity to account for differences in potency among stereoisomers, and (3) amphiphillicity of binding site to accommodate weakly polar anesthetic molecules.

If anesthesia occurs purely at a single protein binding site, then the site must have incredibly broad specificity (i.e., almost no specificity). A site fulfilling predictions 1–3 above could potentially accommodate all of the known anesthetics while excluding known non-anesthetics, but it is difficult to reconcile such a site with the relatively inflexible nature of protein structure *(71)*. On the other hand, proteins with very broad substrate binding capacities do exist. For example, the *OppA* protein of *E. coli* binds tripeptides containing each of the 20 amino acids at the middle position in a single, adaptable binding site *(72)*. Crystallographic analysis of the *OppA* protein complexed with Lys-X-Lys tripeptides (where X denotes each of the 20 naturally occurring side chains found in proteins) reveals that a conformationally constrained, high affinity fit can be made with each of 20 different amino acid side chains. The protein's broad substrate binding repertoire is accomplished by alternate arrangements of polar and electrostatic interactions between binding site residues and bound water molecules *(72)*.

Proteins such as the OppA binding protein are rare exceptions. Most protein ligand binding sites are quite specific. This specificity also extends to the cavities with proteins and between protein molecules in crystals. The protein anesthetic binding sites characterized to date are best described as "hard" sites, in that they are small and accommodate very few anesthetics. For example, the anesthetic binding cavity in myoglobin is quite selective *(73,74)*. A natural cavity exists in certain crystal forms of insulin that binds small haloalkanes *(75)*. This cavity is also quite selective on the basis of molecular size, shape, and halogenation *(75)*. When anesthetics bind to such "hard" sites little if any structural perturbation of the proteins is observed. For example, in a 2.4Å resolution study of halothane bound to human serum albumin (HSA), no changes were noted in the structure *(76)*. Similarly, bromoform binding to luciferase has minimal impact on the crystallographic structure *(77)*. These results are consistent with the elastic solid character of proteins described previously and are at odds with the notion of a distensible binding site that can accommodate a wide range of anesthetics. However, anesthetic interactions with proteins do alter their conformational dynamics. For example, isoflurane and halothane stabilize the folded form of BSA with respect to thermal denaturation *(78)*, presumably by binding specifically to the folded form. Thus, most of the characterized ligand binding sites and cavities in proteins are not good candidates for a promiscuous anesthetic binding site, but rather argue in favor of specific and structurally selective interactions.

It is imaginable that anesthetic binding between subunits or domains of large, multidomain or multisubunit proteins might provide a suitably promiscuous site. A subunit or domain interface site is attractive because it could explain anesthetic effects in terms of allosteric modulation of large proteins whose function is governed by the equilibrium between multiple conformations. However, such interfaces are usually tightly packed and ordered, much the same as the protein interior *(79)*.

Another conceptual approach to the promiscuous binding site notion is to infer that anesthetics alter the conformational equilibrium between native and relatively unstructured protein conformers by binding preferentially to the unstructured species. This theory would allow for the possibility that anesthesia results from interactions with a relatively small number of targets because interaction with an unstructured conformer presumably would have relatively low structural specificity. Hence, binding affinity and anesthetic potency would be dominated by nonspecific interactions such as the hydrophobic effect and the Meyer-Overton correlation could be readily explained. Although conceptually attractive, the hypothesis that anesthetics act by recruiting unstructured forms of their protein targets is supported by little data. For example, changes in protein secondary and tertiary structure are typically accompanied by observable changes in properties such as circular dichroism, UV, and fluorescence spectra, but such changes have not been reported. even when proteins are exposed to high concentrations of anesthetic agents. In fact, specific anesthetic-protein interactions stabilize the folded conformation of proteins and reduce the dynamic fluctuations of protein structure *(80,81)*.

Multiple Protein Targets

A conceptual alternative to the single-site model is to propose multiple distinct but related binding sites on the same protein (or on a family of related proteins), each capable of binding to a few anesthetics. Such related protein families are common in nature. The immunoglobulins and the P-450 cytochromes are examples of proteins (or families of proteins) with broad substrate specificity. The cytochrome P-450 system is a large family of homologous heme proteins that metabolize drugs as well as hydrocarbon compounds from dietary and endogenous sources. This family of enzymes is characterized by broad substrate specificities for each member and a large number of related subtypes with partially overlapping but distinct substrate preferences. Thus, the P-450 monooxygenases are a conceptually attractive model of a protein site of action for the general anesthetics, in that the multiplicity of binding sites found throughout the family could accommodate the diversity of anesthetic structures *(69,82)*. The P-450 monooxygenases are competitively inhibited by alcohols, and inhibitory potency is directly correlated with lipophilicity (estimated by the number of carbon atoms in each alcohol, Fig. 5A) *(82)*. Furthermore, K_i for P-450 inhibition shows a 1:1 correlation with EC_{50} (the concentration of alcohol for general anesthesia in 50% of a group of animals) for tadpoles (Fig. 5B) *(82)*. This has led to the speculation that anesthesia may result from generalized, reversible inhibition of heme proteins (with selective sparing of heme proteins required for cell respiration) and the consequent changes in the levels of their second messenger products *(69,82)*.

Invoking multiple sites on one (or multiple) protein(s) to account for the variety of compounds that produce anesthesia is a modification of the unitary hypothesis of anesthesia. This modified hypothesis is unitary in the sense that all anesthetics are proposed to produce an identical end result (anesthesia) via similar actions on one or more protein targets, mediated through multiple possible sites. For example, even within the GABA receptor, different subunit compositions confer differing responses to anesthetics. Anesthetic efficacy and potency can be modulated by subunit composition, with responses to volatile anesthetics differing from responses to structurally distinct non-volatile drugs *(83)*. This implies different loci for the actions of these two classes of anesthetics. Similarly, the direct and indirect actions of the anesthetic etomidate on the GABA receptor can be separated by mutation, implying that the two effects arise from different loci within the protein *(84)*. The effects of long and short chain alcohols on the nAChR (ion flux enhancement and channel blocking, respectively) appear to occur at distinct sites on that receptor as well *(85)*. Covalent labeling studies with photoactivatable anesthetics confirm multiple sites of anesthetic interaction with the nAChR *(86)*. The long chain alcohol analog 3-azi-octanol can be photoactivated when bound to its target to covalently label and identify anesthetic binding sites. Using this photolabel, Glu262 in the nAChR α subunit (αGlu262), a putative channel lining residue, is preferentially labeled. Labeling is also readily identified at αHis408 and αHis412, residues thought to reside at the lipid protein interface, and at αTyr190 and αTyr198 in the agonist binding site *(86)*. This result indicates at least three distinct binding sites for a single anesthetic on the receptor.

Given the multiplicity of effects on one example of ligand gated channels and the number of such channels of this type found in the central nervous system that are sensitive to anesthetics in vitro, it is unlikely that only one receptor type is critical for the production of anesthesia. This argument can be

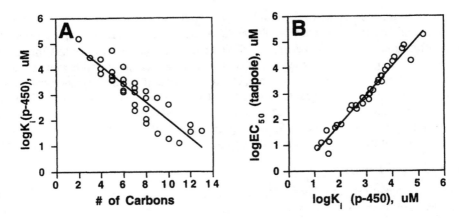

Fig. 5. The correlation of the anesthetic potency of alkanols with cytochrome P-450 inhibition. **(A)** Correlation between hydrophobicity affinity for mixed P-450 cytochromes for alkanols. Hydrophobicity is estimated by hydrocarbon chain length, while affinity for P-450 is expressed as the binding constant, K_I, for cytochrome P-450 inhibition. **(B)** Alkanol anesthetic potency in tadpoles is correlated with cytochrome P-450 inhibition. Data were taken from refs. *(69,82)*.

extended to include the multiple classes of proteins (beyond receptors) found to be sensitive to anesthetics as well.

Finally, to sustain a multi-site protein based theory of anesthesia that explains the Meyer-Overton correlation, it is not sufficient to posit a variety of sites for different shapes/sizes of anesthetic molecules. It is also necessary to propose that the affinities of the various sites are ordered in such a way across targets that the correlation between potency and hydrophobicity is observed.

INTERACTIONS BETWEEN ANESTHETICS AND THE LIPID BILAYER REVISITED

As described above, it is conceptually simplest to explain the Meyer-Overton correlation in terms of anesthetics interacting with a target or targets with lax specificity. This, in turn, implies a relatively unordered target site. One might ask: how unordered is enough? For example, although lipid bilayers are considerably more ordered than the apolar solvents used to derive the Meyer-Overton correlation, they do have liquid-like properties. Membrane-only theories of anesthetic action are clearly inadequate. However, it is reasonable to propose that anesthetics act within the membrane to alter the functions of proteins such as ligand gated ion channels. Thus, the Meyer-Overton correlation might in fact describe the propensity of an anesthetic to reach its target, rather than the end effect of the anesthetic on the target itself.

Lipid is intrinsically less ordered than protein and could be sufficiently like an apolar liquid to be accurately described by the M-O relationship. Several observations suggest that the role of the lipid bilayer in anesthetic mechanisms should be re-examined, even though proteins are likely to be the ultimate target.

For example, molecules predicted to be anesthetics achieve high concentrations in membranes, and their locations within the lipid bilayer may hold important clues about how they function and where they exert their effects. General anesthetics vary tremendously in their polarity and the arrangements of their polar atoms. Similarly, the environment offered by the bilayer ranges from polar to almost completely non-polar (Fig. 6). As expected, alcohols spend much of their time in the bilayer oriented, presumably with their hydroxyl groups in the more polar region *(87,88)* while alkanes are found in the central hydrocarbon chain region *(87–89)*.

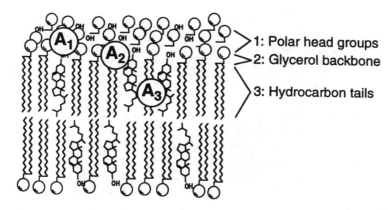

1: Polar head groups
2: Glycerol backbone
3: Hydrocarbon tails

Fig. 6. An illustration of anesthetic position with the lipid bilayer. A hypothetical anesthetic is shown dissolved in the phospholipid charged headgroups (A_1), within the moderately polar glyerol backbone (A_2), or in the nonpolar hydrocarbon tails (A_3). Recent evidence indicates that anesthetics reside preferentially within region 2, while non-immobilizers are found in region 3.

Molecular dynamics simulations modeling the interactions between anesthetics, the bilayer, surrounding water and the solvent-bilayer interface reveal a picture of anesthetic-membrane interactions consistent with the recent discoveries described above. Briefly, the nonimmobilizers as a class, are almost completely non-polar, whereas full anesthetics are amphiphillic. Simulations of the two classes of compounds in water-bilayer systems predict that amphiphillic compounds achieve high concentrations at the lipid-water interface, while the completely non-polar nonanesthetics do not *(90)*. This prediction has been confirmed by NMR studies *(91,92)*. In these studies, the halogenated hydrocabon anesthetics, halothane, isoflurane, and enflurane are indeed preferentially located in the shallower portion of the bilayer nearer the glycerol backbone (Fig. 6), with some in the interior and virtually none in the headgroup region *(93)*. These studies have been extended by comparing the locations of full anesthetics to those of structurally similar compounds that are nonimmobilizers, even at concentrations well in excess of those predicted to be anesthetizing based on their lipid solubility *(57)*. The nonimmobilizers all reside primarily in the deeper layers of the bilayer (region 3 in Fig. 6) *(91,92)*. The resulting hypothesis is that anesthetics act at, or must pass through, an amphiphillic site, and that the nonimmobilizers, lacking any polar character, do not satisfy the requirement for some polar interaction in the site where anesthetics act. Note that the Meyer-Overton hypothesis and its exceptions are both explained by such a theory. All hydrophobic compounds attain high membrane concentrations, but only the full anesthetics achieve suitable concentration within a specific zone of the apolar phase to be biologically active.

Interactions Between Anesthetics and the Bilayer Communicated to Proteins

How might an anesthetic concentrated at the bilayer-water interface exert an effect on membrane proteins? Two general modes are possible: by altering heretofore unappreciated properties of lipid bilayers whose effects are communicated to proteins (an indirect effect), or by direct actions at the bilayer/water/protein interface. Neither possibility has been excluded and both may operate in vivo. Both modes are discussed below, the potential indirect interactions followed by direct actions.

The slight preference of anesthetics for the shallower part of the lipid bilayer (region 2 in Fig. 6) has been invoked to explain the interesting observation that anesthetics reduce the magnitude of the membrane dipole potential *(94)*. Membranes have a large internal potential, perhaps due to a dipole layer at the membrane-solution interface arising from net orientation of water or lipid carbonyl atoms *(95)*. Thus, the hydrocarbon tails of the phospholipids are positive with respect to the shallower, interfacial region. Because the membrane has two such dipole layers with opposite orientation, there is no net transmembrane dipole potential. However, a transmembrane protein will experience a quadrupolar interaction with the bilayer. Anesthetics dissolved in the membrane apparently lower the dipole potential in each leaflet. The change in dipole potential was estimated to be about 10 mV at physiological concentrations *(94)*, a change that could alter the conformational equilibria of voltage sensitive membrane proteins.

Lipid bilayers in water have a large interfacial free energy concentrated over the very narrow membrane thickness, resulting in large lateral pressures within the membrane *(96)*. This pressure is not uniform throughout the membrane, varying systematically from the membrane-water interface to deeper layers in the membrane. Small compounds that dissolve into the membrane with a preference for the membrane-water interface (said to be 'interfacially active') are predicted by modeling studies to cause large increases in the lateral pressure in shallower layers of the membrane, with concomitant decreases in the lateral pressure in deeper layers *(96)*.

Changing the lateral pressure profile within monolayers, either by adding anesthetics (e.g., halothane, isoflurane) or by physical compression influences the activity of membrane proteins. For example, manipulating the lateral pressure profile at first enhanced, then abolished the hydrolysis of dipalmitoylphosphatidylcholine by membrane phospholipase C *(97)*. By affecting the lateral pressure profile, anesthetics (which distribute preferentially to the interface) could conceivably alter ion channel open (or closed) probabilities without directly interacting with the protein *(96)*. This hypothesis has been extended to explain why short chain alcohols are anesthetics, while long chain alcohols are not, assuming that the polar hydroxyl group is preferentially located at the interface (Fig. 7). Short chain n-alcohols are predicted to cause large increases in the lateral pressure at the interface, relative to deeper levels, while long chain n-alcohols have similar effects at all levels *(96)*.

Membrane phospholipids are subject to a variety of attractive and repulsive forces when assembled as a monolayer, and these forces are modified in bilayers *(98)*. In monolayers, the forces between molecules include the van der Waals attractions and steric repulsions in the hydrocarbon portion, with added polar and electrostatic interactions occurring in the head group region. The attractive forces within the two regions are usually not equal in magnitude, and the monolayer curves spontaneously *(98)*. This tendency to spontaneous curvature is a function of phospholipid headgroup size and charge, as well as the composition of the hydrocarbon tails. Upon forming a bilayer (which is locally a planar structure) this curvature must be flattened, requiring the input of energy which is stored in the form of an elastic curvature energy *(98)*.

The elastic curvature energy is related to, but distinct from, the lateral pressure arising from interfacial tension, but it modifies membrane protein activity and can, in turn, be modified by anesthetics. For example, the Ca^{2+} pumping efficiency of the Ca^{2+}/ATPase is greater in membranes possessing high elastic curvature energy than in membranes containing low elastic curvature energy. This behavior is independent of the chemical nature of the lipids in the membrane, but instead is a function of their tendency to curve in monolayers (and hence, of their elastic curvature stress in a planar bilayer) *(99)*. Studies of the effect of membrane curvature on gramicidin A channel assembly show that curvature stress can also influence protein conformation *(100)*. With respect to compounds that cause anesthesia, short chain *n*-alcohols increase the tendency to curve, thus raising the elastic curvature energy within bilayers, and this effect is countered by pressure *(98)*.

Curvature stress and lateral pressure are both likely increase with temperature *(98)*. Hence, both proposed mechanisms predict that the effects of anesthetics should be mimicked by changes in temperature, but these predictions have not been examined experimentally.

Direct Anesthetic-Protein Interactions at the Lipid/Protein/Water Interface

The observation that complete anesthetics have an interfacial preference within the bilayer, while non-immobilizers reside primarily in the deeper regions of membranes may have important functional consequences as a direct result of protein binding in addition to altering the properties of the

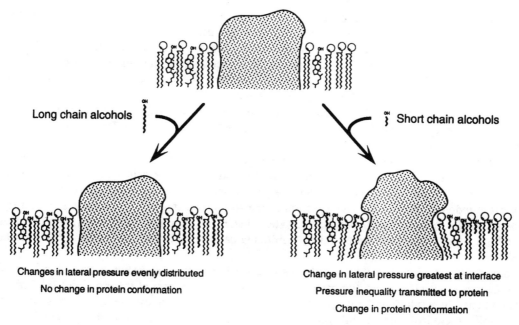

Fig. 7. An illustration of anesthetic effects on the lateral pressure profile within the bilayer. A hypothetical transmembrane protein is shown inserted in a lipid bilayer. In the absence of anesthetic (an alkanol in this example), the lipid bilayer exerts a uniform lateral pressure against the membrane protein. Long chain alcohols preserve the uniform lateral pressure when dissolved in the membrane, which could explain their lack of potency. Short chain alcohols, however, produce changes in the lateral pressure profile that may change protein conformational equilibrium.

bilayer. For example, preferential localization deep in the bilayer suggests that non-immobilizers may simply not reach a suitable concentration at a protein site of action located adjacent to the aqueous interface. Alternatively, complete anesthetics may be effective because they concentrate at the interface and are also capable of some interaction with the interfacial portion of membrane proteins that nonimmobilizers could not satisfy even if they achieved sufficient concentration at the site.

These possibilities have been investigated in some detail in a series of studies of anesthetic and nonimmobilizer interactions with the gramicidin A cation channel by Tang, Xu, and co-workers. Gramicidin A is a small cation channel antibiotic composed of two identical 15 amino acid peptides that assume a right-handed helical structure and assemble head-to-head to form a transmembrane channel in lipid bilayers and SDS micelles *(101,102)*. Each peptide contains four Trp residues located at the end of the peptide found in the headgroup region of the bilayer. These Trp residues are hypothesized to anchor the carboxyl end of the gramicidin A channel within the amphiphillic head group region of the bilayer *(103,104)*. The planes of the Trp indole rings are oriented parallel to the long axis of the lipid hydrocarbon tails. Each ring possesses a cloud of delocalized pi electrons, giving the ring faces a partial negative charge, and the ring edges a partial positive charge. These partial charges are thought to stabilize the interfacial localization by favorable interactions with the polar atoms in the lipid headgroups. The indole N-H of each Trp ring is pointed towards the aqueous solvent, where it makes a hydrogen bond with a water molecule at the bilayer/water interface *(104,105)*.

Clearly gramicidin is not involved in the clinical features of anesthesia. However, this small, structurally characterized and biologically active transmembrane protein can be used to probe the structure-function relationships between anesthetics and proteins. In particular, the effects of two structurally similar compounds on gramicidin A behavior have been extensively studied *(92,106,107)*.

The full anesthetic 1-chloro-1,2,2-trifluorocyclobutane (F3) and the non-immobilizer 1,2-dichloro-hexafluoro cyclobutane (F6) differ by degree of halogenation and partial charge distribution (*see* Fig. 2). F3 has a dipole, with 'acidic' protons that possess some partial positive charge as a consequence of asymmetric fluorine substitution. F6 possesses no such asymmetry or partial positive charge. As expected, F3 preferentially resides at the bilayer/water interface, while F6 is found primarily in the bilayer core *(92)*. Ion flux studies reveal that F3, but not F6 increases the conductance rate for sodium ions through gramicidin. NMR studies of the channels in SDS micelles indicate that F3 but not F6 make a preferential interaction with the indole N-H protons of the Trp residues that anchor the interfacial region of the peptide *(106)*.

Drug-protein interactions between F6 or F3 and gramicidin do not alter the secondary structure of the channel at the concentrations studied *(107)*. Instead, a partial mechanism of action based on modulation of Trp indole-water interactions has been suggested. F3 but not F6 induce chemical shifts in the Trp indole N-H protons. The direction of the shifts indicates that F3 facilitates the ability of these protons to make hydrogen bonds with water. This, in turn, is proposed to account for the change in sodium conductance induced by F3 by stabilizing cation binding to the entrance of the channel *(107)*.

Importantly, binding between anesthetics and the interfacial Trp residues was shown to be a consequence of specific interaction with the membrane channel form of the protein *(108)*. This was accomplished by exploiting the propensity of gramicidin A to adopt different structures depending on its solvent environment. In bilayers or SDS micelles, the channel form of right handed head-to-head dimers predominates. In ethanol, the peptide forms an intertwined left handed antiparallel double helix of two monomers *(109)*. Using halothane, the Trp indole N-H proton chemical shifts were again perturbed by the anesthetic, but this was only observed for the channel form of the peptide (in SDS micelles). The ethanol dissolved form, in which the Trp residues are found in an apolar environment (but not a bilayer/water interface) does not have any interaction with halothane as evidenced by N-H proton chemical shifts. Finally, the ability of halothane to photolabel adjacent atoms after UV irradiation was used to demonstrate that the Trp residues in gramicidin A were preferentially labeled when the bilayer-channel form predominated. The hypothesis resulting from this work is that the pi electron cloud of the aromatic Trp rings when placed in the amphiphillic environment of the lipid/water interface forms part of a specific binding site preferred by the partially positively charged full anesthetics, and that such specific binding mediated by the bilayer underlies the effect of anesthetics on membrane proteins *(108)*.

Modulation of Lipid-Protein Interactions

Interaction between membrane proteins and their surrounding lipids is an inescapable consequence of their transmembrane structure. The lipid-protein interface is an obvious potential target for specific interactions between membrane dissolved anesthetics and membrane proteins. Lipid-protein interactions can be conceptually divided into those arising from bulk properties of the membrane phospholipids (i.e., relatively nonspecific interactions), and those involving specific interactions between protein and lipid. Nonspecific interactions can be modulated by mechanical properties of the membrane, such as thickness (a manifestation of hydrocarbon chain length and order), asymmetry, lateral pressure within the membrane, and the membrane's tendency to curve. Membrane charge, internal dipole potential, headgroup size, and hydrocarbon unsaturation are all properties that could affect protein function in relatively nonspecific ways, and these chemical properties give rise to the mechanical characteristics of the membrane.

Specific lipid-protein interactions imply the existence of a lipid binding sites which clearly would be potential targets for anesthetics. Specific lipid interactions with transmembrane proteins can be classified as annular (meaning between the receptor and the annulus of immobilized lipids surrounding it *[110, 111]*) or non-annular (meaning at sites distinct from the protein-lipid interface). Annular binding sites may be less structurally selective because they occur in the part of the protein exposed to bulk lipids, but this is not necessarily so, because membrane phospholipids are chiral and are capable of specific interactions.

Lipid-protein interaction studies require large quantities of protein and in the ligand-gated ion channel superfamily only the *Torpedo* nAChR is sufficiently abundant. Negatively charged lipids such as phosphatidylserine have a preference over phosphatidylcholine for the lipid annulus of the nAChR *(112,113)*. On the other hand, cholesterol and fatty acid spinlabeled analogs bind much less effectively to the receptor after proteolytic removal of the extracellular regions. Under these conditions, the secondary structure of the remaining transmembrane portion of the protein appears to be preserved, and phospholipid interaction is preserved (although somewhat reduced). Keeping in mind that 'shaving' the receptor almost certainly alters the remaining structure, this result suggests that cholesterol and fatty acids bind to the extracellular portion of the protein (i.e., in a non-annular position) *(112)*.

Although non-annular lipid-protein interactions have been well established, their functional role is still being elucidated. In the case of the nAChR, cholesterol is required in the membrane for activity *(114)*, but the site of cholesterol's effect on the protein has not been established. Indirect evidence that cholesterol acts at non-annular sites on the nAChR comes from combining the results of two studies. In the first *(115)*, quenching of the receptor's fluorescence by brominated cholesterol could be attributed to cholesterol binding at non-annular sites. In the second study, rapid conformational changes during activation of the receptor were also found to require cholesterol *(116)*, with a concentration dependence similar to that of dibromocholesterol quenching. This suggests that cholesterol's functional effect may be at a nonannular binding site. On the other hand, other neutral lipids (even structurally dissimilar compounds such as tocopherol) can be substituted for cholesterol, and also support nAChR activation in reconstituted vesicles *(117)*. This observation requires that either the nonannular sites for cholesterol have fairly lax structural specificity, or suggests that cholesterol and neutral lipids exert their effects elsewhere. A competing hypothesis is that cholesterol, because it can flip from one membrane leaflet to the other, serves to relieve curvature stress induced in the membrane during receptor conformational cycling *(118)*. However, this appears not to be the case, as cholesterol analogs bearing standing charges support nAChR activation despite their inability to flip between leaflets *(119)*. In fact, cholesterol tethered to a phospholipid backbone by a short spacer also supports nAChR activation. Thus, the cholesterol site required for activation appears to be non-annular, but it must not be deep in the receptor, because cholesterol analogs with bulky substituents and standing charges are functional *(119)*.

If non-annular binding proves to be functionally important for ligand gated ion channel functioning, then the lipid binding site clearly deserves scrutiny as a potential site for anesthetic effects. A non-annular lipid binding site with a large, amphiphillic natural ligand, lax selectivity requirements and a strong effect on protein function certainly meets the criteria for a plausible protein site of anesthetic binding, in that it would likely obey the Meyer-Overton rule. As mentioned previously, 3-azi-octanol photolabels the nAChR at αHis408 and αHis412, residues thought to reside at the lipid protein interface, suggesting that such binding sites may exist on ligand gated ion channels.

SUMMARY

The Meyer-Overton relationship is still important because it establishes the key role of hydrophobicity in determining anesthetic potency. Unfortunately, this seminal observation for a time dominated mechanistic thinking about theories of anesthetic action. The correlation between anesthetic potency and solubility in apolar solvents is simply an observation, and no inferences about the site or mechanism of anesthetic action can properly be made from it. However, any theory of anesthetic action must account for the Meyer-Overton relationship. Meanwhile, a case for protein sites of anesthetic action on transmembrane ion channels has accumulated. Anesthetics clearly affect the function of these receptors, and these effects have been elegantly manipulated by reverse pharmacology. This indirect evidence for anesthetic binding to membrane ion channels has recently been complemented by direct labeling of protein anesthetic binding sites, both within the channel and at the lipid-protein interface *(86)*.

While our knowledge of anesthetic-protein interactions has grown, developments over the past decade indicate that a role for the lipid bilayer in the mechanism of general anesthesia cannot be written off entirely. As a relatively non-ordered bulk material, the membrane provides a seductively simple explanation for the remarkable lack of selectivity seen for most general anesthetics, while accounting for the behavior of hydrophobic non-anesthetics. Anesthetics are present in the membrane at high concentrations under clinical conditions, and exert major influences on membrane behavior even though their structural effects are small. There is an emerging body of evidence that general anesthetics exert their bilayer effects at the outer end of the acyl chains and the glycerol backbone region (region 2; Fig. 6). The putative protein targets of anesthetics are integral membrane proteins, whose function is dependent to some degree on the surrounding lipid bilayer, and it seems likely that the mechanism of general anesthesia will involve both components. All of the data can be qualitatively accounted for within the context of such a model by two proposals:

1. Anesthetics act within the membrane (explains hydrophobicity/potency correlation) on membrane proteins (explains cutoff and stereospecificity).
2. The significant interaction occurs at a region of the protein-bilayer interface just below the lipid headgroups.

An experimental demonstration that the small perturbations that general anesthetics induce in bilayers can indeed modulate membrane protein function is only now developing, but the renewed appreciation of a potential role for the lipid bilayer in anesthetic action promises to enrich our understanding of anesthetic action.

REFERENCES

1. Bernard, C. (1875) Lecons sur les Anesthetiques et sur l'Asphyxie., Paris: Bailliere.
2. Kita, Y., Bennett, L., and Miller, K. (1981) The Partial Molar Volumes of Anesthetics in Lipid Bilayers. *Biochim. Biophys. Acta* **647,** 130–139.
3. Miller, K., et al. (1973) The Pressure Reversal of General Anesthesia and the Critical Volume Hypothesis. *Mol. Pharmacol.* **9,** 131–143.
4. Seeman, P. (1969) Temperature Dependence of Erythrocyte Membrane Expansion by Alcohol Anesthetics. Possible Support for the Partition Theory of Anesthesia. *Biochim. Biophys. Acta* **183,** 520–529.
5. Melchior, D., Scavitto, F., and Steim, J. (1980) Dilatometry of Diplamitoyllecithin-Cholesterol Bilayers. *Biochemistry* **19,** 4828–4834.
6. Rand, R. and Pangborn, W. (1973) A Structural Transition in Egg Lecithin-Cholesterol Bilayers at 12°C. *Biochim. Biophys. Acta* **318,** 299–305.
7. Metcalfe, J., Seeman, P., and Burgen, A. (1968) The Proton Relaxation of Benzyl Alcohol in Erythrocyte Membranes. *Mol. Pharmacol.* **4,** 87–95.
8. Trudell, J. R. (1977) A unitary theory of anesthesia based on lateral phase separations in nerve membranes. *Anesthesiology* **46,** 5–10.
9. Mountcastle, D., Biltonen, R., and Halsey, M. (1978) Effect of Anesthetics and Pressure on the Thermotropic Behavior of Multilamellar Dipalmitoylphosphatidylcholine Liposomes. *Proc. Nat. Acad. Sci. USA* **75,** 4906–4910.
10. Kamaya, H., et al. (1979) Antagonism Between High Pressure and Anesthetics in the Thermal Phase-transition of Dipalmitoyl Phosphatidylcholine Bilayer. *Biochim. Biophys. Acta* **550,** 131–137.
11. Lieb, W., Kovalycsik, M., and Mendelsohn, R. (1982) Do Clinical Levels of General Anaesthetics Affect Lipid Bilayers? Evidence form Raman Scattering. *Biochim. Biophys. Acta* **688,** 388–398.
12. Pang, K.-Y., et al. (1980) The Perturbation of Lipid Bilayers by General Anesthetics: A Quantitative Test of the Disordered Lipid Hypothesis. *Mol. Pharmacol.* **18,** 84–90.
13. Bradley, D. and Richards, C. (1984) Temperature Dependence of the Action of Nerve Blocking Agents and Its Relationship to Membrane-buffer Partition Coefficients: Thermodynamic Implications for the Site of Action of Local Anesthetics. *Brit. J. Pharmacol.* **81,** 161–167.
14. Eger, E., 2nd, Saidman, L., and Brandstater, B. (1965) Temperature Dependence of Halothane and Cyclopropane Anesthesia in Dogs: Correlation with Some Theories of Anesthetic Action. *Anesthesiology* **26,** 764–770.
15. Steffey, E. and Eger, E., 2nd (1974) Hyperthermia and Halothane MAC in the Dog. *Anesthesiology* **41,** 392–396.

16. Johnson, S. and Bangham, A. (1969) The Action of Anesthetics on Phospolipid Membranes. *Biochim. Biophys. Acta* **193**, 92–104.

17. Johnson, S., Miller, K., and Bangham, A. (1973) The Opposing Effects of Pressure and General Anesthetics on the Cation Permeability of Liposomes of Varying Lipid Composition. *Biochim. Biophys. Acta* **307**, 42–57.

18. Bangham, A., Standish, M., and Miller, N. (1965) Cation Permeability of Phospolipid Model Membranes: Effect of Narcotics. *Nature* **208**, 1295–1297.

19. Bangham, A. and Mason, W. (1980) Anesthetics May Act by Collapsing pH Gradients. *Anesthesiology* **53**, 135–141.

20. Akeson, M. and Deamer, D. (1989) Steady-State Catecholamine Distribution in Chromaffin Granule Preparations: A Test of the Pump-Leak Hypothesis of General Anesthesia. *Biochemistry* **28**, 5120–5127.

21. Raines, D. E. and Cafiso, D. S. (1989) The enhancement of proton/hydroxyl flow across lipid vesicles by inhalation anesthetics. *Anesthesiology* **70**, 57–63.

22. Raines, D. E. and Miller, K. W. (1994) On the importance of volatile agents devoid of anesthetic action. *Anesth. Analg.* **79**, 1031–1033.

23. Pringle, M., Brown, K., and Miller, K. (1981) Can the Lipid Theories of Anesthesia Account for the Cutoff in Anesthetic Potency in Homologous Series of Alcohols? *Mol. Pharmacol.* **19**, 49–55.

24. Raines, D. E., et al. (1993) Anesthetic cutoff in cycloalkanemethanols. A test of current theories. *Anesthesiology* **78**, 918–927.

25. Liu, J., et al., (1994) A Cutoff in Potency Exists in the Perfluoroalkanes. *Anesth. Analg.* **79**, 238–244.

26. Liu, J., et al. (1993) Is There a Cutoff in Anesthetic Potency for the Normal Alkanes. *Anesth. Analg.* **77**, 12–18.

27. Franks, N. and Lieb, W. (1986) Partitioning of Long-chain Alcohols into Lipid Bilayers: Implications For Mechanisms of General Anesthesia. *Proc. Natl. Acad. Sci. USA* **83**, 5116–5120.

28. Miller, K., et al. (1989) Nonanesthetic Alcohols Dissolve in Synaptic Membranes without Perturbing Their Lipids. *Proc. Natl. Acad. Sci. USA* **86**, 1084–1087.

29. Bull, M., Brailsford, J., and Bull, B. (1982) Erythrocyte Membrane Expansion Due to the Volatile Anesthetics, the 1-Alkanols, and Benzyl Alcohol. *Anesthesiology* **57**, 399–403.

30. Franks, N. and Lieb, W. (1984) Do General Anaesthetics Act by Competitive Binding to Specific Receptors? *Nature* **310**, 599–601.

31. Alifimoff, J., Firestone, L., and Miller, K. (1989) Anesthetic Potencies of Primary Alkanols: Implications for the Molecular Dimensions of the Anesthetic Site. *Brit. J. Pharmacol.* **96**, 9–16.

32. Eckenhoff, R. G., Tanner, J. W., and Johansson, J. S. (1999) Steric hindrance is not required for n-alkanol cutoff in soluble proteins. *Mol. Pharmacol.* **56**, 414–418.

33. Alifimoff, J., Firestone, L., and Miller, K. (1987) Anesthetic Potencies of Secondary Alcohol Enantiomers. *Anesthesiology* **66**, 55–59.

34. Franks, N. and Lieb, W. (1991) Stereospecific Effects of Inhalational General Anesthetic Optical Isomers on Nerve Ion Channels. *Science* **254**, 427–430.

35. Dickinson, R., Franks, N. P., and Lieb, W. R. (1994) Can the stereoselective effects of the anesthetic isoflurane be accounted for by lipid solubility? *Biophys. J.* **66**, 2019–2023.

36. Lysko, G., et al. (1994) The Stereopecific Effects of Isoflurane Isomers In vivo. *Eur. J. Pharmacol.* **263**, 25–29.

37. Dickinson, R., et al. (2000) Stereoselective loss of righting reflex in rats by isoflurane. *Anesthesiology* **93**, 837–843.

38. Eger, E. I., 2nd, et al. (1997) Minimum alveolar anesthetic concentration values for the enantiomers of isoflurane differ minimally. *Anesth. Analg.* **85**, 188–192.

39. Harris, B. D., et al. (1994) Volatile anesthetics bidirectionally and stereospecifically modulate ligand binding to GABA receptors. *Eur. J. Pharmacol.* **267**, 269–274.

40. Moody, E., Harris, B., and Skolnick, P. (1993) Stereospecific Actions of the Inhalation Anesthetic Isoflurane at the GABA$_A$ Receptor Complex. *Brain Res.* **615**, 101–106.

41. Olsen, R. W., Fischer, J. B., and Dunwiddie, T. V. (1986) Barbiturate enhancement of γ-aminobutyric acid receptor binding and function as a mechanism of anesthesia, in *Molecular and Cellular Mechanisms of Anesthesia* (Roth S. H., and Miller, K. W., eds.) Plenum, NY, pp. 165–178.

42. Huang, L.-Y. M. and Barker, J. L. (1980) Pentobarbital: Stereospecific Actions of (+) and (−) Isomers Revealed on Cultured Mammalian Neurons. *Science* **207**, 195–197.

43. Akaike, N., et al. (1985) γ-Aminobutyric-acid- and Pentobarbitone-gated Chloride Currents in Internally Perfused Frog Sensory Neurones. *J. Physiol.* **360**, 367–386.

44. Roth, S. H., et al. (1989) Actions of pentobarbital enantiomers on nicotinic cholinergic receptors. *Mol. Pharmacol.* **36**, 874–880.

45. Miller, K., Sauter, J., and Braswell, L. (1982) A Stereoselective Pentobarbital Binding Site in Cholinergic Membranes from Torpedo californica. *Biochem. Biophys. Res. Comm.* **105**, 659–666.

46. Ashton, D. and Wauquier, A. (1985) Modulation of a GABA-ergic inhibitory circuit in the in vitro hippocampus by etomidate isomers. *Anesth. Analg.* **64**, 975–980.

47. Tomlin, S., et al. (1998) Stereoselective Effects of Etomidate Optical Isomers on Gamma-aminobutyric Acid Type A Receptors and Animals. *Anesthesiology* **88**, 708–717.

48. Taheri, S., et al. (1991) What solvent best represents the site of action of inhaled anesthetics in humans, rats, and dogs? *Anesth. Analg.* **72**, 627–634.

49. Taheri, S., et al. (1993) Anesthesia by n-alkanes not consistent with the Meyer-Overton hypothesis: determinations of the solubilities of alkanes in saline and various lipids. *Anesth. Analg.* **77**, 7–11.

50. Liu, J., et al. (1994) Effect of n-alkane kinetics in rats on potency estimations and the Meyer-Overton hypothesis. *Anesth. Analg.* **79,** 1049–1055.

51. Fang, Z., et al. (1996) Anesthetic and convulsant properties of aromatic compounds and cycloalkanes: implications for mechanisms of narcosis. *Anesth. Analg.* **83,** 1097–1104.

52. Fang, Z., et al. (1997) Anesthetic potencies of n-alkanols: results of additivity and solubility studies suggest a mechanism of action similar to that for conventional inhaled anesthetics. *Anesth. Analg.* **84,** 1042–1048.

53. Koblin, D. D., et al. (1998) Minimum alveolar concentrations of noble gases, nitrogen, and sulfur hexafluoride in rats: helium and neon as nonimmobilizers (nonanesthetics). *Anesth. Analg.* **87,** 419–424.

54. Eger, E. I., 2nd, et al. (1999) Minimum alveolar anesthetic concentration of fluorinated alkanols in rats: relevance to theories of narcosis. *Anesth. Analg.* **88,** 867–876.

55. Koblin, D. D., et al. (1999) Polyhalogenated methyl ethyl ethers: solubilities and anesthetic properties. *Anesth. Analg.* **88,** 1161–1167.

56. Zhang, Y., et al. (2000) The anesthetic potencies of alkanethiols for rats: relevance to theories of narcosis. *Anesth. Analg.* **91,** 1294–1299.

57. Koblin, D., et al. (1994) Polyhalogenated and Perfluorinated Compounds that Disobey the Meyer-Overton Hypothesis. *Anesth. Analg.* **79,** 1043–1048.

58. Eger II, E., et al. (1994) Molecular Properties of the "Ideal" Inhaled Anesthetic, Studies of Fluorinated Methanes, Ethanes, Propanes and Butanes. *Anesth. Analg.* **79,** 245–251.

59. Franks, N. and Lieb, W. (1978) Where Do General Anesthetics Act? *Nature* **274,** 339–342.

60. Janoff, A., Pringle, M., and Miller, K. (1981) Correlation of General Anesthetic Potency with Solubility in Membranes. *Biochim. Biophys. Acta* **649,** 125–128.

61. Johansson, J. S. and Zou, H. (1999) Partitioning of four modern volatile general anesthetics into solvents that model buried amino acid side-chains. *Biophys Chem.* **79,** 107–116.

62. Sandberg, W. S. and Terwilliger, T. C. (1989) Influence of interior packing and hydrophobicity on the stability of a protein. *Science* **245,** 54–57.

63. Sandberg, W. S. and Terwilliger, T. C (1991) Energetics of repacking a protein interior. *Proc. Natl. Acad. Sci. USA* **88,** 1706–1710.

64. Sandberg, W. S. and Terwilliger, T. C (1991) Repacking protein interiors. *Trends Biotechnol.* **9,** 59–63.

65. Xu, J., et al. (1998) The response of T4 lysozyme to large-to-small substitutions within the core and its relation to the hydrophobic effect. *Protein Sci.* **7,** 158–177.

66. Eriksson, A. E., et al. (1992) Response of a protein structure to cavity-creating mutations and its relation to the hydrophobic effect. *Science* **255,** 178–183.

67. Zhang, H., et al. (1996) Context dependence of mutational effects in a protein: the crystal structures of the V35I, I47V and V35I/I47V gene V protein core mutants. *J. Mol. Biol.* **259,** 148–159.

68. Tilton, R. F., Jr., et al. (1988) Protein-ligand dynamics. A 96 picosecond simulation of a myoglobin- xenon complex. *J. Mol. Biol.* **199,** 195–211.

69. LaBella, F. and Queen, G. (1993) General Anesthetics Inhibit Cytochrome P450 Monooxygenases and Arachidonic Acid Metabolism. *Can. J. Physiol. Pharmacol.* **71,** 48–53.

70. Slater, S., et al. (1993) Inhibition of Protein Kinase C by Alcohols and Anesthetics. *Nature* **364,** 82–84.

71. Richards, F. M. (1977) Areas, Volumes, Packing, and Protein Structure. *Ann. Rev. Biophys. Bioeng.* **6,** 151–176.

72. Sleigh, S. H., et al. (1999) Crystallographic and calorimetric analysis of peptide binding to OppA protein. *J. Mol. Biol.* **291,** 393–415.

73. Tilton, R. F., Jr., Kuntz, I. D., Jr., and Petsko, G. A. (1984) Cavities in proteins: structure of a metmyoglobin-xenon complex solved to 1.9 A. *Biochemistry* **23,** 2849–2857.

74. Tilton, R. F., Jr. and Petsko, G. A. (1988) A structure of sperm whale myoglobin at a nitrogen gas pressure of 145 atmospheres. *Biochemistry* **27,** 6574–6582.

75. Gursky, O., et al. (1994) Stereospecific dihaloalkane binding in a pH-sensitive cavity in cubic insulin crystals. *Proc. Natl. Acad. Sci. USA* **91(26),** 12,388–12,392.

76. Bhattacharya, A. A., Curry, S., and Franks, N. P. (2000) Binding of the General Anesthetics Propofol and Halothane to Human Serum Albumin. HIGH RESOLUTION CRYSTAL STRUCTURES. *J. Biol. Chem.* **275,** 38,731–38,738.

77. Franks, N. P., et al. (1998) Structural basis for the inhibition of firefly luciferase by a general anesthetic. *Biophys. J.* **75,** 2205–2211.

78. Johansson, J. S., Zou, H., and Tanner, J. W. (1999) Bound volatile general anesthetics alter both local protein dynamics and global protein stability. *Anesthesiology* **90,** 235–245.

79. Chothia, C. (1976) The Nature of the Accessible and Buried Surfaces in Proteins. *J. Mol. Biol.* **105,** 1–14.

80. Eckenhoff, R. G. and Johansson, J. S. (1997) Molecular interactions between inhaled anesthetics and proteins. *Pharmacol. Rev.* **49,** 343–367.

81. Eckenhoff, R. G. and Tanner, J. W. (1998) Differential halothane binding and effects on serum albumin and myoglobin. *Biophys. J.* **75,** 477–483.

82. LaBella, F., et al. (1997) The Site of General Anaesthesia and Cytochrome P450 Oxygenases: Similarities Defined by Straight Chain and Cyclic Alcohols. *Brit. J. Pharmacol.* **120,** 1158–1164.

83. Harris, B., et al. (1995) Different Subunit Requirements for Volatile and Nonvolatile Anesthetics at γ-Aminobutyric Acid Type A Receptors. *Mol. Pharmacol.* **47,** 363–367.

84. Moody, E., et al. (1997) Distinct Loci Mediate the Direct and Indirect Actions of the Anesthetic Etomidate at GABA$_A$ Receptors. *J. Neurochem.* **69,** 1310–1313.

85. Wood, S., Forman, S., and Miller, K. (1991) Short Chain and Long Chain Alkanols Have Different Sites of Action on Nicotinic Acetylcholine Receptor Channels from Torpedo. *Mol. Pharmacol.* **39,** 332–338.
86. Pratt, M. B., et al. (2000) Identification of Sites of Incorporation in the Nicotinic Acetylcholine Receptor of a Photoactivatible General Anesthetic. *J. Biol. Chem.* **275,** 29,441–29,451.
87. Colley, C. and Metcalfe, J. (1972) The Localisation of Small Molecules in Lipid Bilayers. *FEBS Lett.* **24,** 241–246.
88. Pope, J., Walker, L., and Dubro, D. (1984) On the Ordering of N-Alkane and N-Alcohol Solutes in Phospholipid Bilayer Model Membrane Systems. *Chem. Phys. Lipids* **35,** 259–277.
89. Jacobs, R. and White, S. (1984) Behavior of Hexane Dissolved in Dimyristoylphosphatidylcholine Bilayers: An NMR and Calorimetric Study. *J. Amer. Chem. Soc.* **106,** 915–920.
90. Pohorille, A., et al. (1998) Concentrations of anesthetics across the water-membrane interface; the Meyer-Overton hypothesis revisited. *Toxicol. Lett.* **100–101,** 421–30.
91. North, C. and Cafiso, D. S. (1997) Contrasting membrane localization and behavior of halogenated cyclobutanes that follow or violate the Meyer-Overton hypothesis of general anesthetic potency. *Biophys. J.* **72,** 1754–1761.
92. Tang, P., Yan, B., and Xu, Y. (1997) Different distribution of fluorinated anesthetics and nonanesthetics in model membrane: a 19F NMR study. *Biophys. J.* **72,** 1676–1682.
93. Baber, J., Ellena, J., and Cafiso, D. (1995) Distribution of General Anesthetics in Phospholipid Bilayers Determined Using 2H NMR and 1H-1H NOE Spectroscopy. *Biochemistry* **34,** 6533–6539.
94. Qin, Z., Szabo, G., and Cafiso, D. (1995) Anesthetics Reduce the Magnitude of the Membrane Dipole Potential. Measurements in Lipid Vesicles Using Voltage Sensitive Spin Probes. *Biochemistry* **34,** 5536–5543.
95. Cafiso, D. (1995) Influence of Charges and Dipoles on Macromolecular Adsorption and Permeability, in *Permeability and Stability of Lipid Bilayers* (Disalvo, E. and Simon, S., eds.) CRC Press, Boca Raton, FL, pp. 179–195.
96. Cantor, R. (1997) The Lateral Pressure Profile in Membranes: A Physical Mechanism of General Anesthesia. *Biochemistry* **36,** 2339–2344.
97. Goodman, D., et al. (1996) Anesthetics Modulate Phospholipase C Hydrolysis of Monolayer Phospholipids by Surface Pressure. *Chem. Phys. Lipids* **84,** 57–64.
98. Gruner, S. and Shyamsunder, E. (1991) Is the Mechanism of General Anesthesia Related to Lipid Membrane Spontaneous Curvature? *Ann. NY Acad. Sci.* **625,** 685–697.
99. Navarro, J., Toivo-Kinnucan, M., and Racker, E. (1984) Effect of Lipid Composition on the Calcium/Adenosine 5'-Triphosphate Coupling Ratio of the Ca^{2+}-ATPase of Sarcoplasmic Reticulum. *Biochemistry* **23,** 130–135.
100. Lundbaek, J., Maer, A., and Anderson, O. (1997) Lipid Bilayer Electrostatic Energy, Curvature Stress, and the Assembly of Gramicidin Channels. *Biochemistry* **36,** 5695–5701.
101. Killian, J. A. (1992) Gramicidin and gramicidin-lipid interactions. *Biochim. Biophys. Acta* **1113,** 391–425.
102. Ketchem, R. R., Hu, W., and Cross, T. A. (1993) High-resolution conformation of gramicidin A in a lipid bilayer by solid-state NMR. *Science* **261,** 1457–1460.
103. Hu, W. and Cross, T. A. (1995) Tryptophan hydrogen bonding and electric dipole moments: functional roles in the gramicidin channel and implications for membrane proteins. *Biochemistry* **34,** 14,147–14,155.
104. Hu, W., Lee, K. C., and Cross, T. A. (1993) Tryptophans in membrane proteins: indole ring orientations and functional implications in the gramicidin channel. *Biochemistry* **32,** 7035–7047.
105. Woolf, T. B. and Roux, B. T (1997) The binding site of sodium in the gramicidin A channel: comparison of molecular dynamics with solid-state NMR data. *Biophys. J.* **72,** 1930–1945.
106. Tang, P., et al. (1999) Distinctly different interactions of anesthetic and nonimmobilizer with transmembrane channel peptides. *Biophys J.* **77,** 739–746.
107. Tang, P., Simplaceanu, V., and Xu, Y. (1999) Structural consequences of anesthetic and nonimmobilizer interaction with gramicidin A channels. *Biophys J.* **76,** 2346–2350.
108. Tang, P., Eckenhoff, R. G. and Xu, Y. (2000) General anesthetic binding to gramicidin A: the structural requirements. *Biophys J.* **78,** 1804–1809.
109. Langs, D. A., et al. (1991) Monoclinic uncomplexed double-stranded, antiparallel, left-handed beta 5.6-helix (increases decreases beta 5.6) structure of gramicidin A: alternate patterns of helical association and deformation. *Proc. Natl. Acad. Sci. USA* **88(12),** 5345–5349.
110. Marsh, D. and Barrantes, F. (1978) Immobilized Lipid in Acetylcholine Receptor-Rich Membranes from Torpedo marmorata. *Proc. Natl. Acad. Sci. USA* **75,** 4329–4333.
111. Antollini, S., et al. (1996) Physical State of Bulk and Protein-Associated Lipid in Nicotinic Acetylcholine Receptor-Rich Membrane Studied by Laurdan Generalized Polarization and Fluorescence Energy Transfer. *Biophys. J.* **70,** 1275–1284.
112. Dreger, M., et al. (1997) Interactions of the Nicotinic Acetylcholine Receptor Transmembrane Segments with the Lipid Bilayer in Native Receptor-Rich Membranes. *Biochemistry* **36,** 839–847.
113. Raines, D. and Miller, K. (1993) The Role of Charge in Lipid Selectivity for the Nicotinic Acetylcholine Receptor. *Biophys. J.* **64,** 632–641.
114. Fong, T. and McNamee, M. (1986) Correlation between Acetylcholine Receptor Function and Structural Properties of Membranes. *Biochemistry* **25,** 830–840.
115. Jones, O. and McNamee, M. (1988) Annular and Nonannular Binding Sites for Cholesterol Associated with the Nicotinic Acetylcholine Receptor. *Biochemistry* **27,** 2364–2374.
116. Raines, D. E. and McClure, K. B. (1997) Halothane interactions with nicotinic acetylcholine receptor membranes. Steady-state and kinetic studies of intrinsic fluorescence quenching. *Anesthesiology* **86,** 476–486.
117. Sunshine, C. and McNamee, M. (1992) Lipid Modulation of Nicotinic Acetylcholine Receptor Function: the Role of Neutral and Negatively Charged Lipids. *Biochim. Biophys. Acta* **1108,** 240–246.

118. Rankin, S., et al. (1997) The Cholesterol Dependence of Activation and Fast Desensitization of the Nicotinic Acetyl-choline Receptor. *Biophys. J.* **73,** 2446–2455.
119. Addona, G., et al. (1998) Where Does Cholesterol Act During Activation of the Nicotinic Acetylcholine Receptor? *Biochim. Biophys. Acta* In Press.
120. Firestone, L. L., Miller, J. C., and Miller, K. W. (1986) *Tables of Physical and Pharmacological Properties of Anesthetics, in Molecular and Cellular Mechanisms of Anesthetics* (Roth, S. H. and Miller, K. W., eds.) Plenum, NY 455–470.

23

Protein Models

Jonas S. Johansson and Roderic G. Eckenhoff

THE RATIONALE UNDERLYING THE CURRENT USE OF MODEL PROTEINS TO STUDY GENERAL ANESTHETIC ACTION

The mechanisms of action of the inhaled general anesthetics remain poorly understood despite extensive studies over the past century *(1–4)*. There is abundant functional (electrophysiological) evidence that favors both ligand- and voltage-gated ion channels as potential in vivo targets for the volatile general anesthetics *(5–8)*. For example, the γ-aminobutyric acid type A receptor (GABA$_A$R) chloride conduction is enhanced by enflurane (0.23–0.46 mM) in the presence of low levels of the endogeneous neurotransmitter GABA (3 μM), suggesting that anesthetics might depress neuronal activity by enhancing synaptic inhibition *(5)*. However, functional studies are unable to directly test whether anesthetics indeed bind to the proteins in question, or whether they alter their activity by changing the physical properties of the membrane environment. Indeed, lipid theories of anesthetic action remain viable *(9–12)*, albeit difficult to test experimentally at present. The only direct evidence to date that volatile general anesthetics actually bind to membrane proteins is derived from photoaffinity labeling studies with ^{14}C-halothane and the *Torpedo nobiliana* nicotinic acetylcholine receptor *(13)*, rabbit skeletal muscle sarcoplasmic Ca^{2+}-Mg^{2+}-ATPase *(14)*, and bovine retinal rhodopsin *(15)*. The photoaffinity results indicate that halothane does indeed interact directly with these different types of membrane proteins, which are representatives of the families of ligand-gated ion channels, P-type ATPases, and heterotrimeric guanine nucleotide-binding protein (G-protein) coupled receptors, respectively. Furthermore, there are several anesthetic binding sites on each nicotinic acetylcholine receptor, and on the Ca^{2+}-Mg^{2+}-ATPase, suggesting that volatile anesthetic binding sites are widespread, and presumably have fairly generic architectural features.

A molecular understanding of volatile anesthetic mechanisms of action will require structural descriptions of anesthetic-protein complexes, which will in turn provide the further understanding required for a rational approach to drug design. A 2.6 Å resolution X-ray crystal structure of the rabbit sarcoplasmic reticulum Ca^{2+}-Mg^{2+}-ATPase has been reported recently *(16)*. The transmembrane region of the Ca^{2+}-Mg^{2+}-ATPase is composed of a series of ten α-helices of different lengths, showing varying inclinations to the membrane Z (normal to the bilayer) direction. The activity of this Ca^{2+}-Mg^{2+}-ATPase is altered by halothane and diethyl ether *(17–20)*, making it an attractive candidate for crystallization in the presence of anesthetic molecules, in order to deepen our understanding of how anesthetics might alter macromolecular function.

An X-ray crystal structure of bovine rhodopsin at 2.8 Å resolution (Fig. 1) has also been reported recently showing that the transmembrane domain consists of seven α-helices, arranged as a seven-helix bundle *(21)*. This structure is of considerable interest because it predicts the overall architecture

From: *Contemporary Clinical Neuroscience: Neural Mechanisms of Anesthesia*
Edited by: Joseph F. Antognini et al. © Humana Press Inc., Totowa, NJ

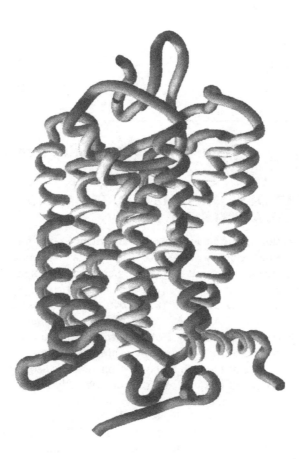

Fig. 1. The X-ray crystal structure of bovine rhodopsin in mixed micelles at 2.8 Å resolution (Protein Data Bank access code 1F88). For clarity, only a trace of the C$^{\alpha}$ positions is shown. The extracellular side is at the top of the Figure.

of the large number of membrane proteins that comprise the G-protein-coupled receptor family (estimated to comprise 3% of the human genome). This also represents an attractive membrane protein for crystallization studies in the presence of anesthetics because m1 muscarinic receptor signaling is inhibited by halothane *(22,23)*, and photoaffinity labeling with halothane suggests a direct interaction with rhodopsin *(15)*.

However, despite these recent successes in defining atomic-level membrane protein topology, there is still no high-resolution structure available for any mammalian voltage- or ligand-gated ion channel. The architecturally best understood ligand-gated ion channel, the nicotinic acetylcholine receptor from *Torpedo nobiliana* postsynaptic membranes, has an electron cryomicroscopy structure solved to 4.6 Å resolution at 4 kelvin *(24)*. At this level of refinement, it is not possible to make definitive statements about protein secondary structure *(25)*, far less to probe the topology of any small molecule binding sites that may be present. Furthermore, the large size of the ligand-gated ion channels makes it impossible to use many of the biophysical techniques that can provide high-resolution structural information on ligand-protein interactions as outlined below.

In the interim, the binding of anesthetics to proteins is being explored using well-characterized model systems such as the firefly luciferase enzyme *(26,27)*, albumin *(28–31)*, gramicidin A *(32,33)*, and synthetic four-α-helix bundle proteins *(34–38)*. These smaller proteins and peptides are amenable to structural analysis using X-ray crystallography, various spectroscopic approaches (NMR, circular dichroism, and fluorescence), and molecular dynamics simulations. Studies with these model proteins should provide guidelines regarding the general architecture of volatile anesthetic binding sites on central nervous system proteins, and are expected to furnish important clues for how anesthetic binding might alter protein function.

BINDING SITE ARCHITECTURE

Nature of Volatile General Anesthetic Binding Sites

What are the architectural features of volatile general anesthetic binding sites on proteins? There are relatively few X-ray crystal structures that have been solved to date that involve a protein with a bound anesthetic. All involve model proteins such as myoglobin, haloalkane dehalogenase from *Xanthobacter autotrophicus* GJ10, human serum albumin, and the enzyme firefly luciferase. There is no high-resolution structure to date that involves any of the modern halogenated ether anesthetics. However, very recently an X-ray crystal structure of human serum albumin with several bound halothane molecules has been published *(31)*. An atomic-level resolution NMR structure of halothane interacting with the gramicidin A channel in sodium dodecyl sulfate micelles has also been reported *(33)*, which indicates that the anesthetic interacts preferentially with the indole amide protons of the four tryptophan residues (W9, W11, W13, and W15). This finding was supported by photoaffinity labeling results using halothane, which again showed a preferential interaction of the anesthetic with the four tryptophan residues present in gramicidin A.

The binding of xenon, which has a minimum alveolar concentration of ca. 0.7 atm *(39)* to crystals of sperm whale myoglobin has provided some high (2.8 Å) resolution data. Xenon forms weak Debye- and London interactions with a number of proteins, and therefore has utility for phase determination in X-ray crystallography as the xenon-protein complex is highly isomorphous with the native protein structure *(40)*. At 2.5 atm, xenon was noted to bind at a single site equidistant from the proximal histidine and one of the heme pyrrole rings in myoglobin *(41)*. Further studies indicated that cyclopropane and dichloromethane also bound to the same site in crystals of sperm whale myoglobin, using X-ray diffraction at 2.8 and 2.7 Å resolution, respectively *(42,43)*. The recruitment of additional lower affinity binding sites became apparent on sperm whale myoglobin with X-ray diffraction data at 1.9 Å resolution when the xenon pressure was raised to 7 atm *(44)*.

X-ray crystallography at 2.7 Å resolution has demonstrated a single binding site for xenon and cyclopropane on each of the α and β chains of equine hemoglobin *(45)*. The sites in hemoglobin are located more peripherally (distant from the heme) than in myoglobin, with xenon making van der Waals contacts with valine, leucine, and phenylalanine side-chains. Dichloromethane was shown to bind to hemoglobin at three or four sites, each of which lies in the hydrophobic core with adjacent aromatic residues, such as W14α or F71β, or at the interface between subunits close to Y145 *(46)*.

X-ray diffraction (at 2.1–2.5 Å resolution) has also been used to study the binding of xenon to a number of previously crystallized proteins—porcine pancreatic elastase, subtilisin Carlsberg from *Bacillus licheniformis*, cutinase from *Fusarium solani*, collagenase from *Hypoderma lineatum*, hen egg lysozyme, the lipoamide dehydrogenase domain from *Neisseria meningitides* outer membrane protein P64k, urate-oxidase from *Aspergillus flavus*, mosquitocidal δ-endotoxin CytB from *Bacillus thuringiensis* sp. *kyushuensis*, and the ligand-binding domain of the human nuclear retinoid-X receptor RXR-α *(47)*. The side-chains that were most frequently in contact with the bound xenon atoms in these nine different proteins were aliphatic (A, L, V, and I) and aromatic (F).

Xenon binding to an engineered cavity in the hydrophobic core of phage T4 lysozyme has also been analyzed using X-ray crystallography at 1.9 Å resolution *(48)*. This packing defect in the hydrophobic core was created by replacing a leucine residue with the smaller alanine at position 99 (L99A). The cavity has a molecular volume of 178 Å^3 and accomodates two xenon atoms (van der Waals vol 45 Å^3). The dissociation constant for xenon binding was estimated to be ≤2 atm. Binding of xenon to this site in the phage T4 lysozyme hydrophobic core did not alter the average *B*-factors (related to the mean-square atomic mobility) of the residues lining the cavity wall. This site also bound krypton (van der Waals volume 35 Å^3), which has a MAC value of 3 atm *(39)* with a lower affinity (dissociation constant estimated to be ≈8 atm).

The binding of 1,2-dichloroethane to crystals of haloalkane dehalogenase from *Xanthobacter autotrophicus* GJ10 at 1.9 Å resolution *(49)* and to bovine insulin at 2 Å resolution *(50)* has been reported using X-ray diffraction. In haloalkane dehalogenase, 1,2-dichloroethane binds in a hydro-phobic pocket forming weak polar interactions between its chlorines and two tryptophan and two phenylalanine side-chains. The chlorines are acting as hydrogen bond acceptors and providing some specificity to the interaction. Similar interactions between bound halolkanes and the haloalkane dehalogenases from *Rhodococcus rhodocrous* and *Sphingomonas paucimobilis* have also been reported *(51,52)*. In addition, chlorine acting as a hydrogen bond acceptor has been observed crystallographically in the dichloromethane dehalogenase enzyme from *Methylophilus* sp. DM11 complexed with dichloromethane, where H116 and W117 interact with the halogen *(53)*. Similarly, for *p*-bromobenzoyloxyacetic acid complexed with the α chain of hemoglobin, the bromine atom contacts one of the aromatic ring hydrogens of a phenylalanine side-chain *(54)*. The site in haloalkane dehalogenase is able to accommodate smaller haloalkanes such as methyl- and ethyl chloride, but with lower K_m values, suggesting that less optimal van der Waals contacts are achieved with the smaller ligands. The insulin 1,2-dichloroethane binding pocket is located at the protein-protein interface in the crystal, lined with serine, valine, glutamate, and tyrosine, and is unable to complex either larger or smaller haloalkanes. The insulin interfacial binding pocket is occupied by five water molecules in the absence of 1,2-dichloroethane, and their release should contribute a favorable entropic term to the overall haloalkane binding energetics *(55)*. The presence of water molecules in hydrophobic pockets and clefts on proteins may facilitate the conformational changes associated with function *(56)*. Replacement of disordered water molecules normally present in hydrophobic pockets and clefts by anesthetics might therefore be responsible for changes in protein activity.

A 2.2 Å resolution X-ray crystal structure of the firefly luciferase enzyme from *Photinus pyralis* has been reported with two complexed bromoform molecules *(26)*. One of the bromoform molecules bound to this low-affinity conformation of the enzyme at the luciferin substrate-binding site, whereas the other bromoform bound to a pocket on the protein surface. At the location where luciferin nor-mally binds, the bromoform interacts with G315, A313, R218, and E311. In the groove located on the luciferase surface, the second bromoform interacts with H310, E311, E354, T352, and R337.

A 2.4 Å resolution X-ray crystal structure of human serum albumin with up to eight bound halothane molecules has very recently been reported *(31)*. Six of the binding sites involve a combination of aliphatic and charged residues, such as arginine or lysine, with the remaining two composed of aliphatic and somewhat polar residues such as serine, phenylalanine, and asparagine. The crystallographic results are in accord with the earlier solution studies using fluorescence and photoaffinity labeling that indicated that halothane bound in close proximity to W214 in human serum albumin *(30,57)*.

These high-resolution structural studies indicate that these weakly interacting ligands bind to preexisting cavities (a region not occupied by protein atoms that is inaccessible from the solvent phase in the static structure) in the hydrophobic core of a water-soluble protein, at a hydrophobic interface formed by a protein dimer, or in a groove, or pocket, on the surface of a protein (that is solvent accessible). Access of the ligand to the hydrophobic cavity requires concerted protein domain movements. The presence of a pocket or cavity that can accommodate the anesthetic will favor bind-ing because (1) the formation of van der Waals interactions between the anesthetic and protein will be energetically favorable, and (2) the overall transfer free energy from water to the protein is not compromised by the enthalpic cost of creating such a cavity for the anesthetic in a well-packed region of the protein. Indeed, attempts to bind halothane to a native-like three-α-helix bundle, α$_3$-1 *(58)*, with a well-packed hydrophobic core, resulted in a K_d in excess of 12 m*M* *(59)*, suggesting that this enthalpic cost is prohibitive. Further, aromatic side-chains (tryptophan, tyrosine, phenylalanine, and histidine) appear to form energetically favorable interactions with these ligands, in agreement with solvation studies *(60)*.

This concept of what an anesthetic binding site might look like has been tested using a relatively simple model system consisting of a water-soluble four-α-helix bundle with a hydrophobic core *(34–36)*. Introducing a binding pocket into the hydrophobic core of the four-α-helix bundle by replacing three leucine residues with smaller alanines led to the creation of a binding site for halothane with a $K_d = 0.71 \pm 0.04$ mM. Packing defects on proteins, if of the appropriate size, are therefore predicted to represent likely binding sites for anesthetic molecules in vivo. Cavities, or packing defects, are ubiquitous on natural proteins as determined by X-ray crystallography *(61–69)*, although they vary considerably in size. The presence of cavities (although energetically costly due to the loss of favorable side-chain van der Waals contacts) are thought to be necessary in order to allow proteins to undergo the conformational changes required for their normal function *(70)*. In the absence of packing defects, proteins would simply be too stable from a thermodynamic standpoint, and would be functionally inert.

Binding Constants

Volatile general anesthetics are only capable of relatively weak interactions with macromolecules, compared to conventional ligands such as the opiates, the benzodiazepines, and the neuromuscular blocking agents. Because of this, it has been difficult to directly examine binding of volatile general anesthetics to proteins. Traditional pharmacological radioligand binding assays *(71)* are not applicable because the mean lifetime (τ) of the volatile general anesthetic-protein complex is so short (on the millisecond timescale) that it is not possible to separate bound and free ligand. Other approaches for monitoring anesthetic binding have therefore been developed that rely on manometry *(72)*, ^{19}F-NMR *(28,73–75)*, photoaffinity labeling with halothane *(13,29,57)*, quenching of the emission of intrinsic or added fluorophores *(30,76,77)*, isothermal titration calorimetry *(78)*, and [129]Xe-NMR *(79,80)*.

Manometric Determination of Xenon Absorption by Myoglobin

The absorption of xenon by 10% aqueous solutions of equine myoglobin was estimated using manometry *(72)*. The amount of xenon taken up by the protein was quantified based upon measured pressure changes in the gas phase above the protein solution. The K_d for xenon binding to myoglobin at 25°C was estimated to be 10 mM. A van't Hoff analysis indicated that the enthalpy of xenon absorption was $\Delta H° = -5.1$ kcal/mol, suggesting fairly tight bonding for such a simple ligand.

^{19}F-NMR Spectroscopy

The volatile general anesthetics that are currently in clinical use in the United States (halothane, isoflurane, sevoflurane, and desflurane) are heavily fluorinated in order to decrease both metabolism and flammability. Because fluorine is present in biological systems in negligible amounts, the ^{19}F isotope on the anesthetic molecule can be studied using NMR with minimal background noise *(81,82)*. Isoflurane and halothane have been reported to bind to the native pH 7.0 form of bovine serum albumin with K_d values of 1.4 mM and 1.3 mM, respectively *(28,73)*.

In addition, the ^{19}F-NMR measurements have allowed an estimation of the time constant, or mean lifetime ($\tau = 1/k_{-1}$), of the anesthetic–albumin complex, which is 200–250 µs for isoflurane *(28,74)*. Because the dissociation constant is equal to k_{-1}/k_1 (where k_{-1} and k_1 are the off- and on-rate constants, respectively), the kinetic results indicate that the association rate constant, k_1, is $3 \times 10^6/M$ s. This value for k_1 is approximately three orders of magnitude less than that expected for a diffusion-controlled on-rate constant ($10^9/M$ s). It is of interest that this estimate of the volatile general anesthetic on-rate constant is comparable to those (10^4 to 10^7 M s) measured with more conventional ligands *(83–85)*. The on-rate constants measured for anesthetic binding to albumin are therefore compatible with the presence of a limited number of discrete binding sites on the protein, and render the concept of non-specific (interfacial) binding less likely. Similarly, kinetic analysis of isoflurane binding to *Torpedo nobiliana* membranes rich in nicotinic acetylcholine receptors using ^{19}F-NMR revealed off- and on-rate constants of 1.7×10^4/s and 4.8×10^7/M s, respectively, with an average dissociation constant (for 9–10 sites) at 15 °C of 0.36 ± 0.03 mM *(75)*. Again, this on-rate constant suggests that there exist a discrete number of binding sites on the nicotinic acetylcholine receptor for isoflurane.

Halothane Direct Photoaffinity Labeling

Halothane direct photoaffinity labeling *(29,86)* effectively converts the rapid kinetics of general anesthetic equilibrium binding into a chemically stable covalent interaction. The carbon-bromine bond of halothane is cleaved with ultraviolet radiation to yield the reactive chlorotrifluoroethyl radical, which covalently attaches to amino acid side-chains in the local binding environment (Fig. 2). Following photolabeling of the sample with halothane, the location of the adduct can be determined by including the radioisotope ^{14}C as the trifluoroethyl carbon and performing microsequencing *(36,57)*, or by monitoring regional protein molecular weight with mass spectrometry *(87,88)*. Of note is that photoaffinity labeling is one of the few techniques available that is capable of separating specific from nonspecific binding, because unlabeled halothane can be used as a competitive ligand. In addition, photoaffinity labeling allows for the separation of binding targets from complex mixtures, such as synaptosomal membranes *(89)*.

Two specific binding sites were identified in bovine serum albumin *(57)*, and these correspond approximately to the locations of the two tryptophan residues (W134 and W212) in the protein, in agreement with the fluorescence quenching results *(30)*. The ^{14}C-chlorotrifluoroethyl adduct attaches to several amino acids in the large IIA pocket on bovine serum albumin (W214–R219), suggesting that halothane experiences considerable translational and rotational freedom at this binding site. Photoaffinity labeling of the four-α-helix bundle (A-α$_2$-L38M)$_2$ designed to bind halothane, followed by microsequencing also resulted in preferential labeling of the W15 residue in the hydrophobic core *(36)*, in good agreement with fluorescence quenching data.

In addition, photoaffinity labeling has allowed the initial assignment of halothane binding domains in membrane proteins. In the nicotinic acetylcholine receptor from *Torpedo nobiliana*, halothane photolabeling revealed that each of the five subunits is labeled in a saturable manner to comparable degrees *(13)*. After digesting the α-subunit with V8 protease, more than 90% of the label was found in the fragments containing the four putative transmembrane domains, indicating that these hydrophobic regions of the receptor represent attractive anesthetic binding targets. The inability of isoflurane to inhibit halothane photolabeling suggests that protein binding sites for different classes of anesthetics (halogenated alkanes vs halogenated ethers) are likely to be distinct. This is in agreement with radiographic studies on rat brain slices following ^{14}C-halothane photolabeling *(89)* that reveal distinct binding sites for halothane and chloroform compared to isoflurane. Thus, the photolabeling results with this member of the ligand-gated ion channel family suggest that there are a number of specific halothane binding sites, and that the majority may be found in the transmembrane region. This indicates that anesthetics are preferentially binding at interprotein (interhelical?) sites or at the lipid-protein interfaces. Other evidence that the lipid-protein interface may be an attractive site for general anesthetic molecules has been reported, using X-ray diffraction on the purple membrane of *Halobacterium halobium*, electron spin resonance spectroscopy on nicotinic acetylcholine receptor-enriched membranes from *Torpedo nobiliana*, and a ^{1}H-NMR study of gramicidin A *(33,90,91)*.

Halothane has also been found to bind specifically to the G protein coupled receptor rhodopsin in bovine retinal membranes using photoaffinity labeling *(15)* with an IC$_{50}$ of 0.9 mM. This membrane protein is a representative of the ubiquitous seven-helix G-protein coupled receptor family, whose

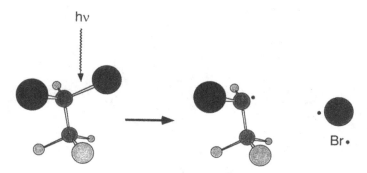

Fig. 2. Direct photoaffinity labeling with halothane. Ulraviolet light of wavelengths ≤260 nm results in cleavage of the C-Br bond to produce chlorotrifluoroethyl and bromine radicals. The chlorotrifluoroethyl radical covalently attaches to neighboring amino acid side-chains in the binding pocket. The number two carbon of halothane (*) is radiolabeled as ^{14}C to allow quantification of bound chlorotrifluoroethyl groups.

members are involved in signal transduction in the central nervous system and at numerous other locations. Binding to, and modulating the activity of this group of membrane proteins may underlie many of the widespread and diverse clinical effects of general anesthetics.

Fluorescence Quenching

Anesthetics that contain chlorine and bromine atoms, such as halothane (Fig. 3), will quench the fluorescence of tryptophan residues provided binding occurs in close proximity to the indole ring *(30,92)*. Monitoring the fluorescence yield as a function of added anesthetic concentration therefore allows determination of dissociation constants and binding energetics *(30,34,77)*. In addition, since tryptophan is the least commonly occurring amino acid in proteins *(93)*, the finding that the fluorescence is quenched provides information on where in the protein matrix the anesthetic is actually binding.

Using intrinsic tryptophan fluorescence quenching, halothane was shown to bind to at least two sites (in subdomains IB and IIA) in bovine serum albumin with an average dissociation constant of 1.8 ± 0.2 mM at 25°C *(30)*. The structurally related halogenated alkane anesthetic chloroform also bound to the same general sites in bovine serum albumin with an average dissociation constant of 2.7 ± 0.2 M at 25°C *(77)*. Designing tryptophan residues into the hydrophobic core of a four- α -helix bundle scaffold has allowed determination of the energetics of halothane complexation, following the introduction of a binding cavity, and in response to the incorporation of potentially favorable polar interactions *(35,36)*. The four-α-helix bundle (Aα$_2$-L38M)$_2$ binds halothane with a dissociation constant of 0.20 ± 0.01 mM, quite comparable to its clinical EC$_{50}$ value of 0.25 mM, indicating that such relatively high affinity sites may indeed exist on in vivo proteins.

Halothane probably quenches tryptophan fluorescence by spin-orbital coupling of the excited (singlet) indole ring and the 2-bromo atom, leading to intersystem crossing to an excited triplet state *(92,94,95)*. The 2-chloro atom may also contribute to the observed quenching of tryptophan fluorescence. Quenching of fluorescence by chloroform is thought to involve electron transfer *(96,97)* and heavy atom perturbation *(98)*. It has been proposed that the electronic orbitals of chromophore and quencher need to overlap for heavy atom spin-orbit coupling to occur *(99–103)*. However, bromine atoms have also been reported to quench fluorophores in other systems at distances of 3–5 Å *(104–106)*. Therefore, the ability of halothane to quench tryptophan fluorescence would indicate that it is binding at least within a few angstroms of the indole ring. This is supported by work with the firefly luciferase enzyme, where halothane binding failed to change the fluorescence quantum yields of the two tryptophan residues *(27)*, since the proposed anesthetic binding site *(26)* is more than 10 Å

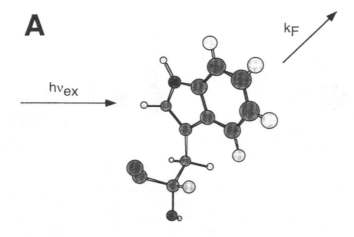

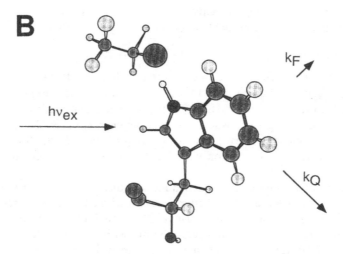

Fig. 3. Deactivation processes affecting the excited state of a tryptophan residue in the absence (**A**) and presence (**B**) of bound halothane. k_F, decay rate of fluorescence; k_Q, rate of intersystem crossing.

distant from the two indole rings. Fluorescence quenching therefore represents an accessible approach for determining anesthetic binding to protein that also provides some structural information.

^{129}Xe-NMR

The magnetic resonance properties of the xenon 129 nucleus are sensitive to its chemical environment *(79)*. Measuring the ^{129}Xe chemical shift has allowed quantification of the dissociation constant for xenon binding to horse skeletal muscle myoglobin *(80)*. Using up to 7 atm of xenon, a relatively high affinity site with a K_d of 7.1 mM (corresponding to 3.4 MAC) was detected (comparable to that measured using manometry), along with a number of lower affinity sites. These lower affinity sites were interpreted as being present on the surface of the protein, and were treated as nonspecific weak binding sites. It was postulated that such weak interactions between xenon, in particular, and volatile anesthetics, in general, may play a role in the action of these drugs.

Isothermal Titration Calorimetry

In isothermal titration calorimetry small aliquots of ligand are sequentially introduced and mixed with the solution containing the protein, and the resulting heat flux is measured and converted to an integrated binding enthalpy *(107)*. Ueda and Yamanaka *(78)* reported on the use of isothermal titration calorimetry for the analysis of chloroform binding to bovine serum albumin. The dissociation constant for chloroform binding was 0.47 ± 0.03 mM, corresponding to a free energy of binding of -4.6 kcal/mol at 25 °C. The enthalpy of chloroform binding was calculated to be -2.5 kcal/mol, indicating that chloroform forms polar interactions (van der Waals and electrostatic) with albumin at its binding sites.

The thermodynamics underlying this interaction is an example of enthalpy-entropy compensation (or an isoequilibrium relationship), which is a general feature of biological processes *(108)*. Because the free energy of binding is composed of enthalpic and entropic components ($\Delta G = \Delta H - T\Delta S$), it follows that as ΔH becomes more negative (stronger binding), ΔS will tend to decrease in magnitude because the ligand becomes more oriented in its binding site. Conversely, as ΔH becomes less negative (weaker binding), ΔS will increase as the ligand becomes more mobile at its binding site.

EFFECTS OF BOUND ANESTHETIC ON THE STRUCTURE, STABILITY, AND DYNAMICS OF PROTEINS

Protein Structure

Once a volatile general anesthetic molecule binds to a protein, how does its presence lead to a reversible change in protein function? The anesthetic may cause a structural change in the target protein, but this has been difficult to detect experimentally since it is likely to be quite subtle given the relatively weak molecular associations that are characteristic of these drugs *(2)*. For example, binding of the small hydrophobic ligands dimethyl sulfoxide and methyl sulfinyl-methyl sulfoxide to the FK506 binding protein (the water-soluble receptor for the immunosuppressant drug FK506) causes root mean square displacements of the backbone C$^\alpha$ atoms of only 0.12–0.16 Å *(109)* as detected by X-ray crystallography at 2.0 Å resolution. However, small structural changes involving side-chain movements of <1 Å can have profound functional effects on proteins because of the enormous amplification of stimulus to response that is a hallmark of biological systems *(110)*. The 2.2 Å X-ray crystal structure of the firefly luciferase enzyme with two bound bromoform molecules revealed that anesthetic binding caused minimal overall protein structural changes *(26)*. The limited information on protein architectural changes induced by bound anesthetic molecules indicates that secondary structure is not altered *(26,30–32,34,77)*. It is therefore likely that a bound anesthetic instead perturbs the tertiary structure of the protein, or perhaps the quaternary structure. Only very high resolution X-ray crystallography will be able to detect the small topological changes that are likely in the case of weakly interacting ligands, such as the volatile general anesthetics.

Examples of changes in quarternary structure are the effects of halothane and diethyl ether on the aggregation state of the membrane-bound skeletal muscle sarcoplasmic reticulum Ca^{2+}-Mg^{2+}-ATP ase *(17–20,111)*, and the effect of halothane on the oligomerization state of the skeletal muscle ryanodine receptor *(112)*. Halothane causes stimulation of the sarcoplasmic reticulum Ca^{2+}-Mg^{2+}-ATPase activity by favoring monomer formation from larger oligomers, which is thought to occur secondary to changes in the physical properties of the lipid portion of the membrane *(17–20)*. However, a recent study *(111)* reported that halothane instead inhibited rabbit sarcoplasmic reticulum Ca^{2+}-Mg^{2+}-ATPase activity by favoring oligomer (tetramer) formation. Similarly, halothane causes oligomer (hexamer) formation by the skeletal muscle ryanodine receptor 1 Ca^{2+}-release channel, which is involved in excitation-contraction coupling *(112)*. More work will be needed to clarify the effects of anesthetics on membrane protein oligomerization states, and the underlying mechanisms involved.

Protein Stability

The majority of proteins adopt a unique three-dimensional structure (the native state) under physiological conditions. The native structure is maintained by the hydrophobic effect and electrostatic contributions, with entropic terms tending to favor unfolding of the polypeptide *(113–115)*. The balance between these opposing energetic components is responsible for the overall stability of the native folded protein conformation. The effect of halothane binding to $(A\alpha_2)_2$ on the four-α-helix bundle scaffold stability was examined using chemical denaturation with guanidinium chloride, monitored by circular dichroism spectroscopy *(116)*. The bound anesthetic stabilized the native bundle conformation by -1.8 kcal/mol at 25°C (corresponding to a 20-fold increased stabilization of the folded form of the protein), and increased the *m* value from 1.6 ± 0.2 to 2.0 ± 0.1 kcal/mol. The latter effect is compatible with improved hydrophobic core packing *(117)*, and supports anesthetic binding to the cavity in the core of $(A\alpha_2)_2$. Using hydrogen exchange *(36)*, halothane was also shown to stabilize the folded conformation of the four-α-helix bundle $(A\alpha_2\text{-}L38M)_2$ by approx -0.9 kcal/mol (representing a 4.6-fold increase in the fraction of the fully folded conformation in the presence of the anesthetic). Thus, binding of anesthetic to the four-α-helix bundle scaffolds is associated with a stabilization of the folded conformation of the protein.

Halothane has been shown to increase the stability of the native folded conformation of bovine serum albumin using differential scanning calorimetry and hydrogen exchange *(118,119)*. Further, both halothane and isoflurane stabilize the native folded state of albumin to thermal denaturation as followed by circular dichroism spectroscopy *(120)*. In contrast, in the case of the firefly luciferase enzyme and myoglobin, there is evidence that anesthetic agents (halothane, isoflurane, chloroform, and enflurane) destabilize the protein and bind most favorably to a partially unfolded conformation *(27,118,121)*. Thus, partial unfolding of proteins in the presence of anesthetics, to yield a higher free energy conformation, remains a plausible mechanism whereby function is altered *(122)*.

Protein Dynamics

Another possibility is that anesthetics change protein activity by modifying amino acid side-chain dynamics. The effect of a bound anesthetic molecule on protein dynamics has been examined, because of the intimate link between protein flexibility and function *(123,124)*. Bovine serum albumin is one of the most extensively studied anesthetic binding proteins *(28–30,77,120)*. One of the anesthetic binding sites is located in a pocket in subdomain IIA, that contains the conserved W212 residue *(30,77)*. Binding of either halothane or isoflurane to bovine serum albumin is associated with attenuation of indole ring mobility as determined using fluorescence anisotropy measurements *(120)*. Anesthetic binding therefore has a stabilizing effect on albumin, in terms of local dynamics and global stability. Halothane bound in the hydrophobic core of the four-α-helix bundle $(A\alpha_2\text{-}L38M)_2$ has also been reported to limit the indole ring mobility as followed during a 1 ns molecular dynamics simulation *(38)*. Similarly, binding of bromoform to crystals of the low-affinity form of the firefly luciferase enzyme caused a neighboring histidine residue (H310) to become less mobile as determined by an improved ability to identify the electron density associated with this side-chain *(26)*.

Molecular Dynamics Simulations

A promising alternative approach for examining the effect of a bound anesthetic molecule on protein structure is to perform molecular dynamics simulations, which can reveal the atomic motions in a macromolecule and a bound ligand as a function of time *(125)*. Large-scale simulation techniques that reproduce biological processes at the molecular level have been made possible by the explosive growth in computational power over the past two decades *(126)* coupled with advances in the quality of force fields and molecular dynamics methodology. No experimental technique is able to reveal as much detailed information about individual molecules and their interactions as can be provided by computer modeling. In particular, the static three-dimensional spatial arrangement of the atoms provided by X-ray crystallography is not by itself sufficient to allow an understanding of function because proteins are extremely complex dynamic systems *(127)*.

Performing 1 ns molecular dynamics simulations on halothane bound to a small four-α-helix bundle reveals some of the details of how an anesthetic might alter protein structure and dynamics *(36–38,128)*. Halothane orients itself in the hydrophobic core of the four-α-helix bundle in such a way that its bromine atom is aligned towards the W15 side-chain, in good agreement with the fluorescence quenching studies *(35,36)*. In addition, the presence of halothane in the hydrophobic core of the four-α-helix bundle attenuates the motions of the W15 side-chain, which is in line with fluorescence anisotropy measurements on albumin *(120)*. Finally, halothane makes a favorable interaction with the C41 side-chain in the hydrophobic core of the four-α-helix bundle, which is in accord with the solvation studies predicting that halothane should interact favorably with cysteine residues *(60)*. Good agreement between experimental data and molecular dynamics simulations lends strong support to the validity of results obtained with the latter technique.

The complex of phage T4 lysozyme L99A with xenon has also been examined during both 1.75 and 6 ns molecular dynamics simulations *(129)*. The less detailed 6 ns simulation allowed detection of domain motions (with relaxation times on the order of 1 ns) associated with opening and closing of the active site, that provide a description of how ligands reach buried cavities in protein hydrophobic cores. A mixture of one- and two-xenon complexes with the protein were detected at 8 atm of xenon, in good agreement with the experimental findings *(48)*. This hydrophobic cavity is apparently not normally occupied by a water molecule owing to an unfavorable entropic contribution dominating the overall binding energetics.

PROPOSED ANESTHETIC MECHANISMS OF ACTION BASED ON MODEL PROTEIN RESULTS

The effect of anesthetic agents on protein motions and stability suggest potential mechanisms for how anesthetic binding may reversibly alter protein function (Fig. 4). The folded, biologically active, conformations of proteins are only marginally more stable (5–10 kcal/mol) than their unfolded counterparts *(130)*, a situation believed to have evolved in order to allow the structural changes to occur at ambient temperatures required for normal protein function *(70)*. In addition, the native structure is the lowest free energy conformation *(131,132)*. The ability of both protein receptors to bind ligands, and for enzymes to transform substrates, is dependent on protein motion *(123,133)*. Any alteration in the stability of a given conformational substate (different substates have the same general structure but differ in local configurations) will alter the equilibrium between the different conformations, by raising or lowering the free energy barriers for subsequent structural changes required for function. By limiting or promoting protein dynamics, volatile general anesthetics might alter the binding of native ligands to their receptors and thus disturb the function of central nervous system proteins. Experimental evidence for these concepts is provided by work on the *Torpedo nobiliana* nicotinic acetylcholine receptor showing that general anesthetic agents increase the proportion of receptors in the desensitized state *(134,135)*. Bound volatile general anesthetic agents may therefore perturb the equilibrium between conformational substates of the protein, which then leads to a change in function.

Anesthetic agents have previously been shown to have fluidizing effects on lipid bilayers *(136–138)*. The finding that halothane and isoflurane have the opposite effect on local protein dynamics and global protein stability *(120)* suggests that the interaction with certain protein targets may be fundamentally different. Protein stability is generally increased following ligand binding, as demonstrated by approaches that measure dynamics, such as fluorescence anisotropy *(139)*, hydrogen-deuterium exchange *(140)*, NMR relaxation rates *(141)*, and crystallographic Debye-Waller or isotropic temperature (B) factors *(142,143)*. In this regard, halothane and isoflurane appear to behave like conventional ligands. Furthermore, anesthetic-induced attenuation of protein dynamics is compatible with the clinical observations that (1) hypothermia decreases anesthetic requirements *(144–146)*, and

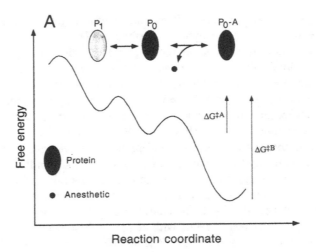

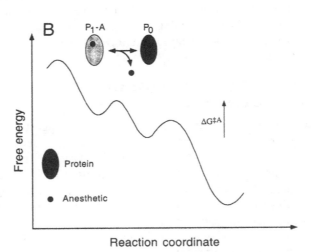

Fig. 4. Schematic depiction of anesthetic-induced stabilization **(A)** and destabilization **(B)** of the native uncomplexed protein, P_0. A is the anesthetic bound to the protein and P_1 is the active form of the protein. In panel **(A)**, $\Delta G^{\ddagger A}$ and $\Delta G^{\ddagger B}$ are the activation energies required to transform the protein conformation to its active state, from the unliganded condition and after binding a single anesthetic molecule, respectively. In **(B)**, anesthetic binding raises the free energy of the protein (partial unfolding), by adding $\Delta G^{\ddagger A}$, which is sufficient to favor the activated protein conformation. Binding of anesthetic to the *N*-methyl-D-aspartate- and the $GABA_A$ receptor, would be examples of **(A)** and **(B)**, respectively.

(2) increased pressures, which denature proteins *(147–149)*, reverse the effects of anesthetic agents *(150–153)*.

However, in the case of the firefly luciferse enzyme, anesthetics preferentially bind to a partially unfolded conformation in solution *(27,121)*. Under these conditions, the motions of a portion of the amino acid residues are enhanced and the overall free energy of the protein will be increased (Fig. 4B). In effect, the anesthetics are acting on this protein in a manner analogous to that observed with the lipid bilayer, with a net increase in fluidity.

CONCLUSIONS

In summary, model proteins are allowing predictions to be made concerning the general topology of in vivo anesthetic binding sites, and have enabled a direct test of the hypothesis that the clinical EC_{50} for halothane ($250\ \mu M$) might equal the K_d of a single protein target. It should be noted, however, that a clinical EC_{50} value is unlikely to correspond to the K_d of a binding site on a protein, since the relationship between the ligand concentration that produces a functional effect and the target dissociation constant is typically disparate *(2,154)*. Taken together, the results with these model proteins suggest that volatile general anesthetics will occupy preexisting appropriately-sized hydrophobic cavities and pockets on proteins, and that the presence of somewhat polar residues lining the binding site will favor anesthetic binding.

In two of the cases studied to date (bovine serum albumin and the synthetic four-α-helix bundles), volatile general anesthetic binding leads to a stabilization of the native folded conformation of the protein. Stabilization of selected protein substates may increase the free energy barrier that must be overcome in order to allow a protein to convert to its functional form. Sufficient stabilization by the bound anesthetic will at some point render thermally-induced fluctuations in protein structure insufficient to allow conversion into the active substate. This may explain how volatile general anesthetics cause reversible protein inhibition, as in the case of the N-methyl-D-aspartate receptor *(6)*, the m1 muscarinic receptor *(23)*, central nervous system Na^+ channels *(155)*, or voltage-gated neuronal Ca^{2+} channels *(156)*.

In the cases of the $GABA_A$ receptor *(157,158)* or neuronal protein kinase C *(159,160)*, where volatile general anesthetics enhance activity, the equilibrium may be shifted so that the active substrate conformation is favored instead. This may represent examples of anesthetic-induced destabilization of the protein as modeled by the firefly luciferase enzyme in the presence of anesthetic. Studies with model proteins are therefore beginning to provide a mechanistic understanding of how bound anesthetics might alter protein activity. With technical advances, such hypotheses will eventually be testable on the much larger ligand-gated ion channels that are currently in favor as the in vivo targets for these widely used clinical compounds.

ACKNOWLEDGMENT

Supported by National Institutes of Health Grant GM55876.

REFERENCES

1. Franks, N. P. and Lieb, W. R. (1994) Molecular and cellular mechanisms of general anesthesia. *Nature* **367,** 607–614.
2. Eckenhoff, R. G. and Johansson, J. S. (1977) Interactions between inhaled anesthetics and proteins. *Pharmacol. Rev.* **49,** 343–367.
3. Belelli, D., Pistis, M., Peters, J. A., and Lambert, J. J. (1999) General anaesthetic action at transmitter-gated inhibitory amino acid receptors. *Trends Biochem. Sci.* **20,** 496–502.
4. Krasowski, M. D. and Harrison, N. L. (1999) General anaesthetic actions on ligand-gated ion channels. *Cell. Mol. Life Sci.* **55,** 1278–1303.
5. Mihic, S. J., Ye, Q., Wick, M. J., et al. (1997) Sites of alcohol and volatile anaesthetic action on $GABA_A$ and glycine receptors. *Nature* **389,** 385–389.
6. Jevtovic-Todorovic, V., Todorovic, S. M., Mennerick, S., et al. (1998) Nitrous oxide (laughing gas) is an NMDA antagonist, neuroprotectant and neurotoxin. *Nat. Med.* **4,** 460–463.
7. Neumahr, S., Hapfelmeier, G., Scheller, M., Schneck, H., Franke, C., and Kochs, E. (2000) Dual action of isoflurane on the γ-aminobutyric acid (GABA)-mediated currents through recombinant $\alpha_1\beta_2\gamma_{2L}$- $GABA_A$-receptor channels. *Anesth. Analg.* **90,** 1184–1190.
8. Ratnakumari, L., Vysotskaya, T. N., Duch, D. S., and Hemmings, H. C. (2000) Differential effects of anesthetic and nonanesthetic cyclobutanes on neuronal voltage-gated sodium channels. *Anesthesiology* **92,** 529–541.
9. Enders, A. (1990) The influence of general volatile anesthetics on the dynamic properties of model membranes. *Biochim. Biophys. Acta* **1029,** 43–50.
10. Jørgensen, K., Ipsen, J. H., Mouritsen, O. G., and Zuckermann, M. J. (1993) The effect of anaesthetics on the dynamic heterogeneity of lipid membranes. *Chem. Phys. Lipids* **65,** 205–216.

11. Cantor, R. S. (1997) The lateral pressure profile in membranes: A physical mechanism of general anesthesia. *Biochemistry* **36**, 2339–2344.
12. Cantor, R. S. (1999) The influence of membrane lateral pressures on simple geometric models of protein conformational equilibria. *Chem. Phys. Lipids* **101**, 45–56.
13. Eckenhoff, R. G. (1996) An inhalational anesthetic binding domain in the nicotinic acetylcholine receptor. *Proc. Natl. Acad. Sci. USA* **93**, 2807–2810.
14. Kosk-Kosicka, D., Fomitcheva, I., Lopez, M. M., and Eckenhoff, R. G. (1997) Heterogeneous halothane binding in the SR Ca^{2+}-ATPase. *FEBS Lett.* **402**, 189–192.
15. Ishizawa, Y., Sharp, R., Liebman, P. A., and Eckenhoff, R. G. (2000) Halothane binding to a G protein coupled receptor in retinal membranes by photoaffinity labeling. *Biochemistry* **39**, 8497–8502.
16. Toyoshima, C., Nakasako, M., Nomura, H., and Ogawa, H. (2000) Crystal structure of the calcium pump of sarcoplasmic reticulum at 2.6 Å resolution. *Nature* **405**, 647–655.
17. Bigelow, D. J. and Thomas, D. D. (1987) Rotational dynamics of lipid and the Ca-ATPase in sarcoplasmic reticulum. *J. Biol. Chem.* **262**, 13,449–13,456.
18. Karon, B. S. and Thomas, D. D. (1993) Molecular mechanism of Ca-ATPase activation by halothane in sarcoplasmic reticulum. *Biochemistry* **32**, 7503–7511.
19. Karon, B. S., Mahaney, J. E., and Thomas, D. D. (1994) Halothane and cyclopiazonic acid modulate Ca-ATPase oligomeric state and function in sarcoplasmic reticulum. *Biochemistry* **33**, 13,928–13,937.
20. Kutchai, H., Geddis, L. M., Jones, L. R., and Thomas, D. D. (1998) Differential effects of general anesthetics on the quaternary structure of the Ca-ATPases of cardiac and skeletal muscle sarcoplasmic reticulum. *Biochemistry* **37**, 2410–2421.
21. Palczewski, K., Kumasaka, T., Hori, T., et al. (2000) Crystal structure of rhodopsin: A G protein-coupled receptor. *Science* **289**, 739–745.
22. Aronstam, R. S. and Dennison, R. L. (1989) Anesthetic effects on muscarinic signal transduction. *Int. Anesthesiol. Clin.* **27**, 265–272.
23. Durieux, M. E. (1995) Halothane inhibits signaling through m1 muscarinic receptors expressed in *Xenopus* oocytes. *Anesthesiology* **82**, 174–182.
24. Miyazawa, A., Fujiyoshi, Y., Stowell, M., and Unwin, N. (1999) Nicotinic acetylcholine receptor at 4.6 Å resolution: Transverse tunnels in the channel wall. *J. Mol. Biol.* **288**, 765–786.
25. Koning, R. I., Keegstra, W., Oostergetel, G. T., Schuurman-Wolters, G., Robillard, G. T., and Brisson, A. (1999) The 5 Å projection structure of the transmembrane domain of the mannitol transporter enzyme II. *J. Mol. Biol.* **287**, 845–851.
26. Franks, N. P., Jenkins, A., Conti, E., Lieb, W. R., and Brick, P. (1998) Structural basis for the inhibition of firefly luciferase by a general anesthetic. *Biophys. J.* **75**, 2205–2211.
27. Eckenhoff, R. G., Tanner, J. W., and Liebman, P. A. (2001) Cooperative binding of inhaled anesthetics and ATP to firefly luciferase. *Proteins* **42**, 436–441.
28. Dubois, B. W. and Evers, A. S. (1992) ^{19}F-NMR spin-spin relaxation (T_2) method for characterizing anesthetic binding to proteins: Analysis of isoflurane binding to albumin. *Biochemistry* **31**, 7069–7076.
29. Eckenhoff, R. G. and Shuman, H. (1993) Halothane binding to soluble proteins determined by photoaffinity labeling. *Anesthesiology* **79**, 96–106.
30. Johansson, J. S., Eckenhoff, R. G., and Dutton, P. L. (1995) Binding of halothane to serum albumin demonstrated using tryptophan fluorescence. *Anesthesiology* **83**, 316–324.
31. Bhattacharya, A. A., Curry, S., and Franks, N. P. (2000) Binding of the general anesthetics propofol and halothane to human serum albumin. *J. Biol. Chem.* **49**, 38,731–38,738.
32. Tang, P., Simplaceanu, V., and Xu, Y. (1999) Structural consequences of anesthetic and nonimmobilizer interaction with gramicidin A channels. *Biophys. J.* **76**, 2346–2350.
33. Tang, P., Eckenhoff, R. G., and Xu, Y. (2000) General anesthetic binding to gramicidin A: The structural requirements. *Biophys. J.* **78**, 1804–1809.
34. Johansson, J. S., Rabanal, F., and Dutton, P. L. (1996) Binding of the volatile anesthetic halothane to the hydrophobic core of a tetra-α-helix bundle protein. *J. Pharmacol. Exp. Ther.* **279**, 56–61.
35. Johansson, J. S., Gibney, B. R., Rabanal, F., Reddy, K. S., and Dutton, P. L. (1998) A designed cavity in the hydrophobic core of a four-α-helix bundle improves volatile anesthetic binding affinity. *Biochemistry* **37**, 1421–1429.
36. Johansson, J. S., Scharf, D., Davies, L. A., Reddy, K. S., and Eckenhoff, R. G. (2000) A designed four-α-helix bundle that binds the volatile general anesthetic halothane with high affinity. *Biophys. J.* **78**, 982–993.
37. Davies, L. A., Klein, M. L., and Scharf, D. (1999) Molecular dynamics simulation of a synthetic four-α-helix bundle that binds the anesthetic halothane. *FEBS Lett.* **455**, 332–338.
38. Davies, L. A., Zhong, Q., Klein, M. L., and Scharf, D. (2000) Molecular dynamics simulation of four-α-helix bundles that bind the anesthetic halothane. *FEBS Lett.* **478**, 61–66.
39. Kennedy, R. R., Stokes, J. W., and Downing, P. (1992) Anaesthesia and the "inert" gases with special reference to xenon. *Anaesth. Intens. Care* **20**, 66–70.
40. Vitali, J., Robbins, A. H., Almo, S. C., and Tilton, R. F. (1991) Using xenon as a heavy atom for determining phases in sperm whale metmyoglobin. *J. Appl. Crystallogr.* **24**, 931–935.
41. Schoenborn, B. P., Watson, H. C., and Kendrew, J. C. (1965) Binding of xenon to sperm whale myoglobin. *Nature* **207**, 28–30.
42. Schoenborn, B. P. (1967) Binding of cyclopropane to sperm whale myoglobin. *Nature* **214**, 1120–1122.

43. Nunes, A. C. and Schoenborn, B. P. (1973) Dichloromethane and myoglobin function. *Mol. Pharmacol.* **9,** 835–839.
44. Tilton, R. F., Kuntz, I. D., and Petsko, G. A. (1984) Cavities in proteins: Structure of a metmyoglobin-xenon complex solved to 1.9 Å. *Biochemistry* **23,** 2849–2857.
45. Schoenborn, B. P. (1965) Binding of xenon to horse haemoglobin. *Nature* **208,** 760–762.
46. Schoenborn, B. P. (1976) Dichloromethane as an antisickling agent in sickle cell hemoglobin. *Proc. Natl. Acad. Sci. USA* **73,** 4195–4199.
47. Prangé, T., Schiltz, M., Pernot, L., et al. (1998) Exploring hydrophobic sites in proteins with xenon or krypton. *Proteins* **30,** 61–73.
48. Quillin, M. L., Breyer, W. A., Griswold, I. J., and Matthews, B. W. (2000) Size versus polarizability in protein-ligand interactions: Binding of noble gases within engineered cavities in phage T4 lysozyme. *J. Mol. Biol.* **302,** 955–977.
49. Verschueren, K. H. G., Seljée, F., Rozeboom, H. J., Kalk, K. H., and Dijstra, B. W. (1993) Crystallographic analysis of the catalytic mechanism of haloalkane dehalogenase. *Nature* **363,** 693–698.
50. Gursky, O., Fontano, E., Bhyravbhatla, B., and Caspar, D. L. D. (1994) Stereospecific dihaloalkane binding in a pH-sensitive cavity in cubic insulin crystals. *Proc. Natl. Acad. Sci. USA* **91,** 12,388–12,392.
51. Newman, J., Peat, T. S., Richard, R., et al. (1999) Haloalkane dehalogenase: Structure of a Rhodococcus enzyme. *Biochemistry* **38,** 16,105–16,114.
52. Marek, J., Vévodová, J., Smatanová, I. K., et al. (2000) Crystal structure of the haloalkane dehalogenase from Sphingomonas paucimobilis UT26. *Biochemistry* **39,** 14,082–14,086.
53. Marsh, A. and Ferguson, D. M. (1997) Knowledge-based modeling of bacterial dichloromethane dehalogenase. *Proteins* **28,** 217–226.
54. Perutz, M. F., Fermi, G., Abraham, D. J., Poyart, C., and Bursaux, E. (1986) Hemoglobin as a receptor of drugs and peptides: X-ray studies of the stereochemistry of binding. *J. Am. Chem. Soc.* **108,** 1064–1078.
55. Dunitz, J. D. (1994) The entropic cost of bound water in crystals and biomolecules. *Science* **264,** 670.
56. Romero, P., Obradovic, Z., Li, X., Garner, E. C., Brown, C. J., and Dunker, A. K. (2001) Sequence complexity of disordered protein. *Proteins* **42,** 38–48.
57. Eckenhoff, R. G. (1996) Amino acid resolution of halothane binding sites in serum albumin. *J. Biol. Chem.* **271,** 15,521–15,526.
58. Johansson, J. S., Gibney, B. R., Skalicky, J. J., Wand, A. J., and Dutton, P. L. (1998) A native-like three-α-helix bundle protein from structure based redesign: A novel maquette scaffold. *J. Am. Chem. Soc.* **120,** 3881–3886.
59. Johansson, J. S., Gibney, B. R., Skalicky, J. J., Wand, A. J., and Dutton, P. L. (1998) A designed three-α-helix bundle scaffold for incorporating volatile anesthetic binding sites. *Anesthesiology* **89,** A100.
60. Johansson, J. S. and Zou, H. (1999) Partitioning of four modern volatile general anesthetics into solvents that model buried amino acid side-chains. *Biophys. Chem.* **79,** 107–116.
61. Rashin, A. A., Iofin, M., and Honig, B. (1986) Internal cavities and buried waters in globular proteins. *Biochemistry* **25,** 3619–3625.
62. Hubbard, S. J., Gross, K.-H., and Argos, P. (1994) Intramolecular cavities in globular proteins. *Protein Eng.* **7,** 613–626.
63. Scapin, G., Young, A. C. M., Kromminga, A., Veerkamp, J. H., and Sacchettini, J. C. (1993) High-resolution X-ray studies of mammalian intestinal and fatty-acid-binding proteins provide an opportunity for defining the chemical nature of fatty-acid-protein interactions. *Mol. Cell. Biochem.* **123,** 3–13.
64. Williams, M. A., Goodfellow, J. M., and Thornton, J. M. (1994) Buried waters and internal cavities in monomeric proteins. *Protein Sci.* **3,** 1224–1235.
65. Hubbard, S. J. and Argos, P. (1994) Cavities and packing at protein interfaces. *Protein Sci.* **3,** 2194–2206.
66. Bianchet, M. A., Bains, G., Pelosi, P., et al. (1996) The three-dimensional structure of bovine odorant binding protein and its mechanism of odor recognition. *Nat. Struct. Biol.* **3,** 934–939.
67. Tegoni, M., Ramoni, R., Bignetti, E., Spinelli, S., and Cambillau, C. (1996) Domain swapping creates a third putative combining site in bovine odorant binding protein dimer. *Nat. Struct. Biol.* **3,** 863–867.
68. Liang, J., Edelsbrunner, H., Fu, P., Sudhakar, P. V., and Subramanian, S. (1998) Analytical shape computation of macromolecules: II. Inaccessible cavities in proteins. *Proteins* **33,** 18–29.
69. Wu, S.-Y., Pérez, M. D., Puyol, P., and Sawyer, L. (1999) β-Lactoglobulin binds palmitate within its central cavity. *J. Biol. Chem.* **274,** 170–174.
70. Richards, F. M. and Lim, W. A. (1994) An analysis of packing in the protein folding problem. *Q. Rev. Biophys.* **26,** 423–498.
71. Weiland, G. A. and Molinoff, P. B. (1981) Quantitative analysis of drug-receptor interactions: I. Determination of kinetic and equilibrium properties. *Life Sci.* **29,** 313–330.
72. Ewing, G. J. and Maestas, S. (1970) The thermodynamics of absorption of xenon by myoglobin. *J. Phys. Chem.* **74,** 2341–2344.
73. Dubois, B. W., Cherian, S. F., and Evers, A. S. (1993) Volatile anesthetics compete for common binding sites on bovine serum albumin: A ^{19}F-NMR study. *Proc. Natl. Acad. Sci. USA* **90,** 6478–6482.
74. Xu, Y., Tang, P., Firestone, L., and Zhang, T. T. (1996) ^{19}F nuclear magnetic resonance investigation of stereoselective binding of isoflurane to bovine serum albumin. *Biophys. J.* **70,** 532–538.
75. Xu, Y., Seto, T., Tang, P., and Firestone, L. (2000) NMR study of volatile anesthetic binding to nicotinic acetylcholine receptors. *Biophys. J.* **78,** 746–751.
76. Johansson, J. S. and Eckenhoff, R. G. (1996) Minimum structural requirement for an inhalational anesthetic binding site on a protein target. *Biochim. Biophys. Acta* **1290,** 63–68.

77. Johansson, J. S. (1997) Binding of the volatile anesthetic chloroform to albumin demonstrated using tryptophan fluorescence quenching. *J. Biol. Chem.* **272,** 17,961–17,965.
78. Ueda, I. and Yamanaka, M. (1997) Titration calorimetry of anesthetic-protein interaction: Negative enthalpy of binding and anesthetic potency. *Biophys. J.* **72,** 1812–1817.
79. Miller, K. W., Reo, N. V., Schoot Uiterkamp, A. J. M., Stengle, D. P., Stengle, T. R., and Williamson, K. L. (1981) Xenon NMR: Chemical shifts of a general anesthetic in common solvents, proteins, and membranes. *Proc. Natl. Acad. Sci. USA* **78,** 4946–4949.
80. Rubin, S. M., Spence, M. M., Goodson, B. M., Wemmer, D. E., and Pines, A. (2000) Evidence of nonspecific surface interactions between laser-polarized xenon and myoglobin in solution. *Proc. Natl. Acad. Sci. USA* **97,** 9472–9475.
81. Wyrwicz, A. M. (1991) Applications of ^{19}F NMR spectroscopy to studies on intact tissues. *Bull. Magn. Reson.* **12,** 209–217.
82. Danielson, M. A. and Falke, J. J. (1996) Use of ^{19}F NMR to probe protein structure and conformational changes. *Annu. Rev. Biophys. Biomol. Struct.* **25,** 163–195.
83. Eigen, M. and Hammes, G. G. (1963) Elementary steps in enzyme reactions. *Adv. Methods Enzymol.* **25,** 1–38.
84. Gutfreund, H. (1987) Reflections on the kinetics of substrate binding. *Biophys. Chem.* **26,** 117–121.
85. Sklar, L. A. (1987) Real-time spectroscopic analysis of ligand-receptor dynamics. *Annu. Rev. Biophys. Biophys. Chem.* **16,** 479–506.
86. El-Maghrabi, E. A., Eckenhoff, R. G., and Shuman, H. (1992) Saturable binding of halothane to rat brain synaptosomes. *Proc. Natl. Acad. Sci. USA* **89,** 4329–4332.
87. Lindeman, J. and Lovins, R. E. (1976) The mass spectral analysis of covalently labeled amino acid methylthiohydantoin derivatives derived from affinity labeled proteins. *Anal. Biochem.* **75,** 682–685.
88. Grenot, C., Blachére, T., de Ravel, M. R., Mappus, E., and Cuilleron, C. Y. (1994) Identification of Trp-371 as the main site of specific photoaffinity labeling of corticosteroid binding globulin using Δ6 derivatives of cortisol, corticosterone, and progesterone as unsubstituted photoreagents. *Biochemistry* **33,** 8969–8981.
89. Eckenhoff, M. F. and Eckenhoff, R. G. (1998) Quantitative autoradiography of halothane binding in rat brain. *J. Pharmacol. Exp. Ther.* **285,** 371–376.
90. Fraser, D. M., Louro, S. R. W., Horvath, L. I., Miller, K. W., and Watts, A. (1990) A study of the effect of general anesthetics on lipid-protein interactions in acetylcholine receptor enriched membranes from *Torpedo nobiliana* using nitroxide spin-labels. *Biochemistry* **29,** 2664–2669.
91. Nakagawa, T., Hamanaka, T., Nishimura, S., Uruga, T., and Kito, Y. (1994) The specific binding site of the volatile anesthetic diiodomethane to purple membrane by X-ray diffraction. *J. Mol. Biol.* **238,** 297–301.
92. Lakowicz, J. R. (1999) *Principles of Fluorescence Spectroscopy*, Second Edition, Kluwer Academic, New York, N Y, pp. 238–264.
93. McCaldon, P. and Argos, P. (1988) Oligopeptide biases in protein sequences and their use in predicting protein coding regions in nucleotide sequences. *Proteins* **4,** 99–122.
94. Kasha, M. (1952) Collisional perturbation of spin-orbital coupling and the mechanism of fluorescence quenching. A visual demonstration of the perturbation. *J. Chem. Phys.* **20,** 71–74.
95. Turro, N. J. (1978) *Modern Molecular Photochemsitry*, University Science Books, Sausalito, CA.
96. Steiner, R. F. and Kirby, E. P. (1969) The interaction of the ground and excited states of indole derivatives with electron scavengers. *J. Phys. Chem.* **73,** 4130–4135.
97. Eberson, L. (1982) Electron transfer reactions in organic chemistry. II. An analysis of alkyl halide reduction by electron transfer reagents on the basis of the Marcus theory. *Acta Chem. Scand. Ser. B. Org. Chem. Biochem.* **36,** 533–543.
98. Cowan, D. O. and Drisko, R. L. E. (1970) The photodimerization of acenaphthylene. Heavy-atom solvent effects. *J. Am. Chem. Soc.* **92,** 6281–6285.
99. Siegel, S. and Judeikis, H. S. (1968) Relative interaction radii for quenching of triplet-state molecules. *J. Chem. Phys.* **48,** 1613–1619.
100. Berman, I. B. (1973) Empirical study of heavy-atom collisional quenching of the fluorescence state of aromatic compounds in solution. *J. Phys. Chem.* **77,** 562–567.
101. Cha, T.-A. and Maki, A. H. (1984) Close range interactions between nucleotide bases and tryptophan residues in an *Escherichia coli* single-stranded DNA binding protein-mercurated poly(uridylic acid) complex. *J. Biol. Chem.* **259,** 1105–1109.
102. Lam, W.-C., Tsao, D. H. H., Maki, A. H., Maegley, K. A., and Reich, N. (1992) Spectroscopic studies of arsenic (III) binding to Escherichia coli RI methyltransferase and to two mutants, C223S and W183F. *Biochemistry* **31,** 10,438–10,442.
103. Sasaki, S., Katsuki, A., Akiyama, K., and Tero-Kubota, S. (1997) Spin-orbit coupling induced electron spin polarization: Influence of heavy atom position. *J. Am. Chem. Soc.* **119,** 1323–1327.
104. Tsao, D. H. H., Casa-Finet, J. R., Maki, A. H., and Chase, J. W. (1989) Triplet state properties of tryptophan residues in complexes of mutated *Escherichia coli* single-stranded DNA binding proteins with single-stranded polynucleotides. *Biophys. J.* **55,** 927–936.
105. Bolen, E. J. and Holloway, P. W. (1990) Quenching of tryptophan fluorescence by brominated phospholipid. *Biochemistry* **29,** 9638–9643.
106. Basu, G., Anglos, D., and Kuki, A. (1993) Fluorescence quenching in a strongly helical peptide series: The role of noncovalent pathways in modulating electronic interactions. *Biochemistry* **32,** 3067–3076.
107. Fisher, H. F. and Singh, N. (1995) Calorimetric methods for interpreting protein-ligand interactions. *Methods Enzymol.* **259,** 194–221.

108. Dunitz, J. D. (1995) Win some, lose some: Enthalpy-entropy compensation in weak intermolecular interactions. *Chem. Biol.* **2,** 709–712.

109. Burkhard, P., Taylor, P., and Walkinshaw, M. D. (2000) X-ray structures of small ligand-FKBP complexes provide an estimate for hydrophobic interaction energies. *J. Mol. Biol.* **295,** 953–962.

110. Koshland, D. E. (1998) Conformational changes: How small is big enough? *Nat. Med.* **4,** 1112–1114.

111. Brennan, L. K., Froemming, G. R., and Ohlendieck, K. (2000) Effect of halothane on the oligomerization of the sarcoplasmic reticulum Ca^{2+}-ATPase. *Biochem. Biophys. Res. Comm.* **271,** 770–776.

112. Frömming, G. R. and Ohlendieck, K. (1999) Isoform-specific interactions between halothane and the ryanodine receptor Ca^{2+}-release channel: Implications for malignant hyperthermia and the protein theory of anesthetic action. *Naturwissenschaften* **86,** 584–587.

113. Privalov, P. L. and Gill, S. J. (1988) Stability of protein structure and hydrophobic interaction. *Adv. Protein Chem.* **39,** 191–234.

114. Fersht, A. R. (1993) Protein folding and stability: The pathway of folding of barnase. *FEBS Lett.* **325,** 5–16.

115. Lazaridis, T., Archontis, G., and Karplus, M. (1995) Enthalpic contribution to protein stability: Insights from atom-based calculations and statistical mechanics. *Adv. Protein Chem.* **47,** 231–306.

116. Johansson, J. S. (1998) Probing the structural features of volatile anesthetic binding sites with synthetic peptides. *Toxicol. Lett.* **101,** 369–375.

117. Pace, C. N. (1986) Determination and analysis of urea and guanidine hydrochloride denaturation curves. *Meth. Enzymol.* **131,** 266–280.

118. Eckenhoff, R. G. and Tanner, J. W. (1998) Differential halothane binding and effects on serum albumin and myoglobin. *Biophys. J.* **75,** 477–483.

119. Tanner, J. W., Eckenhoff, R. G., and Liebman, P. A. (1999) Halothane, an inhalational anesthetic, increases folding stability of serum albumin. *Biochim. Biophys. Acta* **1430,** 46–56.

120. Johansson, J. S., Zou, H., and Tanner, J. W. (1999) Bound volatile general anesthetics alter both local protein dynamics and global protein stability. *Anesthesiology* **90,** 235–245.

121. Ueda, I. and Suzuki, A. (1998) Irreversible phase transition of firefly luciferase: Contrasting effects of volatile anesthetics and myristic acid. *Biochim. Biophys. Acta* **1380,** 313–319.

122. Eyring, H., Woodbury, J. W., and D'Arrigo, J. S. (1973) A molecular mechanism of general anesthesia. *Anesthesiology* **38,** 415–424.

123. Frauenfelder, H., Sligar, S., and Wolynes, P. G. (1991) The energy landscapes and motions of proteins. *Science* **254,** 1598–1603.

124. Zaccai, G. (2000) How soft is a protein? A protein dynamics force constant measured by neutron scattering. *Science* **288,** 1604–1607.

125. Karplus, M. and Petsko, G. A. (1990) Molecular dynamics simulations in biology. *Nature* **347,** 631–639.

126. Sagui, C. and Darden, T. A. (1999) Molecular dynamics simulations of biomolecules: Long-range electrostatic effects. *Annu. Rev. Biophys. Biomol. Struct.* **28,** 155–179.

127. Bernèche, S. and Roux, B. (2000) Molecular dynamics of the KcsA K$^+$ channel in a bilayer membrane. *Biophys. J.* **78,** 2900–2917.

128. Johansson, J. S. and Scharf, D. (2001) Towards an understanding of how general anesthetics alter central nervous system protein function. *Reg. Anes. Pain Med.* **26,** 267–270.

129. Mann, G. and Hermans, J. (2000) Modeling protein-small molecule interactions: Structure and thermodynamics of noble gases binding in a cavity in mutant phage T4 lysozyme L99A. *J. Mol. Biol.* **302,** 979–989.

130. Pace, C. N., Shirley, B. A., McNutt, M., and Gajiwala, K. (1996) Forces contributing to the conformational stability of proteins. *FASEB J.* **10,** 75–83.

131. Anfinsen, C. B. (1973) Principles that govern the folding of protein chains. *Science* **181,** 223–230.

132. Wolynes, P. G., Onuchic, J. N., and Thirumalai, D. (1995) Navigating the folding routes. *Science* **267,** 1619–1620.

133. Shoichet, B. K., Baase, W. A., Kuroki, R., and Matthews, B. W. (1995) A relationship between protein stability and protein function. *Proc. Natl. Acad. Sci. USA* **92,** 452–456.

134. Young, A. P. and Sigman, D. S. (1981) Allosteric effects of volatile anesthetics on the membrane-bound acetylcholine receptor protein. I. Stabilization of the high-affinity state. *Mol. Pharmacol.* **20,** 498–505.

135. Raines, D. E., Rankin, S. E., and Miller, K. W. (1995) General anesthetics modify the kinetics of nicotinic acetylcholine receptor desensitization at clinically relevant concentrations. *Anesthesiology* **82,** 276–287.

136. Hill, M. W. H. (1974) The effect of anaesthetic-like molecules on the phase transition in smectic mesophases of dipalmitoyllecithin. I. The normal alcohol up to C = 9 and three inhalation anaesthetics. *Biochim. Biophys. Acta* **356,** 117–124.

137. Trudell, J. R. (1977) A unitary theory of anesthesia based on lateral phase separations in nerve membranes. *Anesthesiology* **46,** 5–10.

138. Harris, R. A. and Groh, G. I. (1985) Membrane disordering effects of anesthetics are enhanced by gangliosides. *Anesthesiology* **62,** 115–119.

139. Lee, J., Pilch, P. F., Shoelson, S. E., and Scarlata, S. F. (1997) Conformational changes in the insulin receptor upon insulin binding and activation as monitored by tryptophan fluorescence spectroscopy. *Biochemistry* **36,** 2701–2708.

140. Finucane, M. D. and Jardetsky, O. (1995) Mechanism of hydrogen-deuterium exchange in *trp* repressor studied by ^{1}H-^{15}N NMR. *J. Mol. Biol.* **253,** 576–589.

141. Zajicek, J., Chang, Y., and Castellino, F. J. (2000) The effects of ligand binding on the backbone dynamics of the kringle 1 domain of human plasminogen. *J. Mol. Biol.* **301,** 333–347.

142. Kurumbail, R. G., Stevens, A. M., Gierse, J. K., et al. (1996) Structural basis for selective inhibition of cyclooxygenase-2 by anti-inflammatory agents. *Nature* **384,** 644–648.

143. Vincent, F., Spinelli, S., Ramoni, R., et al. (2000) Complexes of porcine odorant binding protein with odorant molecules belonging to different chemical classes. *J. Mol. Biol.* **300,** 127–139.

144. Vitez, T. S., White, P. F., and Eger, E. I. (1974) Effects of hypothermia on halothane MAC and isoflurane MAC in the rat. *Anesthesiology* **41,** 80–81.

145. Antognini, J. F. (1993) Hypothermia eliminates isoflurane requirements at 20°C. *Anesthesiology* **78,** 1152–1156.

146. Antognini, J. F., Lewis, B. K., and Reitan, J. A. (1994) Hypothermia minimally decreases nitrous oxide requirements. *Anesth. Analg.* **79,** 980–982.

147. Silva, J. L. and Weber, G. (1993) Pressure stability of proteins. *Annu. Rev. Phys. Chem.* **44,** 89–113.

148. Royer, C. A. (1995) Application of pressure to biochemical equilibria: The other thermodynamic variable. *Meth. Enzymol.* **259,** 357–377.

149. Heremans, K. and Smeller, L. (1998) Protein structure and dynamics at high pressure. *Biochim. Biophys. Acta* **1386,** 353–370.

150. Johnson, F. H., Brown, D. E. S., and Marsland, D. A. (1942) Pressure reversal of the action of certain narcotics. *J. Cell Comp. Physiol.* **20,** 269–276.

151. Lever, M. J., Miller, K. W., Paton, W. D. M., and Smith, E. B. (1971) Pressure reversal of anaesthesia. *Nature* **231,** 368–371.

152. Halsey, M. J. (1982) Effects of high pressure on the central nervous system. *Physiol. Rev.* **62,** 1341–1377.

153. Wann, K. T. and MacDonald, A. G. (1988) Actions and interactions of high pressure and general anaesthetics. *Prog. Neurobiol.* **30,** 271–307.

154. Eckenhoff, R. G. and Johansson, J. S. (1999) On the relevance of "clinically relevant concentrations" of inhaled anesthetics in in vitro experiments. *Anesthesiology* **91,** 856–860.

155. Ratnakumari, L. and Hemmings, H. C. (1998) Inhibition of presynaptic sodium channels by halothane. *Anesthesiology* **88,** 1043–1054.

156. Miao, N., Frazer, M. J., and Lynch, C. (1995) Volatile anesthetics depress Ca^{2+} transients and glutamate release in isolated cerebral synaptosomes. *Anesthesiology* **83,** 593–603.

157. Tanelian, D. L., Kosek, P., Mody, I., and MacIver, M. B. (1993) The role of the $GABA_A$ receptor/chloride channel complex in anesthesia. *Anesthesiology* **78,** 757–776.

158. Li, X., Czajkowski, C., and Pearce, R. A. (2000) Rapid and direct modulation of $GABA_A$ receptors by halothane. *Anesthesiology* **92,** 1366–1375.

159. Hemmings, H. C., Adamo, A. I. B., and Hoffman, M. M. (1995) Biochemical characterization of the stimulatory effects of halothane and propofol on purified brain protein kinase C. *Anesth. Analg.* **81,** 1216–1222.

160. Hemmings, H. C. and Adamo, A. I. B. (1996) Activation of endogenous protein kinase C by halothane in synaptosomes. *Anesthesiology* **84,** 652–662.

24

The Opioid Receptors

Gary J. Brenner, Jianren Mao, and Carl Rosow

HISTORICAL PERSPECTIVE

There is little doubt that the use of opiates dates to early human history. There are references to opium in the Ebers Papyrus, and the ancient Sumerians recognized its euphoriant properties when they called the opium poppy the "plant of joy." Despite millenia of compulsive use and abuse, the opiates are still unrivaled as analgesics, and derivatives of opium continue to be indispensable in modern therapeutics.

Morphine was isolated by Sertürner in 1803. This phenanthrene alkaloid constitutes 10% of raw opium, but it accounts for almost all of the characteristic pharmacological effects. After the development of the hollow needle in the mid 19th century, morphine began to be administered parenterally, and undesirable opioid side effects like respiratory depression and physical dependence became much more frequent. The large number of morphine-dependent Civil War veterans increased public awareness about "morphine sickness," and this had important consequences for the fledgling discipline of pharmacology. The search for "non-addictive" opioids motivated much of the opioid research (and a large amount of industrial drug development) for the next century. Since there was no scientific basis for creating new analgesics, the pharmaceutical industry modified existing opioids to create large numbers of opioid agonists, partial agonists, competitive antagonists, and stereoisomers. The serendipitous discovery of compounds like nalorphine, naloxone, and dextromethorphan led eventually to new receptor theories in order to account for their peculiar properties.

While tremendous strides have been made in understanding the molecular biology of opioid receptors, it should be appreciated that most of the opioids currently in clinical use were introduced significantly before anyone could measure specific receptor binding, let alone clone and express receptor proteins. The emphasis in this chapter reflects the fact that all of the currently accepted opioid receptors (and their subtypes) were defined initially by in vivo and in vitro experiments with selective ligands.

STRUCTURE—ACTIVITY RELATIONSHIPS μ, κ, AND σ RECEPTORS

Agonists

How could one make an improved opioid agonist — a "better" morphine? The complete chemical structure of morphine (Fig. 1A) was not defined until 1925, but during the latter half of the 19th century, German medicinal chemists created a number of potent semisynthetic opioids by simple chemical modifications of the parent molecule. The most important of these were heroin (diacetyl-morphine) and hydromorphone. Unfortunately, the clinical and preclinical evaluation of these

From: *Contemporary Clinical Neuroscience: Neural Mechanisms of Anesthesia*
Edited by: Joseph F. Antognini et al. © Humana Press Inc., Totowa, NJ

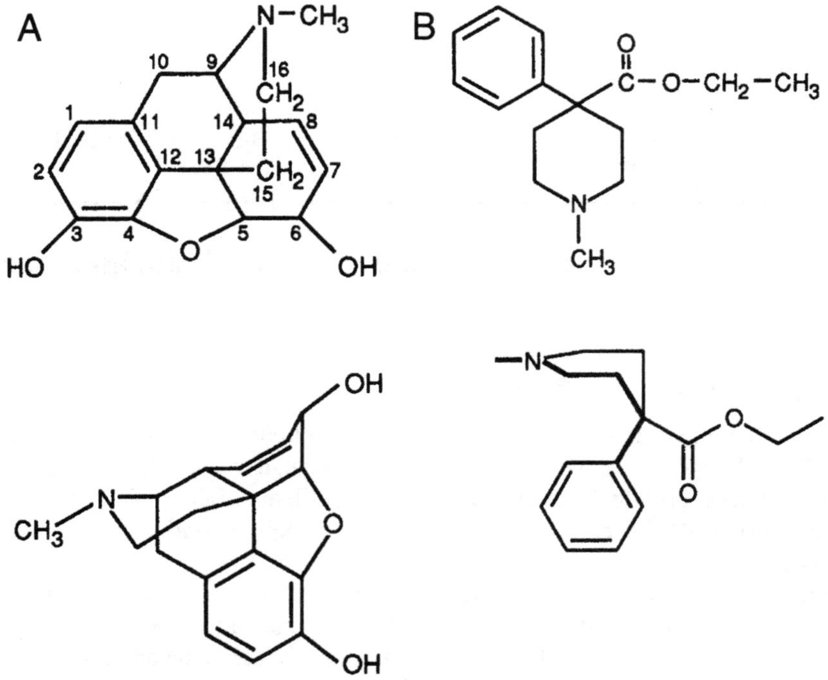

Fig. 1. (A) Planar and stereochemical structures of morphine (*see* text for details). **(B)** Planar and stereochemical structures of meperidine (*see* text for details).

compounds did not live up to the promise of the synthetic chemistry. In 1898, Dreser introduced heroin into clinical practice as a cough suppressant that also cured addiction *(1)*! Opioids were introduced with the same sort of "wishful thinking" several times during the next 50 or 60 yr.

The first totally synthetic opioid agonists, meperidine and methadone, were developed in Germany before and during World War II. Methadone was developed by German Dye Trust chemists in response to the wartime blockade of opium supplies. Meperidine was accidentally discovered by Eisleb and Schaumann in 1939 *(2)*. They were screening congeners of atropine for potential gastrointestinal applications, and meperidine did appear to be weakly atropinic. The circumstances of meperidine's discovery and its planar chemical structure (Fig. 1B) gave no indication that it would be morphine-like, so the drug was introduced and promoted as non-opioid and non-addictive, misimpressions that took years to correct.

As shown in Fig. 1A, morphine is a complex five-ring system consisting of a phenanthrene nucleus, a 5-membered furan ring, and a piperidine ring. Note that there are phenolic and alcoholic hydroxyl groups at positions 3 and 6, respectively, and there is a methyl substitution on the piperidine nitrogen. There is a quaternary carbon at position 13, so morphine is optically active with analgesic activity confined to the levorotatory form.

The opioid analgesics may be categorized into eight related chemical classes that are listed in Table 1. Fentanyl is structurally related to meperidine, but it is still sufficiently different to warrant separate classification. Some newer analgesics (and the opioid peptides) do not lend themselves readily to such a classification scheme.

If we restrict ourselves to consideration of the agonists, these drugs (and several dozen not listed) were the result of an enormous effort to develop an analgesic with a meaningful improvement over morphine in safety and efficacy. Judged by that goal, the effort would have to be considered unsuccessful. Despite substantial differences in chemical structure, all of the pure agonists produce a simi-

Table 1
Chemical Classes of Opioids

Class	Agonists	Antagonists
Opiate	Morphine Codeine	Nalorphine
Oripavine	Etorphine	Buprenorphine Diprenorphine
Morphone	Hydromorphone Oxymorphone Oxycodone	Naloxone Naltrexone Nalbuphine
Morphinan	Levorphanol	Levallorphan Butorphanol
Benzomorphan Diphenylheptylamine	Phenazocine Methadone Propoxyphene	Pentazocine
Phenylpiperidine	Meperidine Alphaprodine	Profadol
Anilidopiperidine	Fentanyl Sufentanil Alfentanil	

Table 2
Depressant and Stimulant Effects of Opioid Agonists

Analgesia	Bradycardia
Respiratory Depression	Nausea and Vomiting
Sedation/Euphoria	Smooth Muscle Spasm
Vasodilation	Skeletal Muscle Hypertonus
Cough Suppression	Miosis

lar set of depressant and stimulant pharmacodynamic effects (listed in Table 2). The major differences between them are in their pharmacokinetics and relative potencies. The therapeutic index is about the same for each of these pure agonist opioids; that is, analgesic potency is an excellent predictor of potency to produce side effects. All of this leads one to conclude two things:

1. The various drugs produce most of their effects by some common receptor mechanism.
2. Because they bind to a common receptor, the drugs must have important structural similarities.

Of course, the common mechanism is now known to be interaction with μ opioid receptors, and extensive work has been done to investigate the common structural features of the different drug molecules. Some of these features can be seen in the stereochemical resprestations in Figs. 1A and 1B. The phenanthrene nucleus is fairly rigid, so the morphine molecule assumes the shape of a T, with the top formed by the piperidine ring and the partially unsaturated ring of the phenanthrene moiety. The other two rings are perpendicular, with the piperidine nitrogen at a maximum distance from the phenolic hydroxyl group. Phenylpiperidines like meperidine, keep only a small portion of this structure, but it can be seen that the piperidine nitrogen and the phenanthrene aromatic ring maintain about the same relationship. The opioid peptides (discussed later) all contain a tyramine residue, and this too, can assume a similar configuration.

Not all classic opioid agonist effects are clearly µ receptor mediated. For example, opioid antitussive effects appear to work by a different mechanism. The potency to produce analgesia is actually a poor predictor of antitussive potency, and some relatively weak analgesics (e.g., codeine) are strong antitussives. The structure activity relationships for this effect have been investigated, and it appears that antitussive activity is increased when a bulky substituent is bound at the 3 position of the phenanthrene nucleus. Thus, cough suppression is stronger with heroin (3-acetoxy) and codeine (3-methoxy) than with meperidine (no functional group) (3). Interestingly, several opioid dextro isomers, (e.g., dextromethorphan) have substantial antitussive effects even though they do not produce analgesia or respiratory depression. It appears that the receptor mechanisms for analgesia and cough suppression involve different stereoselectivity.

Antagonists

Fortuitously, creation of the first opioid antagonists did not require complex chemical synthesis. For the first five chemical classes listed in Table 1, replacement of a methyl group on the piperidine nitrogen by a bulkier substituent (ideally allyl or cyclobutyl) produces a compound with opioid antagonist properties. As early as 1915, Pohl described the opioid antagonist properties of N-allylnorcodeine (4). but the human pharmacology of *N*-allylnormorphine (nalorphine) was not investigated until the early 1950s. Laboratory experiments on nalorphine showed that it could reverse or prevent the effects of morphine in animals, but the traditional analgesic assays like the hot-plate or tail-flick tests had failed to indicate any analgesic activity for this compound. Lasagna and Beecher did the first clinical study of nalorphine in postoperative pain and were surprised to discover that it was approximately equipotent with morphine as an analgesic (5). Wikler and his colleagues showed that administration of nalorphine to morphine-dependent subjects not only failed to produce euphoria, but it actually precipitated withdrawal (6).

Thus, nalorphine was characterized as an "agonist-antagonist" opioid, since it had both analgesic and antagonist effects (7). Nalorphine had high potency but limited efficacy as an analgesic and respiratory depressant (8), so it was also classified as a partial agonist. Lasagna and Beecher noted some important qualitative differences between the agonist effects of nalorphine and morphine. Many of their study patients complained of disturbing mental effects, including auditory and visual hallucinations and severe dysphoria. These reactions made nalorphine unacceptable for clinical use as an analgesic, although it was in widespread use as an antagonist until the introduction of naloxone. Despite its drawbacks, nalorphine generated a good deal of excitement because it provided the first evidence that strong analgesia and addiction liability might be separated.

Nalorphine was also important because it raised the possibility of additional opioid receptor mechanisms. In 1967, Martin postulated that nalorphine was producing its agonist effects by binding to one receptor (later to be called κ), and acting as a competitive antagonist at another (i.e., µ) (9). Martin later expanded his theory to include a third type of receptor, called σ, to account for the stimulant effects produced by some agonist-antagonists (10). As is so often the case, the receptor nomenclature was quite arbitrary and determined by the group of benzomorphan ligands he happened to be testing in his animal experiments: the designations µ, κ, and σ came from morphine, ketocyclazocine, and SKF-10,047 (N-allylnormetazocine). Martin proposed that all opioids could be classified as agonists, partial agonists, or antagonists at each of these receptors. Subsequent work has demonstrated that the σ receptor is not opioid-specific (11), and we now believe that dysphoria and hallucinations may actually be κ effects (12). Dysphoric reactions can be produced in human subjects by enadoline and spiradoline, experimental drugs that are highly selective for the κ receptor.

The clinically available agonist-antagonists can be broadly divided into two classes:

1. Partial agonists at the µ receptor (e.g., buprenorphine, dezocine).
2. Partial agonists at the κ receptor (e.g., pentazocine, butorphanol, nalbuphine).

As one would expect, the µ partial agonists produce analgesia and mood effects that are generally morphine-like, and the κ partial agonists appear different (described below). It is likely that both classes of agonist-antagonists bind to μ receptors with at least some intrinsic activity (i.e., they are all stronger or weaker μ partial agonists), and this accounts for their variable antagonist properties.

Some highly selective and relatively non-selective κ partial agonists have been tested in man, and these give us some insight into the way μ and κ effects differ. The κ-type drugs are strong analgesics that do not usually produce the cloudy dissociation typical of a morphine-like drug. Several of them produce a state that Martin called "apathetic sedation," *(10)* an effect that may reflect the localization of κ receptors in deeper layers of the cerebral cortex *(13)*. Butorphanol, in particular, can produce powerful sedative effects in doses that are subanalgesic *(14)*. Pentazocine and some experimental κ drugs, have produced hallucinations and depersonalization reactions (like nalorphine), and these also occur rarely with butorphanol *(15)*. The κ partial agonists have much less effect on smooth muscle than morphine and therefore appear less likely to produce constipation *(16,17)* or biliary colic *(18)* In contrast to the antidiuretic effects of μ agonists, some κ agonist alkaloids and peptides cause diuresis by complex effects on both brain and kidney *(19,20)*. The κ drugs do not typically produce euphoria, and they have significantly less abuse potential than μ agonists. Although they will not substitute for morphine in a physically dependent subject, κ-type physical dependence and an atypical abstinence syndrome can occur after chronic administration of high doses.

The available agonist-antagonist opioids vary widely in their antagonist potency: nalbuphine is a very strong μ antagonist while butorphanol appears quite weak. Neither the ratio of agonist to antagonist potency, nor the putative receptor interactions have proved to be good predictors for patient acceptance or clinical utility.

ENDOGENOUS OPIOID PEPTIDES AND THE δ RECEPTOR

The endogenous opioid peptides (EOPs) and their synthetic congeners constitute the other major group of opioid ligands. During the 1960s and 70s, Hans Kosterlitz in Aberdeen screened a large number of opioid alkaloids using two in-vitro smooth muscle bioassays, the coaxially-stimulated guinea pig ileum (GPI) and the mouse vas deferens (MVD). A decrease in the amplitude of contractions in the GPI was known to be an excellent predictor for both μ opioid receptor binding and analgesic potency in man. In 1975, Hughes and Kosterlitz extracted two pentapeptides from pig brain, methionine- and leucine-enkephalin (MET-ENK, LEU-ENK), that were also active in these bioassays *(21)*. Morphine was found to have greater activity than the enkephalins in GPI, whereas the opposite was true for the MVD. Kosterlitz therefore proposed that enkephalins were relatively selective for another receptor type that he called δ (for vas deferens) *(22)*.

In 1976, β-endorphin (β-END) was isolated *(23)*. This 31 amino acid polypeptide is a fragment of the pituitary hormone β-lipotropin, and it proved to be a powerful analgesic *(24)*. At about the same time, Avram Goldstein and coworkers isolated another opioid peptide from the pituitary *(25)* that was ultimately shown to be the 17 amino acid polypeptide, dynorphin (DYN) *(26)*. We now know that these peptides (and some 20 additional ones that have been described) are produced from 3 large precursor molecules: proenkephalin, pro-opiomelanocortin, and prodynorphin. These are products of separate genes and have different tissue distributions. DYN is found in widespread locations throughout the brain and spinal cord, as are MET- and LEU-ENK. MET- and LEU-ENK are found in immune cells, in the enteric nervous system, and also co-localized with catecholamines in the adrenal medulla. β-END is found primarily in the pituitary and hypothalamus, although it is also detected in the placenta and pancreas.

The possible function(s) of these peptides is outside the scope of this chapter, but since they are endogenous ligands the EOPs provide additional evidence about the functions of specific opioid receptor populations. Interestingly, the three prototype peptides are relatively selective for the three different opioid receptor types. MET- and LEU-ENK are selective for δ receptors, β-END acts preferentially at μ receptors, while DYN is selective for κ receptors. An ε receptor has been proposed for β-END based on experiments using the rat vas deferens *(27)*, but the significance of this is still uncertain *(28,29)*.

Table 3
Opioid Receptor Subtypes Defined by Selective Alkaloid and Peptide Ligands

Receptor subtype	Agonist	Antagonist
μ_1	Fentanyl	Naloxonazine
	DAMGO[a]	
μ_2	Fentanyl	
	DAMGO[a]	
κ_1	U69,593[b]	Nor-binaltorphimine
κ_2	Ethylketocyclazocine	Nor-binaltorphimine
κ_3	Nalorphine	Naloxone benzoylhydrazone
δ_1	DPDPE[c]	7-benzylidine-7-dehydronaltrexone
δ_2	[D-Pro^2,Glu^4]deltorphin	Naltriben

[a]DAMGO: Tyr-D-ala-Gly-[NmePhe]-NH(CH$_2$)$_2$-OH.
[b]U69,593: 5α,7α,8β-(–)-N-methyl-N-(7-[1-pyrrolidinyl]-1-oxasipiro(4,5)dec-8-yl)benzene acetamide.
[c]DPDPE: cyclic[D-pen^2,D-pen^5]enkephalin

Despite the clinical promise of these peptides, only a few reached the point of human trials *(30)* and they have mainly proven useful as experimental tools. Polypeptides are poorly absorbed, rapidly degraded by plasma and tissue peptidases, and do not readily cross the blood-brain barrier. They also tend to elicit inflammatory and allergic responses. The peptides can be protected from rapid degradation by adding unnatural or D-amino acids or causing the molecule to cyclize. Hundreds of stable experimental peptides have thus been created, and a few of them are highly selective ligands for various opioid receptors (Table 3).

DISTRIBUTION OF OPIOID RECEPTORS

Opioid receptors are found on neurons at virtually all locations from the enteric plexus to peripheral nociceptors to cells of the frontal cortex. They are also located in non-neural tissues such as immune cells *(31)* and are often co-localized with opioid peptides. The distribution of opioid receptors has been investigated using a variety of techniques:

- In vitro tissue assays like the GPI and MVD mentioned previously.
- Microinjection at specific sites in brain and spinal cord.
- Receptor binding studies with radiolabeled ligands. Stereospecific, saturable opioid receptor binding was first described in 1973 by three independent groups using radioactive ligand binding techniques *(32–34)*.
- *In situ* hybridization and autoradiography.

Opioid receptor distribution can be categorized by gross region (supraspinal, spinal, and peripheral) and by function (nociception, respiration, neural-immune interaction, and so on).

Nociception

μ-opioid receptors are found at all levels of the nervous system and are involved in both ascending and descending pathways of pain control. Although μ receptors are found throughout the CNS, they are fairly restricted in their supraspinal distribution. Some of the μ-receptor-expressing supraspinal regions thought to be involved in nociceptive processing include the amygdala, nucleus accumbens, periaqueductal grey (PAG), spinal trigeminal nucleus, mesencephalic reticular formation, cuneate, gracilis, substantia nigra, and thalamic nuclei. μ-opioid receptors involved in pain processing are also found in the substantia gelatinosa of the spinal cord dorsal horn (Rexed laminae I and II). Finally, there are μ-receptors found peripherally on peripheral C-fibers, the unmyelinated nociceptors. The function of these peripheral neuronal opioid receptors is unclear; they may be involved in nociceptive processing utilizing immune cells as a source of endogenous opioids *(35)*.

Respiratory Depression

μ receptors thought to mediate respiratory depression are found in the nucleus of the solitary tract, nucleus ambiguus, and the parabrachial nucleus.

Skeletal Muscle Hypertonus

Rapid administration of opioid agonists can increase tone in skeletal muscle. This effect is thought due to opioid modulation of dopamine and GABA release by actions on presynaptic μ receptors in the striatum and raphe nuclei.

Nausea and Vomiting

The well-known propensity of opioids to induce nausea and vomiting is probably triggered by μ receptors found in the area postrema on the floor of the fourth ventricle.

Bradycardia

The central vagal nuclei contain μ receptors, and the bradycardic effects of fentanyl may be blocked by microinjection of naloxone at those nuclei.

Immunosuppression

Lymphocytes have μ receptors, and chronic administration of opioids in animals can cause lymphoid atrophy and suppression of natural killer cell function.

Smooth Muscle Spasm

The widespread distribution of μ receptors on smooth muscle and in the enteric nervous system accounts for the constipation, urinary retention, and biliary spasm sometimes produced by these drugs.

Like μ opioid receptor binding, δ and κ receptor binding is quite widely distributed, but the relationship of receptor distribution to function has not been as well defined. κ opioid receptor mRNA is expressed in hypothalmus, and this may explain diuresis and other neuroendocrine activity of some κ-selective agonists *(36)*. δ opioid receptor mRNA is found in the dorsal horn and there is good evidence for δ mechanisms in spinal analgesia *(37)*. There is now a substantial amount of in vitro and in vivo data suggesting that δ agonists may function in an allosteric complex with μ receptors *(38)*. The interpretation of this information must be very cautious since some of the results on analgesia are highly dependent upon the ligands selected and the particular method of testing. Additional evidence for μ and δ interaction comes from the recent data on genetic knockouts.

MOLECULAR CLONING

The most convincing evidence for the existence of distinct opioid receptor classes comes from their molecular cloning and subsequent sequencing. Each class of receptors, μ, κ, and δ, has now been cloned from animal and human cDNA *(see* ref. *(39)* for review). Their genes are located on separate chromosomes, have multiple introns, and span large distances on the chromosome. For example, the μ receptor gene has 3 introns and likely spans more than 53 kb. Despite their large size and chromosomal separation, opioid receptor genes have similar genomic structures and there is approx 65% sequence homology between classes. There is also significant conservation of these genes between species; the protein sequence of human and rodent opioid receptors is 85–90% identical.

Recently, a receptor possessing a high degree of sequence homology to the opioid family of receptors has been cloned and named ORL-1 for opioid-like receptor *(40)*. Like the other members of the family it is a G protein-coupled receptor, however, it does not bind opioid agonists or antagonists with high affinity. An endogenous peptide ligand for ORL-1 was identified by two groups simultaneously and named orphanin FQ and nocipeptin; it is considered a new member of the EOP

Table 4
Experiments with μ, δ, and κ Knockout Mice [adapted from (46)]

Opioid	Response	Knockout		
		μ	δ	κ
Morphine (μ)	Spinal Analgesia	ABOLISHED	NO CHANGE	NO CHANGE
	Supraspinal Analgesia	ABOLISHED	–	–
	Reward	ABOLISHED	–	NO CHANGE
	Withdrawal	ABOLISHED	–	DECREASED
DPDPE (δ)	Spinal Analgesia	DECREASED	ABOLISHED	–
	Supraspinal Analgesia	DECREASED	–	–
U50488H[a] (κ)	Spinal Analgesia	NO CHANGE	–	ABOLISHED
	Supraspinal Analgesia	NO CHANGE	ABOLISHED	
	Hypolocomotion	–	–	DECREASED
	Dysphoria	–	–	DECREASED

[a]U50488H: *Trans*-3,4-dichloro-N-methyl-N-(2-[1-pyrrolidinyl]cyclohexyl)benzene acetamide.

family. Although the physiologic function of ORL-1 has yet to be determined, it does seem to be involved in both nociception and a variety of non pain-related functions *(41)*.

As stated previously, molecular approaches have also provided good evidence for functional differences between receptor classes. Knockout mice that lack particular opioid receptor genes have been generated, and antisense oligonucleotides have been used to produce "knockdown," i.e., greatly diminished expression of a specific gene product *(42,43)*. By deleting or decreasing expression of a particular opioid receptor it is possible to reduce or eliminate effects mediated by that receptor without disrupting agonist activity at other opioid binding sites. Knockdown of the μ receptor by injection of antisense oligonucleotide into the periaqueductal gray ablates morphine analgesia *(44)*. Knockout mice deficient in μ receptors do not respond to morphine with analgesia, reward, physical dependence, or the like, while some of the responses to δ and κ agonists are maintained *(45,46)*. Despite the fact that morphine is only moderately selective for μ receptors (perhaps 100-fold relative to κ or δ), the data from μ knockouts indicate that μ mechanisms must account for most of its important properties. The results of several experiments with μ, δ, and κ receptor knockouts are summarized in Table 4.

RECEPTOR SUBTYPES

The genes for the opioid receptors contain multiple introns, and it has been proposed that alternative splicing may yield subtypes of opioid receptors *(47,48)*. The existence of receptor subtypes is supported by a variety of pharmacological data using selective ligands (*see* Table 3). Following the observation of high affinity and low affinity sites for morphine agonists and antagonists, the subtypes, μ_1 and μ_2, were postulated. Using the noncompetitive antagonist, naloxonazine, it was possible to antagonize morphine's analgesic effect while sparing respiratory depression. This suggested that naloxonazine is selective for one subtype (μ_1 receptors), and analgesia is mediated by this subtype *(49)*. A μ_2 antagonist that spared analgesia while antagonizing respiratory depression would have been more helpful, but such a drug has not been developed. More recently, Pasternak has demonstrated incomplete cross-tolerance between morphine, morphine 6-glucuronide, and fentanyl (all nominal μ agonists) and suggested this is further evidence for multiple μ receptors. Selective antagonists have also been used to subtype δ and κ receptors *(50,51)*. At various times, as many as three μ, two δ, and four κ subtypes have been proposed. A large body of animal experimentation suggests that spinal and supraspinal opioid analgesia may involve different opioid receptor subtypes. Thus, μ_1, κ_3, and δ_1 agonists are said to produce mainly supraspinal analgesia, while μ_2, and δ_1 agonists produce

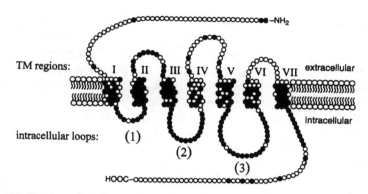

Fig. 2. Amino acid sequences of the cloned mouse κ and δ receptors and the rat μ receptor. Open circles are amino acids that differ among the three receptors, and closed circles are those that are identical. The seven transmembrane (TM) spanning regions (indicated by roman numerals) and the three intracellular loops are very similar in all three. (Reproduced from Blake et al. *(39)* with permission).

spinal analgesia (δ₂ agonists may produce both). It must be emphasized that these results are highly dependent upon the specific agonists selected for testing. The opioids approved for human experiments are not sufficiently selective to confirm these findings in man.

Unlike broad classes of opioid receptors, the existence of subtypes is controversial. The principal objection to the theory is that no cDNA corresponding to receptor subtype has been generated. It has also been argued that the pharmacological evidence for subtypes can be explained by opioid receptor dimerization (*see* ref. *(52)* for review). Direct evidence for dimerization of opioid receptors of different classes (heterodimers) has been generated *(53)*. Further, opioid receptor dimerization is consistent with the finding that several other G-protein coupled receptors exist as dimers. At present, debate continues regarding the existence of subtypes. It is not surprising that those who rely most heavily on the pharmacological data tend to believe in the existence of subtypes while those who place more weight on the molecular evidence do not.

RECEPTOR STRUCTURE

Opioid receptors belong to the superfamily of G-protein coupled receptors (GPCR) and the subfamily of rhodopsin receptors. They are all G_i/G_o protein coupled and possess a degree of homology to a subset of the other GPCR, including those for vasopressin, somatostatin, and substance P. The mRNA for opioid receptors ranges in size from 4.5 kb (δ) to 10–16 kb (μ) and final protein sequences contain between 372 (δ) and 398 (μ) amino acids.

The three classes of receptors share several structural features (depicted in Fig. 2): (1) an extracellular amino terminus with multiple glycosylation sites, (2) seven transmembrane spanning domains, and (3) four extracellular and four intracellular loops including a third extracellular loop with multiple amphipathic α-helixes, and a fourth intracellular loop at the carboxy terminus formed by the putative palmitoylation sites *(54)*. Opioid receptors share approx 65% sequence homology. The regions of greatest homology are the transmembrane domains and the intracellular loops; the regions of least homology are the N-terminus, the extracellular loops, and the C-terminus.

TRANSDUCTION MECHANISMS AND REGULATION OF RECEPTOR ACTIVITY

Second Messengers

Opioid receptors are negatively coupled through pertussis toxin-sensitive GTP-binding ("G_i/G_o-coupled") proteins. Through these G proteins they are coupled to adenylyl cyclase, receptor-operated

K^+ currents, and voltage-sensitive Ca^{2+} currents. Given the structural similarity between the opioid receptor classes, it is not surprising that they possess shared signaling pathways. In general, agonist occupancy of opioid receptors initiates intracellular events that inhibit neuronal activation *(55)*.

Traditionally, activation of the three cloned opioid receptors was thought to inhibit adenylyl cyclase activity, thus depressing cAMP formation. Although such inhibition does occur, the discovery of multiple adenylyl cyclases led to the observation that opioid receptor binding can sometimes produce activation *(56)*. The manner in which cAMP regulation by opioid receptors leads to the observed functional actions of opioids is an area of intense investigation but still poorly understood.

Opioids produce neuronal inhibition by complex effects on ion conductance *(57)*. For example, μ opioid-induced activation of inwardly rectifying K^+ channels increases K^+ conductance and causes hyperpolarization of postsynaptic neuronal membranes. This inhibits neuronal activity by increasing membrane threshold, thus preventing initiation and propagation of action potentials.

Activation of all three types of opioid receptor can inhibit presynaptic N-type and L-type Ca^{2+} channels. The resultant decrease in Ca^{2+} conductance has been demonstrated to inhibit the release of numerous neurotransmitters, including substance P, acetylcholine, norepinephrine, glutamate, GABA, and serotonin. Paradoxically, opioid receptor binding in vitro can transiently increase intracellular Ca^{2+}. This is thought to occur via increases in phospholipase C activity and increased formation of inositol 1,4,5-triphosphate *(58)*. Like the cAMP system, the mechanisms involved in opioid receptor Ca^{2+} modulation are extremely complex. Presumably, this complexity is important for differential regulation of opioid receptor effects between tissues and receptor classes.

Two other important intracellular messengers activated by opioid receptors are the mitogen-activated protein (MAP) kinases, ERK-1 and ERK-2 *(54)*. ERK stands for extracellular-signal-related kinase. These MAP kinases have been shown to be an important component of the pathway through which GPCR's regulate a variety of cellular events including growth and differentiation. Recently, spinal cord neuronal ERK has been shown to be involved in nociceptive-signal processing, highlighting another potential pathway through which opioid receptors may modulate transmission of pain *(59)*.

Receptor Desensitization and Down-Regulation

Tolerance upon repeated exposure to opioids can sometimes be profound, and it is sometimes a barrier to the use of these drugs in chronic painful conditions. In man and experimental animals there seem to be two types of tolerance, acute and chronic *(60)*. Acute tolerance (i.e., tachyphylaxis) can be demonstrated within hours, after a single high dose or a rapid infusion. It occurs in fairly restricted circumstances, and the clinical relevance remains to be proved. Chronic tolerance takes some time to develop (although morphine-pelleted rats and mice can become highly tolerant in a day or two), and it can last a very long time. Tolerance is increased by larger or more frequent dosing and decreased by co-administration of protein synthesis inhibitors. The speed of the changes in acute tolerance suggests rapid cellular autoregulatory responses, while chronic tolerance appears to be a much more permanent alteration in cellular structure and function.

Receptor phosphorylation, G-protein uncoupling, and receptor internalization may all play a role in tolerance *(61)*, although internalization may not be equally important for all opioids *(62)*. The effects of phosphorylation on receptor uncoupling (desensitization) and receptor internalization have been well-described for G-protein coupled receptors like the β adrenergic receptor, and similar mechanisms have been shown for opioid receptors. Agonist-induced phosphorylation of all three classes of opioid receptors has been demonstrated *(63–65)*. Although the precise amino acid residues of the opioid receptor that are phosphorylated have yet to be identified, the major sites appear to be in the intracellular carboxy tails. Several different types of kinases are thought to be involved, including protein kinase C, GPCR kinases, Ca^{2+}/calmodulin-dependent protein kinase II, protein kinase A, and ERK1/ERK2. The kinases involved in phosphorylation-mediated desensitization may be different for each receptor class, thus providing a potential mechanism of differential regulation between classes.

Recent work suggests that another key element in opioid tolerance is the activation of glutamate receptors, particularly the *N*-methyl D-aspartate (NMDA) type. Activation of NMDA receptors is followed by increases in intracellular calcium due to influx as well as mobilization of intracellular stores. Higher intracellular calcium, in turn, leads to kinase activation and tolerance *(66)*. These phenomena are the basis for clinical and experimental efforts to modulate opioid tolerance by administering NMDA antagonists such as dizocilpine (MK801) and dextromethorphan *(67,68)*.

While these post-translational modifications of the opioid receptor are likely to be important for acute changes in opioid receptor activity, transcriptional regulation seems more likely to be the explanation for sustained chronic tolerance. However, there is no consensus that transcriptional down-regulation occurs following chronic opioid exposure or even that agonist potency in the opioid system is receptor-density-dependent. The experimental evidence for transcriptional effects on opioid receptor signaling is presently incomplete. Interestingly, there is good evidence for altered opioid receptor gene expression following acute exposure to other classes of centrally-acting drugs including alcohol and cocaine *(69,70)*. Clearly, further studies will be necessary to elucidate the situations in which altered transcription contributes substantially to regulation of opioid activity.

REFERENCES

1. Dreser, H. (1898) Über die Wirkung einiger Derivate des Morphins auf die Athmung. *Archiv für die Gesamte Physiologie* **72**, 485–521.
2. Eisleb, O. and Schaumann, O. (1939) Dolantin, ein neuartiges Spasmolytikum und Analgetikum. *Deutsche Medizinische Wochenschrift* **65**, 967–968.
3. Parkhouse, J., Pleuvry, B. J., and Rees, J. M. H. (eds.) (1979) Analgesic Drugs. Blackwell Scientific Publications, Oxford, pp.18–19.
4. Pohl, J. (1915) Über das N-allylnorcodein, einen Antagonisten des Morphins. *Zeitschrift für Experimentale Pathologie und Therapie* **17**, 370–382.
5. Lasagna, L. and Beecher, H. K. (1954) The analgesic effectiveness of nalorphine and nalorphine-morphine combinations in man *J. Pharmacol. Exp. Ther.* **112**, 356–363.
6. Wikler, A., Fraser, H. F., and Isbell, H. (1953) N-allylnormorphine: effect of single doses and precipitation of acute "abstinence syndromes" during addiction to morphine, methadone or heroin in man (postaddicts). *J. Pharmacol. Exp. Ther.* **109**, 8–20.
7. Houde, R. W. and Wallenstein, S. L. (1956) Clinical studies of morphine-nalorphine combination. *Fed. Proc.* **15**, 440–441.
8. Keats, A. S. and Telford, J. (1966) Studies of analgesic drugs X. Respiratory effects of narcotic antagonists. *J. Pharmacol. Exp. Ther.* **151**, 126–132.
9. Martin, W. R. (1967) Opioid antagonists. *Pharmacol. Rev.* **19**, 463–521.
10. Martin, W. R., Eades, C. G., Thompson, J. A., Huppler, R. E., and Gilbert, P. E. (1976) The effects of morphine- and nalorphine-like drugs in the non-dependent and morphine-dependent chronic spinal dog. *J. Pharmacol. Exp. Ther.* **197**, 517–532.
11. Chien, C. C. and Pasternak, G. (1994) Selective antagonism of opioid analgesia by a sigma system. *J. Pharmacol. Exp. Ther.* **271**, 1583–1590.
12. Pfeiffer, A., Brantl, V., Herz, A., and Emrich, H. M. (1986) Psychotomimesis mediated by κ opiate receptors. *Science* **233**, 774–776.
13. Goodman, R. R. and Snyder, S. H. (1982) Autoradiographic localization of kappa opiate receptors to deep layers of the cerebral cortex may explain unique sedative and analgesic effects. *Life Sci.* **31**, 1291–1294.
14. Dershwitz, M., Rosow, C. E., DiBiase, P. M., and Zaslavsky, A. (1991) Comparison of the sedative effects of butorphanol and midazolam. *Anesthesiol.* **74**, 717–724.
15. Houde, R. W. (1979) Analgesic effectiveness of the narcotic agonist-antagonists. *Brit. J. Clin. Pharmacol.* **7**, 297S–308S.
16. Shook, J. E., Lemcke, P. K., Gehrig, C. A., Hruby, V. J., and Burks, T. F. (1989) Antidiarrheal properties of supraspinal mu and delta and peripheral mu, delta, and kappa opioid receptors: Inhibition of diarrhea without constipation. *J. Pharmacol. Exp. Ther.* **249**, 83–90.
17. Stanciu, C. and Bennet, J. R. (1974) Colonic response to pentazocine. *Brit. Med. J.* **1**, 312–313.
18. McCammon, R. L., Stoelting, R. K., and Madura, J. A. (1984) Effects of butorphanol, nalbuphine and fentanyl on intrabiliary tract dynamics. *Anesth. Analg.* **63**, 139–142.
19. Leander, J. D. (1983) A kappa opioid effect: Increased urination in the rat. *J. Pharmacol. Exp. Ther.* **224**, 89–94.
20. Salas, S. P., Roblero, J. S., Lopez, L. F., Tachibana, S., and Huidobro-Toro, J. P. (1992) [*N*-methyl-Tyr[1], *N*-methyl-Arg[7]-D-Leu[8]]Dynorphin-A-(1–8) Ethylamide, a stable dynorphin analog, produces diuresis by kappa-opiate receptor activation in the rat. *J. Pharmacol. Exp. Ther.* **262**, 979–986.
21. Hughes, J., Smith, T. W., Kosterlitz H. W., Fothergill, L. A., Morgan, B. A., and Morris, H. R. (1975) Identification of two related pentapeptides from the brain with potent opiate agonist activity. *Nature* **258**, 577–579.
22. Lord, J. A., Waterfield, A. A., Hughes, J., and Kosterlitz, H. W. (1977) Endogenous opioid peptides: multiple agonists and receptors. *Nature* **267**, 495–499.

23. Cox, B. M., Goldstein, A., and Li, C. H. (1976) Opioid activity of a peptide, β-lipotropin-(61–91), derived from β-lipotropin. *Proc. Natl. Acad. Sci. USA* **73,** 1821–1823.
24. Loh, H. H., Tseng L. F., Wei, W., and Li, C. H. (1976) β-Endorphin is a potent analgesic agent. *Proc. Natl Acad. Sci. USA* **73,** 2895–2898.
25. Cox, B. M., Opheim, K. E., Teschemacher, H., and Goldstein, A. (1975) A peptide-like substance from pituitary that acts like morphine; Purification and properties. *Life Sci.* **16,** 1777–1782.
26. Goldstein, A., Fischli, W., Lowney, L. I., Hunkapiller, M., and Hood, L. (1981) Porcine pituitary dynorphin: Complete amino acid sequence of the biologically active heptadecapeptide. *Proc. Natl. Acad. Sci. USA* **78,** 7219–7223.
27. Schulz, R., Wuster, M., and Herz, A. (1980) Pharmacological characterization of the epsilon opiate receptor. *J. Pharmacol. Exp. Ther.* **216,** 604–606.
28. Nock, B., Giordano, A. L., Cicero, T. J., and O'Connor, L. H. (1990) Affinity of drugs and peptides for U-69,593-sensitive and -insensitive kappa opiate binding sites: The U-69,593-insensitive site appears to be the beta endorphin-specific epsilon receptor. *J. Pharmacol. Exp. Ther.* **254,** 412–419.
29. Tseng, L. F. and Collins, K. A. (1991) Involvement of epsilon and kappa opioid receptors in inhibition of the tail-flick response induced by bremazocine in the mouse. *J. Pharmacol. Exp. Ther.* **259,** 330–336.
30. Bloomfield, S. S., Barden, T. P., and Mitchell, J. (1983) Metkephamid and meperidine analgesia after episiotomy. *Clin. Pharmacol. Ther.* **34,** 240–247.
31. McCarthy, L., Wetzel, M., Sliker, J. K., Eisenstein, T. K., and Rogers, T. J. (2001) Opioids, opioid receptors, and the immune response. *Drug Alcoh. Dep.* **62,** 111–123.
32. Pert, C. B. and Snyder, S. H. (1973) Opiate receptor: demonstration in nervous tissue. *Science* **179,** 1011–1014.
33. Simon, E. J., Hiller, J. M., and Edelman, I. (1973) Stereospecific binding of the potent narcotic analgesic [³H]etorphine to rat brain homogenate. *Proc. Natl. Acad. Sci. USA* **70,** 1947–1949.
34. Terenius, L. (1973) Characteristics of the 'receptor' for narcotic analgesics in synaptic plasma membrane fraction from rat brain. *Acta Pharmacol. Toxicol.* **33,** 377–384.
35. Stein, C. (1995) The control of pain in peripheral tissues by opioids. *N. Engl. J. Med.* **25,** 1685–1690.
36. Reisine, T. and Pasternak, G. (1996) Opioid analgesics and antagonists, in *Goodman and Gilman's The Pharmacological Basis of Therapeutics* (Hardman, J.G. and Limbird, L.E., eds.), McGraw-Hill, New York, pp. 521–555.
37. Yaksh, T. L. (1983) In vivo studies on spinal opiate receptor systems mediating antinociception. I. Mu and delta receptor profiles in the primate. *J. Pharmacol. Exp. Ther.* **226,** 303–316.
38. Schoffelmeer, A. N. M., Yao, Y. H., Gioannini, T. L., et al. (1990) Cross-linking of human [¹²⁵I]β-endorphin to opioid receptors in rat striatal membranes: Biochemical evidence for the existence of a mu/delta opioid receptor complex. *J. Pharmacol. Exp. Ther.* **253,** 419–426.
39. Blake, A. D., Bot, G., and Reisine, T. (1997) Molecular pharmacology of the cloned opioid receptors, in *Molecular Neurobiology of Pain: Progress in Pain Research and Management Volume 9* (Borsook, D., ed.) IASP Press, Seattle, WA, pp. 259–273.
40. Meunier, J., Mouledous, L., and Topham, C. M. (2000) The nociceptin (ORL-1) receptor: molecular cloning and functional architecture. *Peptides* **21,** 893–900.
41. Reinscheid, R. K., Nothacker, H., and Civelli, O. (2000) The orphanin FQ/nociceptin gene: structure, tissue distribution of expression and functional implications obtained from knockout mice. *Peptides* **21,** 901–906.
42. Keiffer, B. L. (1997) Molecular aspect of opioid receptors, in *Handbook of Experimental Pharmacology,* Vol 130 (Dickenson, A. and Besson, J. M., eds.), Springer-Verlag, Berlin, pp. 281–303.
43. Law, P. Y., Wong, Y. H., and Loh, H. H. (1999) Mutational analysis of the structure and function of opioid receptors. *Biopolymers* **51,** 440–455.
44. Rossi, G. C., Pan, Y. X., Cheng, J., and Pasternak, G. W. (1994) Blockade of morphine analgesia by an antisense oligodeoxynucleotide against the mu receptor. *Life Sci.* **54,** PL375–PL379.
45. Matthes, H .W. D., Maldonado, R., Simonin, F., et al. (1996) Loss of morphine-induced analgesia, reward effect and withdrawal symptoms in mice lacking the μ-opioid-receptor gene. *Nature* **383,** 819–823.
46. Kieffer, B. L. (1999) Opioids: first lessons from knockout mice. *Trends Pharmacol. Sci.* **20,** 19–26.
47. Pasternak, G. W. (1993) Pharmacological mechanisms of opioid analgesics. *Clin. Neuropharmacol.* **16,** 1–18.
48. Pasternak, G. W. and Standifer, K. M. (1995) Mapping of opioid receptors using antisense oligodeoxynucleotides: correlating their molecular biology and pharmacology. *Trends Pharm. Sci.* **16,** 344–350.
49. Ling, G. S. F., Spiegel, K., Lockhart, S. H., and Pasternak, G. W. (1985) Separation of opioid analgesia from respiratory depression: evidence for different receptor mechanisms. *J. Pharmacol. Exp. Ther.* **232,** 149–155.
50. Sofuoglu, M., Portoghese, P. S., and Takemori, A. E. (1991) Differential antagonism of delta opioid agonists by naltrindole and its benzofuran analogue (NTB) in mice: evidence for delta opioid receptor subtypes. *J. Pharmacol. Exp. Ther.* **257,** 676–680.
51. Portoghese, P. S., Sultana, M., Nagase, H., and Takemori, A. E. (1992) A highly selective delta-1 opioid receptor antagonist: 7-benzylidenaltrexone. *Eur. J. Pharmacol.* **218,** 195–196.
52. Jordan, B. A., Cvejic, S., and Devi, L. (2000) Opioids and their complicated receptor complexes. *Neuropsychopharmacol* **23,** S5–S18.
53. Wessendorf, M. W. and Dooyema, J. (2001) Coexistence of kappa- and delta-opioid receptors in rat spinal cord axons. *Neurosci. Lett.* **298,** 151–154.
54. Law, P. Y. and Loh, H. H. (1999) Regulation of opioid receptor activities. *J. Pharm. Exp. Ther.* **289,** 607–624.
55. North, R. A. (1986) Opioid receptor types and membrane ion channels. *Trends Neurosci.* **9,** 114–117.

56. Law, P. Y., Wong, Y. H., and Loh, H. (2000) Molecular mechanisms and regulation of opioid receptor signaling. *Ann. Rev. Pharmacol. Toxicol.* **40,** 389–430.

57. Duggan, A. W. and North, R. A. (1983) Electrophysiology of opioids. *Pharmacol. Rev.* **35,** 219–282.

58. Smart, D. and Lambert, D. G. (1996) δ-opioids stimulate insositol 1,4,5-trisphosphate formation, and so mobilize Ca^{2+} from intracellular stores, in undifferentiated NG108-15 cells. *J. Neurochem.* **66,** 1462–1467.

59. Ji, R. R., Baba, H., Brenner, G. J., and Woolf, C. J. (1999) Nociceptive specific activation of ERK in spinal neurons contributes to pain hypersensitivity. *Nat. Neurosci.* **2,** 1114–1119.

60. Rosow, C. E. (1987) Acute and chronic tolerance: Relevance for clinical practice, in Problems of Drug Dependence. Research Monograph 76, National Institute on Drug Abuse, U.S. Government Printing Office, Washington, D.C., pp. 29–34.

61. Law, P. Y., Wong, Y. H., and Loh, H. H. (2000) Molecular mechanisms and regulation of opioid receptor signaling. *Ann. Rev. Pharmacol. Toxicol.* **40,** 389–430.

62. Keith, D. E., Murray, S. R., Zaki, P. A., et al. (1996) Morphine activates opioid receptors without causing their rapid internalization. *J. Biol. Chem.* **271,** 19,021–19,024.

63. Pei, C., Kieffer, B. L., Lefkowitz, R. J., and Freedman, N. J. (1995) Agonist-dependent phosphorylation of the mouse delta-opioid receptor: involvement of G-protein-coupled receptor kinases but not protein kinase C. *Mol. Pharmacol.* **48,** 173–177.

64. Arden, J. R., Segredo, V., Wang, A., Lameh, H., and Sadee, W. (1995) Phosphorylation and agonist-specific intracellular trafficking of an epitope-tagged μ-opioid receptor expressed in HEK293 cells. *J. Neurochem.* **65,** 1636–1645.

65. Appleyard, S. M., Patterson, T. A., Jin, W., and Chavkin, C. (1997) Agonist-induced phosphorylation of the κ-opioid receptor. *J. Neurochem.* **69,** 2405–2412.

66. Mao, J. (1999) NMDA and opioid receptors: their interactions in antinociception, tolerance, and neuroplasticity. *Brain Res. Rev.* **30,** 289–304.

67. Trujillo, K. A. and Akil, H. (1991) Inhibition of morphine tolerance and dependence by the NMDA receptor antagonist MK801. *Science* **251,** 85–87.

68. Elliott, K., Minami N., Kolesnikov, Y. A., Pasternak, G. W., and Inturrisi, C. E. (1994) The NMDA receptor antagonists, LY274614 and MK801, and the nitric oxide synthase inhibitor, NG-nitro-L-arginine, attenuate analgesic tolerance to the mu opioid morphine but not to kappa opioids. *Pain* **56,** 69–75.

69. Winkler, A., Buzas, B., Siems, W. E., Heder, G., and Cox, B. M. (1998) Effect of ethanol drinking on the gene expression of opioid receptors, enkephalinase, and angiotensin-converting enzyme in two inbred mice strains. *Alcoh. Clin. Exp. Res.* **22,** 1262–1271.

70. Azaryan, A. V., Coughlin, L. J., Buzas, B., Clock, B. J., and Cox, B. M. (1996) Effect of chronic cocaine treatment on μ- and δ-opioid receptor mRNA levels in dopaminergically innervated brain regions. *J. Neurochem.* **66,** 443–448.

25

Local Anesthetics

Ging Kuo Wang

INTRODUCTION

Local anesthetics (LAs) are drugs primarily utilized in clinic settings to induce local anesthesia. The term *local anesthesia*, unlike general anesthesia, is defined as loss of sensation within a confined region without loss of the patient's consciousness. LAs are purposely used for relief of pain and induction of numbness during surgical procedures and are normally applied by local injection. Selected LAs such as lidocaine may also be used intravenously or taken orally as antiarrhythmics, anticonvulsants, and antiepileptics. The first report of the use of a LA by Carl Koller appeared in 1884 *(1)*. For an operation on glaucoma, Koller applied the only naturally occurring LA, cocaine, topically on the cornea. Cocaine is isolated from the leaves of the coca shrub, *Erythroxylon coca*. His discovery of cocaine as a surface LA for relatively painless surgery was followed by the steady development of novel synthetic LAs spanning the last century. Along the course of this development came various new techniques of local/regional anesthesia.

Traditional LAs can be categorized into two major types, on the basis of structure. The ester-type LAs include benzocaine, procaine, cocaine, and tetracaine, and the amide-type LAs include mepivacaine, lidocaine (*see* Scheme 1 diagram on next page), ropivacaine, bupivacaine, and etidocaine. Lidocaine and bupivacaine are the two most commonly used LAs; both are amide-type compounds, which are much more resistant than ester-type compounds to hydrolysis. In general, traditional LAs consist of a phenyl "hydrophobic tail," an intermediate ester- or amide-containing linker, and a tertiary amine "hydrophilic head." The tertiary amine can be protonated and has a pK_a of ~7.5–9.0 in an aqueous solution with both neutral and protonated forms present. Benzocaine ($pK_a = 3.5$), which does not have a tertiary amine component, is an exception to this rule, and therefore is neutral in aqueous solution, with poor solubility. This neutral drug generally is applied as a topical cream or aerosol formulation.

The primary target of LAs is the voltage-gated Na^+ channel, which is responsible for the generation of action potentials in excitable membranes. LAs also interact with many other types of ion channels (e.g., *2*), and may cause undesirable side effects, particularly in cardiac tissues. Mammalian voltage-gated Na^+ channels exist in different isoforms in various excitable tissues such as skeletal muscles, cardiac tissues, central nervous system (CNS), and peripheral nervous system (PNS) *(3)*. In addition, multiple major isoforms are present in CNS and PNS. Some of these neuronal Na^+ channels are sensitive to tetrodotoxin (TTX) and some are resistant to TTX. TTX is a potent neurotoxin isolated from puffer fish, and has been an invaluable tool for the identification of various neuronal Na^+ channel isoforms. As for differential TTX sensitivity, could the intrinsic potencies of LAs on various neuronal Na^+ channel isoforms also be different? This question remains to be answered. If true, it would then be feasible to target particular isoforms with specific LA drugs.

From: *Contemporary Clinical Neuroscience: Neural Mechanisms of Anesthesia*
Edited by: Joseph F. Antognini et al. © Humana Press Inc., Totowa, NJ

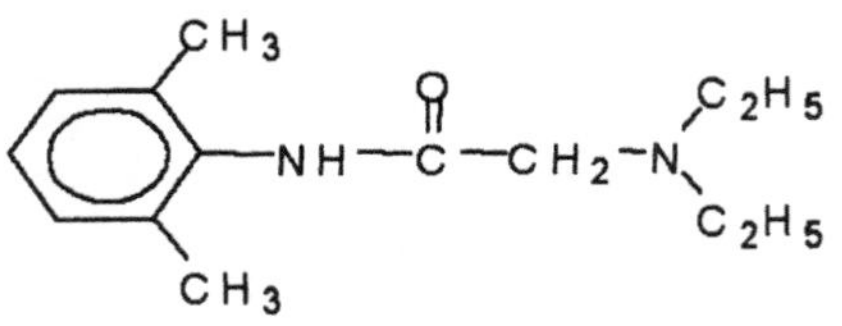

Scheme 1

During the last 25 yr, numerous attempts have been made to develop novel long-acting LAs but, so far, with limited success *(4)*. The aging of the population appears to have increased the demand for new long-acting and ultra long-acting LAs in clinic care. A detailed understanding of the LA receptor in the voltage-gated Na+ channel will be helpful in meeting this demand. The main objective of this chapter is to review our current knowledge of the underlying mechanisms of the LA action with particular emphases on the mapping of the LA receptor in the voltage-gated Na+ channel and on receptor interactions with LAs at the cellular and molecular levels.

CLINICAL APPLICATIONS OF LAS

LAs induce local or regional anesthesia via various injection routes on the basis of the surgical procedure and/or on the requirements of pain management. Among the major techniques that have been developed are surface/infiltration anesthesia; intravenous regional anesthesia; somatic nerve blockade, such as brachial plexus block; and neuraxial blockade (i.e., subarachnoid and extra-dural blockade), such as epidural anesthesia and spinal anesthesia. When injected near specific nerve regions, traditional LAs block action potentials in the nerve conduction pathway that includes pain-related afferent fibers. LAs invariably also block other types of nerve fibers, including motor efferent fibers. Differential block of afferent versus efferent fibers is highly desirable, and such an attribute of LAs, if present, would be beneficial for most patients under local anesthesia. Only bupivacaine and ropivacaine seem to possess a noticeable differential block in practice. Rationales are being provided to develop pain-selective LAs that target the specific Na+ channel isoforms in the afferent nerve fibers or their cell bodies, and this search may identify ideal LAs for pain management in the future *(5)*. Such ideal LAs for pain management, if discovered, would possess desirable attributes such as selective and reversible blockade of sensory nerve fibers but with minimal effects on the motor fibers, heart, and CNS.

The duration of local anesthesia varies greatly depending on the specific LAs used. Benzocaine, chloroprocaine, and procaine are considered to be the short-acting LAs; lidocaine, mepivacaine, and prilocaine the intermediate-acting LAs; and bupivacaine, levo-*(S)*-bupivacaine, ropivacaine, tetracaine, and etidocaine the long-acting LAs. In addition to the intrinsic binding affinities of LA drugs to the Na+ channel, other variables also strongly influence the relative duration of local anesthesia. These include the volume and concentration of drug, the lipophilicity and the pK_a of drugs, the pH of the drug solution, repeated injections, the presence of vasoconstrictors, and the precision of drug injection.

LOCAL ANESTHESIA AND THE VOLTAGE-GATED NA+ CHANNEL

What is the evidence that the neuronal Na+ channel is the primary target of LAs? The block of compound action potentials in frog sciatic nerve fibers by LAs, which was reported very early *(6,7)*, suggests that there is an inverse relationship between action potentials and local anesthesia. These findings enforce the concept that local anesthesia is due to the loss of excitability of nerve fibers. Taylor *(8)* later demonstrated that procaine blocked the propagation of action potentials in squid axons by blocking voltage-gated Na+ channels. Together, these experiments established that the primary mechanism of local anesthesia is via the block of neuronal sodium channels in excitable membranes.

Mammalian voltage-gated Na$^+$ channels are normally activated at a threshold of around -50 mV, and the probability of channels being open is maximal around $+20$ mV. At the single-channel level, the time course of Na$^+$ channel activation is strongly voltage dependent. The open probability during depolarization rises slowly at the threshold and becomes rather fast at the more positive potentials. In contrast, the open Na$^+$ channels inactivate rapidly, with a dwell time that is generally one millisecond or less. Unlike the activation process, the time course of the inactivation of the open Na$^+$ channel is not voltage dependent *(9)*. At the level of macroscopic currents, Na$^+$ currents rise (activate) and decay (inactivate) with overlapping time courses, as would be expected from an ensemble of currents from single channels *(10)*. Detailed kinetic analyses of macroscopic Na$^+$ currents in the presence of various LAs reveal complicated pharmacological profiles under voltage-clamp conditions.

First, LAs reduce peak Na$^+$ currents during the test potential a few minutes after external perfusion of the drug solution at the holding potential. Experimentally the holding potential is usually set at ≤ -100 mV. This reduction in peak current is dose dependent, and the potency ranking of various LAs derived from their dose-response curves correlate well with the relative duration of local anesthesia they elicit in vivo. This LA block of the Na$^+$ channel at resting potential is termed "tonic block." Some LAs also may delay the activation time course and/or accelerate the fast decaying time course (inactivation). However, the level of modification in current kinetics is generally small and is difficult to quantify in native Na$^+$ channels without mathematical modeling *(11,12)*.

Second, most LAs are found to shift the apparent steady-state inactivation curve (h$_\infty$) to the hyperpolarizing direction. Steady-state inactivation measures the availability of resting Na$^+$ channels at various prepulse voltages at which Na$^+$ channels normally do not open *(13)*. The measurement involves a varying prepulse voltage from -120 mV to -40 mV with a duration of 100 ms. Apparently, the resting Na$^+$ channels can enter their inactivated state directly, without opening, during this 100-ms conditioning pulse. This closed-channel inactivation is strongly voltage dependent, unlike the open-channel inactivation *(9)*. A shift of the steady-state inactivation curve by LAs toward the hyperpolarizing direction has significant physiological consequences. To begin with, if the h$_\infty$ is indeed shifted by LAs upon binding, a larger fraction of Na$^+$ channels with LAs bound will be in their inactivated state at the resting potential and therefore will be unavailable to carry currents for the generation of action potentials. Another implication is that the inactivated state of the Na$^+$ channel binds more strongly than other channel states. An elaboration of this concept has evolved into a generalized modulated receptor hypothesis envisioned by Hille *(14)* and by Hondeghem and Katzung *(15)*. They proposed that different states of Na$^+$ channels have different binding affinities for LAs, and that the affinity of the inactivated state is the highest. One obvious drawback in the h$_\infty$ measurement is its rigid two-pulse protocol. A fixed prepulse duration of 100 ms may be not sufficient for the binding of various LAs to reach steady state. This insufficient duration in turn will lead to an underestimation of the degree of shift in the h$_\infty$ curve, particularly by drugs with slower on-rate kinetics. Hence, several LAs do not shift the h$_\infty$ curve according to their intrinsic potency *(14)*. A higher drug concentration will reduce the time to reach steady-state binding but may also eliminate the current for the h$_\infty$ measurement. A longer prepulse duration will allow the binding of selected LAs to reach steady state. Unfortunately, such a pulse protocol also induces a slow inactivation gating process, which progressively reduces the peak current. The slow inactivation occurs when Na$^+$ channels are depolarized for prolonged period of time (i.e., in seconds; *10*). Upon repolarization, Na$^+$ channels recover from their slow inactivated states, but with a slower time course (i.e., in seconds).

Third, repetitive pulses produce an additional block of Na$^+$ currents in the presence of LAs. This additional block of Na$^+$ currents is termed "use-dependent" or "frequency-dependent block," with the two terms used interchangeably. The use-dependent block by LAs may be physiologically important for pain therapy, as many afferent fibers fire action potentials at a high frequency, particularly in the pathological state ($\sim$20 Hz; *[16]*). In theory, LAs with a potent use-dependent attribute will be more effective than LAs without this attribute in blocking the high-frequency abnormal firings of sensory afferent fibers. The interpretation of the use-dependent block within the framework of the modulated

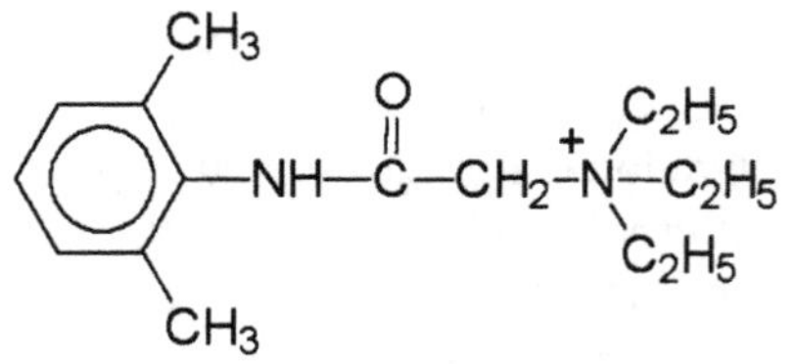

CH₃ ... (chemical structure)

QX-314

Scheme 2

receptor hypothesis is that the inactivated channels populated during repetitive pulses have the highest affinity for LAs. Each pulse therefore enhances an additional fraction of Na$^+$ channels to enter their inactivated states by binding to LAs until steady state conditions are reached. In fact, the modulated receptor hypothesis readily predicts such a use-dependent block phenotype, as long as the drug is dissociated from its receptor with a time constant that is slower than the frequency of the pulse applied. Although the hypothesis that the inactivated state plays a central role in the use-dependent block has been seriously investigated (17,18), the evidence remains inconclusive. The activation process in channel opening may also be essential to the underlying mechanism of the use-dependent block by LAs after repetitive pulses (19,20). Alternatively, LA binding may induce channels to occupy a slow inactivated state, which in turn results in the use-dependent blocking phenomenon (21,22).

A variety of ion channels and receptors other than voltage-gated Na$^+$ channels are also sensitive to LAs. Examples include voltage-gated K$^+$ channels (2), voltage-gated Ca^{2+} channels (23), and ligand-gated channels (24). Under physiological conditions, these proteins may become the unintended targets and may manifest some side effects of LAs both in the CNS and PNS, and in various organs, including the heart and blood vessels. Different LAs may also have different secondary targets and different clinical profiles. For example, in addition to being an LA and a central stimulant, cocaine is a strong vessel constrictor (25).

THE TOPOLOGY OF THE LA RECEPTOR USING DRUGS AS MOLECULAR PROBES

Where is the LA receptor located within the Na$^+$ channel? The short answer to this question is that it is located within the pore region, and is accessible via the intracellular mouth, and probably also via various hydrophobic alleys of the channel protein (for review, *see* ref. 26). Strichartz (27) who used QX-314, a quaternary ammonium (QA) derivative of lidocaine with an additional N-ethyl group as a molecular probe, first addressed this question. He found that QX-314, which bears a permanent positive charge, is inactive when applied externally to a myelinated nerve fiber. However, when QX-314 (*see* Scheme 2 diagram above) is applied intracellularly to the nerve fiber, it behaves as a potent Na$^+$ channel blocker, but only when the channel is first activated by depolarization. Without the channel opening, the site where the LA receptor is located seems inaccessible to QX-314. The results of QX-314 studies and their subsequent interpretations provide crucial information on the relative location of the LA receptor within the Na$^+$ channel permeation pathway (26; *see* Fig. 1). First, a narrow region, previously characterized as a *selectivity filter* near the external surface of the pore, allows Na$^+$ ions to enter the pore but excludes QX-314 ions. Second, an activation gate near the internal surface of the pore modulates the access of the QX-314 molecule within the pore region. Third, the LA receptor, which is located within the inner vestibule of the Na$^+$ channel pore, is accessible to the charged LA drug through the inner mouth of the channel. This general topological arrangement of the Na$^+$ channel (i.e., the selectivity filter, the internal vestibule, and the activation gate) parallels that of the voltage-gated K$^+$ channel, and appears to be well conserved during the evolution of voltage-gated ion channels (26). In support of this general scheme is the finding that raising the external Na$^+$ ion

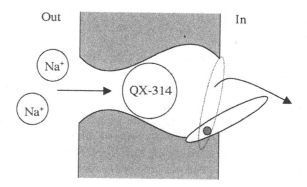

Fig. 1. A cartoon showing the block of the Na$^+$ channel permeation pathway by the lidocaine derivative QX-314. External Na$^+$ ions traverse the channel first through a narrow external aperture named the "selectivity filter," then the internal vestibule and finally the activation gate near the internal mouth. The activation gate (dashed bar) opens when the membrane is depolarized. Permanently charged QX-314 is accessible to the Na$^+$ pore only from the internal mouth and blocks the channel by binding to an LA/QA receptor located within the internal vestibule, perhaps near the selectivity filter region.

concentration reduces the local anesthetic affinity, as if in-flowing Na$^+$ ions remove the QA ions within their path *(28)*. This LA blocking profile is thus similar to the QA block of the K$^+$ channels observed by Armstrong *(29)*.

As tertiary amine-containing compounds, LAs in theory may bind to their receptor in their protonated forms and/or in their neutral uncharged forms. Is the charged form of LAs the active form that binds with the LA receptor? A controversy in 1960 centered on the relative potency of the neutral form versus the protonated form of a tertiary amine LA such as procaine or lidocaine. After reviewing numerous studies, Narahashi and Frazier *(30)* concluded: "It is difficult to exclude the possibility that the uncharged form contributes slightly (e.g., 10%) to the total blockage, the major part of the blockage being caused by the charged form." To this day, their conclusion that the charged form is at least ten times more potent than the neutral form of a tertiary amine LA remains valid. The early assertion that the neutral form is more active than the protonated form can be attributed to the fact that, when the external pH is high, the neutral form of an LA is responsible for the increase in concentration of the LA within the cytoplasm. Only the neutral form can enter the membrane phase of the nerve fiber; the LA then equilibrates into a charged form within the cytoplasm. Hence, the apparent potency of LA drugs increases significantly when the external solution is made more alkaline (i.e., pH $\geq$ 8).

For studies of structure/activity relationships of LAs, inhibition of Na$^+$ currents by various drug concentrations can be measured directly under voltage clamp conditions, and the 50% inhibitory concentration (IC$_{50}$) and Hill coefficient values can be estimated by the dose-response curve. The relative LA binding affinity (IC$_{50}$) can be compared at various voltages with this method. Courtney and Strichartz *(31)* reviewed the roles of the aromatic group, the intermediate linker, and the tertiary amine in LA potency. Unfortunately, the exact contribution of an individual component can not be easily separated from that of the entire LA molecule, from the pK$_a$ of the drug, and from the membrane partition coefficient of the drug. For such information, a series of closely related homologs are needed, e.g., mepivacaine, ropivacaine, and bupivacaine. In this bupivacaine-related series, the potency order is bupivacaine > ropivacaine > mepivacaine, which implies that the N-butyl group (i.e., bupivacaine) interacts more favorably than the N-propyl (ropivacaine) and N-methyl group (mepivacaine) to the Na$^+$ channel. However, these closely related drugs still have different pK$_a$ values and different membrane partition coefficients; both physical properties may make some contribution to their different potencies in the assay.

THE TOPOLOGY OF THE LA RECEPTOR USING TOXINS AS MOLECULAR PROBES

Neurotoxins may also be useful probes for determining the topology of the LA receptor. Batrachotoxin (BTX), a steroidal alkaloid isolated from the skin of *Phylobates* frogs, is one of the most toxic small molecules. In fact, some natives in South America once prepared poisonous blowdarts from these frogs. This toxin hampers both the fast and slow inactivation and therefore keeps the Na^+ channel open throughout the prolonged depolarization. In addition, the voltage dependence of the Na^+ channel activation is shifted toward the hyperpolarizing direction by 30–50 mV. As a result, Na^+ channels are being activated even around the resting membrane potential. In animals the consequences of poisoning by BTX are convulsions, paralysis, and death. Because BTX inhibits the fast inactivation of the Na^+ channel, it also may eliminate the high affinity binding of LAs toward the inactivated state. Indeed, a significant reduction in the LA binding affinity by BTX has been recognized, and such an effect can be explained by an allosteric mechanism between the BTX receptor and the LA receptor *(32)*.

For detailed single channel analysis, Moczydlowski et al. *(33)* first studied the LA block in planar lipid bilayers incorporated with BTX-modified Na^+ channels. This method can be used to obtain the drug-on (LA association) and drug-off (LA dissociation) rate constants at various voltages (e.g., *28*). Cautions should be taken in the interpretation using this assay because the presence of BTX may affect the LA binding. When possible, experiments should be extended to native Na^+ channels for confirmation. One puzzling phenomenon from this type of study is the alteration of the stereoselectivity of cocaine (and bupivacaine) in the open BTX-modified Na^+ channel from a stereoselectivity ratio (−/+ form) of ~0.6 in native channels to a ratio of more than 20 *(34)*. The mechanism(s) and the structural basis for such a drastic alteration in LA stereoselectivity may provide important clues for our understanding of the topology of the LA receptor.

The detailed topology of the LA receptor in the presence of BTX has also been examined in bilayers and/or in cultured cells. The results indicate that one cocaine molecule can block one open Na^+ channel; therefore, there is probably only one receptor per Na^+ channel *(28)*. The LA receptor clearly contains two sub-binding sites: one is the hydrophobic binding domain, which interacts with the aromatic ring of these compounds, and the other is the hydrophilic binding domain, which interacts with the tertiary amine component. A second large hydrophobic binding domain for bupivacaine homologs and for various QA compounds may also be present within the LA receptor *(35–37)*. Another very useful method of ranking the LA potency is to measure the LA displacement of the radioactive [3H]-BTX binding in synaptosomal or skeletal T-tubule preparations. These assays work well because LAs paradoxically inhibit BTX binding in a "competitive" manner and the inhibition is dose dependent, perhaps because BTX and cocaine are mutually exclusive from binding to the resting and to the inactivated Na^+ channel *(38)*. This method can be used to screen a large number of different LA drugs in a given time under identical conditions *(32)*. The LA receptor may accommodate a large variety of compounds other than traditional LAs, e.g., anticonvulsants, antiarrhythmics, antidepressants, antiepileptics, tranquilizers, calcium antagonists, and barbiturates *(39,40)*. The presence of two relatively large hydrophobic binding domains in the LA receptor also may explain why this receptor can accommodate various drugs for binding. The relative LA potency measured by this binding assay correlates well with the IC_{50} measured under voltage-clamp conditions, and with the ranking order of the block duration measured during local anesthesia in vivo.

THE TOPOLOGY OF THE LA RECEPTOR REVEALED BY SITE-DIRECTED MUTAGENESIS

The voltage-gated Na^+ channel is a glycosylated membrane protein with one large α-subunit and one or two smaller β-subunits (β1 and β2). The α-subunit protein contains about 2000 amino acids with four transmembrane repeats (domains 1–4; Fig. 2), each with six transmembrane segments

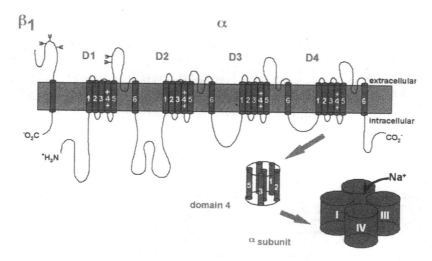

Fig. 2. Putative transmembrane topology of α- and β1-subunits of the Na+ channel. Both subunits are glycosylated. The α-subunit has four repeated domains (D1–D4), each with six transmembrane segments (S1–S6). Multiple positive charges from lysine and arginine residues are present within the S4 segment. The four domains likely arrange in a four fold symmetry about the axis to form a functional channel. The β2-subunit is not shown.

(segments 1–6). At present, nine different α-subunit isoforms of the voltage-gated Na+ channel gene family have been identified (Na$_v$1.1–Na$_v$1.9; *[3]*). Heterologous expression of various Na+ channel clones in mammalian and *Xenopus* oocyte expression systems indicates that the α-subunit alone forms functional Na+ channels with kinetic and pharmacological profiles comparable to those of native Na+ channels. Coexpression of the β-subunit with the α-subunit increases the level of expression in general and somewhat modulates the gating kinetics of Na+ channels *(41)*.

The precise location of the LA receptor within the α-subunit primary structure was first addressed by Ragsdale et al. *(42)*, who found that substitution of several residues within D4–S6 with an alanine residue drastically reduced the LA binding affinities. They proposed that a phenylalanine (F) and a tyrosine (Y) together in the middle of the α-helical D4-S6 segment (Fig. 3; underlined) form a LA binding site; the phenylalanine residue interacts with the charged tertiary amine group, whereas the tyrosine residue interacts with the aromatic group *(43)*. The important roles of these two residues in LA binding have been confirmed, although the contact points of LAs remain unresolved *(44)*. A subsequent study from Catterall's laboratory found that residues in D3-S6 affect the LA affinities significantly, again using the alanine-substitution approach *(45)*. Using a lysine-substitution approach, we have found that both D1-S6 and D3-S6 segments modulate the LA binding affinities (Fig. 3; *[46–47]*). Hence, multiple S6 segments may together form a single LA receptor site. If this is so, the different S6 segments must align in close proximity, so that amino acids residing at different S6 segments may contact the small LA molecule. However, these contact points may not be static and may depend on the resting, open, or inactivated state of the Na+ channel. The fact that multiple S6 segments modulate LA binding may be critical for our understanding of LA action, and this may form the structural basis for the complicated LA blocking profiles. Sunami et al. *(48)* reported that the Na+ channel selectivity filter also regulates LA binding. This region may represent the upper part of the internal vestibule and may be structurally adjacent to the LA receptor.

Unexpectedly, many of the residues critical for LA binding affinities are also critical for the BTX action. In particular, lysine substitutions at the D1-S6, D3-S6, and D4-S6 (Fig. 3; in bold) render these mutant channels completely resistant to BTX at 5 μ*M (38,47,49,50)*. The fact that these residues are important for both BTX and LA actions has several implications. First, it is likely that the

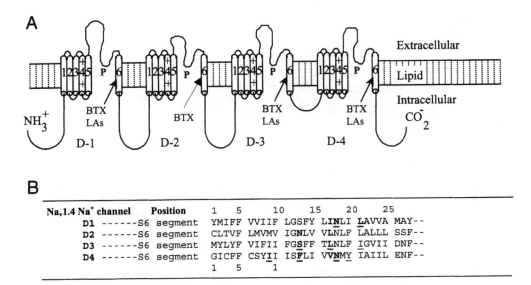

Fig. 3. Putative locations of the LA receptor and the BTX receptor within the Na$^+$ channel α-subunit. **(A)** The positions of residues critical for LA and BTX binding affinities are clustered at the middle of the S6 segment. This region also may form the lining of the internal vestibule of the Na$^+$ permeation pathway in a state-dependent manner. The selectivity filter is located at the P region, which is situated within the S5–S6 linkers. **(B)** Residues within the S6 segments of the rat skeletal muscle Na$^+$ channel α-subunit (Na$_v$1.4) are listed from positions 1–28. Residues critical for BTX binding affinities are shown in bold, whereas residues critical for LA binding affinities are underlined. Two residues at D2-S6 appear to be important for the BTX action but not for the LA action (Wang, S.-Y., and Wang, G. K., unpublished observation).

receptors for BTX and for LAs are overlapped in a state-dependent manner. For the resting state, only one ligand can bind with one channel, whereas for the open state, both ligands can bind simultaneously. This would explain why no block of cocaine was found in the BTX-bound resting channel, since these two ligands are mutually exclusive. In contrast, a time-dependent block developed upon channel opening, since the cocaine binding site becomes available in the open state *(34,38)*. Second, the receptors for BTX and LAs must change their conformation during state transitions, as binding of BTX and LAs with the Na$^+$ channel is highly state dependent. This implies a flexibility of the binding site. Such flexibility might explain why there is little stereoselectivity for LA drugs in native Na$^+$ channels. Receptor flexibility also implies a possible induced fit between ligands and their binding site. Third, bound BTX may alter the stereoselectivity of LAs *in situ*. An overlapping receptor site will bring bound BTX very close to the bound LA *in situ*. Under such conditions, the physical structure of BTX may result in changes in the LA stereoselectivity. The binding affinity of the (−) form of cocaine is 20× higher than that of the (+) form because of the structural hindrance of BTX *in situ*. This would explain the puzzling phenomenon induced by BTX in the altered LA stereoselectivity *(34)*.

HILLE'S MODULATED RECEPTOR HYPOTHESIS AT THE MOLECULAR LEVEL

Hille *(14)* proposed a generalized modulated receptor hypothesis to explain the complicated action of LAs at the macroscopic current level. His hypothesis includes two principal ideas. First, the configuration of the LA receptor is state dependent. Apparently, this LA receptor within the Na$^+$ channel changes its conformation during state transitions from the resting state to the open state and then to the inactivated state. Second, the binding affinity of LAs is state dependent. The inactivated state has the highest affinity for LAs, and is stabilized by the bound drug. Hille's modulated receptor

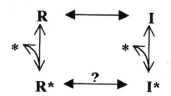

Scheme 3

hypothesis has gained wide support over the last two decades because of its simplicity and because these ideas parallel that of the conformation-dependent binding affinities of allosteric enzymes (51).

One of the defining characteristics of the modulated receptor hypothesis is the prediction of an equilibrium shift in the h_∞ curve by LAs. If LA binding stabilizes the inactivated state of the Na^+ channel, the h_∞ curve should be shifted towards the hyperpolarizing direction. An accurate measurement of this equilibrium shift between the resting state (R^*) (* designated as LAs, *see* Scheme 3 diagram above) and the inactivated state (I^*) by LAs is difficult because of the non-steady state conditions during the measurement. In theory, the apparent affinity for LAs ($1/K_{app}$) will depend strongly on the apportionment of channels between resting and inactivated states (comprising fractions h and 1 − h, respectively; *[52]*). At equilibrium,

$$1/K_{app} = (h/K_R) + (1-h)/K_I \tag{1}$$

where K_R is the resting-state affinity and K_I is the inactivated-state affinity. Even without equilibrium shift induced by LAs, the equation (1) alone will impose an apparent shift in h_∞ curve by

$$\Delta V_h = k \times \ln[(1 + L/K_R)/(1 + L/K_I)] \tag{2}$$

as described by Bean et al. (52) and later by Meeder and Ulbricht (53). An additional shift ($R^* \longleftrightarrow I^*$) must be added to this equation if the inactivated state is stabilized energetically by LA binding. Indeed, an additional shift of about 5 and 10 mV was found for cocaine binding with rat skeletal muscle and human cardiac α-subunit Na^+ channels, respectively (54). This additional shift may represent the direct evidence for the chemical stabilization of the inactivated state provided by the LA binding interactions.

To understand the LA action mechanistically under the framework of Hille's modulated receptor hypothesis, one eventually will need detailed structural information on the LA receptor itself. To date, multiple S6 segments, including D1-S6, D3-S6, and D4-S6, appear critical for the action of LAs. The relative positions of residues within these three segments critical for LA action are clustered near the middle section of the S6 segments (Figs. 3 and 4). The lateral/rotational dynamics of the S6 segments during state transitions have been demonstrated in the K^+ channel, and similar dynamics are expected to occur in the Na^+ channel (45). The implications of a possible LA receptor with residues drawn from multiple S6 segments and a possible S6-segment movement during state transitions seem particularly fitting for the modulated receptor hypothesis (Fig. 4; *[47]*). The movement of S6 segments will likely bring the specific S6 residues either closer or farther away from the drug molecule, and therefore may influence the binding affinity directly during state transitions. If the contact points between the drug and the specific residue in the inactivated state provide additional free energy during their interactions, this additional free energy will in turn stabilize the S6 segment in its inactivated position. Such a state will therefore exhibit a higher affinity for the drug.

The above structural descriptions for the modulated receptor hypothesis are rather crude in molecular terms, and appear overly simplistic. The true picture will certainly be more complicated when the individual contact points are mapped and the precise nature of their interactions with the drug becomes known. We anticipate that the clearer the picture of the LA receptor, the greater the impact on the "receptor-based" development of novel LAs.

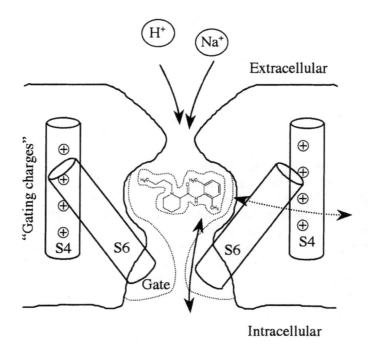

Fig. 4. A possible structural basis for Hille's modulated receptor hypothesis. For clarity, only two of the four S6 segments that form the internal vestibule are shown. The S6 segments are likely in α-helical structures, which are depicted here as cylinders. The lower part of the S6 segments may participate in the channel opening, probably as an activation gate. A bupivacaine molecule is included within the internal vestibule, which is accessible via both the hydrophilic pathway (*solid arrow* via the internal mouth) and the hydrophobic pathway (*dashed arrow* via membrane). Binding of bupivacaine depends on the relative movement of multiple S6 segments. In the inactivated state, the four S6 segments may move toward each other and several residues from three of the four S6 segments together may exhibit stronger binding interactions with bupivacaine. The S4 segments are also shown as cylinders with positive gating charges, which may function as a voltage sensor. Putative signal transduction from the voltage sensor to the activation gate occurs during depolarization. External H^+ ions may reach the internal vestibule to equilibrate with the protonated molecule, bupivacaine.

FUTURE DRUG DESIGN OF LONG-ACTING AND ULTRA LONG-ACTING LAS

Is there a limitation to develop safe long-acting (6–24 h) and ultra long-acting (48–72 h) LAs for clinical uses? Have we already reached the maximal blocking duration by using bupivacaine, the customary yardstick for long-acting LAs? The need for long-acting and ultra long-acting LA drugs with sensory selective attributes is clearly evident as the population of elderly increases. More people in this population will suffer from chronic pain syndromes, neuropathic pain syndromes, rheumatoid arthritis, and cancer-related pain. Additional clinical uses of an ultra long-acting LA for postoperative pain and preemptive analgesia may also be realized when such a drug is developed. Traditional LAs are generally inadequate for prolonged pain syndromes. Opioid tolerance often precludes the use of this type of analgesics for prolonged periods. Repeated injection or continuous delivery of LAs by pumps or catheters may result in plasma levels of drugs that produce CNS disturbances and/or cardiac dysrhythmias.

Before the "receptor-based" design of LAs is possible, what approaches can one take in the interim to develop long-acting and ultra long-acting LAs? One approach is to find a way to extend the time the active drug is trapped within the cytoplasmic region. This, in turn, will make the trapped drug available for a prolonged block of voltage-gated Na^+ channels, as the LA receptor is accessible for

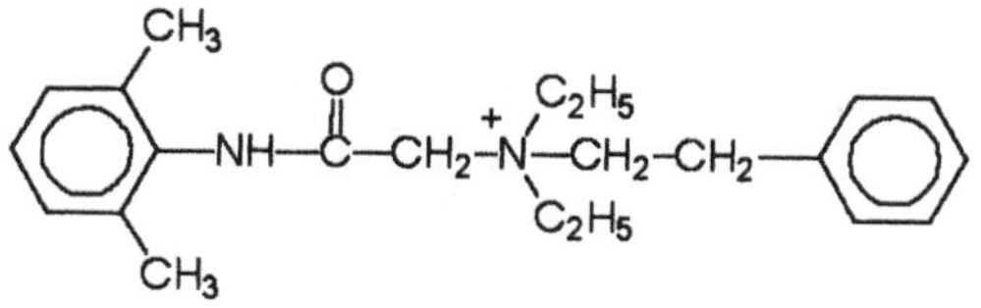

Tonicaine
(N-β-phenylethyl lidocaine QA)

Scheme 4

internal QA compounds. Without trapping, traditional LAs diffuse rapidly through tissue, often enter the vascular systems, and fail to reach the intended target. In fact, less than 2% of lidocaine reaches the inside of the nerve trunk after local injection *(55)*.

One strategy to reduce the drug diffusion rate is the cyclization of LAs. Intramolecular cyclization of amino-amide LAs to promote *in situ* synthesis of a quaternary species was attempted in the early 1970s *(56)*, but this type of LAs has not evolved for clinical uses, probably because cyclization requires a haloalkyl amine component that is also a carcinogen, and the intramolecular cyclization often occurs before penetration of the nerve membrane. An equivalent idea was recently revisited, again with the use of a quaternary species of a lidocaine derivative, N-ethylphenyl lidocaine (i.e., tonicaine; *see* Scheme 4 diagram above), as a possible long-acting LA drug. Being an amphipathic quaternary ammonium, tonicaine also carries a permanent positive charge, is capable of penetrating the cell membrane because of its amphipathic property, and is trapped within the cytoplasmic region for a prolonged period. As a result, tonicaine produces a prolonged sciatic nerve sensory block in vivo that is about 9× longer than that produced by the parent drug, lidocaine *(57)*. In theory, this new strategy should be applicable to other traditional long-acting LAs and their amphipathic QA derivatives should be more potent than their parent drugs. Unfortunately, N-butyl tetracaine was found to be a potent neurolytic agent in rats and caused distal nerve degeneration in vivo *(58)*. This result cautions us about the possible danger of using the same strategy in synthesizing derivatives from different long-acting LAs.

A second approach in the development of long-acting and ultra long-acting LAs is to find a potent Na^+ channel blocker, which has not yet been used as an LA. One such potential drug is TTX, which is at least three orders more potent than bupivacaine (IC_{50}; ~1–10 nM vs ~10–100 μM) in blocking TTX-sensitive Na^+ channels. Although the TTX receptor is located externally and is distinct from the internal LA receptor, the idea of using TTX as an ultra long-acting LA was assessed by Ritchie and Greene *(59)*. Unfortunately, TTX is highly hydrophilic and does not penetrate the nerve sheath readily. Hence, this toxin for the time being appears inadequate for clinical use. Taking this line of approach, we have screened various other drugs reported to be potent Na^+ channel blockers using the rat sciatic nerve block as an in vivo model along with the bupivacaine drug as a yardstick for comparison. A tricyclic antidepressant, amitriptyline, was found to be >5× more potent than bupivacaine in the sciatic nerve sensory block in vivo *(60)*. In rats, no apparent side effects of amitriptyline injection have been found thus far. In fact, intramuscular injections of amitriptyline (*see* Scheme 5 diagram on next page) intended for depressed patients who decline oral treatments were approved by the Food and Drug Administration. In vitro experiments show that amitriptyline is a very potent Na^+ channel blocker that binds to the LA binding site *(61)*. In addition, amitriptyline elicits profound use-dependent block during repetitive pulses, more so than bupivacaine at the same concentration. Clearly, amitriptyline possesses essential attributes as a potential long-acting LA. Future studies on this potential drug are warranted for possible clinic applications. In addition, it may be feasible to modify this potent drug in a manner similar to tonicaine and to use such a quaternary

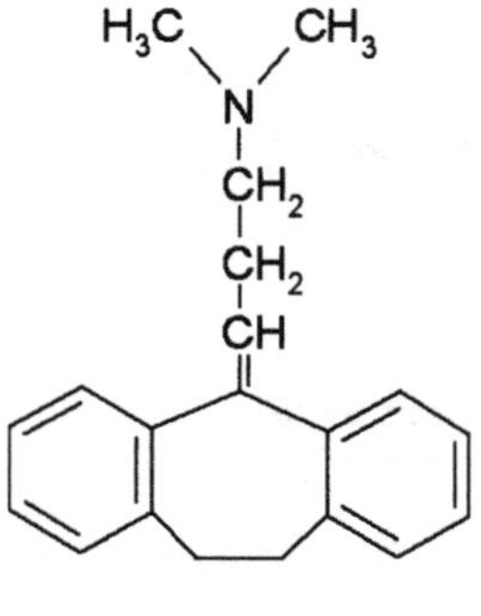

Amitriptyline

Scheme 5

derivative as an ultra long-acting LA. Caution should be taken in developing these QA derivatives, as such compounds may cause neurolysis, as exemplified by N-butyl tetracaine.

SUMMARY

LAs elicit local/regional anesthesia by targeting the voltage-gated Na^+ channels. The LA receptor within the voltage-gated Na^+ channel is currently being mapped by site-directed mutagenesis. Detailed mapping of this receptor within the α-subunit Na^+ channel protein should answer most questions concerning the underlying mechanism of the LA action. First, where are the contact points between LAs and specific residues on the Na^+ channel? Second, how do LAs occlude the Na^+ channel permeation pathway? Third, how do LAs enhance the inactivated state by binding to multiple S6 segments? Fourth, how does Na^+ channel gating (activation, fast and slow inactivation included) affect the LA binding affinities? Fifth, what is the structural basis for the modulated receptor hypothesis? From a broader perspective, LAs are indeed important molecular probes for gaining a clearer understanding of the voltage-gated Na^+ channel in terms of its gating, its permeation pathway, and its receptor dynamics.

With these basic understandings of the LA action, further rational "receptor-based" design of novel long-acting and ultra long-acting LAs should be feasible. It has been a long time since any novel long-acting LA drugs were brought to the market: bupivacaine was first introduced in 1963 and etidocaine in 1971. More recently, sterenantiomers of $S(-)$ bupivacaine and $S(-)$ ropivacaine have been used clinically because of their decreased cardiotoxicity but duration of block by these isomers is not significantly longer than that for their racemic mixtures. This coming decade will be an exciting and challenging time for the LA field and for the pharmaceutical companies, since the need for improved long-acting LA drugs is immense. Clearly, there is a financial incentive for developing such therapeutic drugs, given that the patents for most long-acting LAs have long been expired.

ACKNOWLEDGMENT

I am grateful to Drs. Carla Nau and Peter Gerner who proofread this manuscript. Dr. Nau also contributed Fig. 2 and parts of Fig. 4 used in this chapter. This work is supported by NIH grants (GM-35401 and GM-48090).

REFERENCES

1. de Jong, R. H. (1994) Local anesthetics: from cocaine to xylocaine, in *Local Anesthetics*, Mosby Yearbook, St. Louis, pp. 1–8.
2. Lipka, L. J., Jiang, M., and Tseng, G. N. (1998) Differential effects of bupivacaine on cardiac K channels: role of channel inactivation and subunit composition in drug-channel interaction. *J. Cardiovasc. Electrophysiol.* **9,** 727–742.

3. Goldin, A. L., Barchi, R. L., Caldwell, J. H., et al. (2000) Nomenclature of voltage-gated sodium channels. *Neuron* **28,** 365–368.
4. de Jong, R. H. (1994) On the horizon, in *Local Anesthetics,* Mosby Yearbook, Inc., St. Louis, pp. 381–401.
5. Akopian, A. N., Souslova V., England, S., et al. (1999) The tetrodotoxin-resistant sodium channel SNS has a specialized function in pain pathways. *Nat. Neurosci.* **2,** 541–548.
6. Gottlieb, R. (1923) Pharmakologische untersuchungen über die stereoisomerie der cocaine. *Archiv für Experimentelle Pathologie und Pharmacologie* **97,** 113–146.
7. Skou, J. C. (1954) Local anesthetics: VI. relation between blocking potency and penetration of a monomolecular layer of lipoids from nerves. *Acta Pharmacol. Toxicol.* **10,** 325–337.
8. Taylor, R. E. (1959) Effect of procaine on electrical properties of squid axon membrane. *Am. J. Physiol.* **196,** 1071–1078.
9. Aldrich, R. W., Corey, D. P., and Stevens C. F. (1983) A reinterpretation of mammalian sodium channel gating based on single channel recording. *Nature* **306,** 436–441.
10. Hille, B. (1992) Gating mechanisms, in *Ionic Channels of Excitable Membranes.* Sinauer, Sunderland, Massachusetts, pp. 472–503.
11. Starmer, C. F., Grant A. O., and Strauss H. C. (1984) Mechanisms of use-dependent block of sodium channels in excitable membranes by local anesthetics. *Biophys. J.* **46,** 15–27.
12. Valenzuela, C., Snyders, D. J., Bennett, P. B., Tamargo, J., and Hondeghem, L. M. (1995) Stereoselective block of cardiac sodium channels by bupivacaine in guinea pig ventricular myocytes. *Circulation* **92,** 3014–3024.
13. Hodgkin, A. L. and Huxley, A. E. (1952) A quantitative description of membrane current and its application to conduction and excitation in nerve. *J. Physiol. (Lond.)* **117,** 500–544.
14. Hille, B. (1977) Local anesthetics: hydrophilic and hydrophobic pathways for the drug receptor reaction. *J. Gen. Physiol.* **69,** 497–515.
15. Hondeghem, L. M. and Katzung, B. G. (1977) Time- and voltage-dependent interactions of antiarrhythmic drugs with cardiac sodium channels. *Biochim. Biophys. Acta* **472,** 373–398.
16. Devor, M. (1984) The pathophysiology and anatomy of damaged nerve, in *Textbook of Pain* (Wall P. D. and Melzack R., eds.), Churchill Livingstone, New York, pp. 49–64.
17. Bennett, P. B., Valenzuela, C., Chen, L.-Q., and Kallen, R. G. (1995) On the molecular nature of the lidocaine receptor of cardiac Na⁺ channels: modification of block by alterations in the α-subunit III-IV interdomain. *Circulation Res.* **77,** 584–592.
18. Grant, A. O., Chandra, R., Keller, C., Carboni, M., and Starmer, C. F. (2000) Block of wild-type and inactivation-deficient cardiac sodium channels IFM/QQQ stably expressed in mammalian cells. *Biophys. J.* **79,** 3019–3035.
19. Wang, G. K., Brodwick, M. S., Eaton, D. C., and Strichartz, G. R. (1987) Inhibition of sodium currents by local anesthetics in chloramine-T treated squid axons. *J. Gen. Physiol.* **89,** 645–667.
20. Vedantham, V. and Cannon, S. C. (1999) The position of the fast-inactivation gate during lidocaine block of voltage-gated Na⁺ channels. *J. Gen. Physiol.* **113,** 7–16.
21. Khodorov, B. I., Shishkova, L., Peganov, E., and Revenko, S. (1976) Inhibition of sodium currents in frog Ranvier node treated with local anesthetics. Role of slow sodium inactivation. *Biochim. Biophys. Acta* **433,** 409–435.
22. Ong, B.-H., Tomaselli, G. F., and Balser, J. R. (2000) A structural rearrangement in the sodium channel pore linked to slow inactivation and use dependence. *J. Gen. Physiol.* **116,** 653–661.
23. Guo, X., Castle, N. A., Chernoff, D. M., and Strichartz, G. R. (1991) Comparative inhibition of voltage-gated cation channels by local anesthetics. Ann NY Acad Sci **625,** 181–199.
24. Fodor, A. A., Gordon, S. E., and Zagotta, W. N. (1997) Mechanism of tetracaine block of cyclic nucleotide-gated channels. *J. Gen. Physiol.* **109,** 3–14.
25. Fleming, J. A., Byck, R., and Barash, P. G. (1990) Pharmacology and therapeutic applications of cocaine. *Anesthesiology* **73,** 518–531.
26. Hille, B. (1992) Mechanisms of block, in *Ionic Channels of Excitable Membranes.* Sinauer, Sunderland, MA, pp. 390–422.
27. Strichartz, G. R. (1973) The inhibition of sodium currents in myelinated nerve by quaternary derivatives of lidocaine. *J. Gen. Physiol.* **62,** 37–57.
28. Wang, G. K. (1988) Cocaine-induced closures of single batrachotoxin-activated Na⁺ channels in planar lipid bilayers. *J. Gen. Physiol.* **92,** 747–765.
29. Armstrong, C. M. (1971) Interaction of tetraethylammonium ion derivatives with the potassium channels of giant axons. *J. Gen. Physiol.* **58,** 413–437.
30. Narahashi, T. and Frazier, D. T. (1971) Site of action and active form of local anesthetics. *Neurosci. Res.* **4,** 65–99.
31. Courtney, K. R. and Strichartz, G. R. (1987) Structural elements which determine local anesthetic activity, in *Local Anesthetics* (Strichartz G. R., ed.), Springer-Verlag, New York, pp. 53–94.
32. Postma, S. W. and Catterall, W. A. (1984) Inhibition of binding of H3 batrachotoxin A 20-α-benzoate to Na channels by local anesthetics. *Mol. Pharmacol.* **25,** 219–227.
33. Moczydlowski, E., Uehara, A., and Hall, S. (1986) Blocking pharmacology of batrachotoxin activated sodium channels, in *Ion channel reconstitution.* (Miller C., ed.), Plenum Press, New York, pp. 405–428.
34. Wang, G. K. and Wang, S.-Y. (1992) Altered stereoselectivity of cocaine and bupivacaine isomers in normal and BTX-modified Na⁺ channels. *J. Gen. Physiol.* **100,** 1003–1020.
35. Wang, G. K. (1990) Binding affinity and stereoselectivity of local anesthetics in single batrachotoxin-activated Na⁺ channels. *J. Gen. Physiol.* **96,** 1105–1127.
36. Wang, G. K., Simon, R., and Wang, S. Y. (1991) Quaternary ammonium compounds as structural probes of single batrachotoxin-activated Na⁺ channels. *J. Gen. Physiol.* **98,** 1005–1024.

37. Wang, G. K., Simon, R., Bell, D., and Wang, S. Y. (1993) Structural determinants of quaternary ammonium blockers for BTX- modified Na⁺ channels. *Mol. Pharmacol.* **44,** 667–676.

38. Wang, S.-Y. and Wang, G. K. (1999) Batrachotoxin-resistant Na⁺ channels derived from point mutations in transmembrane segment D4-S6. *Biophys. J.* **76,** 3141–3149.

39. McNeal, E. T., Lewandowski, G. A., Daly, J. W., and Creveling, C. R. (1985) [³H]Batrachotoxinin A 20-alpha-benzoate binding to voltage-sensitive sodium channels: a rapid and quantitative assay for local anesthetic activity in a variety of drugs. *J. Med. Chem.* **28,** 381–388.

40. Ragsdale, D. S., McPhee, J. C., Scheuer, T., and Catterall, W. A. (1996) Common molecular determinants of local anesthetic, antiarrhythmic, and anticonvulsant block of voltage-gated Na⁺ channels. *Proc. Natl. Acad. Sci. USA* **93,** 9270–9275.

41. Catterall, W. A. (2000) From ionic currents to molecular mechanisms: the structure and function of voltage-gated sodium channels. *Neuron* **26,** 13–25.

42. Ragsdale, D. S., McPhee, J. C., Scheuer, T., and Catterall, W. A. (1994) Molecular determinants of state-dependent block of Na⁺ channels by local anesthetics. *Science* **265,** 1724–1728.

43. Catterall, W. A. and Mackie, K. (1996) Local Anesthetics, in *Goodman and Gilman's The Pharmacological Basis of Therapeutics.* (Hardman J. G., Limbird L. E., Molinoff P. B., Ruddon R. W., and Gilman A. G., eds.), Macmillan, New York, pp. 331–347.

44. Li, H.-L., Galue, A., Meadous, L., and Ragsdale, D. S. (1999) A molecular basis for the different local anesthetic affinities of resting versus open and inactivated states of the sodium channel. *Mol. Pharmacol.* **55,** 134–141.

45. Yarov-Yarovoy, V., Brown, J., Sharp, E., Clare, J. J., Scheuer, T., and Catterall, W. A. (2001) Molcular determinants of voltage-dependent gating and binding of pore-blocking drugs in transmembrane segment IIIS6 of the Na⁺ channel α subunit. *J. Biol. Chem.* **276,** 20–27.

46. Wang, G. K., Quan, C., and Wang, S.-Y. (1998) Local anesthetic block of batrachotoxin-resistant muscle Na⁺ channels. *Mol. Pharmacol.* **54,** 389–396.

47. Wang, S.-Y., Nau, C., and Wang, G. K. (2000) Residues in Na⁺ channel D3-S6 segment modulate batrachotoxin as well as local anesthetic binding affinities. *Biophys. J.* **79,** 1379–1387.

48. Sunami, A., Dudley, S. C., and Fozzard, H. A. (1997) Sodium channel selectivity filter regulates antiarrhythmic drug binding. *Proc. Natl. Acad. Sci. USA* **94,** 14,126–14,131.

49. Wang, S.-Y. and Wang, G. K. (1998) Point mutations in segment I-S6 render voltage-gated Na⁺ channels resistant to batrachotoxin. *Proc. Natl. Acad. Sci. USA* **95,** 2653–2658.

50. Linford, N. J., Cantrell, A. R., Qu, Y., Scheuer, T., and Catterall, W. A. (1998) Interaction of batrachotoxin with the local anesthetic receptor site in transmembrane segment IVS6 of the voltage-gated sodium channel. *Proc. Natl. Acad. Sci. USA* **95,** 13,947–13,952.

51. Monod, J., Changeux, J. P., and Jacob, F. (1963) Allosteric proteins and cellular control systems. *J. Mol. Biol.* **6,** 306–329.

52. Bean, B. P., Cohen, C. J., and Tsien, R. W. (1983) Lidocaine block of cardiac sodium channels. *J. Gen. Physiol.* **81,** 613–642.

53. Meeder, T. and Ulbricht, W. (1987) Action of benzocaine on sodium channels of frog nodes of Ranvier treated with chloramine-T. *Pflugers Arch* **409,** 265–273.

54. Wright, S. N., Wang, S.-Y., Xiao, Y.-F., and Wang, G. K. (1999) State-dependent cocaine block of sodium channel isoforms, chimeras, and channels coexpressed with the β-subunit. *Biophys. J.* **76,** 233–245.

55. Popitz-Bergez, F. A., Leeson, S., Strichartz, G. R., and Thalhammer, J. G. (1995) Relation between functional deficit and intraneural local anesthetic during peripheral nerve block. A study in the rat sciatic nerve. *Anesthesiology* **83,** 583–592.

56. Ross, S. B. and Akerman, S. B. A. (1972) Cyclization of three N-ω-haloalkyl-N-methylaminoaceto-2,6-xylidide derivatives in relation to their local anesthetic effect in vitro and in vivo. *J. Pharmac. Exp. Ther.* **182,** 351–361.

57. Wang, G. K., Quan, C., Vladimirov, M., Mok, W.-M., and Thalhammer, J. G. (1995) Quaternary ammonium derivative of lidocaine as a long acting local anesthetic. *Anesthesiology* **83,** 1293–1301.

58. Wang, G. K., Vladimirov, M., Quan, C., Mok, W.-M., Thalhammer, J. G., and Anthony, D. C. (1996) N-butyl tetracaine as a neurolytic agent for ultralong sciatic nerve block. *Anesthesiology* **85,** 1386–1394.

59. Ritchie, J. M. and Greene, N. M. (1985) Local anesthetics, in *Goodman and Gilman's The Pharmacological Basis of Therapeutics.* (Gilman, A. G., Goodman, L. S., Rall, T. A., and Murad, F., eds.), MacMillan, New York, pp. 302–321.

60. Gerner, P., Mujtaba, M., Sinnot, C. J., and Wang, G. K. (2001) Amitriptyline versus bupivacaine in rat sciatic nerve blockade. *Anesthesiology* **94,** 661–667.

61. Nau, C., Seaver, M., Wang, S.-Y., and Wang, G. K. (2000) Block of human heart hH1 sodium channels by amitriptyline. *J. Pharmacol. Exp. Ther.* **292,** 1015–1023.

26

Neuromuscular Blocking Agents and General Anesthesia

Gerald A. Gronert and Timothy Tautz

NEUROMUSCULAR BLOCKERS: DO THEY ALTER GENERAL ANESTHESIA?

The molecules of neuromuscular blocking agents are hydrophilic and ionized, and thus do not generally cross fatty membranes such as the blood-brain barrier to enter the central nervous system or cerebrospinal fluid. Therefore they seem unlikely to directly affect the status imposed by general anesthesia. It seems possible that they might, during light planes of anesthesia, indirectly alter the state of general anesthesia through their relaxation of skeletal muscle and imposed modification of neuronal stimuli returning to the central nervous system. Sensory nerves as well as muscle spindle fibers may in part be responsible for such changes, if indeed they occur. Before examining evidence concerning alteration of general anesthesia, we will review some basic properties of these agents.

BASIC TENETS

The propagated wave of depolarization traveling along the motor nerve toward the neuromuscular junction activates voltage-dependent calcium channels on the presynaptic membrane and increases the concentration of intracellular calcium at the nerve terminal (1). This in turn stimulates release of acetylcholine from storage vesicles (Fig. 1). Quanta of acetylcholine diffuse across the synaptic cleft, bind to the nicotinic acetylcholine receptors, and as chemical agonists, depolarize these resulting in excitatory postsynaptic potentials. These non-selective cation channels activate the inward current primarily carried by sodium, and depolarize the muscle cell membrane. The resulting wave of excitation is actively propagated along the surface membrane and into the transverse tubules. Depolarization of the transverse tubule causes a charge movement within the dihydropyridine receptor to activate the ryanodine receptor to its open position, with release of calcium into the sarcoplasm.

At concentrations greater than the resting level of $10^{-7} M$, usually about $5 \times 10^{-5} M$, calcium removes the troponin inhibition of the myofibrils to cause contraction. Two interactions halt this stimulation and muscle contraction: (1) Junctional acetylcholinesterase rapidly hydrolyses acetylcholine and ends its depolarizing effect, and (2) calcium pumps lower the sarcoplasmic free unbound ionized calcium ion concentration by binding it back into the sarcoplasmic reticulum, thus effecting relaxation. These processes are rapid, and the motor unit is ready for another stimulus within milliseconds.

NICOTINIC ACETYLCHOLINE RECEPTOR BLOCKING AGENTS

The depolarizing skeletal muscle blocker succinylcholine is composed of two molecules of acetylcholine bound by an ester linkage. It is not a competitive neuromuscular blocking agent, but rather an acetylcholine-like agonist with a prolonged effect, because it is hydrolyzed only by plasma cholinest-

From: *Contemporary Clinical Neuroscience: Neural Mechanisms of Anesthesia*
Edited by: Joseph F. Antognini et al. © Humana Press Inc., Totowa, NJ

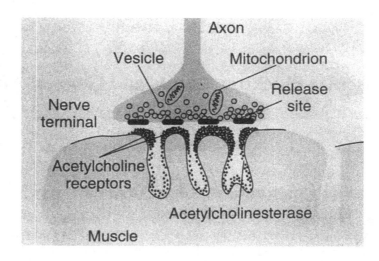

Fig. 1. Schematic of the neuromuscular junction, from Figure 1, Drachman, D. B. (1994) Medical Progress: Myasthenia Gravis, *New Eng. J. Med.* **330,** 1797–1810. Copyright © 1994 Massachusetts Medical Society. Adapted with permission, 2001. All rights reserved.

erase. The ensuing prolonged endplate depolarization delays repolarization of the adjacent skeletal muscle membrane, resulting in paralysis. While its 5–10 min duration of action is far longer than that of acetylcholine (milliseconds), it is still shorter than that of other skeletal muscle relaxants.

Non-depolarizing skeletal muscle blockers comprise the other major category of direct-acting skeletal muscle relaxants (dantrolene, the lipid-soluble hydrophobic intramuscular calcium blocker will not be considered). These curare-type blockers competitively interact with acetylcholine molecules for occupation of the α sub-unit on the shoulder of the acetylcholine receptor (Fig. 1). The action of these blockers is longer than that of succinylcholine, with structure-activity relationship that dictate varying durations of paralysis ranging from 10 min to several hours. Ordered by shorter to longer durations, these include rapacuronium (recently withdrawn from the market, perhaps to be re-introduced later after re-labeling), rocuronium, mivacurium, atracurium, vecuronium, cis-atracurium, pancuronium, doxacurium, pipecuronium; curare, gallamine, and metocurine (dimethyl D-tubocurarine) are longer-lasting, older agents, and generally no longer used clinically.

ABNORMAL RESPONSES TO NEUROMUSCULAR BLOCKING AGENTS

Abnormal responses occur due to dysfunction at the motor nerve, the myoneural junction, the endplate area, the muscle surface membrane, or the muscle contractile apparatus per se. These include upper motor neuron lesions such as stroke or cord disease, motor nerve section or loss of function of the anterior horn cell, altered acetylcholine release, altered endplate receptors, or altered responses of skeletal muscle *(1)*. The latter responses could originate from the dihydropyridine receptor in the wall of the transverse tubule, or the ryanodine receptor in the sarcoplasmic reticulum, to the contractile fibrils themselves, with loss of motor units.

Disorders that include diminished motor nerve function with lessened to absent acetylcholine effects upon skeletal muscle result in upregulation of the postsynaptic nicotinic acetylcholine receptors, i.e., there are increased numbers of receptors, with resistance to competitive antagonists, e.g., curare-like drugs, and sensitivity to agonists, e.g., succinylcholine, with an attendant hyperkalemia *(1)*. Upregulation also occurs when there is pharmacologic denervation due to chronic use of non-depolarizing agents, as in the intensive care unit *(2)*. Downregulation occurs when there are fewer numbers of functioning endplate acetylcholine receptors, e.g., myasthenia gravis. As the opposite of upregulation, this results in diametrically opposing effects of relaxants: there is now the classic sensitivity to non-depolarizing agents, and resistance (although clinically modest) to succinylcholine *(1)*

Myopathies may result in loss of functioning motor units, with sensitivity to relaxants because there are fewer muscle fibers. Frequently, disuse atrophy is an accompaniment of this. There is then an interplay between the situation of fewer fibers, e.g., sensitivity, with that of the upregulatory effects of disuse, e.g., resistance *(1)*.

Finally, it had been demonstrated on several occasions, in parallel studies in geographically widely separated countries, that there is a national variation in potency of non-depolarizing blocking agents *(3–6)*. Some nationalities are more sensitive to non-depolarizing than others. Is this acquired or genetic? Is it related to degree of activity or diet or inheritance? It is unlikely that the people of one nation would in general have greater or lesser activity patterns than those of another. But if so, this would affect national responses. In, addition, dietary habits can alter metabolism of some relaxants, e.g., potatoes and cholinesterase *(7)*. Would this have anything to do with alterations in general anesthesia? If skeletal muscle is different, can the CNS be different? There is no evidence relating differing national responses to general anesthesia, but there are certain species genetic differences, e.g., Drosophila, nematodes *(8,9)*. Should this be investigated by human pharmacokinetic-pharmacodynamic studies in these various countries, with continuing evaluation of potentially altered general anesthesia?

Any of these finding appear to provide little relaxant-related effects as regards central nervous system actions with general anesthesia. Further, any use of relaxants must be accompanied by adequate monitoring with a nerve stimulator, as effects are unpredictable, even in supposedly normal subjects. When abnormalities are known, their precise effect is impossible to determine, as the causative process may be ongoing, worsening, or improving. It is thus difficult to define alterations as regards general anesthesia. So what is the evidence for altered general anesthesia by muscle relaxants?

ALTERED GENERAL ANESTHESIA AND NEUROMUSCULAR BLOCKING AGENTS

The neuromuscular effects of volatile inhalational agents have been known for some time. The ED_{50} of nondepolarizing neuromuscular blockers (that concentration associated with 50% paralysis) is decreased in patients anesthetized with potent inhalational agents. Moreover, both twitch height and ability to sustain tetany exhibit dose-dependent decreases under volatile anesthesia *(10–12)*. These anesthetic action are most probably due to conformational changes in the membrane lipid at the neuromuscular junction, altering channel function and decreasing impulse transmission. These effects, however, are usually observed above 1 MAC (that concentration that eliminates movement in 50% of subjects). Therefore, a direct affect of volatile anesthetics on muscle of the neuromuscular junction cannot account for the ability of these anesthetics to suppress movement.

The possible effects of neuromuscular blockers on MAC is more controversial. Effects on anesthetic requirements can be studied by using the isolated forelimb technique whereby tourniquets are placed on one or more limbs, thus preventing the muscle relaxant from affecting muscles in those extremities. Forbes et al. *(13)* showed an apparent 25% decrease in the MAC of halothane by co-administration of pancuronium; MAC was determined based on the response to skin incision. The authors theorized that, if the isolated limb did not react to surgical stimulation at sub-anesthetic MAC levels, it was due to either a direct CNS effect of pancuronium, or perhaps a deafferentiation effect from deceased muscle spindle activity. A direct effect is unlikely, since pancuronium does not readily cross the blood-brain barrier. Furthermore, muscle relaxants, when directly applied to the cerebral cortex, appear to cause seizures *(14,15)*. However, modification of cerebral input via a decrease in muscle fiber "noise" from paralyzing doses of pancuronium is an intriguing possibility. Subsequent studies have yielded conflicting data. Fahey et al. *(16)* failed to show any clinically relevant alterations in MAC with pancuronium, vecuronium, or atracurium.

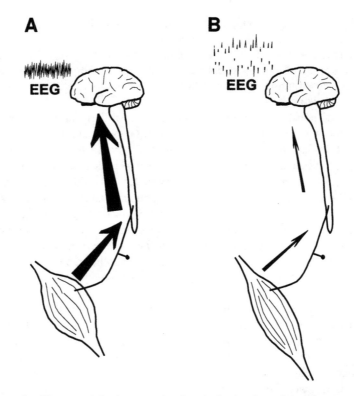

Fig. 2. In **(A)**, muscle afferent activity is transmitted to the brain via peripheral nerves and the spinal cord, resulting in cerebral activation as depicted by a low amplitude, high frequency pattern in the electroencephalogram (EEG). In **(B)**, a muscle relaxant diminishes MAA and this action limits activation influences on the EEG, which has a high amplitude, low frequency pattern.

Lanier et al. *(17–19)* published a series of papers examining the cerebral effects of neuromuscular blockade in a dog model. They measured cerebral metabolic rate, cerebral blood flow (CBF), intracranial pressure (ICP), electroencephalogram (EEG), and cerebral energy state in dogs anesthetized with 1 MAC halothane and the changes induced with succinylcholine, pancuronium, and atracurium. They showed no significant changes in any of the measured parameters with pancuronium *(19)*. EEG evidence of arousal was evident in only one dog (given atracurium). There was good evidence of EEG arousal in the group of dogs receiving atracurium and halothane titrated to sub-MAC end- expired concentrations, without significant increases in cerebral metabolic rate for oxygen, CBF or ICP. This effect was presumed to be due to laudanosine, a metabolite of atracurium. Succinylcholine, however readily and reliably increased CBF, ICP, and Pa CO_2, while changing EEG patterns to an arousal pattern *(17,18)*. These changes began immediately after fasciculation in the dogs, and no change in any measured parameter was noted if the dogs were pretreated with paralyzing doses of pancuronium. They also studied the effect of defasciculating doses of pancuronium followed by succinylcholine on CBF, electromyographic (EMG) activity, and muscle afferent activity (MAA) and found that while changes in MAA were attenuated, significant increases in CBF, Pa CO_2 and ICP occurred *(18)*. They attributed these findings to stimulation of muscle spindle activity by succinylcholine, thereby increasing cerebral activity, and secondarily increasing Pa CO_2, which contributed to changes in CBF and ICP. Defasciculating doses of pancuronium attenuated the responses, while complete abolition of muscle spindle activity via pancuronium abolished these phenomena (*see* Fig. 2). Schwartz et al. *(20)* reported increased duration of EEG burst suppression using pancuronium in dogs anesthetized with isoflurane, that promptly reverted with administration of neostigmine and glycopyrrolate. They concluded that blockade of afferent muscle activity diminished activating influences on arousal and thus increased the amount of time that EEG was isoelectric.

The anatomy and physiology of the muscle spindle may explain these findings *(21)*. Individual muscle spindles are made up of two fibers types. Outer, contractile fibers are termed extrafusal and are innervated by α efferents. Intrafusal fibers are located more deeply in the muscle spindle, are non-contractile, and have α efferent innervation, delivering increased afferent information regarding static muscle length and dynamic muscle stretch to the brain. Extrafusal fiber contraction during fasciculations would increase intrafusal activity, which in turn would increase afferent information to the cortex via the spinal cord, thereby increasing cerebral activation.

There is some evidence of direct intrafusal stimulation by succinylcholine. Lanier reported increased electrical activity in isolated rootlets and cut nerve fibers exposed to succinylcholine *(18)*. Also, the period of cerebral stimulation and increased MAA from succinylcholine outlasted any EMG evidence of activation or fasciculations. Given the above information, paralyzing doses of pancuronium would prevent cerebral stimulation from succinylcholine by abolishing both intra- and extrafusal fiber depolarization. Nonparalyzing doses would be expected to attenuate responses, but direct binding of succinylcholine would still increase MAA and cerebral activity.

Cerebral stimulation from atracurium can be attributed to its active metabolite laudanosine, a known cerebral stimulant. Shi and colleagues *(22)* showed that laudanosine increased MAC requirements in rabbits by up to 30% in concentrations similar to those found buy Fahey et al. in renal failure patients given atracurium *(23)*. Laudanosine also increases cerebral arousal, in addition to its effect on MAC. Hennis et al. *(24)* found that laudanosine was associated with signs of awakening in halothane anesthetized dogs. Laudanosine in higher doses can cause seizure activity.

SUMMARY

Cerebral cortical and neuromuscular activities appear to be linked. Volatile anesthetic agents exert a direct, dose-dependent depressant effect on the neuromuscular junction. The effect of neuromuscular blockade on anesthetic requirements and cerebral cortical activity is more complex. Depolarizing agents affect cortical activity via increased afferent traffic from muscle spindles, while non-depolarizing agents given in paralyzing doses might decrease anesthetic requirements by suppressing those afferent impulses. Although certain factors, e.g., genetic, dietary, activity, alter muscle relaxant responses, only genetic factors (in animals) are known to alter general anesthetic requirements. However, evidence has been gathered more easily in muscle than in the central nervous system.

REFERENCES

1. Martyn, J. A., White, D. A., Gronert, G. A., Jaffe, R. S., and Ward, J. M. (1992) Up-and-down regulation of skeletal muscle acetylcholine receptors. Effects on neuromuscular blockers. *Anesthesiology* **76**, 822–843.
2. Markewitz, B. A. and Elstad, M. R. (1997) Succinylcholine-induced hyperkalemia following prolonged pharmacologic neuromuscular blockade. *Chest* **111**, 248–250.
3. Katz, R. L., Norman, J., Seed, R. F., and Conrad, L. (1969) A comparison of the effects of suxamethonium and tubocurarine in patients in London and New York. *Brit. J. Anaesth.* **41**, 1041–1047.
4. Fiset, P., Donati, F., Balendran, P., Meistelman, C., Lira, E., and Bevan., D. R. (1991) Vecuronium is more potent in Montreal than in Paris. *Can. J. Anaesth.* 38,717–721.
5. Semple, P., Hope, D. A., Clyburn, P., and Robert, A. (1994) Relative potency of vecronium in male and female patients in Britain and Australia. *Brit. J. Anaesth.* 72,190–194.
6. Salib, Y., Frossard, J., Plaud, B., Debaene, B., Meistelman, C., and Donati, F. (1994) Neuromuscular effects of vecuronium and neostigmine in Montreal and Paris. *Can. J. Anaesth.* **41**, 908–912.
7. McGehee, D. S., Krasowski, M. D., Fung, D. L., Wilson, B., Gronert, G .A., and Moss, J. (2000) Cholinesterase inhibition by potato glycoalkaloids slows mivacurium metabolism. *Anesthesiology* **93**, 510–519.
8. Dapkus, D., Ramirez, S., and Murray, M. J. (1996) Halothane resistance in *Drosophila melanogaster*: development of a model and gene localization techniques. *Anesth. Analg.* **83**, 147–155.
9. van Swinderen, B., Galifianakis, A., and Crowder, C. M. (1998) Common genetic determinants of halothane and isoflurane potencies in *Caenorhabditis elegans*. *Anesthesiology* **89**, 1509–1517.
10. Fogdall, R. P. and Miller, R. D. (1975) Neuomuscular effects of enflurane, alone and combined with d-Tubocurarine, pancuronium, and succinylcholine, in man. *Anesthesiology* **42**, 173–178.

11. Miller, R. D., Eger, E. I., Way, W. L., Stevens, W. C., and Dolan, W. M. (1971) Comparative neuromuscular effects of Forane and halothane alone and in combination with d-tubocurarine in man. *Anesthesiology* **35,** 38–42.

12. Caldwell, J. E., Laster, M. J., Magorian, T., et al. (1991) The neuromuscular effects of desflurane, alone and combined with pancuronium or succinycholine in humans. *Anesthesiology* **74,** 412–418.

13. Forbes, A. R., Cohen, N. H., and Eger, E. I. (1979) Pancuronium reduces halothane reguirement in man. *Anesth. Analg.* **58,** 497–499.

14. Cardone, C., Szenohradszky, J., Yost, S., and Bickler, P. E. (1994) Activation of brain acetylcholine receptors by neuromuscular blocking drugs. A possible mechanism of neurotoxicity. *Anesthesiology* **80,** 1155–1161.

15. Szenohradszky, J., Trevor, A. J., Bickler, P., et al. (1993) Central nervous system effects of intrathecal muscle relaxants in rats. *Anesth. Analg.* **76,** 1304–1309.

16. Fahey, M. R., Sessler, D. I., Cannon, J. E., Brady, K., Stoen, R., and Miller, R. D. (1989) Atracurium, veruronium, and pancuronium do not alter the minimum alveolar concentration of halothane in humans. *Anesthesiology* **71,** 53–56.

17. Lanier, W. L., Milde, J. H., and Michenfelder, J. D. (1986) Cerebral stimulation following succinylcholine in dogs. *Anesthesiology* **64,** 551–559.

18. Lanier, W. L., Iaizzo, P. A., and Milde, J. H. (1989) Cerebral function and muscle afferent activity following intravenous succinylcholine in dogs anesthetized with halothane: the effects of pretreatment with a defasciculating dose of pancuronium. *Anesthesiology* **71,** 87–95.

19. Lanier, W. L., Milde, J. H., and Michenfelder, J. D. (1985) The cerebral effects of pancuronium and atracurium in halothane-anesthetized dogs. *Anesthesiology* **63,** 589–597.

20. Schwartz, A. E., Navedo, A. T., and Berman, M. F. (1992) Pancuronium increases the duration of electroencephalogram burst suppression in dogs anesthetized with isoflurane. *Anesthesiology* **77,** 686–690.

21. Guyton, A. C. (1986) Textbook of Medical Physiology, 7th Edition. Philadelphia, WB Saunders, pp. 607–612.

22. Shi, W. Z., Fahey, M. R., Fisher, D. M., Miller, R. D., Canfell, C., and Eger, E. I. (1985) Laudanosine (a metabolite of atracurium) increases the minimum alveolar concentration of halothane in rabbits. *Anesthesiology* **63,** 584–588.

23. Fahey, M. R., Rupp, S. M., Canfell, C., et al. (1985) Effect of renal failure on laudanosine excretion in man. *Brit. J. Anaesth.* **57,** 1049–1051.

24. Hennis, P. J., Fahey, M. R., Canfell, P. C., Shi, W. Z., and Miller, R. D. (1986) Pharmacology of laudanosine in dogs. *Anesthesiology* **65,** 56–60.

VI Future Research

27

The Future of Anesthetic Mechanisms Research

Joseph F. Antognini, Douglas E. Raines, and Earl Carstens

This book began first describing what anesthesia is and is not, and then followed with the history of how prior researchers explored the mechanisms of anesthesia. We end the book with a look forward to what might occur in the future of research into anesthetic mechanism.

ANOTHER LOOK INTO THE PAST

Just as anyone else who tries to predict the future, we take a look at the past, in particular developments during the 1950 and 1960s. Prior to this period, very few anesthetics had been developed. The need to develop nonflammable anesthetics became more pressing as more and more explosions occurred in operating rooms worldwide. Chemists began to realize that substitution of halogens, such as chloride and fluoride, for hydrogen on alkane molecules would render the resulting compound less flammable *(1)*. This chemistry was made possible because of the fluoride chemistry needed for development of explosive-grade uranium used for atomic bombs. Interestingly, the pharmacologists who tested these compounds on animals determined that perfluorcarbons (substitution of all hydrogens with fluoride) had no apparent anesthetic properties. For decades these compounds were a curiosity, with no obvious value to researchers. When the Meyer-Overton hypothesis began to crack, perfluorcarbons were pulled off the shelf, in as much as one would predict that they should have anesthetic properties. In fact, these began to be used as research tools *(2)*. Some had no anesthetic properties, whereas others appeared to have no effect on movement responses, but did appear to have amnestic properties. This led to a change in the classification of these interesting compounds: from nonanesthetics to nonimmobilizers. In any case, the development of the modern anesthetics began in the chemistry laboratory, with very little to guide the chemists as regards potential mechanisms. Through empirical "trial and error," isoflurane, desflurane, sevoflurane, enflurane, and halothane were discovered. Desflurane was discovered years before its introduction into the clinical arena. Its low blood-gas solubility was thought to be detrimental because fast emergence from anesthesia and speedy discharge to home was not economically required at the time. Only when financial pressures dictated faster discharges did desflurane get dusted off from the shelf. Currently, to our knowledge, there is no industrial push to develop newer anesthetics. Has the pharmacuetical industry reached the point of "this is as good as it gets?" We don't know. It behooves us as researchers to continue to promote awareness of the problems associated with anesthesia and how research can solve those problems.

WHAT IS THE DRIVE TO IMPROVE ANESTHESIA?

Why improve anesthetic delivery at all, let alone develop newer anesthetics? This answer might be obvious to those involved in clinical anesthesia, but it is less obvious (or not obvious at all) to those

From: *Contemporary Clinical Neuroscience: Neural Mechanisms of Anesthesia*
Edited by: Joseph F. Antognini et al. © Humana Press Inc., Totowa, NJ

outside this clinical and research discipline. Nonetheless, certain groups will be driving forces for improved anesthetics and anesthetic techniques. Patients might be a driving force, as they seek improved outcomes with fewer and fewer complications. They might not appreciate the ins-and-outs of cardiovascular depressive effects of anesthetics, but they fully understand the nausea and vomiting that occurs after anesthesia. And, despite the very low risk of death due to anesthesia, even one excess death is disastrous for that patient and his or her family.

Surgeons will require improved anesthetic techniques as surgical techniques advance. This might eventually require new anesthetics. Anesthesiologists will also wish to improve and advance the field as well. After all, any professional group seeks to improve its services. This can occur only with continued research. If our techniques and drugs become stagnant, so too will our specialty.

Where will the money come from to fund research of anesthetic mechanisms? The National Institutes of Health, through the National Institute of General Medical Sciences, currently funds a significant portion of anesthetic-mechanisms research occurring in the United States. Around the world, government research institutes likewise fund this research. The total amount of money that the NIH administers for anesthetic mechanisms research is about 50 million dollars, or 0.25% of the total NIH budget. Is this enough? Too little? Too much? As researchers, we are likely to want more. As taxpayers and healthcare consumers, however, we likely want dollars going to fund research of common life threatening diseases. Virtually none of us will die because of an anesthetic mishap; many of us will die of cancer or heart disease.

Aside from clinical influences, there are also scientific reasons to explore anesthetic mechanisms. For example, the mechanisms of consciousness and anesthesia are closely linked. It would be difficult to understand one without understanding the other. Any theory that seeks to explain consciousness must incorporate the effect of anesthetics, and vice versa, a theory of anesthesia must incorporate what is known about consciousness.

SPECIFIC TECHNIQUES

Various chapters in this book have discussed new techniques to explore anesthetic mechanisms, including functional magnetic resonance imaging (fMRI), positron emission tomography (PET), and genetic methods. Imaging techniques hold considerable promise to elucidate mechanisms of anesthesia. As these imaging methods become more and more precise, with better resolution, it will soon become possible to detect changes in activity of just a few neurons. This will permit researchers to correlate anesthetic effects with anatomic sites and physiological changes.

Gene therapy also will further our understanding of anesthesia. Manipulations at the genetic level will help elucidate what genes are responsible for the proteins of interest. This approach is already yielding important information, as explained in Chapter 15. It may be possible to genetically alter patients, at least for a short period during the perioperative setting. For example, transfection with mRNA can lead to upregulation of specific proteins in the rat brain *(3)*. This technique would permit transient expression of desirable proteins, receptors, and the like. Knock-outs and knock-ins allow researchers to determine which receptors and subunits of receptors are important to anesthetic action.

In recent years, great advances have been made in characterizing the ways in which general anesthetics interact with proteins. Such studies have shown that the functions of ligand-gated ion channels, G-protein coupled receptors, and voltage-gated ion channels are perturbed by anesthetics at clinically relevant concentrations, making them all plausible anesthetic targets *(4–10)*. Nonetheless, the $GABA_A$ family of receptors is generally considered to be the most important general anesthetic target in the central nervous system. Although future studies may ultimately confirm this assumption, several recent studies strongly suggest that other targets also play important roles. For example, it has been shown that nonhalogenated alkanes, nitrous oxide, and xenon have little or no effect on the $GABA_A$ receptor even at concentrations that are sufficient to induce immobility *(11–13)*. Amnesia can be induced by general anesthetics at sub-MAC partial pressures that have negligible effects on

GABAergic currents *(14)*. These findings suggest that future studies will necessarily focus on the potential roles of other receptor systems in mediating anesthetic action. What might such studies show? One possibility is that they will reveal that different behavioral endpoints (i.e., immobility, amnesia, analgesia) are mediated by different receptor targets. The significance of such a finding is that it would suggest that anesthetic agents could be designed to act specifically at receptor targets to achieve specific clinical endpoints. This concept is, perhaps, most strongly suggested by studies showing that the major neuronal nicotinic acetylcholine receptor subtype ($\alpha4\beta2$), which is believed to play a central role in memory formation, is inhibited by general anesthetics at the very low partial pressures that induce amnesia *(8)*. These studies might also suggest that specific behavioral endpoints are achievable via interactions with more than one receptor systems. For example, enflurane may be capable of inducing immobility by either potentiating $GABA_A$ receptors or inhibiting NMDA receptors. Such redundancy might explain, in part, why knocking out $GABA_A$ subunits increases MAC only modestly *(15,16)*.

Chimeric receptors and site directed mutagenesis techniques have been used to identify putative anesthetic binding sites at the level of individual receptors *(17,18)*. Such studies have lent strong support to the hypothesis that anesthetics act directly on membrane receptor targets rather than indirectly via the membrane lipid. However, the interpretation of such studies is confounded by the fact that changing even a single amino acid can alter receptor function as assessed, for instance, by the agonist concentration- dependence of channel activation or the rate of agonist-induced desensitization. This raises the possibility that these receptor domains modulate anesthetic sensitivity by altering the channel gating process, but do not actually form part of the anesthetic binding site. In the case of the $GABA_A$ receptor, this possibility is suggested by the observation that mutations that reduce the receptor's anesthetic sensitivity also tend to reduce the concentration of agonist required to open it in the absence of anesthetic *(19)*. Furthermore, ligand-gated ion channels are, by definition, allosterically modulated proteins; agonists bind to one part of the receptor and induce a functionally important structural change (channel opening) in another part. By analogy, it is conceivable that mutating one amino acid allosterically modulates the conformation of an anesthetic binding site located elsewhere on the receptor. Therefore, future biochemical and structural studies will need to confirm the existence and location of putative sites. One approach to locating such sites is to irreversibly photo-incorporate general anesthetics or anesthetic analogs into relevant neuronal membrane proteins and then determine which amino acids are labeled using Edman degradation or mass spectroscopy. This approach will allow the identification of amino acids that actually make contact with general anesthetic molecules, an obvious requirement of any true binding site. To date, this approach has been applied to only one ligand-gated ion channel, the highly abundant *Torpedo* nicotinic acetylcholine receptor *(20)*. In this case, the results of photo-labeling studies using *Torpedo* receptors and mutagenesis studies using closely related mouse muscle nicotinic acetylcholine receptors agreed to the extent that both approaches suggested the existence of a site within the channel lumen itself *(20,21)*. With ongoing advances in the ability to express and purify large quantities of receptors, it should soon be possible to apply these techniques to more relevant anesthetic targets within the central nervous system. An important limitation of this approach, however, is that it yields relatively little information about the physical structure of the binding site. Such structural information will be necessary if an ultimate goal of mechanism research is to use structure-based drug design to develop selectively acting (and presumably safer) anesthetic agents. To acquire such information, X-ray diffraction must be used to define the structures of the anesthetic binding sites on proteins in three-dimensions. Unfortunately, membrane proteins are extremely difficult to crystallize and it is likely to be many years before a high-resolution structure of any relevant membrane protein model is obtained. As an alternative strategy, several groups have succeeded in expressing smaller receptor fragments that may be more amenable to crystallization and eventual structure determination *(22,23)*.

Studies at the molecular level are likely to give us better insight into the forces that govern anesthetic binding to proteins and a better understanding of what anesthetics do once they have bound.

Microscopy techniques are becoming more powerful and individual receptors and molecules can now be visualized. It is not inconceivable that we will be able to observe individual anesthetic molecules interacting with receptors. In addition, we will likely be able to determine the forces of these individual interactions. Atomic and scanning force microscopy are two techniques that are currently used to observe and probe molecular interactions. Classically, hydrophobic interactions have been considered to be the most important interactions. In light of recent studies demonstrating that some highly hydrophobic anesthetics and non-immobilizers fail to potentiate agonist actions on the ligand-gated ion channels, it will be critical to identify the other interactions that govern activity *(11,24,25)*. Interactions that have been suggested to be important include hydrogen bonding and dipolar interactions, but to date, experimental evidence demonstrating their importance is limited *(26,27)*. Continuing advances in computational speed will promote the use of molecular dynamics simulations to help elucidate the nature of interactions between anesthetics and their putative binding sites on relevant proteins, and to provide valuable insights into dynamics of anesthetic binding.

Advances in our understanding of the role that lipids may play in modulating anesthetic action will likely come at a much slower pace as the focus of anesthetic mechanisms research has shifted over the past several years towards proteins. Does this mean that we witnessing the end of lipid studies of anesthetic action? Given the ability of lipid theories to predict much of the phenomenology of anesthesia (Meyer-Overton Correlation, anesthetic cut-off, pressure reversal, and the existence of non-immobilizers), it seems likely that there will continue to be interest in trying to understand any role that lipids might play in modulating anesthetic action. In recent years, theories have been proposed that suggest that anesthetics may alter protein function either by reducing the membrane dipole or changing the lateral pressure profile of lipid bilayers *(28–30)*. Although these theories seem plausible, without experimental evidence demonstrating that the function of relevant membrane proteins is governed by these bilayer properties, it seems unlikely that such theories will gain widespread support.

When considering all the various methods with which to investigate anesthetic mechanisms, we conclude in much the same way we began this book: we will never understand anesthetic mechanisms by examining just one aspect (e.g., receptors). All the data must be integrated to explain what happens in the intact organism.

REFERENCES

1. Vitcha, J. F. (1971) A History of Forane. *Anesthesiology* **35**, 4–7.
2. Sonner, J., Li, J., and Eger, E. I., 2nd. (1998) Desflurane and nitrous oxide, but not nonimmobilizers, affect nociceptive responses. *Anesth. Analg.* **86**, 629–34.
3. Hecker, J. G., Hall, L. L., and Irion, V. R. (2001) Nonviral delivery to the lateral ventricles in rat brain: evidence for widespread distribution and expression in the central nervous system. *Molec. Ther.* **3**, 375–384.
4. Zimmerman, S. A., Jones, M. V., and Harrison, N. L. (1994) Potentiation of gamma- aminobutyric acid A receptor Cl⁻ current correlates with in vivo anesthetic potency. *J. Pharmacol. Exp. Ther.* **270**, 987–991.
5. Banks, M. I. and Pearce, R. A. (1999) Dual actions of volatile anesthetics on GABA(A) IPSCS: dissociation of blocking and prolonging effects. *Anesthesiology* **90**, 120–134.
6. Mascia, M. P., Machu, T. K., and Harris, R. A. (1996) Enhancement of homomeric glycine receptor function by long-chain alcohols and anaesthetics. *Brit. I. Pharmacol.* **119**, 1331–1336.
7. Franks, N. P. and Lieb, W. R. (1994) Molecular and cellular mechanisms of general anaesthesia. *Nature* **367**, 607–614.
8. Flood, P., Ramirez, L. J., and Role, L. (1997) Alpha 4 beta 2 neuronal nicotinic acetylcholine receptors in the central nervous system are inhibited by isoflurane and propofol, but alpha 7-type nicotinic acetylcholine receptors are unaffected. *Anesthesiology* **86**, 859–865.
9. Durieux, M. E. (1995) Halothane inhibits signaling through ml muscarinic receptors expressed in *Xenopus* oocytes. *Anesthesiology* **82**, 174–182.
10. Rehberg, B., Xiao, Y. H., and Duch, D. S. (1996) Central nervous system sodium channels are significantly suppressed at clinical concentrations of volatile anesthetics. *Anesthesiology* **84**, 1223–1233.
11. Raines, D. E., Claycomb, R. J., Scheller, M., and Forman, S. A. (2001) Nonhalogenated Alkane Anesthetics Fail to Potentiate Agonist Actions on Two Ligand-Gated Ion Channels. *Anesthesiology* **95**, 470–477.
12. Yamakura, T. and Harris, R. A. (2000) Effects of gaseous anesthetics nitrous oxide and xenon on ligand-gated ion channels, comparison with isoflurane and ethanol. *Anesthesiology* **93**, 1095–1101.

13. de Sousa, S. L., Dickenson, R., Lieb, W. R., and Franks, N. P. (2000) Contrasting synaptic actions of the inhalational general anesthetics isoflurane and xenon. *Anesthesiology* **92,** 1055–1066.
14. Cook, T. L., Smith, M., Winter, P. M., Starkweather, J. A., and Eger, E. I. (1978) Effect of subanesthetic concentration of enflurane and halothane on human behavior. *Anesth. Analg.* **57,** 434–440.
15. Mihalek, R. M., Banerjee, P. K., Korpi, E. R., Quinlan, J. J., Firestone, L. L., Mi, Z. P., Lagenaur, C., et al. (1999) Attenuated sensitivity to neuroactive steroids in gamma-aminobutyrate type A receptor delta subunit knockout mice. *Proc. Natl. Acad. Sci. USA* **96,** 12,905–12,910.
16. Quinlan, J. J., Homanies, G. E., and Firestone, L. L. (1998) Anesthesia sensitivity in mice that lack the beta3 subunit of the gamma- aminobutyric acid type A receptor. *Anesthesiology* **88,** 775–780.
17. Mihic, S. J., Ye, Q., Wick, M. J., Koltchine, V. V., Krasowski, M. D., Finn, S. E., Mascia, M. P., et al. (1997) Sites of alcohol and volatile anaesthetic action on GABA(A) and glycine receptors. *Nature* **389,** 385–389.
18. Wick, M. J., Mihic, S. J., Veno, S., Mascia, M. P., Trudell, J. R., Brozowski, S. J., Ye, Q., et al. (1998) Mutations of gamma-aminobutyric acid and glycine receptors change alcohol cutoff. evidence for an alcohol receptor? *Proc. Natl. Acad. Sci. USA* **95,** 6504–6509.
19. Koltchine, V. V., Finn, S. E., Jenkins, A., Nikolaeva, N., Lin, A., and Harrison, N. L. (1999) Agonist gating and isoflurane potentiation in the human ganima- an-iinobutyric acid type A receptor determined by the volume of a second transmembrane domain residue. *Mol. Pharmacol.* **56,** 1087–1093.
20. Pratt, M. B., Husain, S. S., Miller, K. W., and Cohen, J. B. (2000) Identification of sites of incorporation in the nicotinic acetylcholine receptor of a photoactivatible general anesthetic. *J. Biol. Chem.* **275,** 29,441–29,451.
21. Fonnan, S. A., Miller, K. W., and Yellen, G. (1995) A discrete site for general anesthetics on a postsynaptic receptor. *Mol. Pharmacol.* **48,** 574–581.
22. Schrattenholz, A., Pfeiffer, S., Pejovic, V., Rudolf, R., Godovac-Zimmerman, J., and Maelicke, A. (1998) Expression and renaturation of the N-terminal extracellular domain of torpedo nicotinic acetylcholine receptor alpha-subunit. *J. Biol. Chem.* **273,** 32,393–32,399,
23. Tierney, M. L. and Unwin, N. (2000) Electron microscopic evidence for the assembly of soluble pentameric extracellular domains of the nicotinic acetylcholine receptor. *J. Mol. Biol.* **303,** 185–196.
24. Raines, D. E. (1996) Anesthetic and nonanesthetic halogenated volatile compounds have dissimilar activities on nicotinic acetylcholine receptor desensitization kinetics. *Anesthesiology* **84,** 663–671.
25. Mihic, S. J., McQuilkin, S. J., Eger, E. I., Ionescu, P., and Harris, R. A. (1994) Potentiation of gamma-aminobutyric acid type A receptor-mediated chloride currents by novel halogenated compounds correlates with their abilities to induce general anesthesia. *Mol. Pharmacol.* **46,** 851–857.
26. Abraham, M. H., Lieb, W. R., and Franks, N. P. (1991) Role of hydrogen bonding in general anesthesia. *J. Pharm. Sci.* **80,** 719–724.
27. North, C. and Cafiso, D. S. (1997) Contrasting membrane localization and behavior of halogenated cyclobutanes that follow or violate the Meyer-Overton hypothesis of general anesthetic potency. *Biophys. J.* **72,** 1754–1761.
28. Qin, Z., Szabo, G., and Cafiso, D. S. (1995) Anesthetics reduce the magnitude of the membrane dipole potential. Measurements in lipid vesicles using voltage-sensitive spin probes. *Biochemistry* **34,** 5536–5543.
29. Cafiso, D. S. (1998) Dipole potentials and spontaneous curvature: membrane properties that could mediate anesthesia. *Toxicol. Lett.* **100–101,** 431–439.
30. Cantor, R. S. (1998) The lateral pressure profile in membranes: a physical mechanism of general anesthesia. *Toxicol. Lett.* **100–101,** 451–458.

INDEX

455